D1613906

GOVERNMENT AND HEALTH SERVICES

*Government's Role
in the Development of
U.S. Health Services 1930–1980*

WILLIAM SHONICK

New York   Oxford
OXFORD UNIVERSITY PRESS
1995

Oxford University Press

Oxford   New York   Toronto
Delhi   Bombay   Calcutta   Madras   Karachi
Kuala Lumpur   Singapore   Hong Kong   Tokyo
Nairobi   Dar es Salaam   Cape Town
Melbourne   Auckland   Madrid

and associated companies in
Berlin   Ibadan

Published by Oxford University Press, Inc.,
200 Madison Avenue, New York, New York 10016

Oxford is a registered trademark of Oxford University Press

Library of Congress Cataloging-in-Publication Data
Shonick, William.
Government and health services : government's role in the
development of U.S. health services, 1930–1980 / by William Shonick.
p. cm.   Includes bibliographical references and index.
ISBN 0-19-506968-4
1. Medical policy—United States—History—20th century.
I. Title.
RA395.A3S49   1995
362.1′0973′0904—dc20   94-11500

9 8 7 6 5 4 3 2 1

Printed in the United States of America
on acid-free paper

To the memory of
Helen Bierman Shonick, MSW

Preface

This book describes the role of government in furthering an acceleration in the development of the system of health services in the United States that occurred mainly during the years 1930 through 1980. In 1935 federal legislation launched the first major systematic support by government for health services and created the network of federal aid to state and local public health departments that has continued to the present. By 1945–46 this system had been operating for some 10 years, government support for hospital construction was imminent, and plans were being made to greatly expand government medical services for veterans. The end of World War II seemed a good time to analyze these developments and a number of books were published, including those by Franz Goldmann (1945), Harry S. Mustard (1945), Bernhard J. Stern (1946), and Joseph W. Mountin (1947).

After the end of World War II, the pace of growth in government support for health services quickened. By 1980 an impressive national system had been built and government's role had become a central factor in the formation of health services policy. By the late 1960s, however, political rumblings presaged a move to halt further expansion of this governmental role. By the 1970s these rumblings had grown and reached a peak in 1981 with the election of Ronald Reagan, whose administration undertook to dismantle as much as possible of the system that had been built. The arguments for this proposed reversal hinged on assertions that while a few of the government programs had done some good at the time they were instituted, most were no longer needed because of changed conditions. In some quarters it was even claimed that many of the programs had never done much good and some were even harmful.

Thus, 1980 was a watershed year in which a fifty-year policy of expanding the role of government in health services development was re-placed by one that sought a sharp reduction of this role. As with 1945, it seems a natural point to pause and consider just what did happen to the relationship between government and health services during the preceding fifty years. Hence the origins of this book.

During these fifty years the U. S. government was transformed from a strongly laissez-faire structure to a cautious version of the modern social welfare state, and the development of health services was an important part of this transformation. Virtually all other developed capitalist nations followed the same route, although starting earlier, so that the changes introduced in this country were in no sense unique or trendsetting. An attempt is made here to view these changes from a more objective perspective than those that reflect mainly the overheated rhetoric of political battle.

An account of how this system was built, of course, must include descriptions of how it looked at different times and especially at the endpoint of the buildup. My intention is to present a view of the salient aspects of the relationships between governmental activities and the health services system that is general enough to offer a reasonably comprehensive picture yet sufficiently detailed to be more than another "introduction to" health service organization.

Although I look upon the previously cited books on government and health services that were issued in 1945–46 as progenitors of this one because of the similarity of their authors' interest in the nature of governmental roles in a predominantly private health services system, there is nevertheless a difference in approach. While the books of Goldmann, Mustard, and Stern were almost entirely descriptive, I pay more attention to policy analysis, as Mountin (1947) did. The governmental health policy formulation is presented in the context of the general development of a modern capitalist social welfare state in this country over this period.

WHAT IS PUBLIC POLICY ANALYSIS?

The term ''policy analysis'' is used today in two main contexts. In the first sense the term refers to a method of prospectively analyzing the implications for policy of a proposed action such as a legislative bill. The professional analyst is expected to give the likely alternative outcomes and to estimate their costs and benefits as a guide to policy formation. This type of probabilistic predictive analysis is done within a framework developed by the discipline of policy analysis. It is what many policy analysts working for government, consulting firms, and other corporate bodies do.

The second meaning refers to a retrospective analysis of policies that have been pursued by an organization. This type of analysis usually includes a description of the policies themselves, the events and forces that led to their adoption, and what the consequences have been. This type of retrospective policy analysis is often done by columnists and academicians in analyzing *public* (that is, governmental) policy. The term policy analysis is used mainly in this second way in this book, which is an analysis of health services policy in the United States.

Just what the content of ''public policy'' research should be has been widely debated by policy analysts, especially those primarily concerned with analyzing government policy on social programs. Should one concentrate on the policy *declaration* made by the government or only on the actual *operation* of programs and their final *outcomes* in terms of the program goals of the declared policy. One writer (Bardach, 1977) suggests that the policy pronouncement is ''only a collection of words'' and that only the implementation is the real policy. I do not hold a policy pronouncement to be ''only'' a collection of words. Many policy declarations that are never or very weakly implemented are nevertheless important to consider, for the very act of making the announcement is itself part of a government's real policy. For one thing, it provides a foundation or rallying cry, as Saul Alinsky never tired of telling us (1945), upon which activists and advocates can, and often do, base many of their demands, proposed programs, and campaigns that may ultimately lead to the implementation of the enunciated policy and turn it into an operating policy.

In this book, then, public policy in the health services field will be treated as consisting of three elements: enunciated policy, de jure policy, and de facto policy. *Enunciated* public policy consists of public pronouncements, such as State of the Union addresses, statements to the media, or preambles to pieces of legislation. It is a statement of intentions—general goals, and possibly also some quantified objectives. *De jure* policy is expressed in existing law. It consists of legislative enactments, judicial decisions on disputed interpretations of legislation, and the executive regulations for implementing the legislation. A de jure policy is often the first step toward implementing an enunciated policy for it is clearly more binding upon a government than enunciated policy. As the law of the land, it provides remedies to citizens who want the policy implemented that is not available for merely enunciated policies. *De facto* policy is the real or actual public policy; it is deduced from observed government actions and their effects on the health system and is the primary type of health services policy discussed in this book. It may or may not coincide with existing enunciated or even de jure policy, as attested by phrases like ''dead letter law.'' The totality of a government's actions constitutes the true or de facto government policy on a particular issue; thus, enunciated and de jure public policy are themselves part of the de facto public policy.

This book is written with no single *discipline* or its paradigms as a primary orientation. Its subject is a subset of the *field* of health services policy analysis. *De facto* government policy on health services, as revealed by government actions, is analyzed to determine what the role of government has been in the development of the health services system. The aim is to describe government actions in this field and show their connection to significant societal trends.

THE QUESTION OF PUBLIC ETHICAL PERCEPTIONS

Two main ethical issues in health policy formulation have been at the center of most differences over its content. One is the basis for access to medical care and the other is the conflict between individual desires for market freedom and the wishes of broader constituencies for improved public health through regulation of entrepreneurial activities. Because at different periods in history the prevailing view of the "correct" answers to these value-system questions determined much of the developmental path that was taken in health services policy, the oscillation over time in their public perception is an important theme throughout the book.

This book is divided into five parts. Part I deals with the government's role in protecting the public against health threats. Chapter 1 discusses the general background of public health services in industrially developed countries, focusing on England and the United States. Chapter 2 is a more detailed account of the U. S. public health effort, particularly early public policy with respect to the organization and function of *local* agencies established to protect the public health. The introduction and development of *state* public health agencies is discussed in Chapter 3, and the entry of the *federal* government into the field of "public health" or disease prevention, as the term was originally understood, is addressed in Chapter 4. Taken together, Chapters 2, 3, and 4 describe the development of a cooperative federal system of public health agencies and analyze the public policy implications of this arrangement.

Part II deals with the *direct* provision of personal health care services (i.e., medical care) by government using its own personnel and resources: by the federal government to particular groups of persons—veterans, members of the merchant marine, and American Indians (Chapter 5); by the state governments to chronically ill long-term patients (Chapter 6); and by local governments to the indigent sick (Chapter 7).

Part III examines the role of government as *payer* for medical care services obtained from nongovernment providers. It describes the increasing participation of the federal government in assuring general medical care for ever widening categories of persons and the stepped up debate of whether this is a bona fide "public health" function.

Chapter 8 deals with government-sponsored medical care for the *poor* before 1965; Chapter 9 discusses attempts to pass *national health insurance* with universal eligibility before 1965; Chapter 10 reviews programs for the *poor*, the *near poor*, and the *elderly* after 1965; and finally Chapter 11 addresses a special type of effort to pay for providing medical care to the poor through support of free-standing *neighborhood health* centers.

Part IV discusses the federal programs that sought to strengthen the resources of the health services system, thereby increasing the *supply* of services as well as their quality. These include federal efforts to increase the supply of medical facilities, mainly the number of hospital beds (Chapter 12), as well as the supply of health services personnel, mainly physicians (Chapter 13).

The development of public policy aimed at improving quality of services by supporting both biomedical and health services research is discussed in Chapter 14, and governmental actions to enhance local areawide planning in the health services system are described and evaluated in Chapter 15.

Finally, Chapter 16 recapitulates the major points of the book and weighs their significance. It summarizes the development of the complex system of health services analyzed in Chapters 2–14 and hypothesizes a theoretic explanation for the unique (among nations) form that the development took, as well as speculates on what some of the events after 1980 might portend for the future of health services in the United States.

Contents

I

Community-Wide Preventive and Control Aspects of Governmental Public Health Activities

Part I deals with the government's role in protecting the public against health threats that are community-wide in nature, or "public health." Such threats have been of two general types: epidemic diseases that spread extensively through a population and diseases caused by environmental factors. These categories are by no means mutually exclusive, for many rapidly spreading epidemic diseases are disseminated through a polluted environment, as in the case of cholera, and a polluted drinking water supply.

Public health services are often distinguished from curative health services (also designated as therapeutic health services, personal health services, or medical care), but this distinction, too, has overlapping elements. Syphilis is often treated in public health facilities, and the prevention of measles epidemics is largely handled by private physicians. What distinguishes public health from other measures taken to protect society's health is that its activities primarily involve organized community action against impending health threats, while medical care activities involve health professionals treating individuals. Another way to put this is that medical care concerns itself primarily with the person as patient receiving the best treatment available when he or she sees the physician, while public health concerns itself with the health status and health service needs of defined populations. From this point of view, assessing the adequacy of the medical care system to provide state-of-the-art medical care to all in the community who need it is a public health responsibility and so is planning to improve the existing medical care system.

By the very nature of these functions government bears the main responsibility for their implementation, and the main governmental role in public health has been played by public health agencies in local, state and federal governments. There are other governmental agencies that perform public health activities, such as medical licensing bodies, and in fact the number of public health activities assigned to agencies other than the official government health agency has been increasing in recent years. Health agencies at the three different levels of government have each had unique roles, both in what they do individually and what is expected of them in making a cooperative system work among the local, state and federal levels.

The three levels of governmental health agencies are dealt with here in the order in which they appeared historically: local health agencies first, state second, and national third. Chapter 1 deals with the European (chiefly British) antecedents of public health in the United States, and Chapters 2, 3, and 4 deal with the development of local, state and federal health agencies in the U.S. as well as the cooperative network linking the three.

1

Society and Health: The Historical Background of Public Health Services Development

Public health services have traditionally focused on the prevention of disease. As a new capitalist society evolved out of the decline of feudalism in Europe, new ways of living and the growth of global exploration and commerce brought with them new contagious diseases that threatened whole communities and regions with severe illness and death. Cities grew rapidly, and worldwide exploration and trade were accompanied or followed by large population movements. Western society and its economy moved inexorably toward the establishment of formidable technology. While these changes improved the economic and social position of many persons and offered the potential for many greater improvements yet to come, they also brought forth an ever-changing set of diseases that posed major threats to the health of different communities as people struggled to adapt to their new environments (Dubos, 1959, 1965). The main health threats during the early stages of capitalism were epidemics of acute, infectious, and quickly lethal disease. Consequently, early efforts in Europe, and later also in America, were directed at preventing or mitigating the outbreaks of acute infectious disease. Foremost among these were smallpox, bubonic plague, cholera, typhus, typhoid fever, malaria, yellow fever, venereal disease, tuberculosis, and the childhood diseases of measles, mumps, scarlet fever, diphtheria, and whooping cough.[1]

As better public health measures and other factors, such as acquisition of immunity by large portions of the population, diminished the threats from these diseases, other threats appeared. These involved the chronic and debilitative diseases like emphysema, asbestosis and other pulmonary diseases, cancer, stroke, heart disease, arthritis, and mental and emotional dysfunctions associated with modern living. Throughout all these changes, public health practitioners, policy makers, and researchers have attempted to learn the nature of the new threats and to organize public measures to combat them. The development of public health services has been a process involving a four-pronged attack: (1) establishing which diseases were the leading causes of death and disability; (2) learning the etiology of each disease, i.e., its causes and/or modes of transmission; (3) finding methods for preventing or controlling disease dissemination; and (4) learning how to organize society to apply the controls effectively. Because this last step usually involved governmental authority in some way, these activities were correctly subsumed under the term "public health."

The development of modern technological society that accompanied the spread of capitalism may be conveniently discussed in terms of three major stages, each accompanied by its own form of environmental changes and corresponding patterns of threats to health. The earliest form was mercantile capitalism. Often called the commercial revolution, it began with trade and small handicrafts practiced in the developing towns. Existing side by side with the final stages of feudalism, it led to the age of exploration, beginning with the early Crusades and culminating in the conquest of foreign lands and colonization. The Italian city-states, Spain, Portugal, the North Sea countries—all sent expeditions to Af-

3

rica, Asia, and the Americas. The noted biologist René Dubos (1959, 1965) has convincingly argued that these excursions to foreign shores were largely responsible for many devastating epidemics. For example, bubonic plague was rampant in Europe during the later Middle Ages (1300–1500) (Tuchman, 1978), and somewhat later, incursions of yellow fever began to decimate the populations of the American port cities at regular intervals. These epidemics only began to abate on a wide geographic scale about 1890 and not until 1920 were they largely controlled in industrialized countries. Dubos postulated that populations living in a locale for many generations develop a genetic immunity to many local diseases, especially the acute ones that kill nonimmune persons early in life. Over the long run those who survive are mostly the naturally immune people who predominantly produce subsequent generations. When people from one locale—sailors from Europe, for example—visited locales in different continents, they easily fell prey to endemic diseases against which they had poor natural immunity. Some of these travelers brought the infective agents back to Europe, and centuries of devastation followed.

The second major stage of technological development, industrial capitalism, consisted of a rapid development of factory-based manufacturing, often called the industrial revolution. The rapid strides made by the physical and chemical sciences, accompanied by widespread application of these sciences to industry, caused a rapid growth of large cities in Europe. To find work in the expanding industries, the population of some European countries, especially England, thronged (not always voluntarily) to the cities, where unsanitary conditions of living and working produced epidemics of cholera, typhus, and typhoid fever.

The third major stage of technological development was characterized by widespread use of high technology. In its current state it is typified by the accelerating use of machines to control machines and by large-scale manufacture of artificial products, such as plastics, made under conditions using intensive concentrations of irritating and even deadly chemicals. Noxious chemicals are widely used to increase agricultural yields, atomic decomposition is used to produce energy with attendant dangers of radi-

ation, and enormous amounts of concentrated fuels are used for industrial power and to achieve high-speed transportation of passengers and freight. These processes produce effects harmful to human tissue and psyche, but the exact extent of the damage and the mechanisms by which the damage is effected are as yet but dimly understood.

As each new threat to the health of populations appeared, it drew a response from professionals and lay persons interested in public health. They organized preventive services to mitigate or eliminate these threats, with varying degrees of success. The following sections describe some major social changes and the pattern of health problems that accompanied them. Although the discussion focuses on what are today called the "industrialized" countries, it generally refers to the European countries and Japan; the United States is only sketchily treated because the remainder of this book is devoted to it. Those countries that until only recently have had a socialist society but are commonly classified as "industrialized" are also included in this discussion because the threats posed by the rise of modern technology have been shown to clearly apply there also. These countries are the Soviet Union, the German Democratic Republic (East Germany), Czechoslovakia, and Hungary.

EARLY CAPITALISM: THE MERCANTILE STAGE

As the new health threats accompanying the progress toward an industrial urban society developed, public figures and health professionals during the mercantile stage of capitalism sought to gain public approval for measures to prevent the spread of disease. The main threats during this stage were diseases that were spread from person to person by animals such as mosquitoes, lice, and rats. Such disease-carrying agents are known to public health professionals as "vectors" (Last, 1980). Because the role of vectors was not recognized until after the germ theory of disease causation was developed in the late 1800s, measures advocated for prevention or control of the vector-borne diseases were based on varying perceptions of the association of certain events with their onset. These were drawn from interpreting observations made by different reporters, physicians, and others. When tried, certain of these disease-prevention measures worked some of the time, but whether they worked or not they exacted a heavy price in human suffering and treasure. The fact that they worked only in some instances and not in others made it clear that the underlying theory of their causes was seriously deficient.

One of the main theories extant during this period was that epidemic diseases were transmitted by dirt and "filth," or by impure air ("miasmas").[2] Since accumulated filth was assumed to produce miasmas, the entire concept of visibly unclean surroundings as a cause of epidemic disease has been referred to as the "miasmatist" theory. This theory provided the rationale for using sanitation methods ("cleanup" activities) of disease control.

The other widely held theory posited that disease transmission occurred by direct personal contact with the infected person or with his or her personal effects such as clothing and dishes ("fomites"). This "contagionist" theory provided the rationale for using quarantine (isolation of patient) methods of disease control. In the Renaissance Italian city-states, for example, persons coming from abroad or from another city where infection was known to exist, and wishing to enter the city, would often be compelled to have all their clothing aired or otherwise cleaned and to live outside the city for a specified period, usually forty days, to make sure that they were not carrying a contagious disease. Similarly, arriving ships were often compelled to keep their passengers aboard for a requisite period to make sure that no contagious diseases were prevalent among them. Also, in some areas, when it was determined that any member of a household had a contagious disease, all its members were forbidden to leave the house until there was no further evidence of disease among them. All other citizens were forbidden to enter the stricken house except for specifically designated agents of help and mercy.

These measures were moderately effective in controlling some diseases but not others, depending on the true mode of transmission for the particular disease. When a disease is in fact transmitted by body lice or the discharges of a sick person, avoiding contact with the person can be effective; but when a disease is transmitted by polluted water, quarantine is only of limited help. In these cases, its imposition led to great cruelties without helping much to curb the spread of the disease. For example, the contagionists wrongly held that cholera and some other dread contagious diseases were spread only by personal contact with the infected person and therefore counseled quarantine. The miasmatists wrongly held that transmission of these diseases was by dirty air ("miasmas") or premises, and they counseled cleanup environmental sanitation that would dispose of visible filth. It was later found that cholera is mainly transmitted by a water supply polluted by human wastes.

Many other epidemic diseases are transmitted in such a way that control cannot be effected by quarantine. Bubonic plague, for example, is transmitted by a microorganism carried by lice, which are in turn transported by rodents. In this case infected rodents are the main means of transmission. Typhus, on the other hand, which is transmitted by human body lice, can more easily be transmitted by direct contact between persons or the use of clothing infested with lice. If typhus were involved, burying the clothes and cleansing the bodies of arriving persons could be effective control measures, but a long period of quarantine might then be an unnecessarily harsh imposition. In contrast, if bubonic plague were involved, none of the known measures would help if rats bearing infected lice were able to get off an arriving ship and into a city.

Speculation about disease transmission was not wholly without empirical foundation. It was noticed, for example, that in some places cholera was associated with failure to dispose of human wastes properly and that carting the wastes away helped control cholera epidemics. Where the disposal of human wastes polluted the local drinking water, the water-borne cholera agent was spread by that process. In such instances the miasmatist theory, which argued for sanitation for all epidemic control, seemed correct. But if the water was polluted by sources far upstream, local sanitation might not help.

To take another example, it was often noticed that yellow fever and malaria were more prevalent in swampy areas. This led to a suspicion, especially in some places in early America, that the swamp air carried yellow fever (the miasma theory), and people were advised to live away from swamps and damp areas. We now know that certain mosquitoes carry the disease-producing mechanisms and breed in swamps and other places with stagnant water. Thus, some of the implications drawn from the observations were justified, and draining swamps to be rid of miasmas would be effective if these insects were the culprits, even though the method of transmission of the disease was thoroughly misunderstood. But quarantining incoming ships in United States ports until all signs of these diseases were gone from the passengers and crew could not be expected to achieve consistent control of these diseases. If infected persons aboard ships were kept out of range of mosquitoes from the shore the measure might be partially effective, but this contingency was highly improbable. Furthermore, quarantining a house that had been stricken by yellow fever would not be effective if a proper mosquito vector (*Aedes* or *Aegypti*) were prevalent in the vicinity and had access to the stricken individuals.

One class of disease for which quarantine is effective is represented by scarlet fever and diphtheria, which are transmitted directly from person to person by nasal or oral sprays and can be transmitted by the medium of infected dishes or other household items. Quarantining the house of a person infected with one of these diseases was found useful in prevention and control and was utilized even before the discovery that a microscopic organism was the agent of transmission.

It is instructive and important for current and future public health practice to realize how many measures did prove to be at least of some use in controlling the spread of certain communicable diseases before their exact cause or method of transmission was known, for we are in a similar situation with respect to many of the chronic and degenerative diseases prevalent today. Still, although measures like quarantine and sanitation were used, and sometimes for the appropriate disease, the choice of the correct control method was generally haphazard. A favorable result occurred partly by chance and partly because of the presence of exceptionally acute local observers who correctly associated the course of certain epidemics with particular changes in the local surroundings, even though the actual method of transmission of these diseases and their causes were unknown. The more definitive determination of disease etiology and methods of dissemination had to await the later findings of bacteriology, pathology, and medical entomology, as well as the development of more rigorous ways of reasoning from observed effect to cause which were to be developed by the science of epidemiology.

In the meantime, furious controversies raged among physicians and lay writers about what caused epidemics and how they could be controlled. The disputants arrived at their strongly held positions in one of two ways. Some generalized from observations that were carefully made but limited to one or a few epidemics. Others jumped to conclusions based on some general impressions and driven by ideological convictions. The latter produced theories blaming all epidemics on shabby housing conditions or improper civic maintenance, for example.

It seems that the less that was actually known about the causes of a particular disease, the more raucously propounded and unyielding were the debaters' assertions. Whatever theory was adopted by a locality as a basis for control action, it worked only if the etiology of the epidemic disease the community was fighting happened to coincide with the theory the action was based on.

INTERMEDIATE CAPITALISM: THE FIRST INDUSTRIAL REVOLUTION STAGE

The intermediate stage of capitalism, often referred to as the industrial revolution, followed the early or mercantile stage, but the two overlapped extensively. Extensive foreign trade expansion to new areas and the development of factory-based manufacturing existed side by side with handicraft and other small-scale manufacturing all throughout the period from 1650 to about 1900. Manufacturing had been carried on during the mercantile period but it then consisted largely of handicraft products, often made in the home ("cottage industry"). What was new in the industrial revolution of 1750–1850 was the application of extra-human power to machines used in manufacturing—first water power and then steam power (especially coal-fired). Because power-driven machines could not be effectively operated in the home, factories grew rapidly. With factories came a need to congregate large numbers of workers in towns, which rapidly expanded into cities. Housing conditions and working conditions in factories crowded with large numbers of operatives—many of them children—worsened rapidly. In England, and later also in the United States, the cities became increasingly congested, leading to serious epidemics of water-borne diseases such as cholera and typhoid fever. Writers on public health matters, public health authorities, and public health advocates in England before the 1880s, and in early America, were divided in their opinions of how the epidemic diseases should be controlled, based on how they believed them to be transmitted. Those who thought that these diseases were transmitted by filth or miasmas advocated sanitary campaigns to keep the cities looking clean and swampy areas drained; those who thought epidemics to be primarily transmitted by personal contact (contagion) advocated quarantine of the infected persons in their homes. Thus, quarantine and a limited type of sanitation became the staples of early public health efforts, but these were of little avail in controlling cholera and typhoid fever.

It remained for two British physicians to demonstrate for the first time that some epidemics were transmitted mainly by polluted drinking water. John Snow in his famous 1854 "Broad Street pump" studies established the fact that the discharge of human wastes from infected persons into the community's water supply was the mechanism for transmitting cholera. And in 1873, William Budd published a summary of his studies of many years showing the same correlation for typhoid fever (Winslow, 1978, p. 271f.). Their discoveries were among the early triumphs of the developing science of epidemiology in its efforts to establish links between factors in the environment and disease. Sanitation methods continued as a mainstay of public health efforts after the water-borne transmission of cholera and typhoid fever was established, but with extended functions. These methods now included monitoring drinking water sources and household waste disposal arrangements to see that disease-producing human wastes were not discharged into the water supply. But even these public health efforts could be effective to only a limited degree until advances in bacteriology enabled accurate monitoring of the water supply. It remained for the later work of bacteriologists to identify the actual organisms causing the water-borne diseases so that water (and food) supplies could be effectively tested for their presence. Public health authorities were then able to detect sources of pollution that they had been unable to uncover by site examination alone.

By the end of the 1800s, when the causes of epidemic disease had become better known and preventive vaccines for them developed, the work of public health agencies had been put on a scientific basis. The severe ravages of acute disease epidemics were largely eliminated in developed countries between 1890 and 1920.

LATE CAPITALISM: THE SECOND INDUSTRIAL REVOLUTION STAGE

The development of mass production techniques after 1900 greatly accelerated urban concentration and the size and complexity of the economies of developed countries. This was particularly true in the United States. First England and later Germany had been the centers of the most rapid progress of the second stage of development, the industrial revolution. As might have been expected, therefore, the development of public health organization took place most rapidly in these two countries, especially England. The third or most advanced stage of the development of modern capitalism was concentrated in the United States, and the discussion of public health activities in this latest period centers on the United States.

Sometimes called the second industrial revolution or the postindustrial society (Bell, 1973), the identifying features of this advanced period, which slowly began about 1900 and exhibited greatly accelerated development after 1945, were the refinement of mass production technology by using processes controlled first by mechanical devices aided by some electronic ones and later by increasingly complex computer-guided control systems; the ever more rapid concentration of industry into national and increasingly into multinational combines; the application of advanced chemical and physical science to uncover new sources of power and fabricate new materials; and the greater growth of service employment in such industries as restaurants, recreation, and computer-related occupations, compared with production ones such as manufacturing and mineral extraction. The essence of the first industrial revolution was the application of extra-human power to run machines; that of the second industrial revolution was the application of extra-human controls to guide the application of power to machines, implying a declining need for workers to control the automation process. These developments exercised a major influence on the course of public health practice.

In the earlier years of the second industrial revolution, 1900–1945, the United States was among the leaders in developing modern mass production. The expansion of its industry resulted in a shortage of workers, which led to a large influx of immigrants who came to work in the factories, mines, and mills—an influx that actually began soon after 1890 and whose main thrust ended in the early 1920s. Immigrants crowded into large cities, where many serious health problems developed. The slums in which many of them lived were unsanitary and often physically unsafe. Since this period coincided with the making of great strides in the discovery of the causes, methods of prevention, and control of many epidemic diseases, public health agencies were able to launch effective programs of prevention and control offering immunization, nutrition, and prenatal care. The need for them was clear-cut and the practice of public health developed rapidly, especially between 1915 and 1945.

In the years just after 1945 the United States industrial system was at its apogee. Its industries had grown spectacularly during the World War II years, both in technological sophistication and productive capacity. Perhaps the most important feature affecting the health services system was the rapid change in the patterns of disease and disability: the principal diseases from which people were suffering and dying now were the chronic and degenerative ones. The acute infectious diseases had been largely controlled by advances in biomedical knowledge and their widespread application, both by public agencies and private physicians. But with the benefits of increased production and easier living brought by the new technology came the usual byproducts of new health risks. The increased prevalence of chronic and disabling diseases was largely due to people living longer, resulting in an older population. But it was also due to increasing threats to healthy living from the noxious effects of the new high technology upon the air, water, land, and the food supply; automobile accidents; the effects of increased speed and other pressures of modern urban living upon behavior and mental health; and the cumulative effects on the human body of sedentary living and unhealthful health habits, many of the latter associated with relative affluence as well as with poverty. A substantial number of these problems are not amenable to amelioration by the eminently successful public health methods of 1890–1950.

What, therefore, was the scope of public health to be in the United States under these new conditions? What should it be? Were there any lessons to be learned from the way public health had organized itself in the past to control outbreaks of acute infectious disease accompanying rapid changes in the methods of producing goods?

It was in Europe that early capitalism had first developed, bringing with it new threats to health and the first formal organization of public health to combat them. And it was European, especially British, public health principles and practices that influenced early United States public health organization. The later development of public health organization, after about 1870, was largely led by the United States, even though it was based on scientific discoveries made mainly in Europe. The major development of formal public health organization took place in the United States during this period largely because there was more to be done here. After 1870 the United States rapidly became the leading example of fast-growing industrial and commercial development and of spreading population settlement and movement. These were arguably the main sources of public health threats needing community action in that period.

THE BRITISH BACKGROUND OF EARLY PUBLIC HEALTH ORGANIZATION IN THE UNITED STATES

A brief account of organized efforts to reduce threats to the public's health in nineteenth-century capitalist Europe may usefully begin with the description of the voluntary public health societies set up in England (and some other European countries) after 1800 (Shryock, 1979, p. 218f). Prompted by the spread of contagious diseases, these societies were formed as local public health councils. They were volunteer bodies usually appointed by local governments, but at different times in different countries they received guidance and supervision from central national offices. For example, the detection of the slow spread of a cholera epidemic that had begun in India in 1819 prompted the formation, by royal proclamation, of a temporary national board of health in England in 1831. Headquartered in London, the board's functions centered on getting town authorities throughout England to appoint local boards of health. (Spain and the German states already had "analogous" local organizations, France was organizing them, and in Sweden "regular town health boards" existed after 1800 (Ashford, 1975).[3] The function of the local boards of health in England was to supervise the keeping of statistics on deaths, particularly during suspected epidemics; to investigate reports of unsanitary conditions or infectious disease; and to advise government officials on "proper" methods of prevention and control.

The nature of the advice offered by a particular board on "proper" methods depended on whether the membership of the board was under the influence of one or the other of the two contending schools of thought, the contagionist or the miasmatist (Winslow, 1978, Chap. 11), for, as has been noted, definitive knowledge about the actual way the epidemic diseases were transmitted had to await later scientific discoveries. Ultimately, the scientific aspect of the problem was solved for most of the communicable diseases by use of vaccines that increased the immunity of populations to infection from them. Except for smallpox, however, these vaccines were not developed until after 1890[4] and therefore, to be on the safe side, earlier public health organization generally attempted to enforce both a relatively rudimentary form of sanitation control *and* the use of quarantine in a broadside manner against all epidemics, although sanitation was more often used. The more comprehensive programs called for the cleanup of wastes and improvement of public water supplies in the best manner then known as well as quarantine of infectious diseases both in dwellings and on board ships in harbors. Organized implementation of these measures was sporadic, however, and done only in some places, largely because of the strictly local basis of most public health organization and the general failure to appoint full-time staff.

Yet many of the local boards established or strengthened by the previously mentioned royal proclamation of 1831 did proceed to act vigorously, using their weapons of simultaneously applied quarantine and sanitation to protect the health of their communities. The improvement of the public's health took on the character of a social movement, with the roster of activists overlapping that of persons seeking to improve the general conditions of the industrial cities, especially the workplaces and dwellings of workers, on social or moral grounds. Local boards also carried out investigations of slum conditions, producing numerous detailed reports leading to public measures for their alleviation.

The composition of the early public health councils and boards—physicians, sanitarians, public officials, public reformers, and other citizens—was an important feature differentiating them from purely professional organizations such as medical societies. It reflected the fact that public health workers made up a goal-oriented team rather than a single discipline, and that interested lay people were in the forefront along with full-time professionals in promoting public health measures. What defined activities and personnel as being engaged in public health was the primacy of the goal of protecting the health of *populations*.

These organizational characteristics of the British public health movement influenced public health organization in the United States and their imprints remain to the present day. For example, the American Public Health Association (APHA), organized in 1872, still reflects this pluralism. Its twenty-three sections represent public health agency workers and social, physical, and natural scientists (both theoretical and applied), public officials, medical and allied medical practitioners, and a host of other disciplines and walks of life. Most American cities or counties with public health departments of any size have also had a citizen board of health that often provided important input into decision processes. Moreover, many voluntary organizations active in promoting public health goals are led by persons of varied backgrounds. Schools of public health teach and train persons for the *field* of public health as opposed to disciplines such as law, medicine, or engineering. Persons who graduate from these schools as specialists in environmental control may have quite different training than those whose specialty was the organization and management of maternal and child care. What unites the specialties under the rubric of "public health" is their goal: to be part of the team that protects the health of the public. It is in this sense that public health often has been called a movement rather than a single profession, a concept inherited from its English ancestry.

With the later biological discoveries of 1890–1945, public health organization in the United States adjusted to incorporate the greater potential for effective prevention and control. Although it always retained some pluralism in its leadership, it became more specialist in the composition of its personnel. Its organization spread from being primarily local to including state and then national public health agencies; and finally international organizations were formed.

Many of the activities that have for years been regarded as "standard" functions of health departments in the United States had their origins in British developments. For example, one of the main weapons of public health advocates in Great Britain was the use of vital statistics. Local data were assembled into reports showing the relationship of mortality rates to bad living conditions, which in turn were shown to be closely associated with extremely unsanitary conditions. One of the most famous of these reports, issued in 1842, was that of Edwin Chadwick, a nonmedically trained sanitarian. He analyzed the data collected and supplied by "poor law physicians" ("welfare" doctors, as we would call them) in a comprehensive survey of the disease conditions in their practice areas. The resulting

Report . . . on an Inquiry into the Sanitary Condition of the Laboring Population of Great Britain is one of the classic documents of the public health movement. Chadwick showed that mortality rates and longevity were strongly related to economic status. In Liverpool, for example, "the average age of 'gentry' at death was 35 years, while that of laborers was only 15" (Shryock, 1979, p. 225). He expressed the opinion that this difference mainly reflected housing conditions.

The desire to have better vital statistics for inferring the causes of disease was a major factor in the decision to establish an office of the Registrar General of Births, Deaths, and Marriages in Great Britain in 1836. A prominent position in this office was held by William Farr, an English physician greatly interested in the use of vital statistics to improve prevention and cure disease. Joining the Registrar General's office in 1841, he became one of the world's leading authorities on vital statistics. His work was instrumental in organizing British public health and collecting census data dealing with disease (and poverty) in British manufacturing towns. Farr's efforts, as well as the work and backing of Chadwick, were important influences in later establishing the importance of vital statistics collection as an important function of local public health departments in the United States.

SUMMARY AND COMMENTS

Organized public health arose as a societal institution to meet newly appearing threats to health. These were epidemics of acute infectious disease that accompanied the global travel, population migration, and industrial development of the rising capitalist system. No cure was known for these diseases. A large number of persons died after contracting them. Nor were any specific substances known that could be administered to individuals to prevent them from contracting one of these diseases.

The only methods for preventing outbreaks and spread of epidemic disease consisted of communal actions, the main ones being quarantine and sanitation. Applying them required social organization and led to the first local public health entities. These first appeared in Europe where commercial and industrial capitalism began and then were taken up in the United States as it grew to be the most developed capitalist country and the center of advanced technological capitalism. Of all the European countries, England had the greatest influence on the development of public health organization in the United States.

NOTES

1. For a description of these diseases see Last, 1980, especially section 4. This work is also an excellent source for terms and concepts used in epidemiology and public health practice.

2. A theory that had some vogue was that they spread during periods when some strange and entirely unknown condition of the atmosphere and the solar system prevailed, a so-called epidemic constitution of the environment. I shall not discuss this theory further, because it never became one of the leading ones on which local action was based.

3. I mention these other countries in passing to show that public health organization was proceeding in countries other than England also. However, the British developments had overwhelmingly the greatest influence on United States public health organization, and the discussion is largely confined to them. In terms of the influence of Europe on the scientific content of United States public health practice, however, France and Germany were at least as important as England, perhaps more so.

4. Shryock, 1979, especially Chapter XII, and Winslow, 1978 discuss these questions in some detail. Much of the factual material cited on these few pages comes from Shryock.

2

The Local Health Department

Until the late 1800s, the function of public health in the United States was necessarily defined almost entirely in terms of controlling epidemics through quarantine and sanitation. The state of medical knowledge such such that the question of curative medical care did not loom large as a problem requiring governmental action. Private physicians, variously qualified, treated the sick who could pay, almost invariably at home. Indigent sick persons were often attended by a physician designated as a health officer or town or county physician; he was paid by the locality to minister to the sick poor in their homes and to inmates of the poor farm or jail (Volkenburg, 1951).

In early America (before 1800), local efforts to protect community health were typically administered by a board of health. It met as occasion required using its powers to decree the isolation of sick individuals (quarantine) or to force compliance with some sanitary code (sanitation) in its attempts to control or prevent an epidemic. With the passage of time, in some places a practicing local physician was officially designated as the local public health officer. He advised the board about health threats to the community and suggested measures for combatting them. Local officials and other citizens often turned to him to investigate a perceived threat to the public health. For his public duties he was paid modestly or not at all. The very composition of the local board of health was often an ad hoc improvisation, its members assembled to meet a particular emergency. During the first half of the 1800s, some boards evolved into more permanent bodies with members appointed for specified terms, and some part-time health officers were replaced by "full-time"[1] departments of health. This development continued through the latter half of the 1800s, and sizable public health departments were organized in a few large cities. These became more sophisticated in their disease control operations as progress in the biological and epidemiological sciences began to be made. The number of "full-time" departments of health grew rapidly from 1900 through 1945, under the stimulus of state health department leadership. Federal funding (beginning in 1935), an increasingly self-conscious public health profession, and some prodding by the American Medical Association in the first two decades of the twentieth century were also stimulants to the proliferation of full-time departments. But perhaps the most important factor was the growing effectiveness of the techniques available to health authorities for controlling the outbreak of many acute, epidemic diseases.

Harry S. Mustard, writing in 1945, described the dynamics of this development vividly:

the responsibility of local health authorities for provision of public health services has developed through a number of fairly definite states. First, in early seacoast towns and frontier settlements, there was no formal provision for meeting public health problems. The situations that made themselves dramatically obvious, as epidemics, were handled as the need arose. Second, as provincial councils or state legislatures got to the matter, it was *permitted* that local jurisdictions might have a board of health. Third, as time passed, it was *required,* in a number of states, that each locality must have a board of health. Coincident with or following this, the requirement went further: each local jurisdiction *must have* a health officer, by custom part-time. Fifth, through existing laws or new ones, local jurisdictions were *permitted* in most states to provide themselves with more nearly adequate health service: full-time personnel and a continuing program. . . .

[D]uring the early part of the fifth phase state health departments took the role of salesmen. They bargained with and cajoled local authorities, all to the end that a local health department be established. . . .

By rule of thumb, the state health departments fought their way on until they had gone about as far as they could in the circumstances. They had established health departments in most jurisdictions where some powerful political figure did not oppose them too vigorously; where the local medical society did not regard the proposal for a health department as a proposal for state medicine; where an entrenched specialized voluntary agency, sometimes subsidized by government funds, did not view the coming health department as a dark shadow; where the incumbent part-time local health officer did not mind yielding up his office [Emphases in the original.] (Mustard, 1945, p. 135)

During this latter period, from about 1900 to 1945, while the states were busy attempting to establish additional local health departments to "cover" their populations, public health professionals were trying to define and gain public acceptance of the need of communities for local public health departments that met approved standards. They faced more than the usual problems of gaining professional legitimacy: to determine the scope of function of such agencies; to formulate qualifications for accrediting or preferably licensing practitioners; and to establish minimal standards by which the adequacy of a public health agency's service could be judged and perhaps accredited.

THE PERIOD BEFORE 1935

Scope of Function

The functions that by 1940 were widely regarded as appropriate and necessary for a local public health department developed out of the experiences of localities struggling to prevent or control the spread of epidemics. Many of the scientific and organizational techniques that had come to be used by American public health were based on applications of European scientific discoveries and, as noted in Chapter 1, on adaptations of European organizational experience, especially British.

Preventive Services: Evolution of the "Basic Six" Functions

The activities that came to be seen as necessary or appropriate for local public health depart-

ments were preventive services and some types of primary medical care. While there was almost unanimous agreement about the strictly preventive functions, however, there was often sharp disagreement over the appropriateness of the delivery of primary medical care by these departments.

Early Developments—Before 1890 The British experience exerted the strongest influence on the *organization* of public health in the United States, especially before the 1800s, largely because the earliest colonial settlements along the East Coast, beginning in Massachusetts and Virginia, were primarily English.

During the colonial period of 1620–1781, the British colonies consisted mainly of small agricultural communities. They did engage in some trade, and a few port towns such as Boston, New York, Philadelphia, and Charleston were beginning to develop into cities. The port towns were the sites of some of the more serious epidemics, which probably resulted in part from poor sanitation and other unhealthy local conditions—unsafe water supplies, swamps, crowding, poor housing—but probably mainly from diseases brought in by ships anchored in the harbors. Local organizations to counter these epidemic threats consisted of British-style voluntary boards of health, most of them assembled on an ad hoc basis to meet particular threats. These ad hoc boards applied what they considered to be the appropriate sanctions to enforce quarantine and sanitation measures. After independence from Britain, local public health services continued much as before. Local community boards, meeting intermittently as occasion required, used their powers of quarantine and of summons to isolate sick individuals and to enforce compliance with a sanitary code. As has been noted, with the passage of time a practicing local physician was in some cases designated as the local public health officer and sometimes paid a small amount for his public duties.

Despite these efforts, the continued development of mercantile capitalism was accompanied by increasingly frequent and severe epidemics in the port cities. These outbreaks were also related to the accelerating development of industrial capitalism, which further increased the size and congestion of manufacturing cities. Since much of the new manufacturing was water powered, factories tended to be established either at the "fall line" where the mountain rivers descending to the ocean achieve major force, or along swift-running rivers that were dammed. Water power, the principal source of industrial power until 1850 (Shannon, 1951, pp. 228–280) enabled cities to grow at places other than the seaports, because early industrial centers, like Lowell, Fall River, and Lawrence, Massachusetts, "were located with reference to the best available water power" (Shannon, 1951, p. 229). Although this also increased the number of places where urban development could give rise to epidemics, by all accounts the epidemics in the port cities continued to be more severe, attesting to the fact that the most serious ones at this time were imported and that urban congestion was not yet the primary health threat it was fast becoming in England.

Yellow fever attacked the port cities in a series of epidemics, many of them severe. For example, the Philadelphia epidemic of 1793 "was in many ways the worst calamity of its kind ever suffered by an American city" (Shryock, 1979, p. 216). It was particularly serious because Philadelphia was then the capital and cultural center of the infant United States and virtually the entire government deserted the city. One-tenth of the population died. The usual measures of quarantine and sanitation were followed, with sanitation being more frequently used. The city fathers were frightened into paving streets, and making Philadelphia the first city in the entire English-speaking world to supply water "pumped by steam at public expense" (Shryock, 1979, p. 216). But this was to little avail, for yellow fever is not a water-borne disease. Other cities, like Savannah, resorted to draining stagnant water and achieved a marked reduction in yellow fever and other "autumnal diseases" without, of course, understanding why. It was not understood why quarantine was sometimes helpful in slowing the spread of yellow fever but more often was not, and why sanitation was also sometimes effective in combatting the spread of yellow fever and sometimes not. Swamp drainage in Savannah helped, but purifying the water supply in Philadelphia did not. Why had applying "sanitation" measures

in these two places had different results? When applying the same measure to control the same disease at different times and difference places produced different outcomes, it was difficult to associate the advent of the disease with a causative agent. But because sanitation and quarantine measures were sometimes effective, they became standard measures used by public health departments, often in tandem. After 1840, as understanding of the etiology of communicable diseases grew, control measures began to be more narrowly targeted to the causative disease, and after 1890 progress along these lines was very rapid.

Ad hoc local boards of health formed to meet outbreaks of pestilential disease continued to be the principal form of public health organization until after the Civil War. The growth and increased centralization of business—especially manufacturing, extraction, and transportation—and the expansion of the country accompanying the construction of railroads led to the formation of state departments of health, a trend parallel to that in England, Germany, and France. The first permanent state department of health was established by Massachusetts in 1869, and by 1890 a number had been organized. (By 1913 every state had one.)[2]

During the years 1840–1890, along with the trend toward organizing state boards of health to certify and develop local public health work, there was also a discernible move to professionalize the staffing, especially the leadership, of local health departments by appointing permanent full-time officials who came to be known as "health officers." The local organizational pattern that developed, especially in large cities, was one of policy-making volunteer boards of health and operating, full-time, professionally staffed health departments, headed by chief health officers (or commissioners) for program administration. The perception of the need for professionally staffed local public health departments grew with the expansion of scientific knowledge about epidemic disease causation and control and led to increased employment of full-time specialists in fields like epidemiology, sanitation, and communicable disease control. A brief review of some of the scientific developments that led to increased professional staffing of public health departments will help clarify and illustrate the connection.

VITAL STATISTICS AND "CORRELATIONAL" EPIDEMIOLOGY. One of the earliest functions of local public health agencies before 1890 was the collection and analysis of vital statistics—again, an American adaption of European public health practice. Among the English formulators of the vital statistics techniques were the physician William Petty, who worked in the mid-1600s, his contemporary, John Graunt, who first formulated life tables, and Edward Holley, who published a usable life table in 1693 (Mountin, Pennell, Flook, 1936, pp. 111–113). The later work of William Farr and Chadwick in the 1840s, noted in Chapter 1, developed methods that were particularly useful to American public health administrators.

Records were kept of deaths classified by cause and demographic strata, and in later years, physicians were required to report the incidence of communicable diseases to the local health authority. Such data were collected by public health nurses in the course of their regular duties in small towns, and in large cities specialists known as registrars began to take over these duties. These data were used to alert governmental authorities to the development of epidemics. They could also be used to establish causes of disease by association with environmental or demographic factors as, for example, the higher prevalence of yellow fever in areas with stagnant water, higher mortality rates in areas where working people lived compared with those where middle-class people lived, or higher incidence of cholera among persons using a particular water supply. The identification of the "correlates" of disease, i.e., the attempt to find associations between environmental and demographic factors on the one hand and the incidence and prevalence of a specified disease on the other is a major task of epidemiology. This technique was sometimes successful in determining the environmental causes of disease before the exact disease-producing organism was identified in the laboratory, as in the case of cholera. It thus enabled public health authorities in certain instances to mount targeted campaigns to prevent and control epidemics earlier than would otherwise have been possible. Epidemi-

ology became one of the basic disciplines used by local public health departments, and correlational methods constituted one of their fundamental techniques.

IDENTIFICATION OF MICROSCOPIC AGENTS OF DISEASE TRANSMISSION AND LABORATORY-BASED EPIDEMIOLOGY. With the development of biological science in Europe, methods of preventing and controlling outbreaks of contagious disease became more effective. The microscopic agents of a number of important epidemic diseases were definitively identified, enabling public health workers to determine the presence or absence of specific contagious diseases in persons and in environmental media like water and food. It enabled verification of previous hypotheses about the method of transmission of some diseases that had been established by correlational methods as well as determining the transmittal routes of others. These scientific advances had an important effect on the functions expected from a local health department and on its staffing patterns. After it was determined that cholera and typhoid fever were primarily water-borne diseases involving human waste disposal, but that diphtheria, measles, and whooping cough were highly contagious and spread by proximity to an infected person, it became clear the sanitation—uncontaminated water supplies—was the key to preventing the spread of water-borne diseases, while quarantine would help abate the spread of the direct contact contagious diseases. It was now important to have staff and facilities that could scientifically determine the identity of any existing disease-carrying organisms, whether in the water supply, in samples taken from humans, or in any other source. In particular, it enhanced appreciation of the importance of appropriate laboratory facilities for correctly analyzing samples. Thus a fourth basic function (after vital statistics, sanitation, and quarantine)[3] was added for local public health departments—laboratory services.

The first bacteriological laboratories dedicated principally to serve active public health practice were established in the United States. In 1892 "the first American laboratories of hygiene ... were established at the University of Pennsylvania and in connection with the New York City health department ..." (Shryock,

1979, p. 283). In New York City, the names of William H. Park[11] (Winslow, 1929, p. 34) and Herman Biggs (Winslow, 1929) stand out as pioneers in introducing the bacteriological laboratory into public health *practice,* a development in which the United States was in advance of Europe.

Herman Biggs is a good example of the young scientists who were going abroad to study and bringing back the latest biological research findings for application to public health practice in the United States. Biggs received his M.D. degree from Cornell in 1882, the year that has been characterized as the beginning of the period of the most rapid development of bacteriology. He visited Europe exclusively and learned of the discoveries of Koch and Pasteur. After a period of work at the Carnegie laboratory that had been established at Bellevue Medical School, he became chief medical officer of the New York City Health Department, where he was instrumental in introducing applied bacteriology to the work of the department.

The bacteriological laboratory set up in the New York City Health Department in 1892 with Biggs as its head was actually called the division of Pathology, Bacteriology, and Disinfection, and had among its duties the disinfection of arriving passengers—that is, the examination for and elimination of lice and other vectors performed on quarantined ships and quarantine holding places on shore. Public support for this laboratory was greatly reinforced by the appearance of a cholera epidemic in Europe that threatened to be transmitted to the United States. Laboratory facilities were needed to diagnose cholera on arriving passengers being held in quarantine in the New York harbor, and Biggs's laboratory was ready and available. The feared outbreak of epidemic cholera did not materialize in New York City, and the health department was credited with having stopped it. The public perception of the proven efficacy of the New York City Health Department laboratory (as well as that of the similar laboratory at the University of Pennsylvania) accelerated the formalization of public laboratory services as a standard item of the "basic" functions of public health departments—mostly, however in large cities. The principal activities of the public health laboratory were to provide diagnoses of

communicable disease in public quarantine situations as well as for doctors in private practice, and to test samples of water and food supplies submitted by sanitarians and other interested persons.

The pioneering work in applying the growing body of bacteriological knowledge to protection of the water supply against contamination by infectious organisms was done by William T. Sedgwick at the Lawrence Experimental Station of the Massachusetts State Board of Health, established in 1887 (Winslow, 1929, p. 97). Sedgwick was a biologist who devoted his major attention to public health matters, spending some forty years as head of the biology department of the Massachusetts Institute of Technology. He studied and taught public health sanitation, concentrating on water supplies, milk, and other problems of food contamination. His focus was different from that of Hermann Biggs in New York. Biggs was more concerned with prevention via laboratory-aided medical diagnosis by analysis of specimens taken from humans and also with promoting immunization, including the distribution of vaccines to private practitioners. Sedgwick concentrated on the treatment of food, water, and sewage:

[T]hrough all these [Sedgwick's] studies there runs a single consistent tendency, the attempt to apply exact laboratory and statistical methods to the study of environmental influences affecting the life and health of man. Bacteriology, as it was introduced by Biggs and Park in New York and by the other early workers in the United States, was largely pathological in its bearing. It was the bacteriology of the human body in health and disease. In this field the Institute of Technology made little or no contributions. Diagnostic procedure, the study of carriers, immunologic control, owe little to the work of Institute laboratories. On the other hand, the microbiology of water supplies was created by Sedgwick and his pupils. The bacteriology of water and sewage owes all its first impetus to them ..." (Jordan, Whipple, and Winslow, 1924, p. 64).

Thus, the initiation of public laboratory services as a local public health function is associated with Biggs and Park with respect to its medical diagnostic and vaccine distribution aspects, and with Sedgwick with respect to its water- and food-testing aspects. Three of the six major "standard" functions that finally came to be widely accepted as basic to a health department (see page 20) were based on bacteriologic applications pioneered by these public health leaders—sanitation, communicable disease control, and laboratory services. The sanitation and communicable disease control functions were recast in their modern forms using the scientific findings of bacteriology instead of more or less informed guesses about miasmas and contagion.

Later Developments—1890–1935 As the end of the 1800s approached, we find local public health agencies using four main lines of attack to detect and abate both the occurrence and spread of acute communicable disease: collection and interpretation of vital statistics, sanitation, quarantine[4] and laboratory services. Although the scientific knowledge supporting these functions grew substantially after 1850 and was changing the content of public health practice in important ways even before 1900, important gaps still remained that limited the degree of control possible for many epidemic diseases. The gaps diminished rapidly after 1900, however, as further scientific discoveries about the cause and spread of these diseases were made from 1900 through 1935.

IDENTIFICATION OF THE VIRUS AS A DISEASE-CAUSING AGENT. Despite the important discoveries of the bacterial causes of many epidemic diseases, there remained some question in the early 1900s about how widespread the microbial agents were as causes of infectious diseases, because many major communicable diseases, like mumps and yellow fever, still had not been shown to be caused by microbial organisms. But this was changed with the discovery of viruses, which were not visible under a light microscope. In 1892, the Russian botanist D. Iwanowski showed that some disease-causing agents could pass through a filter that was impenetrable to any bacterium. With the invention of the electron microscope in 1932, viruses were made visible and in 1935 the American virologist W. M. Stanley shared a Nobel Prize for his work in outlining the structure of virus particles. Some of the contagious diseases caused by viruses are measles, mumps, smallpox, yellow fever, rabies, poliomyelitis, influenza, and the common cold. (The most talked-about current contagious health threat, AIDS, is caused by a virus, HIV.) The viruses produce antibodies as

bacteria do, and vaccines for some of these diseases could therefore be developed (e.g., as in the case of measles, mumps, and poliomyelitis). Because they are not as susceptible to treatment with drugs as bacterial diseases are with antibiotics, they can be devastating when they reach epidemic proportions, as has been the case with certain strains of influenza. Most contagious diseases have been shown to have a microbial causative agent, but the applied research on identifying individual viruses was just beginning in 1935.

IDENTIFICATION OF DISEASE-CARRYING VECTORS. In addition to the bacteriological advances of 1870–1900 that were incorporated into the content of public health practice by public health practitioners, the findings of medical entomologists further increased the ability of public health organization to prevent and control infectious disease. These findings emerged somewhat later than the first bacteriological discoveries, the largest number coming between 1895 and 1920. Until it was established that the great scourges of yellow fever and malaria were carried by insects that transmitted disease-causing agents—whether bacteria, protozoans, or viruses—from infected persons to well ones, effective control measures were usually hit-or-miss. Knowing the culprit organism was not always sufficient to be able to intercept it.

Recognition of insects and other animals as carriers (vectors) of disease-causing microorganisms (pathogens) was the missing link in the chain of knowledge required to control communicable disease effectively, and it proved to be the most stubborn relationship to ferret out. Research on animal vectors was going on all through the 1890s. In 1889, for example, "Texas fever" was shown to be disseminated among cattle by infected ticks; and in 1894 Shibamiro Kitasato demonstrated the rodent and louse to be the carriers of the microorganism causing bubonic plague (the major form of the dreaded Black Death of medieval Europe). But the key discoveries for controlling vector-borne diseases came at the turn of the century. In 1898, Ronald Ross and G. B. Grassi demonstrated the role of the mosquito carrier for malaria, and in 1901 a commission of the U.S. Surgeon General headed by Walter Reed, J. W. Lazear, and James Carrol demonstrated it for yellow fever. These discoveries were followed by a sequence of important research results on this subject. For example, David Bruce of the British Army showed in approximately 1900 that sleeping sickness was carried by the tsetse fly; and the body louse was shown to carry typhus in 1912. By 1920, the method of transmission of many of the leading and highly fatal communicable diseases that had afflicted humanity for thousands of years, producing the most withering epidemics in Europe and America since about 1300, had been identified. Preventive measures had been developed for most of these: water and food sanitation or body decontamination ("delousing," "disinfecting") for some, immunization of potential victims ("population at risk") through the use of vaccines for others, and vector control (principally the mosquito and rat) for still others.[5]

These scientific developments enabled the safeguarding of the health of populations against epidemic assault to take on some characteristics of scientifically based medical practice: keeping track of "symptoms" (vital statistics); making a definitive diagnosis about which epidemic disease, if any, was threatening; and prescribing the appropriate "treatment." Although many of these measures were carried out on aspects of the environment and population aggregates rather than individual patients, the procedures were sufficiently analogous to the practice of medicine for its practitioners to be accepted by the medical profession as constituting a medical specialty—public health officer, later elaborated into a formal residency training program in preventive medicine. The requirements for applying these controls to communities formed the basis of the administrative structures and operational content of local public health departments. With respect to many of the acute communicable diseases, the occurrence of epidemics or the widespread endemic presence of most of these diseases would henceforth be due much more to a failure to organize public health services than to unknown factors about the etiology or method of dissemination of the diseases. The very presence of these diseases was thereafter more properly considered a societal rather than an unsolved scientific or medical problem.

In the face of developments such as these, localities increasingly deemed it necessary, or at least desirable, to employ more full-time, professionally trained staff. As the United States approached the end of the nineteenth century, many large cities had sizable public health departments with a substantial core of personnel trained in various public health specialties. A large city with a fairly adequate public health organization would have a board of health[6] composed of volunteer, policy-making appointees, and a department of public health with a full-time professional staff. It would typically have a large health department with a physician in charge of quarantine and immunization. If the city and the department were not very large, however, this physician would generally also be the administrative head of the agency and in that capacity might be called the chief health officer. Large departments had more than one health officer, each of whom specialized in various aspects of public health work. The head of the agency might then be called the commissioner of health instead of chief health officer. Assisting the health officers in these large departments were public health nurses, who helped administer the immunization or other clinics and made house visits to determine the need for quarantine, encourage immunization, or provide health education to families. They frequently were also the main collectors of the vital statistics.

In a large city, sanitation functions were typically headed by civil engineers who specialized in sanitation or sanitary science and were called sanitary or sanitation engineers. They drafted ordinances and carried much of the responsibility for the water supply and waste disposal systems being designed to assure freedom from contamination. Even when they did not actually plan the system, they were consulted on proposals for sanitation construction. Working under them were specially trained technicians called sanitarians who inspected places of business (especially food establishments), houses, streets, and other sites for violations of the sanitary code, often in response to citizen complaints. They reported such violations to the health department, where the reports were routed to the appropriate health officer or sanitation engineer. Smaller health departments rarely had sanitation engineers on staff, working only with sanitarians.

The vital statistics function in the large public health department, with its complement of specialist public health officers, had to meet staff demands for data appropriate for disease control. Rudimentary collection of birth and death data presented in simple tables was increasingly found to be insufficient. The use of statistical inference, special health indicators, and analyses that correlated disease incidence and prevalence with population factors slowly became more common. The assembly and analysis of these data increasingly required specially trained personnel. At first these were specially trained clerks, but as time went on a class of personnel known as registrars found its way into the formal staff organization chart in large health departments. In smaller departments public health nurses collected and often also assembled the data required by health officers.

Responsibility for communicable disease control either rested in a special division headed by a health officer specialist in large health departments or was supervised directly by the executive health officer in smaller ones. This division ran diagnostic clinics for identifying venereal disease and tuberculosis and also provided some treatment, enforced isolation, or arranged hospitalization for patients with these diseases. It also offered immunizations against those diseases for which vaccines and antitoxins were available and supervised vector control, such as drainage of stagnant water and rat and louse eradication. The functions of quarantine and immunization thus came to be subsumed under the functional category of communicable disease control. After 1900, immunization of children came increasingly under the purview of a special division devoted to maternal and child care. These divisions offered prenatal care and postpartum instruction to pregnant women and new mothers and immunization against childhood acute infectious diseases for children.

There would also be a division of public health laboratories, providing diagnostic testing services for physicians and public health clinics and testing food and water samples for contamination for the sanitarians. Many laboratories also distributed vaccines to private physicians, although this was often done by the division of communicable disease control. This practice had been initiated by Herman Biggs as part of the operations of the public health department laboratory he established in New York City in 1892 (see p. 16). For smaller cities and rural areas,

public health laboratory services were generally available from the state public health department.

Growth of Direct Primary Care after 1890

The changes in local public health practice in evidence around the turn of the century resulted not only from scientific advances but also from changes in the population composition of the United States. Large waves of immigrants arrived in New York and other port cities beginning in 1892, and the immigration did not subside substantially until 1920. Coming to fill the need for operatives in factories and mills, these immigrants were predominantly poor and settled into urban ghettos, particularly in New York City. The resulting slum conditions produced responses similar to those brought forth in Great Britain during the industrial revolution of 1750–1850, when its cities became very unhealthful and unsafe to live in because of massive immigration from the countryside. Reform-minded persons in the United States worked and agitated to alleviate the plight of the tightly packed slums, with the health conditions of the immigrants a principal concern. The reformers took up such problems as communicable disease control and infant mortality; housing conditions, with particular attention to sanitation; and nutrition. As one response, voluntary agencies opened milk stations in slum areas to provide uncontaminated milk and clinics for child care. There was a great need also for general medical primary care. The outpatient departments of public and some not-for-profit private hospitals were inundated with patients seeking such care.

Under the pressure of these needs, the first evidence of a major rift in public health professional circles over the place of personal health care in public health work appeared. As has been noted, the functions of local public health departments up through about 1900 had largely been associated with community-wide environmental control measures—vital statistics, sanitation, quarantine, communicable disease control and immunization, and laboratory services. The administration of these activities generally featured centralized direction and control rather than operations centered on neighborhood clinics or health centers. Collection of vital statistics was an office-based administration activity; sanitation was an engineering and inspection activity; quarantine called for physical examinations at times, but it was basically an administrative and police activity (the government's right to quarantine supersedes even property rights); communicable disease control consisted in large part of tracing contacts, and some treatment, of persons found to be infected with venereal disease who could not afford private physicians, as well as making provision for infectious tuberculosis cases; much immunization was done by private physicians with vaccines obtained from the health department laboratories; and the newer laboratory services function was also a central headquarters rather than a neighborhood clinic operation. Thus, most health departments were operating out of one central location, or perhaps just a few. With the advent of the aggravated problems of slums in the big cities after 1890, many voices in public health were saying that the biggest new health need of these people was to have preventive health centers in their neighborhoods, that is, that the public health department in these large cities should develop chains of neighborhood health centers.[7] Furthermore, it was argued, these centers should offer additional preventive services of a personal kind—in particular, maternal and child health (well-care only), and health education including nutrition, as well as expanded clinics for tuberculosis and venereal disease control. The subject remained controversial[8] until about 1910, when the New York City health department implemented a system of neighborhood health centers in poor areas that offered not only maternal and child health, but also examinations for venereal disease and tuberculosis detection (and even some treatment). These programs used part-time privately practicing clinicians in their clinics, and thereafter these services gained almost unanimous acceptance in professional public health circles as part of the fundamental rubric of public health services.

By 1920, then, the local public health department in the large city was typically performing the following six basic functions:

1. Vital statistics-collection and interpretation.
2. Sanitation.
3. Communicable disease control (CDC), including immunization, quarantine, and other measures such as identifying communicable disease carriers and distributing vaccines to physicians as well as doing immunizations directly.
4. Maternal and child health (MCH), consisting of prenatal and postpartum care for mothers and well babies and supervision of the health of schoolchildren. In some places immunization of children was handled by the MCH programs.
5. Health education, including instruction in personal and family hygiene, sanitation, and nutrition, given in the schools, at neighborhood health center classes, and in home visits.
6. Laboratory services to physicians, sanitarians, and other interested parties.

In addition to health officers and public health nurses, sanitation engineers and sanitarians, registrars and clerks, and a group of assorted supporting personnel, both professional and administrative, the typical health department staff now also included pediatricians and general practitioners in private practice who served part time in the maternal and child care and communicable disease control programs, being paid on the basis of a fixed fee per clinic session. While these were the basic programs in large cities, additional services such as mental health were often offered, particularly in the largest urban centers.

It is important to bear in mind that health departments in rural areas and small cities had few staff and rarely offered anything beyond the basic services, often being unable to cover even those adequately. Small towns and rural areas continued to have public health organization that was very inadequate in the eyes of public health professional leaders. In many there was no access to any local public health services. Among the small communities that did have a local public health organization, resources were often inadequate to bring to the community the benefits of the preventive services made possible by modern science. Local public health services were provided by an assortment of skeletal staffing patterns. Some places had only a local practitioner who served as a part-time health officer, often with no formal training in public health. There might be a public health nurse, sometimes full time, sometimes part time, and there might be a sanitarian. The problem of bringing the full spectrum of public health skills to the many small communities in the United States was never fully solved. Thus, when we speak of the network of effective local public health departments that had arisen by 1935, it is the large cities, and not even all of these, and some medium-sized cities, that we mean.

I shall return in greater detail to the question of what "covering" the entire United States population with adequate preventive public health services means, but it was necessary to mention here the qualifiers that must be borne in mind in connection with the assertion that the advances in bacteriological science in this era were quickly translated into practical application by local public health departments in the United States.

Primary Care in Public Health Departments and Local Medical Societies

The attitude of the organized medical profession was an important factor in determining the functional boundaries of public health departments. Any expansion of local public health departments into an aspect of "curative," i.e., therapeutic general medicine, was closely and nervously watched by local medical societies.

With the improved state of medical knowledge resulting from biological advances, and the better-trained and more scientifically educated physicians who were graduating from the modern post-1920 medical schools with their scientifically based curricula, the value of personal medical care assumed new importance in the public eye. Along with this rise in public esteem came, naturally enough, a sharpening of the question of who was to be permitted to render this service. The scientific wing of American medicine had organized itself into the American Medical Association (AMA) in 1847, and for the ensuing sixty or seventy years fought a tireless battle to establish its brand of medicine (called "allopathic") as the only one that could be legally practiced. In the course of this battle they fought vigorously against competing schools of medical thought whose adherents they labeled quacks and charlatans. After 1870 the allopaths were successful in getting more and more states to pass laws giving the scientifically based medical societies the sole power to determine the requirements for licensing physicians. With the triumps of medical science and the acceptance of the Flexner report calling for allopathically based curricula in all medical schools[9], their position acquired the force of law in all the states. The medical profession, via the American Medical Association and its state and local affiliates, was busy developing standards and defining the qualifications for practitioners of personal, therapeutic medical care, including the only acceptable mode of medical practice organization. The profession was also defining what types of ancillary medical personnel physicians were permitted to work with and to what scope of function these personnel were limited—in short, what services constituted "medical care," how it should be delivered, and by whom. (See Chapter 13.)

Having gone through some seventy years of bitter struggle to establish the hegemony of scientifically based, or allopathic, medicine, and to secure legal sanction for their exclusive right to define all aspects of medical practice, the local and national medical societies jealously guarded their sole right to give medical care. Their opposition to perceived challenges often took on a very truculent tone accompanied by strong proscriptive action. The American Medical Association and its local affiliates, as part of their insistence on their exclusive right to determine what personal medical "treatment" was and under what circumstances it could be dispensed, were largely responsible for the restriction of public health departments to community-wide activities such as communicable disease and sanitation control after 1920.[10] If a patient were completely indigent, then the organized medical profession had no objection to local or other government agencies treating him or her in public clinics or arranging for treatment in the offices of government-reimbursed physicians. In that case, however, the preference was for per session reimbursement to privately practicing physicians rather than the use of on-staff salaried physicians, and for welfare department sponsorship rather than health department. The health department was expected to restrict itself to strictly preventive activities as defined by the medical societies.

Mustering public support for the claim of the licensed medical profession to be the only legitimate healers was facilitated by the historical development of public health practice. Because of the relatively greater importance of "public" health measures as against personal ministrations during most of the 1800s, public health sanitation and quarantine measures were widely respected while medical therapeutic practice was held in widespread disdain. Sarcastic allusions to the undignified public battles among different "schools" of medical thought often appeared in the press (Shryock, 1979, Chap XIII). Many of the most eminent physicians were in the forefront of public health education and writing. This made it easier for medical societies to develop a consensus after 1920 around a concept that amounted to saying, "Let the public health departments continue to do what public health has always done so very well." However, it developed that the medical societies were saying more than that public health departments be *allowed* to continue their traditional functions. They were saying that public health departments should be *restricted* to performing *only* these functions, and many leading public health officers agreed with them. The local health department's functions came to be considered by the medical profession, public health practitioners, and the general public, to lie almost exclusively in the traditionally public domain of preventing and eliminating threats to the health of the community at large via work in sanitation, communicable disease control, health education, and the like. The other part of this consensus was that the private physician should continue to wield his or her traditional authority over the curative and other personal health care areas for patients who could pay for treatment. The public would long continue to regard the private medical practitioner as a free-lance medical consultant entrepreneur whose services were available on the free market for a fee even though the content of practice and its rewards were changing very sharply and had already changed substantially. The traditional free-lancing private physician was being replaced by an organizational monopoly that could dictate all the terms of practice.

Despite this separation of function, it was usually considered appropriate for the local public health department to offer personal diagnostic, and less frequently, treatment services also, for diseases that were contagious and threatened to become epidemic, notably tuberculosis and venereal disease. These services, consisting of case finding and rendering active cases noninfective, were perceived as part of community-wide prevention activities. A similar interpretation was placed on maternal and child health services, which were viewed as safeguarding the future health of the population, or as later economic writers were to call it, investing in human capital. However, the consensus with respect to the provision of these services by health departments was weaker than on the community-wide services, with opposition sometimes coming from some local medical associations and from the AMA in 1920 (Burrow, 1963, 157–158). The operation of local public general hospitals by local public health departments was not strenuously opposed by private medicine, although as previously noted, welfare department operation was preferred. But public operation of general medical clinics for ambulatory patients was another matter, especially if the eligible clients included low-income persons who were economically a notch above official relief recipients—those later called the near poor, working poor, or "medically indigent only."

In general, there was no need for the local medical society to take overt action to prevent local health departments from operating ambulatory general medical care programs. The belief systems instilled in public health personnel by their training, education, and other social conditioning made them willing and cooperative accessories in these arrangements. The health officers were nearly all physicians and were themselves imbued with the prevailing medical-society ethos. For the most part, they shared the medical profession's views of the appropriate boundaries of public health practice. They also knew that employing part-time private physicians to serve in these general medical care clinics would be a near impossibility if the local medical society disapproved of the operation.[11]

When a local medical society did occasionally decide to take openly proscriptive action, such action could be swift and thoroughgoing. A case in point is the fate of the health care clinics of the Los Angeles County Health Department in

1932 (Worcester, 1934). Under the urging of its director, Dr. J. I. Pomeroy, the state law had been amended to permit, and the county board of supervisors persuaded to establish, a network of twelve "completely equipped health centers" that offered both preventive services and personal general ambulatory care. The latter was available only to patients who could not pay the fees requested by locally practicing physicians in private practice, and the local privately practicing physicians manned the clinics. During the relative prosperity of 1920–29 the operation of the clinics was tolerated by the medical profession; but in 1932, after the Great Depression had severely depleted the patient loads of the local practicing physicians, the county medical society forbade its members to serve in the health centers. The centers were left standing unused, and the medical treatment of indigents was turned over the county welfare ("public charities") department for administration. All patients were referred to the outpatient department of the one county hospital, which was as far as eighty miles distant from some parts of the county. Later a new plan was inaugurated to supplement the county hospital outpatient clinic. It called for fee-for-service reimbursement of physicians treating these indigents in their private offices. A three-year residence requirement for eligibility for welfare benefits reduced the county's patient load, and making the eligibility standards for service at the county hospital more stringent curtailed it still further. Interestingly enough, the private physicians did not experience any noticeable increase in their clientele except for the welfare-office-payment patients. The 1934 article describing this incident concludes: "Last summer [1933] the Los Angeles County Medical Association drew up a long document giving their idea of the whole duty of a health department . . . declaring that all treatment whatsoever should be given under the Welfare Department, not the Health Department. . . . 'Treatment' was defined in a most inclusive manner" (Worcester, 1934).

Thus was the public health department's role with respect to direct patient care laid out for it—in the first instance, internalized by tradition, and occasionally more directly by sharp rebuff when it was perceived by medical societies as overstepping prescribed bounds. The bounds were established at first by historically set precedent and later formally articulated by the medical societies. Clearly the dominant ethos of the time saw curative medical care as a commodity to be purchased by those who could afford it and to be dispensed as charity to those who could not. Wherever an interface existed between the services offered by the local health department and those supplied by the private practitioner, it consisted primarily of two interrelationships. The first relationship centered on communicable disease control. The physician helped public health authorities in their efforts to control communicable disease by reporting cases of certain specified (i.e., "reportable") diseases that came to his or her attention. The local health department, for its part, provided certain services to community physicians that they needed in order to cooperate fully in communicable disease control, services that were not feasible for each physician to provide individually. In particular, laboratory services and other diagnostic aids, usually restricted to communicable disease control, were supplied to community physicians. Under the second relationship, which involved personal services, private physicians served as part-time clinicians in health department clinics approved by the local medical society. These were most often tuberculosis, venereal disease, and maternal and child health clinics. These attitudes were the prevailing ones until quite recently, and their influence can be seen in the types of activities to which most local health departments have predominantly confined themselves to the present day.

As an example of the diffusion of these ideas as norms (i.e., de facto policy), I cite a textbook on "administrative medicine," which was how public health administration was commonly designated. Published as late as 1951 and in widespread use for many years thereafter, its editor was Haven Emerson.[12] The book included an article expressing some of these norms in the following terms:

The modern health department . . . should provide the physician with the bacteriologic, serologic and pathologic tests which are so essential to prompt and adequate diagnosis. . . .

[T]he economic burden of these laboratory services cannot always be borne by the patient and certainly should not become an obligation of the physician. An adequate diagnostic service can be made available to all citizens irrespective of the degree of financial self-sufficiency ... without in any way interfering with the personal relationship which has existed between patient and physician. . . .

The health department must assist in serving the needs of the practicing physician; the public should provide a subvention for service given by the physician to the medically indigent (Vaughan, 1951).

The proper role of a local public health department was thus seen primarily as providing community-wide preventive services. By 1935 the functions of a "full service" department had come to consist of the six services listed on page 20, which were later to be defined as "the basic six" functions of a local health department. Other preventive areas were often included, and it was also deemed proper for public health agencies to provide some direct medical care to specified populations for conditions that were communicable. Those portions of maternal and child care that were primarily concerned with health education and preventive measures were also permitted the public health department. Although prenatal and well-baby clinics had become common features of the local public health department, these functions were much more carefully scrutinized by local medical societies than were the other functions. Accepting, and indeed for the most part actively acquiescing in these limitations of its function, the leadership of the public health profession turned to developing professional staffing standards for carrying out its role and to obtaining public support for implementing these standards. How many and what types of public health staff did a community require?

Staffing Standards and Measuring the Extent of Population Covered by Existing Public Health Departments

A substantial professional literature appeared during the most active period in the development of local public health departments (about 1900–1945) devoted to specifying the resources required to "cover" populations of defined geographic areas with adequate public health services. The earlier studies dealt with descriptions of existing resources rather than with sug-

gested norms, and even when normative studies were later done, they were always fewer than those that collected data on existing resources. This is not an uncommon situation. It is apparently easier to count than to achieve a conceptual consensus on how much is enough.

The early pre-1935 studies assembled and published data on such matters as the number of existing local public health departments, the composition of their staffs, the methods by which they were financed, the populations covered by their services, the item distribution of their expenditures, the type of activities they engaged in, and the type of their local sponsoring governments. While these studies were often directed, in the first instance, at investigating the status of state health departments, a good part of the data collected and the conclusions presented concerned local public health departments because the development of good local departments was seen as a central responsibility of state health departments.

One early study was conducted for the American Medical Association in 1915 by Charles V. Chapin and its results published as a *Survey of State Departments of Health.* Somewhat later, another study was done by the Committee on Administrative Practice (CAP) of the American Public Health Association and was published by the U.S. Public Health Service in 1925 as a Public Health Bulletin entitled *Survey of 100 Largest Cities in the United States* (APHA, 1925). The last study made before 1935 was that of Ferrell and his colleagues,[13] which was carried out under the direction of the Surgeon General of the United States and published by the U.S. Public Health Service in 1929 (Ferrell et al., 1929). Data were collected from state health departments for the calendar year 1925. Some of the principal findings and conclusions of this study follow.

The 1925 Situation per the Ferrell Study

The purpose of the study was to identify geographic areas in the United States served by "full-time" health departments, describe certain characteristics of the departments, and estimate the geographic size and population of each such area with the ultimate intention of deriving the total area and population of all these areas served by full-time departments. A "full-time" local health department was defined simply as one that employed at least one full-time health officer, however trained.[14]

One of the descriptive attributes that was presented was the type of sponsoring local government. The study identified four types of local public health units[15] in existence:

1. The municipal health department, which was quite independent of the state, functioning in a city that operated under charter from the state legislature. This type of department was found in the large cities.

2. The town or township local health department, usually consisting of part-time personnel and offering few services. It was deemed, "as a rule . . . [not to afford] . . . a satisfactory unit for local health work. Its limited population and wealth precludes the employment of full-time professional personnel." This characterization applied only to the preponderance of states where the town or township was a very small local community. It did not apply to the New England states, Illinois, Minnesota, Wisconsin, and "a few other states" where the township was the larger and more important unit of local government compared with the county. In these states the town or township health department was analogous to the county health department described below as the third type of local public health unit.

3. The county health department. The county form of local government existed in at least three-fourths of the states. Its health department had traditionally been a part-time service and because of this ". . . as a rule [it] accomplished little and has not satisfied the State health officers." However, between the period of the earlier study by Chapin (1915) and the year covered by the Ferrell study (1925), the number of full-time county health departments was found to have risen from 13 to 303. It was noted that:

Generally there is intimate cooperation, involving joint administrative and financial responsibilities between the State and county health officials . . . [but] the relationship between State and local health services varies widely. Usually if the local health organization, whether city, county or township, fails to function, particularly during an emergency, the State health officer may assume charge of the situation, do what to him seems necessary, and require the local government to pay the cost. (Ferrel et al., 1929)

In many counties that contained one or more large cities, there were both a county health department and city health departments. The large city health departments served their populations with a range and depth of services that was nearly always much greater than those offered by the county health departments to the residents outside the city. The relationships between the city and county public health departments were often complicated, especially in the area of financing, because the city dwellers paid taxes to both the city and the county but received services only from their city department. Systems of rebates as well as contractual agreements for the exchange of services between city and county governments had arisen in many localities.

4. The district plan. This form of organization was found to exist in two main forms: (a) the state health district plan, under which the state was divided into districts and employees of the state carried out local public health work. The study found the local health work in these districts uncoordinated. Each district had on its staff representatives of different functional or professional divisions of the state health department who looked to the professional specialty-oriented leadership of their division in the state office for guidance, rather than to the community health problem-oriented leadership of their local district chief health officer. (b) The multi-county local health district plan, in which several counties, each often having its own county health department, were loosely grouped together for administrative purposes into a multi-county district under a single district officer who exercised overall supervision over the local health district's employees. Each of the participating counties would then claim to have a full-time, medically trained chief public health officer, even though the same person was being named by the several counties.

With the growth of full-time county health departments, the states increasingly came to administer state health districts only in those areas where full-time local departments did not exist. The perception of the key to good local public health department coverage outside large urban centers came to focus on the concept of *full-time* staffing. The percentage of the state's population that was judged to have access to full-time service varied from less than 1 percent in Massachusetts to 82 percent in Ohio. (A list of all the states may be found in Ferrell et al., 1929, Table 8.)

The division of the funding of local public health departments between state and local sources also varied greatly from state to state. In some states the funds came almost exclusively from the state, while in others the localities contributed more or less substantially. (An idea of the divergence in degree of local contribution to such funding may be gleaned from the examples taken from Table 2–1, Ferrell et al., 1929). Whether the variations from state to state in the proportion of health expenditures met locally reflected primarily differences in local interest, differences in local taxing power vis-à-vis state taxing power, or other factors was not evident from the report.

Although the federal government did not enter substantially into the local public health picture until 1935, the early years of the twentieth century did witness the introduction of some federal participation in funding local public health work, foreshadowing the complicated patchwork quilt that was later to become the predominant pattern. Three important instances of federal financial assistance for local public health work in these earlier years were grants-in-aid to the states under the Kahn-Chamberlain Act of 1918, providing funds for venereal disease control; the Shepherd-Towner Act of 1921, making grants available to states providing funds for maternal and child health care through 1929; and U.S. Public Health Service grants for studies and demonstrations in rural sanitation beginning with 1914. Much of the federal funds granted to the states under these acts found their way to local public health departments.

Later studies gave the total number of counties (areas outside large cities only—large cities

Table 2–1. Local Share of Total State Public Health Expenditures

State	Total public health budget in state	From local funds	Percent local funds of total
Alabama	$732,083	$430,971	58.87
Arizona	32,405	—	0.00
Arkansas	116,113	8,882	7.65

nearly all had full-time departments) covered by full-time local public health departments as having risen to 762 by 1935. These "covered" 37 percent of the population outside the large cities; the total population covered, including the large cities, was 74 million, or about 56 percent of the nation's population. This compares with only fifteen counties that had been found to have full-time local county health departments in 1915 (Kratz, 1962; Sanders, 1959).

THE PERIOD 1935 AND AFTER

Growth in Local Health Department Coverage During 1936–45

The ten-year interval 1936 through 1945 was characterized by growth in local and state public health departments financed substantially with newly introduced federal assistance.[16] The programs appropriate for a state-of-the-art health department were defined by leading members of the American Public Health Association working in committees, and the new financial aid made available through federal funds was used to expand the coverage of the United States population by professionally staffed health departments.

The Social Security Act and Public Health

The Social Security Act of 1935 established annual grants-in-aid from the federal government to the states. Part of the purpose of these grants was to further the development of full-time local public health departments. The passage of the Social Security Act marks the beginning of the period that is the principal subject of this book, 1935–1980. I identify this period as the era of transformation of the United States government from a laissez-faire to a social welfare state. Because I shall refer to this landmark act subsequently in many places, and in connection with topics other than public health departments, it may be useful to outline its original provisions briefly here.

Passed on August 14, 1935, as Public Law No. 271 of the Seventy-fourth Congress (i.e., P.L. 74–271), the Social Security Act consisted

of eleven titles and addressed four principal areas of social legislation. These areas and the
numbers of the titles applying to them were as
follows:

1. Social insurance.
   a. Establishment of Retirement Benefits—
      Titles II and VIII, to be administered by
      an independent agency, the Social Secu-
      rity Board.
   b. Establishment of Unemployment Insur-
      ance Benefits—Titles III and IX, to be ad-
      ministered by the states.
2. Cash assistance for categorically[17] indigent
   persons (''public welfare'' or ''public assistance''). Matching grants were provided to
   the states for:
   a. Old Age Assistance—Title I.
   b. Aid for Dependent Children—Title IV.
   c. Aid to the Blind—Title X.
3. Public health work to be administered by the
   U.S. Public Health Service.
      Grants were provided to the states for aid-
   ing the work of state and local public health
   departments—Title VI (see also Title V, part
   1, under No 4.a. immediately below). The
   states were required to match the federal
   grants with specified contributions of their
   own. These have therefore been designated
   as ''matching grants.''
4. Maternal and Child Welfare to be administis-
   tered by the U.S. Children's Bureau.
   a. Matching grants were provided to the
      states for aiding state and local health de-
      partments in providing maternal and child
      health services—Title V, part 1.
   b. Matching grants were provided to the
      states for services to crippled children—
      Title V, part 2.
   c. Matching grants were provided to the
      states for child welfare services—Title V,
      part 3.

Other titles and provisions dealt with definitions of terms and with augmenting federal support for the Vocational Rehabilitation Act,
passed originally in 1920.

The Social Security Act was the first substantial entry of the national government into the
general field of social welfare and may be
viewed as its founding charter. It was, for so

technologically developed a country, very late
in arriving. Germany had legislated major social
insurance provisions in the 1880s, a point that is
discussed more fully later when we turn to medical care services. In addition to the lateness in
our history of federal entry into the social welfare arena, it should be noted that the four components of social welfare included in the act,
retirement pensions, cash assistance, unemployment insurance, and public health, are
treated quite differently in important respects.
This reflects fundamental differences in policy
conceptions about these social welfare measures.

The centerpiece of the Social Security Act
was the establishment of what most people today
regard as *the* ''social security system''—
namely, old age retirement pensions. It was established as a uniform system across the nation,
involved no state participation and no contributions to the retirement fund from general taxes
such as the income tax. The financing was solely
by employer and employee contributions, and
eligibility for benefits was on the basis of having
paid into the fund for a requisite number of specified time periods (''quarters''). Thus, collecting
one's retirement check was clearly recognized
as a *right* because the money had come from
worker and employer contributions expressly
made for this purpose. These special taxes were
placed into an earmarked reserve fund, a so-
called trust fund, which was not subject to congressional appropriate action or discretionary
presidential disbursement actions. The fund was
administered by a specially created Social Security Board not lodged within any cabinet department. The Social Security Board was responsible for collecting the taxes, putting them
into the proper trust funds, and paying out the
benefits according to the stipulations of the
act.

The provisions for general public health services, Title VI, and for maternal and child
health, Title V, part 1, were quite different.
While the retirement provisions constituted an
insurance scheme conferring personal pension
rights on its beneficiaries based on *special* taxes
paid by them and their employers and laid away
in special trust funds, the money for public
health and maternal and child health was allotted

to state governments in the form of congressionally appropriated grants from *general* tax revenue for state and local government-operated health services. It was true that persons wishing to use public health services, now to be partially subsidized by the federal government, were all eligible without proof of having paid into any fund. In this sense, use of available public health services was a right rather than an earned privilege. However, the amount of money available was subject to annual appropriations by Congress; and the state and local administration of the program meant that the available services would vary greatly in quality and population coverage from region to region, again differentiating it from the pension system, which was strictly federal and uniform across the nation. It was expected that this variability in public health services would be reduced over time by the setting of uniform standards by the national government. It was, to a degree, but federal support of the programs was never great enough to enable it to effectively mandate a uniform national system of high-quality public health services, as we shall see. The public health grants did not guarantee directly to individual persons the national availability of a specified level of maternal and child health or other public health services. They only offered support (matching) for the efforts a state wished to make up to a specified level of expenditure. The retirement program, on the other hand, nationally guaranteed uniform pensions directly to individual persons.

The fact that the federal public health money came out of the national general tax fund has implications for policy that are worth noting carefully. On the one hand, the general tax fund, or more simply the general fund, consists of money collected by the government for the general purpose of running the government. At the time of collection it is not earmarked for any specific governmental functions. Its disposition is decided by legislative appropriation and by the presidential budgeting and disbursing processes. By contrast, earmarked or trust fund taxes are collected for a special purpose and can be used only for this purpose. Congress determines what amounts shall be collected and paid out and how the agency administering the trust fund shall operate, but the funds cannot be used for any purpose other than that for which it was

collected. Examples of other programs for which taxes are often collected on a trust fund or earmarked basis are those for highways and schools. The amount of public health and maternal and child health money available under the Social Security Act was, therefore, subject both to congressional appropriation and presidential disbursement processes because it came from the general fund. Presidential disbursement procedures can seriously affect how a congressional appropriation is spent during the implementation process through the various types of executive orders and regulations issued. In the sequel we shall see how the president was able to substantially thwart congressional intent by using these devices when the majority in Congress and the president disagreed on a program at different times in subsequent years. It should also be noted that the payment of the federal grants allocated to any one state was contingent on the state matching the expenditures. Although this never became a major problem with respect to public health grants, the policy position implied by this difference in treatment was that retirement benefits for employed persons were perceived as too great a national concern to be left to the vagaries of state-by-state variation or the changing moods and views of different Congresses or presidents. Public health,[18] on the other hand, was left as an unsettled *national* priority, to be battled over perennially in the political arena.

On the other hand, the income tax, which is the main component of federal general revenues is, to some degree at least, a progressive tax. That is, the tax rate is positively related to a person's income. By contrast, the pension fund's earmarked tax was a flat rate on earnings and was capped at a fixed maximum income. That is, a working person paid no further pension (Social Security) tax after a specified income. If the maximum for a particular year were $10,000 for example, a person earning $10,000 and one earning $100,000 paid the same Social Security tax. From the point of view of progressivity, then, the financing of the public health grants was more equitable than that of the pension fund. Thus, the funding of the pensions was more secure, but the funding of the public health grants was more equitable in social welfare point terms.

Effects of the Social Security Act on Public Health Organization: Findings of the Mountin Report

The portions of the act that concern us most at this point are Title VI and Title V, part 1, as listed in numbers 3 and 4 above. Federal support providing for local public health departments was based on these two titles. Much of the progress in the development of these departments through 1946 was described by Joseph W. Mountin and his associates in a noteworthy Public Health Bulletin (Moutin, Hankla, and Druzina, 1947). Dr. Mountin was an assistant Surgeon General of the United States Public Health Service, well known for his work in health policy analysis during this period, and a substantial expansion of local and state services is detailed in that report.[19]

Further consideration of these federal grants-in-aid to public health departments will be given under the discussion of the role of the federal government in Chapter 4, but a brief overview of some of these reported changes in the local health department picture during the first ten years, 1936–1946, is pertinent here. It may safely be presumed that many of these changes flowed from the federal funds pumped into local health departments as "pass throughs" by the states, for, as Mountin noted, "Large portions of the grants-in-aid distributed to States by the Public Health Service . . . have been reallocated to local health units or expended for the provision of direct local services by the State health agency itself (Mountin, Hankla, and Druzina, 1947).

Local Health Department Growth During 1936–45, Excluding Cities[20] The Mountin report,[21] indicated that the number of counties covered by full-time local public health services grew from 762 in 1935, to 1,577 in 1940, and to 1,851 in 1946, and that the proportion of the population outside the cities covered by public health services rose from 37 percent in 1935 to 72 percent by 1946. The growth in number of counties covered was not paralleled by a proportionate increase in the number of public health organizational "units," for the structural form of local health department organization was shifting in favor of more multicounty units, either locally controlled or organized as state districts. A

"unit" is any one of the four local public health organizational forms described on pages 25 through 26. (See also note 15.) The number of units was 561 in 1935 and 980 in 1946, an increase of only 75 percent compared with an increase of 143 percent in the number of counties covered. (The percentage of the total population, *including* cities, covered by full-time local health services also increased: from 56 percent in 1935 to 82 percent in 1946.)

The influence that Mountin presumed these funds to have had on the staffing growth in local health departments, exclusive of the independent urban centers, was equally marked. Total full-time personnel, excluding cities, increased from 3,435 to 10,320 and more rapidly in nonmedical than in medical personnel. The relative increases are shown in Table 2–2. This improvement was accomplished in face of the fact that "a considerable proportion of established positions for medical—and others—were vacant for war-related reasons . . ." (Mountin et al., 1947).

The Municipal Health Department As has been noted, the local organizations delivering public health services that fully reflected the scientific advances made in determining the cause of disease and the way it spread were largely to be found among the municipal health departments. Mountin defined municipal health departments as "those city health units which operate under full-time technical direction and are independent of county or district organization" (Mountin et al., 1947). The data he presented indicated that during the period from 1936 through 1945 at least sixty cities with populations of 10,000 or over were added to the list of cities with "some type of full-time official public health organization."

He also noted that "all data on units reported

Table 2–2. Increases in Full-time Health Personnel 1936–49 (County or Multi-county Health Organizations)

Type of personnel	Percent increase
Medical	25.95
Nursing	170.12
Sanitation	225.12
Clerical	297.74
Other	450.88
Increase in total personnel	200.44

in both years seem to indicate a tendency for municipal health departments to combine with single county organizations or to become part of State or local districts.'' The trend toward combining county health departments with city health departments continued beyond 1946 and was very much in evidence in the 1960s and 1970s. It was an important phenomenon and is discussed further at the end of this chapter where the general question of mergers of local government public health agencies is addressed.

Yet, in 1946 approximately 30 percent of the nonmetropolitan, and almost 20 percent of the total population, still remained without full-time local health coverage. Perhaps more importantly, an undetermined amount of the expanded ''full-time'' coverage was of questionable quality and often came close to being a reporting artifact. Mountin noted that much of the increase in ''percent of rural population covered by full-time health departments'' resulted from simply bringing additional areas into the jurisdiction of an existing public health unit by consolidating counties into local multicounty or state health districts. In Mountin's words:

The organization of two or more counties, especially those forming natural social and economic districts, into larger public health units in order to use combined resources and personnel more effectively has many advocates. It should be pointed out, however, that the present organizations have frequently resulted somewhat haphazardly from deficiencies in personnel. Some units cover such vast areas that adequate local service cannot be maintained with the staff available (Mountin et al., 1947).

In other words, if public health ''coverage'' was unacceptably thin, it was hardly coverage at all. But just what must public organization consist of if its coverage was not to be considered too thin? The Emerson Report attempted to answer this question.

The Emerson Report

By 1940 public health professional leadership and analysts were already asserting with growing insistence that extending coverage by ''full-time'' local public health services of at least minimally acceptable quality to the entire population was an important and perhaps the over-

riding goal of public health. The public health they were talking about was government-owned and -operated health services restricted in scope to preventive measures, control of communicable disease, and allied matters.[22] In the words of one of their main spokesmen, Haven Emerson: ''We know now that we can afford nothing less than coverage of every population and area unit of our nation with competent local health service'' (foreword to Emerson Report, 1945). It was becoming increasingly evident, however, that if the term ''full-time coverage'' were to be really meaningful for making comparisons among areas or measuring change over time, it would have to be defined just what services and personnel constituted acceptable ''coverage.'' Certainly greater specificity was needed than merely having at least a full-time chief.

The growth of local public health departments brought about with the aid of federal grants was accompanied by a heightened interest in defining minimally adequate quality, which was formulated largely in terms of establishing ''adequate'' staffing per population. The practice cited by Mountin of increasing the reported ''population covered'' by merely extending the geographic jurisdiction of existing personnel, and thereby spreading them too thin, was only too well known. A number of annual meetings of the American Public Health Association issued policy statements redefining the standards for staffing local departments in the hope that the quantity ''percent population covered'' would come to represent a well-defined minimum standard of depth of coverage. A special committee of the APHA working on this question had by 1945 prepared and issued a carefully defined set of minimum staffing standards for judging whether a local public health department was at least structurally ''competent.'' Applying these minimum staffing standards to local health departments would make possible a valid judgment of just how well the country was covered by adequate public health services and enable an effective campaign to be waged for complete coverage. These standards were embodied in what has come to be known as the ''Emerson report.''

Issued in January 1945, the report was the result of a study by the Subcommittee on Local Health Units of the Committee on Administrative Practice (CAP) of the American Public Health Association, chaired by the well-known public health administrator and writer Haven Emerson. The report (1945) presented data describing the existing situation in 1942 with respect to public health personnel, expenditures, and the number and types of governmental units in charge of local public health work. Alongside these numbers detailing the existing situation for each state were figures representing the "required" resources, personnel, and expenditures deemed necessary to provide for "basic and reasonably adequate local health services." Jurisdiction boundaries were prescribed for local public health units across the entire country as were the organizational forms of local health department units. The report focused on two inadequacies of local public health services in the United States: (1) As of 1942, the committee estimated that 40 million persons, or about 30 percent of the population, lived in communities that were not served by full-time local public health services, even when the "full-time" continued to be defined merely as a service in charge of a full-time health officer (however trained). The complete discontinuance was recommended of public health departments headed by a part-time health officer who often was also in private medical practice. (2) In many supposedly covered communities the existing "full-time" services were staffed and supported at levels below those the subcommittee considered minimally adequate. A national total of 40,782 public health personnel and an average expenditure of 61 cents per capita were the conditions existing in 1942, compared with the committee's suggested minimum of 63,865 personnel and 97 cents per capita. Applying their norms for minimum staffing for "adequate" services to the local populations the committee found that the percentage coverage in 1942 of the population by *adequate*local public health services was substantially less than the commonly used 70 percent derived by using the weak standard of "at least one full-time health officer" as the criterion for defining *full-time* coverage.

Personnel Standards The Emerson Report's recommendations included detailed specifications of personnel standards and a definition of the scope of function of public health depart-

ments that was to serve as the basis for determining adequate staffing criteria. For example, the minimum staffing specification for a public health unit of acceptable quality included a full-time, professionally trained and experienced medical officer of health and a full-time public health or sanitary engineer at the top. There was also to be, for each 50,000 persons covered, one full-time sanitarian of nonprofessional grade, ten public health nurses (1 per 5,000 persons), and three clerical workers (1 per 17,000 persons). All clinicians needed for diagnosis and control of tuberculosis and venereal disease and for prenatal, infant, preschool, and school health services were to be part-time consultants in private practice.

For places with larger populations, additional full-time health officers heading up divisions (e.g., communicable disease control, maternal and child hygiene, etc.) would be feasible, and it was suggested that special personnel such as health educators and nutritionists be employed. Whenever the community would go along, staffing and programming richer than the "minimally adequate" levels were recommended, but always within the limits of the standard public health scope of function.[23] When these recommended minimal staffing standards were applied to the 1,197 suggested local public health jurisdictions, a total of some 55,000 full-time positions was projected.

Clearly, had some form of these standards been widely adopted and applied, it would have reduced the statistical legerdemain used in reporting what percent of the population has "full-time coverage,"[24] but as we shall see, widespread implementation was never achieved. The standards set by the Emerson Report and adopted by the full APHA constituted a privately enunciated policy formulated by a private association of professionals. They never became either enunciated or de facto public policy.

It is noteworthy that the subcommittee recommended the elimination of all part-time employees except privately practicing clinical physicians and dentists who came in for clinical sessions. It recommended that the existing 5,966 other part-time positions, in particular those of the 4,316 part-time health officers, be abolished and that the numbers of part-time clinicians be sharply increased from 5,615 in 1942 to 9,508, with the most dramatic increase being suggested for dentists.[25]

One of the most important recommendations was for an increase in public health nurses from the then existing ratio of 1 per 8,900 population to 1 per 5,000.

Scope of Function The section of the report that proved to have the greatest longevity in terms of public perception of what public health departments do was the subcommittee's definition of the six basic functions of a local health department which came to be known as the "basic six" (see page 20). It is evident that the definition had not broadened from the pre-1920 conceptualization that I call "standard public health".[26] It also was substantially, though not completely, in agreement with the formulation of the medical societies. The official national position of organized medicine generally granted these functions to the local health department, but did not do so unqualifiedly even as late as seventeen years after the Emerson report. For example, the official policy recommendation on the scope of public health services adopted by the 1962 meeting of the American Medical Association House of Delegates stated:

(1) That the state and county medical societies be encouraged to evaluate periodically their public health department's activities in terms of local health needs, programs, and resources.[27]

(2) That state and county medical societies ascertain and acknowledge that public health departments should include at least the following basic services:

(a) Vital Statistics
(b) Public health education
(c) Environmental Sanitation
(d) Public health laboratories, *if private facilities are unavailable*
(e) Prevention and control of communicable disease
(f) Hygiene of maternity, infancy, and childhood, *if private facilities are unavailable.*

(3) That the policy statement of the American Medical Association be as follows: Public health is the art and science of maintaining, protecting, and improving the health of the people through organized community efforts. It includes those arrangements whereby the community provides medical services for *special groups* of persons and is concerned with the *prevention or control of disease*, with persons *requiring hospitalization to protect the community*, and with the *medically indigent.*

(4) That state and county medical societies should collaborate with departments of public health in the interest of community health, always keeping in mind the need for a prope balance between local public health programs and the private practice of medicine (AMA, 1962). [Emphasis added.]

This statement, while more restrictive in its view of the scope of public health functions than the APHA position of the Emerson report (as indicated by the italicized phrases), was already an expanded view of the functions allowed to the public health department in prior AMA positions. More important than the nature of any differences in policy between the APHA and the AMA is the fact that while APHA policy pronouncements generally remained *enunciated* private policy, representing expressions of desires of public health professionals, AMA policy declarations were very often enforced as de facto public as well as private policy. Thus, the role of public health vis-à-vis offering personal general medical services was more effectively shaped by the organized medical profession than by the public health profession. The enforcement and conversion to de facto public policy by the general medical profession of its *enunciated* policies was accomplished through its lobbying powers in government, control of hospital privileges, licensing bodies, and other such means. It is an instructive example of how the health care system works, illustrating where many of its power centers lie and how they are largely hidden from view. In contrast to the political power wielded by a highly organized medical profession to convert its enunciated policies into de facto ones, the public health profession could only offer professional opinions by people who, on the one hand, were anxious not to offend their medical colleagues in private medical practice, and on the other, had to contend with their local government employers who were vulnerable to the lobbying of the powerful local, state, and national medical societies.

Jurisdictional Boundaries Another subject on which the Emerson Report had much to say was the drawing of jurisdictional boundaries defining catchment areas of local public health departments. In attempting to survey the public health needs of the nation, the Emerson committee used the methodology that was later followed by the Hill-Burton program (see Chapter 12) to assay the national "need" for hospital beds. It was one of the early examples of population-based planning for small areas. After boundaries of catchment areas were delineated, the fixed per capita standards for personnel that the subcommittee had formulated were applied to the population of the defined catchment areas and a "requirements" figure derived.[28] The establishment of mutually exclusive catchment areas, or jurisdictions, has always proved to be one of the most difficult problems in population-based health services planning, and this case was no exception. The area had to be small enough for a health department to minister to the local client population and large enough to contain sufficient population to warrant employing the recommended minimal staff.

The subcommittee found that in 1942 there were "38,000 local jurisdictions of civil government within the 48 states," including 3,070 counties. Of these, there were 18,500, apart from school districts,

which may be responsible for local public health service. . . . In addition, in most states school health service [was] the responsibility of school boards in either the entire state or in parts of it. . . . In most of the southern, western and midwestern states, the county has been the local unit of government, but in many of the New England and North Atlantic states each town, village or city traditionally had its own board of health and health officer. Working state by state and considering such factors as natural trading areas, geographic and topological characteristics, disposable income, number of practicing physicians and number of hospital beds available, the Committee arrived at a total of 1,197 units of local health jursdiction.

The health officers of thirty-seven states and the District of Columbia approved these boundaries "in principle"; the rest offered various objections or did not reply to the request for their approval.

The Local Board of Health The Emerson Report also concerned itself with the definition of the desirable structure and functions of the local board of health.

It is suggested that where permissive or at least no inhibitory legislation is in effect there be a board of health appointed by the executives of the local government included within the unit of health administration, such a board to have not less than five nor more than seven members, to be approximately representative of the counties and cities within a unit, but to be selected from among persons with knowledge of public health, either professionally or from public service or civic interest. It is desirable that at least two or three of the board members be physicians. Others should by laymen, men or women from any walk of life, persons of ability and known to have a broad social viewpoint and a serious interest in the health protection of their community.

The terms of members of such a board should be of about five years duration and overlapping so that not more than two members retire or are replaced or re-elected in any one year.

The functions of such a board should be advisory to the health officer, who should be the secretary of teh board but without a vote, policy-forming in respect to the functions of the department of health, legislative with respect to local ordinances not inconsistent with the public health law of the state, and quasi-judicial in the matter of hearings where citizens complain of arbitrary action of the officer of health in enforcing sanitary law. The members of the board of health should serve without pay. Travel expenses to attend meetings of the board should be met (Emerson, 1945).

It should be noted that the later idea of "consumer" representation in the sense of "typical" and "representative" community persons is not stressed. Instead, the more traditional idea of "public member" is stressed in describing the lay representatives; the emphasis is on persons of "ability" and civic prominence "with knowledge of public health either professionally or from public service or civic interest." The qualifications speak to obtaining board members with expertise,[29] power, and prominence in the community. These ideas were different from the thinking about the composition of public boards that was to arise in the 1960s and 1970s when emphasis was in almost the opposite direction: that the board not be dominated by technical expertise and thus insufficiently represent the needs of the nonexpert constituent public. The later idea was that consumer representatives should be "experts" in knowing what the community wants and needs, rather than knowing only what the community should have from a technically professional expert assessment. The report presents the board as a policy-forming, legislative and quasi-judicial appointive body—typical of many regulatory bodies in governmental functioning today. The question of who should make up boards of health was later "solved" by their total disappearance in many places. This was even more true of state health boards levels and is discussed in Chapter 3.

Financing Also interesting, especially in light of subsequent developments, is a recommendation about continuing need for state and federal subsidies to local public health departments as an equalizing factor:

It is taken for granted that, by state and federal subsidies or grants, indispensible health protective services will be provided for those units of local health jurisdictions which cannot from their own tax resources meet the cost.

In support of the contention that the relative per capita expenditure for public health had continued to be quite uneven among the different states, even after six years of federal support under the Social Security Act of 1935, the report exhibited data that clearly indicated the pattern of wide divergence among states in expenditures relative to ability to pay (expressed as the ratio of per capita expenditures to per capita spendable income). The states that could afford it least were often paying more for public health, relative to their per capita incomes, because they needed public health services the most; yet there was every reason to believe that these states were not spending enough despite the fact that they were straining their budgets more than many less needy states.

For example, Mississippi, which had the lowest estimated per capita spendable income of any state ($238), spent more per capita for local health services (57 cents) than 27 other states including Delaware, Illinois, Indiana, and Pennsylvania, all of which are among the 16 states having the highest per capita spendable income in 1941. In Mississippi 24 cents of $100 per capita spendable income was spent for local health service; in no other state was more than 18 cents spent, in 30 states less than 10 cents, and in Indiana and Iowa only 4 cents.

These observations were offered to support the continued need for federal grants that would be structured to equalize the burden of per capita expenditure for "public health work" among the states. At the time this notion elicited no significant opposition from any segment of public opinion, given acceptance of the assumptions about appropriate scope of function of local health departments.[30]

Comments The report gave the goals of public health for the future in these terms:

The Committee is of the opinion that a present goal should be the creation of such number and boundaries of areas of local health jurisdiction in every state in the Union as will bring within the reach of every person and family the benefits of modern sanitation, personal hygiene, and the guidance and protection of trained professional and accessory personnel employed on a full-time basis at public expense, selected and retained on a merit or civil service basis, and free from disturbance by the influence of partisan politics.

(The emphasis on the merit civil service system of personnel practice, a recurring theme in public health policy literature of the time, is worthy of note.)

The importance that this committee and the American Public Health Association attached to the goals enunciated in their report may be inferred from their aforementioned efforts to obtain approval of the professional and political organizations whose cooperation would be needed to implement the recommendations. In addition to the previously noted approval by the health officers of thirty-seven states, endorsers of the principles included the House of Delegates of the AMA, the American Public Health Association, and the State and Provincial Health Authorities of North America.

By 1945 the Mountin study had documented the gains made in organizing public health department work in the first ten years after the passage of the Social Security Act. It had also pointed to the remaining deficiencies. The Emerson Report had made specific the requirements for an adequate local public health department and laid out the boundaries of some 1200 local public health units that would cover the entire nation with adequate public health services if each unit would meet the minimum standards prescribed in the report. Written approval for this plan was obtained from important bodies and individuals. Thus armed and motivated, the public health profession set forth after 1945 to complete its mission of bringing at least minimally adequate public health services to all the American people. We turn now to an examination of how this "movement" fared.

Developments After the Emerson Report: The Period 1946–1965

Development of the "Standard" Local Public Health Department Reaches its Zenith

The period 1936–1945 had been one of consolidating the position of local health departments. With the new federal Social Security Act Title V and Title VI funds and the matching state contributions, local public health departments performing the standard "basic six" functions became better established in many localities. The careful formulations of the Emerson Report testify to the efforts put into planning and to the intellectual vitality of the national professional leadership and of the chief executives of these public health departments. Moreover, the staff leadership of the federal government's health activities was in general accord with the goals of the Emerson Report and worked hand-in-glove with local and state leaders to develop public health departments with greater depth of personnel and wider geographic coverage.

But dissenting voices were beginning to be raised—some had even been heard in the earlier pre-1946 period—about the inadequacy of the scope of function of these departments, noting that times were changing and the "basic six" functions would no longer suffice to discharge the public health department's duty to protect the health of the public. Two main themes dominated these critiques: one called for more attention to controlling the incidence and progression of chronic and degenerative diseases; the other for providing general medical ambulatory care in public health department clinics. These jarring notes began to be widely and loudly heard during the period after World War II. The Mountin study, while generally lauding the progress made in public health organization, had nevertheless warned in 1946 that the emergence of chronic disease as an increasingly important public health problem necessitated a reorientation of priorities for public health work. Also, the growing social and economic problems in the large cities, the growth of a system of private health insurance that covered only the nonpoor, and the social reformism of the national administrations combined to put pressure on local public health departments to deliver types of services that were essentially alien to the spirit expressed by the Emerson Report's recommendations. Fundamentally, these had been limited to calling for improved preventive services directed at controlling acute infectious disease.

By 1960, it appeared that the development of the local public health department had gone about as far as it was to go. Federal funding was declining, and expansion of the departments, either in the percentage of the population covered or in the depth of services offered, had reached a peak and was remaining static or even declining. An analysis made in 1957 by Barker S. Sanders (1959), a technical consultant for the U.S. Public Health Service, indicated that the percentage of the total population covered by full-time local health services had risen from 75 percent in 1946 to 86 percent by 1950. Thereafter, its annual rate of increase was slow, reaching about 90 percent in 1957. The number of counties with full-time health departments rose from about 1,850 in 1946 to 2,100 in 1950 and thence to about 2,300 in 1957. Similarly, expenditures, when adjusted for population changes in the areas affected and by a wage and price index specially constructed to reflect changes in value of the dollar for those items for which local health departments spent most of their money (i.e., real per capita expenditures), showed an increase between 1946 and 1950, and thereafter remained static or declined slightly. The same was true of the percentage of the gross national product spent by local health departments, and a similar pattern was shown in the number of full-time public health workers employed.[31] The analysis also indicated a sharp decline in the contribution of federal funds to the cost of local public health department operations from $15 million (19 percent) in 1947 to $9 million (5 percent) in 1956 (Sanders, 1959), so that the brunt of the total expenditures fell increasingly on state and especially local sources. The decline in the federal contribution was made up by increases in the local contribution from $54 million to $127 million, and in the state contribution from $10 million to $40 million over the span of the indicated years. The reduction in the relative contribution from federal sources, therefore, was even greater than the reduction measured in absolute dollar amounts. Had the federal contribution increased proportionally as much as the state and local did, it would have added some $30 million additional dollars, and the resulting picture would have been quite different from what it actually was. The decline in federal contribution reflects, in part, increases in funds spent directly by the states and by federal agencies instead of being channelled through grants to local public health departments. Sanders speculated on the possible causes for this slowdown in rate of increase:

[It] could mean that other agencies are taking over certain needed health services, or that American communities are not so much interested in health, or perhaps health needs that can be dealt with effectively by local health departments have diminished. (1959)

The causes for this declining federal contribution to local public health departments have not been widely investigated, but the first and third of Sanders's suppositions seem reasonable and explain the subsequent course of events rather well. It can be cogently argued that many of the functions of protecting the public's health had become increasingly less amenable to local control, and it is a fact that regional, state and federal agencies have been performing them more and more. These functions include such matters as pollution control, safety, food and drug regulation, and a host of others, discussed in Chapters 3 and 4.

By 1960, some 94 percent of the population was judged to have access to the services of full-time health departments (Greve and Campbell, 1961). There were 1,557 such departments and they included 2,425 of the 3,072 counties in their jurisdictions. But the 94 percent coverage was still being measured under the less than satisfactory definition of "full-time" as having "at least one full-time health officer" rather than by some more meaningful measure like the "recommended per capita" personnel standards of the Emerson Report. Thus, one of the main goals of the APHA as voiced in that report—to change the commonly accepted way of computing public health coverage to consider only departments that were adequate, i.e., staffed to APHA minimal standards—was not realized. Although, in an arbitrarily narrow sense, widespread coverage had been achieved, the depth or quality of

coverage recommended by the Emerson Report was lacking, as may be seen by comparing the staffing levels recommended by the report with actual numbers in 1960. Table 2–3 compares the full-time personnel levels per population existing in 1942, the recommendations of the Emerson report, and the actual situation as of January 1, 1960.[32] The data clearly indicate that the per capita personnel implied in the Emerson Report recommendations had not been achieved by 1960. In the all-important categories of public health nurses and dental personnel, the staffing remained far short of the recommendations; dental hygienists and public health nurses per population actually declined from the 1942 ratios. Indeed, the overall staff to population ratio was somewhat lower in 1960 than in 1942.

Furthermore, the concern of Joseph Mountin expressed in 1946 that "Some [public health] units cover such vast areas that adequate local service cannot be maintained with the staff available," had also not been addressed. This applied particularly to areas of the country where a number of counties, each with its own public health department, would band together into a loosely confederated multicounty health district headed by a single district health officer. Each of the counties was listed as having "full-time" health departments in national tallies. It had been a central purpose of the Emerson Report to call attention to this thinness of staffing by establishing staff/population ratios; but a 1978 study (Shonick and Price, 1978) found that as late as 1975, 9.2 percent of the 545 local public health units reporting "full-time" public health officers as their head were sharing the same person with one other unit and 16.9 percent of the reporting units had public health officers that were in charge of three or more units. Of the total 721 units reporting, 26 percent had "full-time" public health officers who were shared with other jurisdictions. Furthermore, 24 percent of these units still had only part-time chiefs, and 22 percent of all the units having part-time chiefs shared them with other jurisdictions. Only 203 of 746 reporting agencies (27.2 percent) were headed by what the Emerson Report called "a professionally trained . . . medical officer of health" and a number of these were part-time with some serving more than one local government jurisdiction.

Table 2–3. Comparison of Local Health Department Personnel: Actual for 1942, Recommended by the Emerson Report, and Actual for 1960 (per 100,000 population)

	1942 actual per Emerson Report			Min. recommended in Emerson Report			1960 actual per Greve & Campbell		
	Full time	Part time	Total	Full time	Part time	Total	Full time	Part time	Total
Physicians	2.24	4.28	6.52	1.53	—	1.53	0.79	4.87	5.66
Part-time clinicians	—	4.61	4.61	—	4.56	4.56	—	—	—
Public health nurses	13.61	0.53	14.14	19.60	—	19.60	8.13	0.25	8.38
Clinic nurses	—	—	—	—	—	—	0.37	0.20	0.57
Sanitary personnel									
professionally trained	0.53	0.04	0.57	1.40	0.01	1.41	3.84	0.27	4.11
others	4.63	0.25	4.88	2.91	—	2.91	1.37	0.17	1.54
Laboratory personnel	1.19	0.15	1.34	2.62	—	2.62	0.84	0.05	0.89
Clerical and administrative workers	4.79	0.44	5.23	6.64	—	6.64	5.99	0.06	6.05
Dentists	0.30	0.95	1.25	0.33	2.48	2.81	0.17	0.87	1.04
Dental hygienists	0.32	0.05	03.7	3.17	—	3.17	0.22	0.01	0.23
Health educators	0.04	—	0.04	0.40	0.01	0.41	0.16	0.00	0.16
Maintenance, custodial, and service	—	—	—	—	—	—	1.04	—	1.04
Others:									
Nutritionists	—	—	—	—	—	—	0.08	0.00	0.08
Medical & Psychiatric Social Workers	—	—	—	—	—	—	0.24	0.03	0.27
Psychologists	—	—	—	—	—	—	0.06	0.04	0.10
Public health investigators	—	—	—	—	—	—	0.22	0.01	0.23
X-ray technicians	—	—	—	—	—	—	0.20	0.04	0.24
Physical therapists	—	—	—	—	—	—	0.09	0.07	0.16
Medical aides and assistants	—	—	—	—	—	—	0.46	0.04	0.50
Technicians & therapists	—	—	—	—	—	—	0.16	0.09	0.25
All others	1.27	0.17	1.44	1.78	—	1.78	0.43	0.00	0.43
TOTALS	29.82	11.47	40.39	40.38	7.06	47.44	24.86	7.08	31.94

Source: Adapted from Haven Emerson: Local Health Units for the Nation, p. 14, Table C; and Greve and Campbell, 1961. Organization and Staffing for Local Health Services, Public Health Publication #682 (1961 Revision).

Note: The entry "—" signifies that data were not given in the source in the detail indicated by the line title. I presume that the data for these cells are included in the "All others" category.

And yet, the development of the "standard" local public health department had gone about as far as it was to go and seemed to have reached a peak. A study by Jack Haldeman cited in Hanlon (1969, 216) indicated that the counties remaining without full-time service were mostly in the sparsely populated western Great Plains and Rocky Mountain areas. Their populations were older than those in other areas, employed more in agriculture than in manufacturing, had relatively few members of nonwhite ethnic groups, and enjoyed a high family income and educational level.

According to these indications, it would appear that by 1960 most of nonurban America had access to full-time local health department services as defined in national surveys, and the small part that did not appeared to perceive little need for it. (Of course, the cities had for many years been deemed to be "covered.") The "full-time" criterion was evolving to simply requiring a separate public health department address (i.e., not a physician's private-practice office) and one full-time employee, even if only a clerk.[33] Far from being an advance over the previous requirement that the *head* be "full-time," this was a step backward. But publicly evident or politically effective sentiment for enriching staff in rural and semirural areas was not very strong. The politically discernible pressures for improvement in publicly provided health services were coming from another quarter, the metropolitan areas; and the pressures were not so much for more depth in standard public health services as they were for more medical care, especially primary care, and for more environmental protection along newer, more extended dimensions. In these areas, defined here similarly to the Census Bureau's Standard Metropolitan Statistical Area (SMSA) as consisting of a large city and its surrounding trading area, two postwar civilizations that are of particular interest to us here were developing: the central or inner city, and the relatively affluent suburbs. These two cultures, while developing in distinctively different fashions, also interacted with each other, usually to the detriment of the inner-city population. In terms of requirements for publicly provided health services, each culture was expressing a different need.

New Health Service Needs and the Public Health Response

The Urban Inner Cities As noted, the inner-city populations (and their advocates) were pressing for more and better public medical services, especially primary care. Although in many places they also campaigned for better protection against unsafe and unclean dwellings and streets, the push for medical care was politically predominant.

The need for medical care in the inner cities had been exacerbated by the economic expansion of 1946–1960. This period of growth was marked by the increasing dominance of large oligopolistic industry (Galbraith, 1968) and furthered the division of the business economy into a dominant or oligopolistic sector and a subsidiary or competitive sector.[34]

Much has been written about these two sectors (Beck, Horan, and Tolbert, 1978), but the aspect of this bifurcation important to note here is the greater security and superior economic position enjoyed by those working for the dominant corporations, such as International Business Machines (IBM), International Telephone and Telegraph (ITT), and General Motors (GM). Compared with those working in the subsidiary sector (e.g., retail trade, furniture and fixtures manufacturing, repair services, personal services) the employees in the dominant sector were better paid, and—most important here—had much better fringe benefits, including good private health insurance. Large numbers of people remained effectively outside the dominant economic sector during the entire post–World War II period. These "outsiders" consisted of employees in the subsidiary sector, who had much less adequate health insurance, if any; unemployable persons living in the public welfare (or assistance) economy; and many of the unemployed who, like the unemployables, depended on public programs for medical care. (The unemployables and the unemployed together constitute the nonemployed.) A sizable population fluctuated between being employed in the subsidiary economy and being in the public assistance economy, depending on the current unemployment rate. With respect to health care, many persons were in both the subsidiary and assistance economies simultaneously. These people had some medical insurance that enabled them to use private-sector medical care for some routine problems but were dependent on public medical care programs for serious episodes.[35] (See Chapter 9 for further discussion of this group of persons.) The generous benefits provided under the private health insurance held by dominant-sector employees helped increase the demand for services from existing sources of medical care. It thereby also bid up the price of these services and made it more expensive to provide care under public programs for lower-income working people and the nonemployed poor. The inner cities, where most of these people lived, found themselves with even fewer physicians than before as physicians followed the more affluent population to the suburbs, and the cost of publicly provided medical care soared.

Many urban areas had for a long time had public health departments that met or exceeded the minimum recommended standards of the Emerson Report. There was generally no problem of adequate full-time coverage in these areas, adequate by the Report's limited view of public health department function, but neither the organization nor the functioning of the standard public health department was structured to cope with the postwar inner-city needs. Provision of general medical care was by longstanding tradition alien to it. Fighting for improved sanitation in housing *was* part of the traditional scope of function of the standard local public health department (Terris, 1946), but the mammoth proportions of the deterioration of the inner cities overwhelmed their resources. The widespread physical devastation of the slum areas and the fiscal pligut of the cities were simply too much for these departments to cope with.[36] Local public health departments were unable to respond adequately to the two major needs of the inner city for publicly provided health services: medical care and aggressive enforcement of sanitation (including home safety).

The Suburban Expansion The demands of the suburban populations were different. They were concerned about the quality of life that their affluence was buying. For many of these people the affluence was new and its fruits disappointing, while the older, previously established affluent population was finding its comforts and amenities diluted by the recently arrived nouveaux riches. Their dissatisfaction with the growing deterioration of the environment was being articulated by writers like Rachel Carson (1962), who lamented the poisoning of the earth, water, and air and the befouling of the planet; Ralph Nader and his confreres, who were proving that large industries were producing unhealthy and shoddy, indeed lethal (1972) products; and the economist John Kenneth Galbraith, who argued that the overly rapid expansion of private development along with insufficient provision for appropriate public services and facilities was making it impossible to enjoy much of what the newly developed communities had been expected to offer. The intellectual spokespersons for this population as well as publicists dealing with these concerns expressed a need for control of environmental threats to health, both old and new: air pollution, radiation emissions, solid waste disposal, automobile accidents, and similar matters. The relatively feeble local public health departments that existed in these newly developed suburban and exurban areas were often holdovers from what had been rural environments. They were ill equipped to handle the new demands accompanying the rapid surge of development.

In many places the county public health department, which had been serving the areas of the county outside the city, merged with the city public health department, which had been operating autonomously and serving only the city's inhabitants. During these years there was a proliferation of the "urban county" form of locality as the developed suburbs pushed steadily out into the previously rural sections and urbanized them. One of the aims of this type of merger was to bring the richer staffing and greater sophistication of the city department to bear on the urban type of public health problems that were growing in the previously rural areas of the county. In the 1950s and 1960s a large number of these "city-county" merged public health departments were established or the merger process begun.

However, even those local public health departments that were among the best, those operating efficiently under knowledgeable leadership and organized in accordance with current state-of-the-art public health thinking, found that most of the large-scale environmental problems resulting from the activities of large and powerful national industries such as the automotive, petrochemical, and extractive corporations, could scarcely be controlled by any local health department. And it had long been the case that even many smaller and more localized businesses could threaten to move to a more congenial regulatory climate. Barry Rabe, who had studied government environmental management from a political scientist's perspective, writes:

Political economists have long noted the implausibility of locally-based regulatory strategies that threaten the abiding local government interest in economic development. Given the potential loss of productive industries, local governments are poorly equipped to undertake any unilateral regulatory or redistributive initiatives. They will instead cultivate cordial public-private relations by emphasizing services that foster economic development and meeting basic housekeeping needs. Applied to environmental protection, this argument can help explain the historic caution of local governments, including their health departments, to take any action that would significantly damage their relations with industry or other pollution sources that contribute to the local economy.

Further:

In such a setting [i.e., local health departments playing a leading role in environmental protection] informal negotiation prevailed over adversarial proceedings. And in the absence of strict federal and state oversight and forceful pro-regulatory pressure groups, local health departments were largely free to chart their own course in working with industry. . . .

In the view of many analysts . . . this corporatist style of regulation resulted in neglect of many severe environmental problems and ultimately required vigorous regulatory approaches (1987).

Only the jurisdictions of regional, state, and in many cases nothing less than federal agencies[37] were adequate in scope to deal with these problems.

An additional factor also played a significant role in the disappointment of middle-class environmentalists with the efforts of both state and local health departments to protect the environment. The environmentalists were interested in protecting the environment qua environment, not only in cases where dire health consequences could be proved to accompany its destruction. Such issues as preserving endangered species, limiting the proliferation of billboards, and controlling commercial development of natural recreation areas were important to them but were not widely taken up by health departments.[38]

The Search for Mission Redefinition The confluence of these two sets of issues in the metropolitan areas—medical care in the inner city and environmental deterioration in the suburbs (and for the affluent middle class in city areas)—worked to diminish the public standing of the public health departments, neither problem proving very amenable to its standard ministrations as they had developed historically. In the process of decrying the failure of the local public health department to expand its functions, critics often unjustifiably belittled the importance of maintaining the basic six functions. As is so often the case with campaigns of this type in the United States, it seemed as if it were necessary to deprecate older and still needed services in order to emphasize more strongly the need for newer and additional services. The diminished appreciation of the standard public health functions led to reduced federal support for the public health departments, to perform them and their effectiveness in these areas declined. Immunization rates fell, public health nurse staffing shrank, and community health surveillance was curtailed.

Congress and the federal executive were being pressed to consider means of using governmental powers more effectively to make adequate medical care available to all and to improve the quality of the environment. The leadership of many a local public health department, finding itself faced with a changed and seemingly intractable set of problems as well as rapid alterations in the composition of its constituent populations, was disoriented as it was pushed from all sides to do different things. Different "experts" counseled a wide variety of courses. Some writers and practicing professionals advised local public health departments to maintain the status quo and stick to prevention, as defined in the Emerson Report. Others called for a bold expansion into delivering primary medical care. Still others sought to define the fundamental role of the local public health department as one of oversight, surveillance, and areawide health planning. Examples abound of the probing, questioning, and exhortation, often bordering on hectoring, that were appearing everywhere in reflection of the malaise about the "true" role of local public health departments. (Similar questions were being raised about the role of state health departments.) A choice few will illustrate their tone and content.

As a first example, consider the inaugural address of Dr. Knutson, a public health oriented dentist and the incoming president of the American Public Health Association (1957):

[T]here is a ferment in public health that greatly enhances the chances of success in meeting this challenge [of the future road public health is to take]. The ingredients of this ferment are the disappointments, dissatisfactions, frustrations, and discontentments which have been the common lot of the thoughtful public health administrator since World War II.

He has been disappointed with his professional performance in attacking newer health problems. He has been dissatisfied with his efforts to shift emphasis from programs of diminishing relative importance to those designed to meet the new responsibilities. He has been frustrated because he was able to make only imperceptible progress in bringing his program abreast of the times. And he has been discontented and unsettled by the attitudes of disregard or distrust which the general public often seemed to adopt toward his pronouncements. Despite the mounting public interest in health and medical affairs, his recommendations have not been universally heeded—as for example, in the case of water fluoridation. . . .

The role of the forthright, vigorous public health leader, therefore, is to prepare and present the facts needed for the solution of public health problems. He does this from one broad viewpoint—that of the adequacy of health services. This is a great responsibility and how well it is discharged by the leadership in public health will largely determine where we as a nation will go in public health.

Thus, the future mission of public health was seen by the speaker as one of assessing the adequacy of local health services in light of the relevant facts. This would involve community health assessment, service need assessment, and perhaps monitoring and evaluation of existing services. Expanded versions of this view later came to be held by many writers and groups concerned with formulating the mission and functions of public health departments.[39]

At about the same time as Dr. Knutson's address another example testifying to the concern with mission definition for public health departments was provided in November 1957, when the *American Journal of Public Health* issued a special supplement entitled *A Critique of Community Public Health Services.* It was a report of a working conference of the National Advisory Committee on Local Health Departments of the National Health Council, an association of voluntary social service agencies involved in health work. Speaker after speaker at the conference sounded a recurrent theme: the problems facing local health departments had greatly broadened in scope and new approaches were needed.

A third and final example is a report issued by the National Commission on Community Health Services, organized jointly by the American Public Health Association and the National Health Council, which attempted to wrestle with the broader problem of the proper organization of community health services. In 1966, it set up six task forces to study various aspects of the problem. The titles of the subjects assigned to these task forces indicate the areas in which new problems for local health bodies were seen to lie. These were:

1. Environmental Health
2. Comprehensive Personal Health Services
3. Health Manpower
4. Health Care Facilities
5. Financing Community Health Services and Facilities
6. Organization of Community Health Services.

Each task force issued a report on its findings, and these were published together as the collective report of the four-year investigation (1967). One section of the report on organization of community health services is of particular interest here:

The Emerson Report was a landmark in the development of public health programs in the United States, but its span of usefulness was short. In the years immediately following 1945, dramatic increases in shifts in population, changes in health needs, planning techniques, and health and medical knowledge radically changed the conditions the Emerson Report had been designed to deal with.

By the mid-fifties, it had become apparent that the very thing that had made the Emerson Report so important at the time of its publication—its firm structural dogma—*had actually become a hindrance* [emphasis added] in meeting the changing health needs of the fluid and mobile community populations of the United States. The force of these changing needs in such a brief period produced chaotic conditions in community health service organization, chiefly in the lack of pattern—particularly in planning—for interagency relations, the lack of effective organization, and the "overlap and gap" in services which stem from these lacks.

Perhaps the most cogent indication of the widespread concern with redefining the functions of public health departments was to be found within the ranks of the public health leadership itself. The efforts of the governing bodies of the American Public Health Association to rethink and redefine the local department's proper scope of function are evidenced in official policy statements issued at various annual meetings of the association. The changes over time in the way the role of the local public health department was formulated are revealed by a comparison of three policy statements of the American Public Health Association, issued at different times, on the functions and mission of the local health department. These were adopted at annual conventions spaced ten and thirteen years apart: 1940[40], 1950, and 1963.[41] The positions taken on those occasions with respect to the functions and responsibilities of the local public health department (summarized in Table 2–4) may be characterized as following under nine general functional areas:

1. Measurement of population characteristics
2. Communicable disease control
3. Sanitation and environmental control
4. Laboratory services
5. Maternal and child health
6. Health education
7. Operation of health facilities
8. Chronic disease control
9. Areawide planning and coordination.

Only the first six appear in the 1940 statement. Items 7, 8, and 9 were added in one or both of the later two statements. The general direction of the changes is toward expanding and broadening the scope of the functions. A related feature is the changing style of naming the functions. In 1940 these were enumerated as operationally and narrowly defined tasks—

"control of communicable disease." The method of specification immediately pointed to a specific organizational form and its task definition. By contrast, in 1963 they were more likely to be defined as generalized goals—"The attack on disease, injury and disability." The specific tasks were listed under the goals as prerequisite objectives required for achieving a particular generalized goal, but the fact that they appeared as subtopics under a more general goal implied that the achievement of the goal was the central point and that there might be many ways needed to achieve it in addition to the tasks specifically listed.

This trend toward describing local public health department functions in terms of broad goals rather than merely issuing a small set of very specific tasks, such as *the* basic six functions, was a recognition of the large variability among localities, with respect both to the speed with which public health needs were changing as well as the nature of these needs. It also reflected the spread of increased formalization of program planning methodology, which called for first setting generalized goals and then listing specific, measurable objectives suitable for achieving the more general goal (see Chapter 15.) Underlying these changes was the realization among many practicing public health administrators that it had not proved possible to implement the specific blueprint of the Emerson Report everywhere, and that setting more general goals to be implemented with variable local conditions in mind was a more useful and prudent approach. By focusing a definition of scope of function on a list of required minimal functions expressed as narrowly specified tasks, an unjustified verdict of "failure" may be arbitrarily and perhaps unjustifiably written into future program evaluations by the semantics of the goal definition. (See the discussion of the federal OEO health center program in Chapter 11 for a fuller treatment of this point.)

The 1963 statement continued to stress the importance of maintaining the basic "standard" functions at a high level of efficiency, but it now included a strong health department responsibility for community leadership in moving toward the achievement of a coordinated, nonredundant, and comprehensive health services system in its jurisdiction. The importance of integrating elements of behavioral science and statistical disciplines (e.g., surveys and sampling) into the activities of the local health department was noted. Research development and evaluation of methods for efficient provision of population-wide health care coverage were recommended. (It is instructive to compare this view of the wide-ranging responsibilities of local health departments with that of the official position taken by the American Medical Association in 1962, as described on p. 76.)

As noted in note 41, an APHA policy statement issued in 1970 essentially reiterated the functions of the local public health department listed in the 1963 statement, but it did add a specific definition of its role in the work of comprehensive state and regional planning. Although this particular formulation was primarily a response to the growing prominence of the federally subsidized health planning program of that time, described in Chapter 15, it also reflected the position of those who thought that a primary mission, perhaps *the* primary mission, of the local (and state) public health departments should increasingly be the coordinating, monitoring, and assessing of the adequacy of the health services system in its jurisdiction. More than twenty years later, a report by the Institute of Medicine (1988) examined the concept of the functions of local public health departments in greater detail. This report is further discussed in Chapter 4.

Concern over Local Boards of Health and Staffing of Departments of Health Changes were also taking place in the official stance of the American Public Health Association with respect to the organization of local boards of health and the staffing of local health departments, although these changes were not as extensively discussed as were those in functions. The main position change was a recommendation for broadening the composition of the board. For example, while the 1940 statement recommended that at least a specified *minimum* number of physicians be on the board, the later statements stressed that there *not be too many* board members from any single profession, one of Shattucks recommendations in his famous report of 1850.[42] The 1970 statement recommended that the board's composition "ideally

. . . represent the professional, governmental and consumer backgrounds and interests found in the local health jurisdiction."

With respect to staffing, the fixed ratios of the 1940 statement were replaced by a call for flexibility[43] in meeting local needs. There was also the usual recommendation that all staff be hired in accordance with APHA specifications, namely, that in general they be full-time and that a merit system be employed.

Developments after 1965

Changes in Federal Grant Structure The preoccupation of public health leaders during the years between 1950 and 1970 with redefining the functions and mission of the local public health department was largely in response to widely expressed criticisms from many quarters that the local agencies were not meeting the needs of the times. Perhaps the most important of these critiques came from the federal government and was reflected in changes in the federal mechanisms for giving health grants to local governments, as well as in the amounts granted. (This will be discussed in greater detail in Chapter 4.) Those federal grants-in-aid to states which had been used since 1936 to a large extent to help local public health departments develop and maintain their "traditional" functions, the so-called formula grants for general health purposes, declined while the formula grants earmarked for specifically defined service categories and the even more specially targeted project grants increased. The latter were aimed at promoting carefully focused demonstration projects to encourage an innovative approach to expanding public health functions in directions desired by the federal government—medical care to inner-city poor, enforcement of local environmental health protection in the ghettos, broader environmental protection work such as the hazardous waste control being pressed primarily by the middle classes, and greater attention to chronic disease and areawide planning. Writing in 1966, Berdj Kenadjian, an HEW analyst, stated:

Which form of Federal grants-in-aid is desirable depends on the types of need to be served . . . there is a great need for the public health family in the United

Table 2–4. Comparison of positions taken by the American Public Health Association at three different time periods on the functions and responsibilities of local health departments.

Goal	1940—An official declaration of attitude (about the same as the Emerson Report—1945)	1950—An official statement of the American Public Health Association	1963—Policy statement
I. Measurement of population characteristics	1.* Vital statistics Collection, tabulation, analysis, interpretation, and publication of births, deaths, and notifiable disease	1* Recording and analysis of health data both on Disease incidence and resources of health care	*An adequate system of data collection and analysis is basic to most health department functions." Registration and survey are the two basic techniques. Surveys based on sampling can establish baselines on which programs can be developed and from which trends can later be measured. They "will tell health officer how much various health services are used in relation to needs, health insurance coverage, etc." (The statement above is included in position statement but not in the four summary "points.") 4.* Research, development, and evaluation Continual evaluation of health department's programs Special projects; field trials of prophylactic, diagnostic, and therapeutic measures, administrative research on financing, servicing combinations, staffing, etc.
II. Communicable disease control	2.* Control of communicable diseases	4.* Provision of direct environmental health services Communicable disease control and 5.* Administration of personal health services Immunization and innoculation Diagnostic tests and clinics Case finding Diagnostic and treatment services for specific diseases, e.g., VD, TB, special children's diseases	3.* The attack on disease, injury and disability a.* communicable disease control b.* Continue traditional ambulatory and inpatient facilities for VD, TB, and other special diseases
III. Sanitation and environmental control	3.* Environmental sanitation Milk, food processing Public eating places Waste disposal Housing supervision for adequate light, air, water, sanitary necessities, and overcrowding" public places and places of employment	3.* Supervision and regulation of Food, water, milk Nuisances and waste disposal Occupational diseases and accidents Inspection of hospitals and nursing homes Regulation of housing 4.* Provision of direct environmental health services. Waste disposal Rodent and insect control	2.* Maintenance of a healthy environment Food, water, milk Insecticides, herbicides, food additives, drugs Safe home, work, play environment Disposal of solid wastes Radiation, air pollution, street pollution control Conservation of water resources Participation in planning new developments

	1940	1950	1963
IV. Laboratory services	4.* Public health laboratory services	5.* Administration of personal health services. Provision of diagnostic aids to the physician such as laboratory services and crippled children's, cancer, cardiac, and other diagnostic and consultation clinics (see also under Section II above)	Not specifically mentioned but assertions made that "It is necessary ... to continue at an appropriate level the basic health department activities listed in the 1940 and 1950 statements."
V. Maternal and child health	5.* Maternal and child hygiene	5.* Administration of personal health services. Diagnostic and treatment services for defects in children and expectant mothers; orthopedic, cardiac, and other cripplers of children	See remarks in Section IV above.
VI. Health education	Health education	2.* Health education and information	1.* Promotion of personal and community health a* Personal an authoritative source of health information Health education; stimulate "a desire to maintain the best possible health and an understanding of the individual action necessary to achieve this goal."
VII. Operation of health facilities		6.* Operation of health facilities. "should" operate one or more health centers and "may" directly administer hospitals	3.* The attack on disease, injury, and disability b.* Community Play a leadership role in community-wide organization and planning of health resources Promote full use by providers of care of community health resources
VIII. Chronic disease control, health promotion, and mental health			1.* Promotion of personal and community health b.* Community Play a leadership role in community-wide organization and planning of health resources Promote full use by providers of care of community health resources
IX. Local areawide planning and coordination		7.* Coordination of activities and resources. Encourage coordination of all official and voluntary agencies to assure complete health coverage and avoid overlapping maintain close liaison with other agencies: water, sewage, housing, hospital planning, etc. recommend a broad community health council	3.* The attack on disease, injury, and disability b.* "Should" promote and develop resources "for the care of the sick that meets community needs; develop and encourage prepayment plans; supervise hospitals and other health care facilities" "Almost surely" develop an organized home care program c.* Improve use of existing services and facilities; prevent unnecessary duplications of competition among facilities; interpret to public the program of existing facilities to encourage continuity of care

Source: 1940, Amer. Public Health Association (1940); 1950, Amer. Public Health Association (1951); 1963, Amer. Public Health Association (1964).
*These numbers and letters correspond to the numbering of the summary points in the original APHA documents.

States to reorient both public and private leadership and resources in order to make the existing structures for providing health services to entire communities, States, and the nation more optimal. When preventive, diagnostic, therapeutic, and restorative services are not properly related to each other, the total price tag on health care is much higher than it would be in a better integrated system. Moreover, the preventable sickness and premature death that result from imbalances in health systems impose unnecessary burdens on the persons and families least able to bear them at the same time as they limit the production of the nation's labor force.

The diversity of the unmet needs suggests that, if a comprehensive attack on the nation's health problems is to be mobilized, more than one form of Federal assistance will continue to be required.

Historically, the Federal Government has moved to a more categorical and selective approach in assisting the health programs of States and communities (1966).

Obstacles to Mission Redefinition Many in the public health field were keenly aware of the implications that analyses and caveats such as the above held for local public health departments, especially for their future viability. The many articles and speeches by public health figures and the changing positions of the American Public Health Association show that changing social conditions were placing a set of demands before city public health departments that were widely perceived, especially in Washington, as not being met to any great degree. This was so despite the redirection of federal and state monies; the time and effort expended by leading members of the APHA in reformulating its policy on the mission, structure, and function of local health departments; and the goading reflected in the writings of professional public health administrators, academics, journalists, and a wide assortment of general pundits. What was preventing the needed changes?

For one thing, the money available through federal incentive grants for motivating local departments to introduce the new programs was far too little. It was insufficient to provide for all health departments willing to establish the desired programs. The funding was available mostly on a project grant basis to be awarded only to some departments and was time delimited. Renewal was by reapplication. Thus, a department that accepted such a grant was likely to find itself without funding after the program had been installed and a local demand for it established. By contrast, the old general-purpose money was available year after year to all departments. To compound the effects of underfunding, the appropriations for new programs were to some degree made at the expense of general-purpose money. The latter was a funding mainstay for maintenance of the standard functions, especially communicable disease control and maternal and child health, which needed to be maintained with unflagging energy. The reduction in these funds was disturbing to health officers, especially the more experienced ones.

Another problem was that the advanced positions taken by the American Public Health Association about how local public health departments should change did not always originate with the local health officers section of the APHA and in many cases received but lukewarm support or even direct opposition from many of its members (Roemer, 1973). Thus, the people who would be responsible for implementing proposed new programs of primary care, chronic disease control, and wider environmental control were often not the chief movers in getting these positions adopted and frequently did little to push them in their communities. Partly this was because many of the health officers were still imbued with the older "basic six" conception of public health. But another, more important, factor was the health officers' knowledge of the political situation in their respective communities. They knew that proposals to expand public health functions would face opposition from local government officials afraid of the budgetary consequences, of medical societies afraid of competition for patients, of political conservatives who feared or disliked the notion of expanding government influence, and of business groups who feared the possibility of increased control and regulation of their business activities as well as increased taxes to pay for the increased public medical services and regulation.

However, the unenthusiastic response—and even opposition—of many local public health officers to the new calls for public health activism was more a symptom than a cause of the general failure to implement them. More important was the underlying fact that solutions to these problems involved tackling adversaries for which the local public health department was no match politically. It really meant nothing less than taking on the entire problem of the deterioration of the inner city. Meeting the problem of the unhealthy conditions of ghetto life meant fighting the slum landlords, the urban redevelopers, and the city political machines to obtain adequate and meaningful inspection and to enforce compliance. It also meant obtaining more tax money for functions such as trash and garbage removal. Providing adequate medical care for the poor in the cities involved confronting the entire system of medical care distribution, including the traditional treatment of the public medical care sector as a charity, second-class "track." And the environmental decay problem affecting the sensibilities of sections of the middle classes was really not a problem amenable to local solution. The large corporations and their polluting activities, as well as the attendant problems of automobile transportation and housing sprawl, could scarcely be tackled by the states, let alone local governments. The battle to preserve the environment was shifting, in the 1960s, to the federal arena (see Chapter 4), and the problem of medical care for low-income groups was assuming a state and national focus (see Chapters 8–11). Thus, despite all the prodding and hectoring by pundits in their speeches and writings, the pressures exerted by federal program supervisors, and the manipulation of grant mechanisms by the federal and some state governments, local public health departments were slow to depart from their well-beaten paths.

This is not to say that no attempts were made to meet some of these problems. There was the previously described trend across the nation to consolidate county and city health departments. A number of health departments also attempted to supply care on a more comprehensive basis than called for by the "basic six." For example, Mytinger (1968, 1967) studied program innovation in local public health departments and developed models for measuring it. When he applied the models to California health departments, he found varying degrees of innovation in effect. He also chronicled innovation within thirteen local health departments throughout the country. The fact that this research was published and disseminated by HEW is an indication of federal attempts to broaden the work of neighborhood public health centers through wider diffusion of the experience with such efforts. But these remained realtively isolated examples. The fundamental problems of the health delivery system interacting with those of the inner cities could not be solved by individual local public health departments, although vigorously and skillfully led ones could do better than others.

The Public Hospital/Health Department Merger as a Solution to Implementing Mission Redefinition In addition to these examples of some public health department attempts to reorganize their internal structure and functions, either individually or by consolidation with other health departments, there were instances of valiant efforts made by some local governments to meet new demand, by reconfiguring some of their health service agencies into unified systems that might better meet the needs of the poor for general medical care. Beginning with the 1960s, the governments of some large cities and urban counties looked at their two principal health agencies and saw a combination of unsatisfactory service by their public hospital (Cooney, Roemer, and Ross, 1971) and insufficiently rapid response from their health department to local demands for more and better primary care. Some of these governments sought solutions in administrative reorganizations that aimed to merge the two agencies into a unified and coordinated system.

Complaints about large urban public hospitals (Hoffer et al., 1950) were often centered on their geographic inaccessibility, and when they were affiliated with a teaching institution, on their inadequate orientation to the ordinary patient load of everyday complaints. The public health department, on the other hand, although often maintaining neighborhood health centers in low-income areas, was widely regarded as lacking the medical expertise and facilities required for comprehensive primary health care. It was hoped that merging the two departments into a single health services system would combine the best of both worlds—the geographic accessibility and "people" orientation of the public health department with its neighborhood health centers, and the medical expertise technology, and facilities backup of the public hospital (Shonick and Price, 1977; Shonick, 1980). A fuller accounting of such mergers in places like Boston, Denver, and Los Angeles will be given Chapter 7, but for the present the outcomes of these mergers may be summarized by saying that one was entirely successful and a few others moderately so in providing a better system of ambulatory care for the poor. Although public health professionals working in the merged agency generally complained that the hospital was using ''their'' funds, the validity of this complaint could not be established because the merger period (1965–1975) coincided with the beginning of serious overall reductions in public funds in large cities. Public health departments in cities that did not merge their two agencies suffered as much or more retrenchment than those in cities where they were merged. Most cities whose agencies were merged have, either in fact or by actual legislation, dissolved the mergers. It seems clear that while some mergers may have helped to improve the public ambulatory care problem at least temporarily, they did not answer the overall question of what, if anything, a ''modern'' local public health department should do in addition to the basic six functions.

COMMENTS

In retrospect, the turbulent course of the local health department from 1950 onward appears to have been less due to recalcitrance on the part of public health administrators than their detractors asserted. The vision of the public health system put forth in the Emerson Report was, with the addition of some of the emendations suggested in later APHA statements, a good one, and it did not deserve the sharp criticism that the National Health Council and others directed toward it. A national network of effective and financially secure local public health departments, accountable to and adequately supported primarily by the states and federal governments but also responsive to special needs of the localities, seems to have had, and still has, great potential for improving the health services—and the

health—of the United States. Concentrating their scope of function on but not limiting it to environmental protection, prevention campaigns, areawide health planning and evaluation, and the monitoring of the local medical care system need not make them powerless or peripheral to the central issues of medical services improvement. Had such a system been able to mature into a powerful and well-supported organization, had it become the de facto government policy in the United States, it might ahve been one of a kind in the capitalist world and served as a model for other countries.

However, because universal access to needed medical care was an overriding issue during the entire post–World War II period, a major, perhaps the principal, impediment to the development of such a public health system was the failure to establish a universal, comprehensive national health insurance system for personal medical care. Frustrated by the lack of access to adequate medical care by poor people, and in the case of expensive treatment, also by many middle-class persons, socially humanitarian professional health personnel, writers, public figures, and activists cast about for anything that might possibly alleviate the suffering and deprivation. The neighborhood health centers of the larger public health departments had physicians, nurses, and other health care personnel. They seemed to be a readily available solution, however partial, to the shortage of primary-care resources for uninsured persons, if only local health officers would cooperate and loosen their rigid stand on offering only preventive services. We have seen that the budgetary constraints of the local government, and for a long time the opposition of the local medical society, prevented any substantial effort by local health departments to offer general medical care, and that efforts that were undertaken in some cities after 1970 were under constant budgetary atack with much accompanying attrition.

In view of the serious gaps in access, it was laudable for people to campaign for the provision of general medical care in public health centers. But the health officers knew that in addition to the earlier medical society problem, any resources spent on more medical care would often mean reductions in funds for the required maintenance of preventive services, given the "finiteness"[44] of resources available for public health represented by the overall health line in the budget.[45] The well-intentioned critics did not pay sufficient mind to these matters; indeed for many years the humanist proponents of better medical care for all seemed to undervalue the need for adequate preventive health services. The point is simply that increasing access to medical care would require *additional* resources; and the local government, having none available, could only respond by juggling existing resources.

It seemed reasonable that because publicly administered preventive services and publicly provided medical care for the poor were both part of publicly provided health services, they should be reorganized as identifiable components of an overarching local department of health services. But attempts to implement this idea could only succeed if the resources allotted were sufficiently adequate so that neither set of services, particularly the preventive ones, were shortchanged. The latter development did eventuate in many of the mergers that were tried, and that was perhaps the single most important reason for their failure. In fact, there was never any federal support for the main local institution that delivered medical care to low-income persons, the local general public hospital (see Chapter 7), and as a result the local public hospital–local public health department merger placed the federal funds available for the public health department at risk of being put to public hospital use if the latter were badly starved for funds.

Beginning in 1970 the federal government began to enter the field of environmental protection more actively. This changed the role of local public departments in this area, and under the Carter administration (1976–1980) the priorities of local public health departments to some extent shifted away from expanding general medical care and back to traditional services. A combination of the development of community health centers (see Chapter 11) and an increased emphasis on prevention as interpreted by the Surgeon General to include an expanded form of health education called health promotion (see Chapter 4), modified the federal grant structure to favor standard preventive service grants. Under the Reagan administration, federal policy led to even greater changes in program focus and

extent among local public health departments as well as changed relationships with the state.

The preceding pages of this chapter dealt with the growth of local public health departments, with occasional reference to state and federal policies that affected the local departments. During this period, important developments were taking place at the state and federal levels that increasingly enhanced their roles in public health, especially that of the federal government. The more important changes began about 1950 and reached a first climax in the virtual shower of social legislation that emanated from the federal government during 1965–67. They reached a second climax in the Omnibus Budget and Fiscal Responsibility Act of 1981 under the Reagan administration, which began an unraveling of the service net woven in the years between 1950 and 1964. To obtain a better view of these changes, it is necessary to leave our discussion of the local public health department and turn to the state health department and then to the role of the federal government in public health. I shall return to the local public health department after looking at state health departments and the federal effort and shall then be better able to discuss the interactive effect among these governmental levels and the place and future of the local public health agency.

Notes

1. The word "full-time" did not mean that all employees of the department were indeed working full time. The particular meaning of this term when applied to local health departments is discussed later in this chapter.
2. Although the state health department is the subject of the next chapter, these facts are noted here because the formation of state health departments strengthened local public health services throughout a state and worked to standardize their practice.
3. Another aspect of the effect of biological advances on public health practice was the growth of knowledge about the human immune service and the associated development of vaccines. But although the vaccine against smallpox was developed by the English physician Edward Jenner in 1796 and was widely used by early public health departments in the United States, it was the only one. It would not be until 1900 that vaccines would be developed for diptheria, typhoid, and rabies, whose spread could only be controlled by quarantine before then. After

the development of these and other vaccines, immunization became a standard and important function of local health departments. Quarantine and immunization were later to disappear as specifically designated special major functions in public health literature, to be subsumed under the global categories of communicable disease control and maternal and child health. The classification typology formerly based on type of procedure was thereafter based on the type of health threat being addressed.

4. See note 3, above.

5. The statements made here about later knowledge of epidemic disease refer generally to the state of knowledge from about 1920 to 1945. They do not imply that this is the current state of knowledge, which is more sophisticated and detailed. The reader interested in the current state of knowledge should consult the latest edition of Last, 1980, or a comparable work.

6. The policy issues dealing with the structure of the board of health are discussed more fully in Chapter 3, which deals with the state health department. For the present it is sufficient to note that typically the board of health has been a citizen body and the department of health an operating agency of local government. The board of health and the head of the department of health have usually been appointed by the chief executive of the local government with some provision for approval by the local legislature, very often the city council. The staff of the health department has usually been hired, since about 1940, through civil service procedures. Civil service hiring and retention was an ever-present feature in any reasonably complete model of an adequate local public health department formulated by the American Public Health Association.

7. The public health neighborhood health center was in some ways the forerunner of the free-standing, independent comprehensive community health centers that were developed later in the 1960s as part of a national federal program. Chapter 11 is given over to this development and also contains a more detailed discussion of the public health department neighborhood health center as part of the background of the community health center. Here, only the portion of that background that impinges on the development of the typical urban public health department is treated to maintain continuity.

8. The nature of this controversy is discussed in the next section on "Primary Care in Public Health Departments and Local Medical Societies."

9. See Chapter 13 for a discussion of the Flexner Report.

10. See Starr, 1981, especially Chapters 3 and 5, for an excellent sociologically oriented account of some of the interplay of social forces that helped bring this about.

11. The discipline exercised by the local medical society over any of its members who might wish to act contrary to its principles and decisions was also

rarely publicly evident. The need for practicing physicians to be voted admitting privileges by the medical staff of at least one local hospital and to receive referrals from or be able to make referrals to other physicians was a sufficiently strong lever to keep any but the most determined recalcitrant in line in the infrequent instances in which a practicing physician's own inner impulses to agree with medical society principles or decisions might falter. The situation was a good example of the way in which de facto health care policy for important segments of our national health care system has been made in private meeting rooms and other gathering places to produce a medical care system remarkably uniform in its major contours across the country, reflective of tight control and regulation, albeit nongovernment—that is, nonpublic—in nature.

12. Dr. Emerson was a prominent public health leader and the director of the APHA committee that issued the Emerson report in 1945 setting forth proposed norms and standards for an "adequate" local public health department (See Emerson, 1945).

13. The authors were on the staff of the International Health Division of the Rockefeller Foundation, and the study was made at the behest of the Conference of State and Provincial Health Authorities of North America.

14. Joseph Mountin and associates, writing in 1936, felt it necessary to explain that "The employment of a full-time professional health officer to administer a countywide program of public health services constitutes a distinctive feature of modern public health administration (Mountin, Pennell, and Flook, 1936, p. 1). The question of what constitutes a "full-time" local public health department has for many years been a topic of considerable discussion among public health theorists and practitioners.

15. Only three of the four organizational forms listed as doing local public health work represent local health departments in the sense of being a department of the local government. The "district plan" is either jointly sponsored by several local governments or is an office of the state department of health doing local public health work. The latter is clearly not a local public health department in the sense of being an organ of local government but provides the same type of service.

16. The nature of this federal assistance is discussed more fully in Chapter 4, but a brief summary is given here because it is indispensable to consideration of local public health departments after 1935. As noted in the Introduction, the local, state and federal roles need to be looked at simultaneously, but we can only talk about them one at a time in any detail.

17. That is, indigent persons who come under the three categories of person enumerated in the act: the aged, families with dependent children, and the blind.

18. This was also and especially true of cash assistance ("welfare" or "relief") where states often appropriated less than the federal government was

willing to match. While this area is not within our direct purview at this time, the attitudes prevailing on health care for the poor are closely linked with the fate of cash assistance programs. This is treated more fully in Chapters 8 and 9.

19. The data used by Joseph Mountin came from the reports sent to the Public Health Service by state health departments. These were required under the law, and Dr. Mountin, as an assistant surgeon general of the Public Health Service, had access to them. These data were only required to cover expenditures under Title VI. Reports of maternal and child health expenditures under Title V were mandated to be sent to the Children's Bureau, which, it will be recalled, was given administrative responsibility for the disbursement of Title V funds. While some reports to the Public Health Service may have been complete, covering programs supported both by Title VI and Title V funds, Dr. Mountin notes in the monograph that not all were. I shall return to this point in the text later on.

20. The term "cities" used in this context refers to incorporated cities having their own "municipal" health departments. Since the populations of these cities were, by definition, all covered by full-time public health services, the percentage of persons "outside" cities is the crucial indicator of progress along this line.

21. Some of the data I cite are, however, based on more complete data supplied by later United States Public Health Service (USPHS) reports, numbers 47 and 194.

22. Hereafter, whenever this restricted meaning of the term public health services is intended, I shall refer to it as "standard public health" services. By contrast, whenever the term is intended to encompass a wider scope of function, usually including "newer" and more extensive environmental controls and operation or supervision of general medical care services, I shall call it "extended public health." These qualifiers will not be used when the meaning is apparent from the context.

23. The absence of any recommendation that *general* medical clinics be operated by local public health departments or that medical practitioners work for them as full-time clinicians is significant. Medical practice under health department auspices was envisioned as consisting of sessions limited in scope to standard public health and run by private practitioners working part-time for the health department, usually on a free or per-session fee basis. It should be noted that the views of Dr. Emerson and of those he represented were in sharp opposition to those of other writers and public figures who strongly advocated the widespread introduction of *general* medical care programs into the health department (Roemer, 1973).

24. In fact, the entire thrust of the report with respect to this point is the substitution of the concept of measuring coverage in terms of the capacity to deliver "adequate services" rather than merely "full-

time" employment, no matter hos "full-time" is defined. Of course, the degree to which staff is full-time is relevant, but it is only one aspect of measuring staffing adequacy. It must be defined on the basis of what functions a public health department *should* perform in the face of community health needs. The notion of basing local programs on assessments of community health needs was to become increasingly prominent in later years, and development of the idea is still in its infancy with some public health leaders struggling to refine and implement it. Its implementation awaits development of public health assessment methodology, and especially provision of increased funding to support such development.

25. See note 23.

26. See note 22.

27. It is interesting that the AMA should have considered the state and local medical societies competent to assess local health needs, programs, and resources, when the state and local public health agencies have always found this so difficult.

28. It is one thing to make global national estimates of requirements for health services by multiplying some estimated appropriate national per capita average by the total population. It is quite another to make locally specific, directly obtained estimates of requirements for small areas, *taking into account regional differences in needs* from area to area with the total national requirement derived by summing all the local estimates. A national estimate obtained in this manner may yield the same national total as one estimated from a global national sample. The important difference between the two methods is that the global method does not yield estimates than can safely be used to assess the adequacy of services in a region or locality, the regional (local) estimates being obtained by simply multiplying the national per capita figure by the region's (locality's) population. On the other hand, the national estimate derived by aggregating locally derived small area estimates has, by its nature, immediately available directly obtained regional (local) data and valid local estimates. In this respect, the Emerson Report methodology did not meet the standards of modern true "small area" planning any better than the later Hill Burton program did.

29. Note the suggestion in the quoted paragraph that some of the seven board members be physicians (two or three) but that the others be "laymen," i.e., nonphysicians.

30. These notions were soon to be challenged, however. Types of grants more directed at promoting programs that the federal government wanted rather than at equalizing efforts across states became predominant. Many of these federally desired programs involved activities outside the scope of the Emerson Report's recommendations, and most local public health departments did not institute them readily. This is discussed in some detail in Chapter 4.

31. Tables 1–6 of Sanders, 1959, provide details illustrating these points.

32. The latter data are from a study prepared for the U.S. Public Health Service by Greve and Campbell (1961).

33. Later data indicate that this situation continued. An ongoing data collection program assembling annual information from state health departments, known as the National Public Health Program Reporting System (NPHPRS) was begun in 1970 by the Association of State and Territorial Health Officers (ASTHO). These reports contain data on local public health departments or LHDs (Local Health Department). ASTHO's own definition of an LHD required only one full-time professional public health employee who did not need to be a physician.

34. These have been variously designated by names such as the planning and market sectors (Galbraith, 1968), or core and peripheral (Beck, Horan, and Tolbert, 1978). I use "dominant" and "subsidiary" because these terms seem to me to describe their economic and political roles better than other designations I have seen.

35. In health insurance parlance such episodes are called "catastrophic." The "catastrophe" is the economic impact on a family's finances—the medical prognosis may actually be quite good. With respect to such serious episodes these persons were *medically* indigent. The point at which a person becomes medically indigent depends on his or her available income and insurance coverage and the costliness of the treatment required to treat the medical condition. There are few people who would not be medically indigent in the face of some illness requiring very expensive and poorly insured treatment.

36. Not only were the local public health departments unable to assist or materially slow the growing inadequacy of housing conditions for the residents of the inner city, they were also forced to curtail their standard public health services because of conditions brought about by this very deterioration. Detroit, for example, whose health department had been regarded as the best in the country by the APHA, which awarded it first prize for excellence year after year, had to discontinue home visits by public health nurses because of the threats to the safety of the nurses that such visits entailed.

37. As this is being written, one is tempted to add "international agencies" for many important problems.

38. This factor applies more strongly to the activities of state health departments than those of local ones, but it does apply to both. The question is discussed more fully in Chapter 3.

39. The recommendations of a two-year study, *The Future of Public Health,* published by an Institute of Medicine (IOM) study committee in 1988, agreed with the general views expressed by Dr. Knutson in 1957 but extended them to the implementation stages.

It defined "the core function of public health agencies at all levels of government [to be] assessment, policy development, and assurance" (1988).

40. The 1940 official policy statement and the 1945 Emerson Report are henceforth used interchangeably in this discussion because they were identical in the points of interest here.

41. There was a policy statement in 1970 also, but it was so like the 1963 statement that I have omitted it from Table 2-4 and from most of this discussion about the changing nature of these APHA formulations.

42. See Chapter 3 on the State Health Department.

43. Of course, "flexibility" in standards is often a code word for permitting the *lowering* of standards. Despite the opportunity for abuse that flexible standards provide, again the large variability in conditions among localities makes it a necessary condition for appropriate staffing. Flexible standards do not have to be lax ones, however. The fundamental criterion is whether a staffing pattern meets the local health service needs.

44. There was much talk during the years under discussion about the fact that health care expenditures were rising very rapidly while resources were "finite." Therefore, the argument went, restricting health services to fit existing allotments rather than thinking of any further increases in health services loomed as an inevitable eventuality in the near future. Of course, in a theoretical sense resources are always finite, but in the context in which this term has been used, the "finiteness" referred only to the funds actually allocated for health services, which were a function of the tax policies and budgetary allocations that were then in place. The latter included subsidies for growing tobacco and tax deductions for advertising it, not to speak of very controversial budget items dealing with foreign policy and defense. People who advocated more spending for health services, therefore, were far from advocating a flouting of a physical law about making infinite demands upon finite resources. They were only "impractical" when the discussion was confined to a short-term decision that took the existing tax laws and budget as givens.

45. A similar concern was later expressed in the 1988 IOM report, on *The Future of Public Health.* "[T]he responsibility for providing medical care to individuals—precisely because it is so compelling—has drained vital resources and attention away from disease prevention and health promotion efforts that benefit the entire community. These latter efforts encounter great difficulty in competing for policy attention with personal health services. The U.S. failure to find a society-wide answer to the question of financial access to needed care has seriously strained the public health system" (1988).

3

The State Health Department

Permanent state health departments were organized later than local health departments. They came into being as the changes stemming from economic and population growth began to press the states to exercise their "police" powers under the Constitution with respect to safeguarding the public's health. Whereas the local health department has been the main agency carrying the responsibility for the day-to-day local operation of local health programs, the state health department of recent years may be characterized as a supervising, coordinating, equalizing, and mediating agency. As Hanlon (1969, 221) wrote in his textbook on public health:

In all except a few states the direct personal service functions of State health departments are decidedly few and are limited largely to the provision of traveling specialized personnel and mobile equipment to local areas unable to afford them. Many state health departments, for example, staff, equip, and maintain mobile chest X-ray units, dental clinics, and facilities for the examination and treatment of venereal disease.

There have been exceptions but generally the state agency has directly provided a complete set of personal public health services only when local organization was lacking or inadequate, and then usually as an interim measuring pending local organization.[1] More often it has engaged in only a few direct special services, if any. This division of responsibility with respect to public health services is similar to that observed in other public service areas like education and social welfare, where the service programs are generally operated by local government entities but are supervised, standardized, and coordinated by state agencies. For some health programs the state agency is the final authority with respect to statewide supervision and coordination, and for others it is largely a mediating

agency administering federal funds that "pass through" the state to support local programs. In the latter case the complexity of the shared monitoring and supervision that results when local programs operate with both state *and* federal support is formidable (see Chapter 4). The quality of local public health work throughout the United States is strongly influenced by the quality of the state health department leadership, operating within the constraints of the budget, responsibilities, and authority assigned to it by the state government. This is particularly true outside the big cities in counties that are not highly urbanized. In urbanized areas the local health department often depends less on the state health department for guidance and leadership, has more direct ties with Washington, and is often lax in reporting its activities to the state health agency as required under statewide plans for coordination.

The health protection function is not explicitly assigned to the federal government by the United States Constitution, a fact that historically proved to be a fundamental determinant of the pattern of development of state public health authorities. In fact, the Constitutional responsibility and authority for safeguarding the health of the residents within its borders rests with the individual state. The power of the state to carry out functions such as protecting the health of its citizens "is generally referred to as the state's police power . . . i.e., the power 'to enact and enforce laws to protect and promote the health, safety, morals, order, peace, comfort, and general welfare of the people' . . . and local agencies, including state and local public health departments and agencies, derive their power by delegation from the state legislature" (Grad, 1970, 5–6).

Many of the functional areas covered by local

public health department operations, such as sanitation and maternal and child health, are also those most frequently assigned by state law to the state health department for oversight and co-ordination. Because of the breadth of the state's police powers, however, many state health departments engage in health-related functions that are rarely, if ever, practiced by local public health departments, such as licensing and accreditation of health professionals and health facilities, standard setting for automobile safety devices, and supervision of the quality of public medical payment programs like Medicaid. In some states, the department of health services serves as a single umbrella health agency and contains different divisions to carry out health-related functions, one of which is public health.

THE PERIOD BEFORE 1935

Early Organization of State Boards of Health

Local action preceded statewide programs because the early activities were organized in response to emergency conditions, and these were generally local rather than statewide. Only when emergent health problems affected a large proportion of a state's area and population were state health authorities organized and mobilized for action. "Thus yellow fever was probably responsible for the creation of the first state board of health in the United States, when Louisiana established such a board in 1855"[2] (Mustard, 1945, 91). Other temporary and in effect ad hoc organizations had sporadically come into being: some antedated the American Revolution and were thus "colony-wide" rather than "statewide." For example, the General Assembly of Carolina appointed a health officer in 1712 to supervise quarantine activities in the port of Charleston.

The permanently organized state board of health and its health department did not become a familiar part of the state governmental landscape until the years 1870–1910, when it became increasingly apparent that many health problems extended beyond the geographical scope of the local community. A contributing factor to this diffusion of health problems was the rapid growth and dispersion of population and industry, with all its attendant housing, environmental, and workplace conditions. The organization of state boards[3] of health was part of a general tendency to establish uniform standards with respect to governmental functions over ever wider areas, both as an aid to the geographic spread of commercial and industrial enterprise and as a way of controlling its deleterious side effects.

I have previously noted that the origins of modern public health lie in the health problems brought about by early commercial and industrial development. Both of these types of business expansion were associated with urbanization—the development first of seaport cities and later of inland manufacturing towns. It was the health problems of the seaport cities that brought forth the early local public health efforts in the form of maritime quarantine measures. The challenge of maintaining the health of the urban populations of both types of cities quickly began to have ramifications for public health services in their surrounding semirural and rural areas as well. One main factor leading to the formation of a state public health organization was requests "from a comparatively large number of localities which shared a common problem or when some powerful local jurisdiction such as a large city, demanded state action ..." (Mustard, 1945, 91). As the cities grew it became increasingly clear that assuring the provision of safe water supplies and guaranteeing the purity of milk and other food products for use in the city often involved statewide monitoring of milk producers and water sources by a state agency. The needs of the developing urban economy, both mercantile and industrial, for a healthful hinterland that furnished its food and water was a factor inducing the establishment of state health departments. That this phenomenon stemmed from the stage of industrial development rather than idiosyncrasies of American history is supported by parallel developments in Great Britain and Germany (Shryock, 1979, 233). In Europe, however, the drive was directed primarily at achieving national rather than intraprovincial coordination and supervision of local public health organization. In the United States the movement for increased central coordination first turned to intrastate organization rather than moving directly toward a national system stressing interstate coordination, a result of the federalist form of governmental structure and the emphasis on state sovereignty provided by the Constitution.

Although foreign commerce was the mainstay of the economic life of the port cities, such as Boston, New York, and Philadelphia, these cities also developed manufacturing and domestic commerce. But it was the inland industrial cities like Lowell, Massachusetts, that developed factory industry most intensively. The growth of manufacturing in these cities led them, as well as the older port cities, to take on the characteristics of English manufacturing cities—including the public health problems attendant on poor working conditions and crowded, unsanitary living quarters. The power of local public health organization to enforce improvement in these conditions was weak, and state regulation seemed increasingly necessary.

The first state board of health that went on to become a permanently established government entity was organized in 1869 in Massachusetts. It is not surprising that this should have happened in Massachusetts, because the pioneer formulation of the functions and structure of a state board and department of public health was made in that state by Lemuel Shattuck. The imprint of his ideas was indelibly stamped on the organizational design and conception of the functions of state departments and boards of health and persists to the present day. A student of the work of the English public health reformer Edwin Chadwick, Shattuck had been campaigning for the improvement of public health measures in Massachusetts when in 1849 he was named chairman of the Massachusetts Sanitary Commission, which had been appointed by the governor to make a "sanitary survey" of the state.

The report of this commission, issued in 1850, "has become a classic in public health literature and documents" (Mustard, 1945, 93) with many of its recommendations serving as guides for the organization of subsequent state and local public health agencies. The principles of organization and the comprehensive list of recommended public health functions given in the Shattuck report became the core of the principles and the accepted traditional (standard) public health services and remain largely so to the present day. In fact, some of the organizational principles are still regarded as desirable goals even though they continue to remain largely unrealized. Among them[4] are the suggestions that no one profession should completely control or overwhelmingly dominate the composition of the board of health and that the board should employ at least one full-time "secretary." Yet in 1972, doctors of medicine were in the majority on the boards of twelve states and in two of these all the members were physicians (Gossert and Miller, 1973), while the standard of a full-time, fully qualified chief health officer has not been reached in all local public health jurisdictions.

However, no permanent state boards of health were formed immediately following the issuance of the Shattuck report. Instead, between 1857 and 1860 a series of "sanitary conventions" was held, sponsored by local medical and sanitary associations whose representatives met with city officials of eastern seaports to exchange views about common public health problems. Also in 1857, Dr. Wilson Jewell of the Philadelphia health board persuaded the board to call a meeting of state authorities to discuss common sanitary problems. This was followed by another meeting in Baltimore—"The Great American Congress for Hygiene Reform" (Shryock, 1979, 235). With the coming of the Civil War, further progress toward the formation of permanent state public health boards was suspended, but shortly after the end of the war, Massachusetts organized its board of health in 1869 based on Shattuck's recommendations. By 1900, forty states had state boards of health, and by 1909 all the states had organized some form of state board of health. The founding dates of the various boards of health are shown in Figure 3–1.

The Ferrell Report of 1925

For a long time, however, many of these boards were a far cry from the Shattuck model; some of them still are. Using data for 1925, the previously cited study (see Chapter 2) by Ferrell

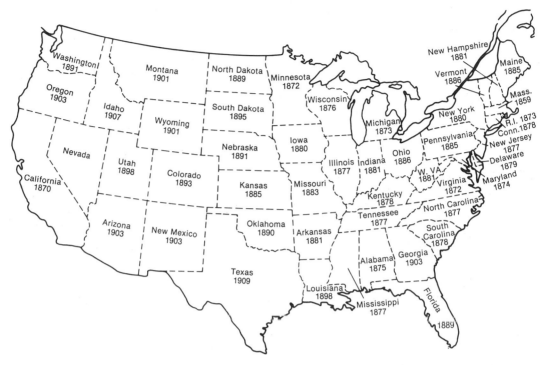

Fig. 3–1. Date of creation of each state board of health for the purpose of promoting public health work. *Source*: Ferrell et al., 1929, figure 1, p. 7.

and associates (1929) reported that eleven states had only public health councils acting in an advisory capacity in place of a board of health. Three states had no state boards or councils of any kind. The remaining thirty-four states had state boards of health that had "supervisory power over the State health activities and . . . legislative authority to make and enforce rules and regulations concerning contagious disease, quarantine, and the health of the people of the State." In two states, Alabama and South Carolina, the state board of health was composed primarily of the medical association; in eleven states, all members of the board were required to be physicians. (As I have noted above, similar conditions still prevailed in 1972.)

Overall, "the most common method of appointment (of board members) [was] either by the governor or by the governor with the consent of the senate." Most states required that the chief executive officer of the health department be a physician, and the two methods of selection in most common use were appointment by the

governor (twenty-four states) and by the state board of health (twenty-one states). In some states where appointment was by the governor, consent of some legislative body was also required. In just over half the states, the executive operating officer was a member of the board, while in only nine of the states were the employees of the state board of health under civil service.

In a total of seventeen states the health department had a separate bureau of county health work headed by a full-time director. This was singled out for note because of the special importance attached by the authors to the promotion of local public health work as a function of the state health department, a function that remains perhaps the most important aspect of the state health agency's public health responsibilities to the present day. Of the total funds used for operating local full-time public health departments, the proportion provided by the states varied greatly from state to state—again, a condition that still prevails. One state met 48 percent of the total expenses for full-time county health service, and in ten states the state's share in the county budgets ranged from 20 percent to 30 percent of the total. The study found that "the trend toward increasing the aid from the state is growing."

Functions most often found to be performed or promoted by state health departments were:

rural or district health work; development of local health units
communicable disease control, particularly tuberculosis and venereal disease
vital statistics
public health laboratories
sanitary engineering
child hygiene
public health nursing
public health education
food and drug regulation and control.

In many states, special divisions headed by outstanding specialists were organized in the state health department to deal with some of these functions.

Because the Ferrell report was the last to describe in detail the existing situation before the federal government began in 1935 to inject federal monies into the states to expand state and local public health department facilities and functions, its data were (with some adjustment) used as a benchmark from which to measure later progress ascribed to the infusion of such funds.

THE PERIOD 1935 AND AFTER

Changes Brought about from 1936 to 1945 under Social Security Act Funding

The Social Security Act, described in Chapter 2, also provided major federal funding for state public health departments, and the analysis by the Mountin study of 1947 described in Chapter 2 analyzed the effect after ten years (1936–1946) of these federal monies on expanding the state health department activities. The federal allotments and health department expenditures described by Mountin referred primarily to funds allocated to the states by the U.S. Public Health

Service for public health work under Title VI of the Social Security Act. Only fragmentarily did he have access to data on the Title V funds, which were transmitted through the Children's Bureau of the Labor Department. It may be presumed, therefore, that the degree to which these funds sparked the observed expansion of activities, particularly in the early years after passage of the Social Security Act, was, if anything, understated by Mountin's analysis.

Using as a baseline the classification schema supplied by the Ferrell report for 1925, but with the data updated to 1930, Mountin found that expenditures of the forty-eight states for their public health departments went from $12.9 million in 1930, to $18.7 million in 1940, to $37.0 million in 1946. The breakdown of these expenditures by categories of activity showed that

such activities as communicable disease control (including tuberculosis and venereal disease control), sanitation, laboratory services, and maternal or child hygiene, which accounted for a majority of State expenditures in 1930, still received more than half of the funds available in 1946. . . .

At the same time, the growth of newer programs is illustrated by such figures as these for dental hygiene: 37 thousand (dollars) in 1930, 227 thousand in 1941 and 708 thousand in 1946 [see Table 3–1].

The fact that the data indicating increased public health expenditures were not merely due to price increases but represented real expansion of services was shown by the corresponding increase in full-time personnel from 4,672 in 1930, to 10,128 in 1940, to 12,414 in 1946.

Additional evidence put forth by Mountin that the expansion in the years 1936–1946 was real and not merely an artifact of price increase was the number of activity types reported as an "identified project" by state health departments. While this sort of measure taken alone does not necessarily imply an increase in total volume of services, it was used by Mountin as one indicator of an increase in the number of different types of function offered in many states. Out of the total of forty-six states reporting, thirty-nine listed communicable disease control for 1935, forty-three in 1940, and forty-five in 1946. The number of state health departments showing tu-

Table 3–1. Estimated Expenditures from All Scoures by the 48 State Health Departments for Specified Health Activities, Excluding Hospitals and Sanatoria Grants to Local health Units, in 1930, 1940, and 1946

| | Expenditures by designated fiscal year | | | | | |
| | Thousands of dollars | | | Percent of total | | |
Specified	1930[a]	1940[b]	1946[b]	1930	1940	1946
Total estimated expenditures	12,882	18,694	36,985	100.00	100.00	100.00
Communicable disease control	1,286	1,397	1,233	9.98	7.47	3.31
Tuberculosis control (excluding hospitals)	680	677	3,104	5.28	3.62	8.39
Veneral disease control	442	740[c]	941	3.43	3.96	2.54
Sanitation	1,828	2,852	4,517	14.19	15.26	12.21
Industrial hygiene	36	421	832	0.28	2.25	2.25
Laboratory services	2,115	4,045	7,198	16.42	21.64	19.46
Public helath nursing[d]	613	526	1,005	4.76	2.81	2.72
Maternity and/or child hygiene[d]	1,643	1,044[e]	5,013	12.75	5.58	13.55
Public health education	160	366	1,085	1.24	1.96	2.93
Dental hygiene	37	227	708	0.29	1.47.21	1.91
Cancer services	292	274	408	2.27		1.10
Mental hygiene	128	39	131	0.99	0.21	0.35
Nutrition	—	—	269	—	—	0.7
Personnel administration	—	—	191	—	—	0.52
Personnel training	—	1,138	1,015	—	6.09	2.74
Surveys and studies	—	38	147	—	0.20	0.40
Other central services	3,423	4,155	8,450	26.57	22.23	22.85
Miscellaneous	199	755	748	1.54	4.04	2.02

Source: Public Health Bulletin No. 300, Table 4, p. 22 (Mountin et al., 1947).

[a]Totals for 1930 were obtained by adding amounts appropriated by the respective state governments as shown in Public Health Bulletin 184, 1932. Comparable data for 1935 are not available.

[b]For 1940 and 1946, expenditures by states as reported to the Public Health Service have been used. Especially in the earlier year, some states reported only programs that received some aid from funds allotted by the Public Health Service. Moreover, assignments of expenditures to activities have not been entirely consistent from state to state nor from year to year.

[c]For tuberculosis and veneral disease control. Federal grants-in-aid alone were considerably more than the amounts shown. Assignment of funds to other services, especially laboratories, accounts for part of the difference. Moreover, the states reallotted a considerable proportion of such funds to localities and they appear in the reports as expended for local health services.

[d]Including aid to crippled children when expenditures for this activity were reported by the state health department.

[e]Federal funds specifically for maternity and child hygiene activities have been allotted by the Children's Bureau, and expenditures for such activities were frequently not reported to the Public Health Service especially in the first years after passage of the Social Security Act.

berculosis control programs had risen from nineteen in 1935, to thirty-two in 1940, and forty-five in 1946. Virtually all the traditionally accepted public health functions showed similar increases in the number of state health departments performing them. Mental hygiene[5] and cancer control, however, showed only seven and twenty-seven states, respectively, listing these activities as "identified projects" in 1946. Planning, chronic disease work, and other more "modern" functions did not appear as "identified projects" at all. If any were in place, they are subsumed under the catchall category "other central services." Thus the increase in number of "new" functions shown by some state public health departments as measured by number of "identified projects" was not, for the most part, in areas new to "public health." It therefore did not represent a widespread expansion of the scope of function beyond the "basic six." Instead it mainly represented the entry into some "standard" areas by departments that had not engaged in them before.

A notable exception to this generalization is the striking increase in the number of states operating industrial hygiene programs. In 1935 only four states engaged in this activity as an "identified project" compared with twenty-six states in 1940 and thirty-eight in 1946. In addition, the two states that did not respond to the question about "identified projects" did in fact have industrial hygiene units in both 1940 and 1946, and New York and Massachusetts provided industrial hygiene units through their departments of labor. By 1946, then, forty-two states had such units covering 96 percent of the country's labor force, but in two states the program was not lodged in the health department. The services most commonly supplied by such units were "general surveys or inspection of plants for occupational health hazards with recommendations for improvement'' (Mountin et al., 1947, 25). Thus, as early as 1946 the rising importance of occupational safety and health was reflected in state health department functions. This increase in what is today called ''occupational health'' projects was undoubtedly due in large part to the rising strength of the labor unions during these years. Further national recognition of this area of public health came in 1970 with the passage of the Occupational Health and Safety Act. This law is treated in Chapter 4.

Trends in Organization and Function Definition 1946–1970

State Boards of Health in 1972

A study of the composition of state boards of health by Gossert and Miller completed in 1972 provided insight into how far the standards of Shattuck still were from having been met. Alaska and Rhode Island had no statutory boards. In Illinois and Delaware there was statutory provision, but no members were currently appointed in Illinois, and the Delaware board consisted entirely of two state officials. Appointments to the board were almost always made by governors, with some form of legislative approval being required in half the states. Only 12.5 percent of the 433 seats in forty-six states were occupied by persons identified as consumers in 1972. In thirty-two of the forty-six states with functioning boards, the membership consisted of at least one-third medical doctors, and in twelve they constituted a majority of the board. In two states, Alabama and South Carolina, the state medical society was the board of health. There was a discernible trend to merge state health departments with other departments. In 1969 there were eight states with such mergers, and in 1972 there were sixteen; four states had a single conglomerate human resources agency.

Changes in APHA Positions on Functions of State Health Departments

In 1968 the functions recommended as appropriate for the state health department were outlined in a policy statement of the governing council of the American Public Health Association and adopted at its 96th annual meeting (1969). The main points were:

1. Health surveillance, planning, and program development.

   the state health department must engage in a continuing agency program-planning process based upon its own continuing surveillance and appraisal of health problems, needs, and resources, and relate these to the comprehensive health plan of the state. . . . [Carrying out] epidemiological, administrative, clinical, behavioral, and laboratory research.

   Stressed under this category are information gathering and analysis, assistance to communities on local areawide planning, and financial aid and consultation.
2. Promotion of local health coverage.
3. Setting and enforcement of standards. This category includes state certification for federally assisted health services—''audit of medical-care services and . . . the administration of medical-care programs.'' The program areas involved are personal health services, control of the environment, research, professional education, public health education, and administration.
4. Personal health services. (See excerpt cited on page 60)
5. Environmental protection.

   The state's obligation to maintain a wholesome living environment devolves largely upon the State health department. . . .

These formulations indicated that some of the same trends in the thinking of leading public health professionals with respect to the functions of the local health department were also operating at the state level. The direction of the change over time was away from a conception of the health department's function that stressed a few community-wide preventive measures, for the most part directly provided by health departments, toward a conception of responsibility for the total system of health services, including personal health care. For example, the 1953 position of the American Public Health Association had enumerated the responsibilities of the state health department for personal health services as ''diagnosis, care and treatment of tuberculosis; immunization procedures; rehabilitation of the disabled [this already was a broadening of scope over previous positions]; maternal and child health services; ... discovering early cases of cancer'' (1954). In contrast to this 1953 statement, the 1968 APHA position stated that under the category of personal health services,

the state agency's responsibility for personal health services is to insure that standards of care and completeness of services are adequate to the personal health needs of the citizens in every part of the state. In meeting these objectives, the state health agency ... will oversee and assist local public health agency medical services; regulate institutions providing medical care; seek to improve the quality of medical care generally, and provide some direct medical services.

Again, while in 1953 the APHA had stated simply that the "health department must coordinate the work of all agencies dealing with public health in the state," the 1968 statement asserted more firmly that "the APHA recommends that the state health department *assume the leadership* [emphasis added] in a multi-agency framework of health services ... that will coordinate the efforts of all agencies." The 1968 statement also asserted the necessity for consumer participation in health planning.

However, these bold and forward-looking pronouncements were the enunciated policy. Their transformation into real, de facto, policy was at best tentative and partial. Comparison of the 1968 statement of policy with the activities actually found to be carried out in the years after 1960 by state health departments reveals that performance of the traditional ("standard") functions continued to predominate with the "newer" ones of community coordination for total health care, particularly medical care, continuing to be much less in evidence. In a 1961 study summarized in Hanlon (1969), Shubick and Wright (1961) listed the principal types of state health activities in terms of the number of the fifty states that were engaging in them. Some of the most frequently listed activities of state health departments and the number of states in which they were encountered are summarized in Table 3–2.[6] These are, for the most part, either the traditional programs or the "programs which are categorically funded by the federal government (Hanlon, 1969). On the other hand, newer

programs such as "program planning, development, and evaluation" appeared as activities in only seven state health departments; "radiologic health" in eleven; and "heart disease control" in twenty-five.[7]

A More Recent Picture

State Boards of Health in 1980

The essence of the Shattuck conception of a state board of health was a body that, once appointed, was significantly independent of legislative and gubernatorial short-term electoral politics, was not dominated by provider interests, and had strong powers to formulate health policy by promulgating regulations and ordinances. The state health agency and its chief were to serve as expert advisers to the board and executors of its policies. But a study published in 1982 (Gilbert, Moose, and Miller, 1982) found that the trend away from having Shattuck-model state boards of health shown in the 1972 study (Gossert and Miller, 1973) had accelerated. The 1982 study found that twenty-two states had disestablished their boards of health since 1900, thirteen in the 1970s alone. The disestablished boards were replaced with bodies that had less power than a full-fledged board of health. By about 1980, twenty-seven states still had boards of health, nine had only bodies that were advisory to the state health agency, four had boards that

Table 3–2. The Activities of State Health Departments in 1961

Type of activity	No. of states practicing the activity
Environmental health	50
Health education	50
Maternal and child health	50
Nursing	50
Vital statistics	49
Laboratories	47
Dental health	46
Communicable disease	45
Engineering	43
Tuberculosis control	43
Hospital survey, planning, and construction licensure	42
Local health services	42
Industrial health	36
Personnel	34
Cancer control	31
Chronic disease control	30

served an entire umbrella agency of which the health agency was but a part, and ten states had no board of any kind. The writers of this report saw this situation as a matter for concern, arguing that

State boards of health represent a potential source of influence for public health policy, rules and regulations, and budgeting. That potential has declined dramatically in recent years. The functions of state boards of health, and the agencies for which they are responsible, have been placed to a large extent under direct control of the executive offices of state government. The potential for such boards to exercise independent and non-partisan influence has been greatly reduced (Gilbert, Moose, and Miller, 1982).

The IOM 1988 report noted that "the disbanding of state boards has meant the loss of an important resource for public health policy," and recommended the formation of state health councils with broad policy development responsibilities. This was very similar to the recommendations of the Shattuck report.

As I have noted previously, the early literature dealing with the growth of state public health organization spoke almost exclusively of state boards of health. Some time soon after 1900 the references began to allude more to state health departments than to state boards of health, and by about 1950 the discussions were almost exclusively concerned with state health departments, or more generally, state health agencies (SHA). I am not aware of any studies tracing this transition. Although there is a revival of interest in whether a citizen board should be regarded as the basic policy-making body for a state's public health operations, with the state health agency being advisory to it, or whether the converse is desirable, is a question with profound implications. Yet the subject of the state board of health and its role remains one of the least investigated in health services literature—either on an empirical or theoretical basis.

The NPHPRS-PHF Data on State Health Agency Functions after 1970; the 1978 Picture

Beginning with 1970, annual statistics on state health departments were assembled via a questionnaire by the National Public Health Program Reporting System (NPHPRS),[8] an arm of the

Association of State and Territorial Health Officials (ASTHO). The data of the first comprehensive NPHPRS published report covered 1974 experience. With the publication of the 1980 report, covering data for fiscal 1978 (Assn. St. & Terr Hlth Officials, 1980), five consecutive years of comprehensive data were made available. This data described the status of the state health departments, or state health agencies (SHAs)[9] as they are called in this reporting system.

In fiscal year (FY) 1978,[10] all fifty-seven "states" (fifty states, six territories, and the District of Columbia) had state health agencies. Together they spent $3.26 billion dollars on their public health programs, of which $2.52 billion or 77 percent was spent on personal health services and the rest on other program categories.[11]

Table 3–3 shows these expenditures by "program category"[12] for the year 1978.

Over the years 1974–1978 there was a marked shift from state and local to federal sources of financing. In 1974, 25.7 percent of the funds were of federal origin; by 1978 this had grown to 34.8 percent. It is worth noting that despite the wide discussion accorded public health issues in the late 1970s, only 2.6 percent of the total $192.4 billion spent for health in 1978 was for operating state and local public health agencies.[13] This small percentage has not grown materially to the present day.

It is clear from Table 3–3 that the main functional categories ("program areas") of the activities performed continued for the most part unchanged. The emphases were largely where Mountin had found them to be in 1946, and Shubick-Wright in 1961. This was clearly true in terms of the relative distribution of the *dollar* but only partly true in terms of the number of SHAs that were performing these functions. For example, in 1978 all fifty-seven agencies reported providing some services in chronic disease, and fifty-six out of fifty-seven were active in mental retardation and developmental disability, while in 1961 these services were not in the top ten of the list shown in Table 3–2 as being provided by forty-three (86 percent) or more of the fifty agencies surveyed. There was thus a marked increase in the *number of agencies* operating programs in chronic disease control, mental retardation, and developmental disabilities.

Table 3–3. Public Health Expenditures of State Health Agencies: Total and by Program Area and Category, Fiscal Year 1978

Program area and selected program categories	Public health expenditures (thousands of dollars)
Total	$3,257,548
Personal health (excluding SHA-operated institutions)	1,666,923
General and supporting	261,659
General and child health	769,807
Crippled children	181,142
Communicable disease	112,832
Dental health	28,053
Chronic disease	76,307
Mental health and related programs	166,426
Other personal health	70,697
SHA-operated institutions	666,477
Environmental health	237,676
Consumer protection and sanitation	84,350
Water quality	55,834
Air quality	23,833
Waste management	13,047
Occupational health and safety and related areas	10,800
Radiation control	11,370
General environmental health	38,422
Health resources	298,737
Planning	19,755
Development	17,989
Regulation	157,164
Statistics	46,883
Genral health resources	56,496
Laboratory	131,127
General administration and services*	195,720
Funds to LHDs not allocated to program areas*	60,888

Source: Adapted from Assocation of State and Territorial Health Officials, 1980, Table II-4, p. 27

*Note that these lines are conceptually allocable to program lines but are not presented that way in the origianl table of the report.

In the main, however, the data indicate again that the state *public health* departments did not enlarge their scope of function very much over the years, especially as measured by the allocation of the dollar resources.[14] It is clear that local consumer protection and sanitation were still their leading environmental protection functions, and that maternal and child health and communicable disease control were still the mainstays of the functional scope of most state health departments in the area of *personal* services in 1978. (That the longstanding principal functions should have remained so predominant in the balance of activities of the state public health department in the face of the growing recognition of ''newer'' health threats reflects important political developments that will be discussed later in this chapter and in Chapter 4.)

In fact, measured in terms of dollars spent, the dominance of a single function (''program cat-

egory''), maternal and child health (MCH), is striking. Expenditures of the state health agencies (SHAs) for this program category made up almost a fourth of total outlays and over 45 percent of their personal health care expenditures (excluding SHA-operated institutions). The percentages are even higher if one includes crippled children programs. The dominant position of expenditures for maternal and child health is in turn largely due to a single item, Women and Infant Care (WIC) nutrition, a diet supplement program supported by the Department of Agriculture. In 1978, $286 million (37 percent) of the $770 million MCH expenditures went for this single program. The predominance of the MCH and crippled children's programs, even without the WIC component, raises provocative questions about the future role of the state health department. If a national medical care program with universal eligibility and comprehensive benefits were implemented, it presumably would include prenatal care, mother and infant care, and care of crippled children. It would, parenthetically, also include much of the care now provided under categorical programs for venereal disease, and to some degree also dental health, chronic disease, and other personal health programs. Unless the state health departments were in some way assigned functions under the national medical care program, it is reasonable to suppose that their direct personal health care functions would then be much reduced, perhaps even eliminated. In that event, what might be left? The environmental, planning, regulation, and monitoring (''statistics'') programs category in Table 3–3) functions are likely candidates to become the most important functions, in addition to the ongoing task of promoting and maintaining local public health departments for local implementation of public health programs. It is instructive, therefore, to pay special attention to the status of these four program types in state health agencies in 1978.[15]

Environmental protection most clearly exemplifies the widespread use of agencies other than the SHA to administer health protection functions. (See Fig. 3–2 and Table 3–4.) In Idaho, Pennsylvania, and the District of Columbia all environmental services were provided by agencies other than the SHA during 1974–1978.[16] The remaining fifty-four state health agencies provided varying mixes of the program categories classified under the environmental program area with just over one-third of the $238 million expenditures going for consumer protection and sanitation programs, as shown in Table 3–3. Another 23 percent went for water quality programs. Thus, most of the environmental health activities were of the standard type that state health departments had been engaged in for many years, largely through their supervision of the direct service activities of local public health departments. The ASTHO report for 1978 put it well:

All of the SHAs reporting environmental health programs provided *consumer protection and sanitation* [emphasis in original] services, including food or milk control, substance control and products safety, sanitation of health care facilities and other institutions, housing and recreational sanitation, or vector and zoonotic disease control. *Water quality* services, provided by 51 SHAs, were usually related to public drinking water, individual water supply, and individual sewage disposal. Public water pollution control services were more often provided by an agency other

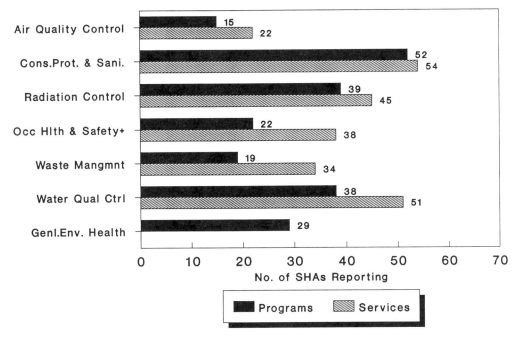

Fig. 3–2. Number of state health agencies reporting specified environmental health programs in 1978. *Source*: Association of State and Territorial Health Officials, 1980, p. 70.

Table 3–4. Environmental Health Expenditures of 54 State Health Agencies, Fiscal Year 1978

Program category	Number of SHAs reporting programs	Expenditures (million of dollars)	Percent of total
Total	54	$237.7	100.0
Consumer protection and sanitation	52	84.5	35.5
General consumer protection and sanitation	45	39.2	16.5
Food and milk control	24	25.0	10.5
Drugs, narcotics, cosmetics, toxic substances, and pesticide control	20	4.3	1.8
Sanitation of health care facilities and other institutions	6	0.3	0.1
Housing, hotel motel, and recreational sanitation	18	4.2	1.8
Vector and zoonotic disease control	18	11.5	4.8
Water quality	38	55.8	23.5
General water supply and pollution control	38	20.8	8.8
Public water supply	18	12.7	5.3
Individual water supply and sewage disposal	9	6.0	2.5
Air quality	15	23.8	10.0
Waste management	19	13.0	5.5
Occupational health and safety and related areas	22	10.8	4.5
Radiation control	39	11.4	4.8
General environmental health	29	38.4	16.2

Source: Association of State and Territorial Health Officials (1980, p. 70).

than the SHA. *Radiation control* services were offered by 45 SHAs. Fewer SHAs provided other environmental health services: *occupational health and safety and related services* (38 SHAs), *waste management* (34), and *air quality* (22).

The funding sources of the environmental health expenditures of state health agencies were predominantly state monies, 57 percent. Twenty-six percent came from federal sources (a bit over half of the federal money was from the national Environmental Protection Agency) and the rest from local government, fees, and other sources (Association of State and Territorial Health Officials, 1980, 71). (See Table 3–5.)

The provisions of the Environmental Protection Act of 1970[17] called for the governor and/or the legislature of each state to designate a "lead environmental agency" to have overall responsibility for environmental activities. There are three generally recognized types of state agencies from which lead agencies for federal environmental protection programs have been selected: a state health agency, a state environmental protection agency, and a state natural resources agency (Council of State Govts., 1976). In 1978, only nineteen of the fifty-four SHAS that had environmental health programs were designated as lead environmental agencies.[18] The four services that a lead agency generally supervised were air quality control, noise

pollution control, solid waste management, and water pollution control. By contrast, as noted in the ASTHO statement above, the services most often assigned by a state government to an SHA that was not a lead agency were consumer protection and sanitation, individual use water quality excluding general water pollution control, and radiation control.

Turning to the role of SHAs in statewide health planning we find a picture similar to that in environmental health but with some differences worth noting. As with environmental health services, many states designated another agency as the principal one for overall health planning, but not as many as in environmental health. During the years 1966 through 1986 the federal government supported a program establishing local area-wide health planning agencies to coordinate all health services in local communities. Two acts, one passed in 1966 and one in 1974, formed the main legislative basis for this program, which is discussed in detail in Chapter 15. Under the later of these acts, the Health Planning and Resource Development Act of 1974 (P.L. 93–641), each state was to appoint a single agency as the State Health Planning and Development Agency (SHPDA), one of whose responsibilities was the submission of an annual state plan for improving all health services in the state. Of the fifty-seven "states," thirty-six had

Table 3–5. Funding Sources of Expenditures of State Health Agenices for Environmental Services in 1978

Funding source	Number of SHAs reporting	Expenditures (million of dollars)	Percent of total
Total	54	$237.7	100.0
Total non-federal	54	176.0	74.0
State	54	134.9	56.8
Local	9	18.2	7.7
Fees and reimbursements	17	15.2	6.4
Other	17	7.7	3.2
Total federal grants and contracts	52	61.7	26.0
Department of Health, Education and Welfare	46	17.8	7.5
PHS Act Section 314(d)(7)(A)	38	9.2	3.9
Center for Disease Control	12	5.7	2.4
Other DHEW	27	2.9	1.2
Environmental Protection Agency	40	33.6	14.1
Department of Agriculture	5	4.6	1.9
Department of Labor	13	3.1	1.3
Other	17	2.6	1.1

Source: Association of State and Territorial Health Officials (1980, p. 71).

designated their state health agency as the State Health Planning and Development Agency by 1978, not much different from the number that did so under the earlier Comprehensive Health Planning Act of 1966 but almost double the nineteen states that did so for environmental health. Furthermore, in fifteen of the states where the main statewide planning function was lodged in another state agency, the SHAs performed planning functions for their official state planning agency to help it meet the P.L. 93–641 requirements, including one SHA (Tennessee) that actually prepared the entire required state plan for the SHPDA.

It should be noted that virtually all SHAs also were active in drawing up state plans of some kind outside the national health planning structure provided by P.L. 93–641. The administration of the national health planning program confined itself primarily to coordinating and monitoring the work of the 205 (in 1978) federally financed local health planning agencies, the so-called Health Systems Agencies (HSAs), and with statewide administration of federal guidelines under that law. And, although the expressed intent of the law was that the local planning work on rationalizing the entire local system (public and private) of health services, their emphasis devolved to a one-sided focus on controlling the expansion of acute-care hospital beds and big-ticket hospital equipment expen-

ditures (see Chapter 15). Many state health agencies that were not chosen as the state's lead agency for overall health planning, continued to be involved in drawing up statewide plans for the state's own health activities, standard *categorical* programs like MCH and family planning, as well as for Emergency Medical Services (EMS), health manpower regulation and development, facilities monitoring and development, direct services, and financing. The number of SHAs engaged in developing statewide plans for categorical services, quite aside from their work in thirty-six states as SHPDAs under P.L. 93–641, varied according to the nature of the service. By way of example, the SHAs of forty-five states were developing statewide categorical health plans for emergency medical services, but only thirteen were doing so for drug abuse (Association of State and Territorial Health Officials, 1980, 89). (Of course, some of the work performed under the two roles of SHA or SHPDA necessarily overlapped where the SHA was the SHPDA.)

With respect to regulation and monitoring we find that in 1978, forty-six out of fifty-four responding agencies reported having programs in this area. Their total expenditure of $158 million for regulation, however, was only about 5 percent of the total public health expenditures of state health agencies, and the amount spent by the fifty-three agencies with monitoring (''statistics'') programs was $47 million, less than 1.5 percent of the total public health state agency expenditures.

I have frequently alluded to the drive of the public health profession for full "coverage" of the entire population by the services of a "qualified" local public health department and to the corollary efforts to define standards for determining what minimal depth and quality of services such "coverage" implies. I have also noted that one of the most important activities of state health departments has always been considered to be development of local public health departments so that they are at least up to standards and the supervision and monitoring of their work. It is interesting to see, therefore, how these matters stood in 1978 according to the National Public Health Program Reporting System data and the interpretations of its sponsoring body, the Association of State and Territorial Health Officials.

We find that the definition of a local public health department (with its implication of what constitutes at least minimal public health "coverage") to have been relaxed in at least one respect from previous definitions by not requiring medical leadership. The NPHPRS defined a local health department (LHD) to be

an official (governmental) public health agency which is in whole or in part responsible to a substate governmental entity or entities. The latter may be a city, county, city-county, federation of counties, borough, township, or any other type of substate governmental entity. In addition, a local health department must meet these criteria: (A) It has a staff of one or more full-time professional public health employees (e.g., public health nurse, sanitarian); (B) it delivers public health services; (C) it serves a definable geographic area; and (D) it has identifiable expenditures and/or budget in the political subdivision(s) which it serves.

Three "generic" types of LHD are identified: an LHD operated by the SHA as part of a centrally directed state system of local public health agencies;[19] a largely autonomous local health department receiving some technical assistance and consultation from the SHA; and a partly autonomous local health department that shares control with the SHA, with the latter having direct operating authority in some areas. Clearly, ASTHO meant a local public health department meeting the conditions of the cited definition to

be the current analogy to what was referred to as "full-time" public health departments in the earlier literature (see discussions of Ferell et al., 1929; Mountin et al., 1947; and Emerson, 1945, in Chapter 2).

Dropping the requirement for a medically trained full-time health officer may not have been only a compromise with unpleasant reality. Some of the literature in the intervening period (Shonick, 1980; Cameron and Kobylarz, 1980) had suggested, and at times even strongly advocated, the discontinuance of this requirement as being desirable, not just expedient. The position was seen by some as largely administrative, requiring more a knowledge of overall public health and administration principles than a medical training. Shonick and Price (1978) found that in 1976 only an estimated 63 percent of local public health agency heads had M.D. degrees. Although there may be considerable merit in the contention that medical training is not by itself a sufficient or even a necessary preparation for properly leading a modern public health department, it is difficult to see how a minimum requirement of only one "public health employee" raises the previous standard. If the aim were to improve on the old standard of "at least one full time medically trained officer of public health," it is reasonable to have expected a substitution of some other requirement for the head of the department, such as a stipulation about training in public health management and in planning and policy analysis (in addition to education on the health services system and in epidemiology). As it stands, the ASTHO requirement for identifying a bona fide LHD can only be seen as a relaxation rather than a rectification of standards unless further stipulations about adequate coverage in rural areas are made.

In 1978 there were 2700 LHDs meeting the definition of the National Public Health Program Reporting system. Ten "states" (four states, the District of Columbia and five territories) had no LHDs by the NPHPRS definition.[20] In thirty-five of the forty-seven states with LHDs, 90 percent of the population lived in areas served by the LHDs (i.e., were "covered" by "full-time" public health services); in eleven of the twelve remaining states the SHA provided all the local public health services and in New Mexico they were provided by the Indian Health Service in some districts.

About 30 percent of State Health Agency money spent on public health went to the LHDs in the forty-two states reporting dollar amounts for this item for 1978. Most of this money was spent for local personal health programs (public health nursing, health education, maternal and child health, chronic disease, etc.) (Association of State and Territorial Officials, 1980, 37). A bit over half the money originated with the state itself and 31 percent was federal money transmitted to the local government via the SHA. The $215 million in federal funds that were part of the SHA funds distributed to LHDs included $62 million from Title V (MCH) funds and $23 million from section 314d (subsection 7A) Public Health Service Act funds, the successor to the old Title VI of the original Social Security Act, described in Chapter 2.

The proportion of local public health services funded by the SHA, some from the state's own budget and some from federal money disbursed by the state as a conduit between the federal and local governments, continued to vary greatly from state to state. Of the forty-seven states with ASTHO-defined LHDs, three (Virginia, Florida, and Mississippi) operated their LHDs entirely with funds from the SHA. For the remaining forty-four states, the NPHPRS estimated that on average about 42 percent of LHD funds came from the SHA. (See Table 3–6—693/1644.) This was an increase in proportion of LHD funds supplied by the SHA over the percentages for 1925 given by the Ferrell study (1929) cited in Chapter 2 which found percentages ranging from 20 to 30 percent to be most common. Furthermore, there were only seventeen states with separate "bureaus of county health work" then. The remark in the 1925 report that "the trend to increasing the aid from the state is growing" would seem clearly to have been pertinent and prescient, but there is uncertainty about the reliability of the present estimates. The indicated 42 percent may be a substantial overestimate, because the reporting of "funds from other sources" by LHDs to the NPHPRS was fragmentary for many states, thus understating the denominator of the 42 percent estimate.[21]

For the twenty-five states from whom the NPHPRS received "reasonably accurate" estimates of *total* LHD expenditures (that is, including good estimates of local non-SHA funds), it was found that the non-SHA funds were one and one half times the SHA funds on average, but the variability was great from state to state. For these twenty-five states, the average percentage of LHD funds supplied by the state was 40 percent, still considerably higher than in 1925, and the total public health expenditure of state and local official health agencies per capita ranged from $9.00 to $68.50, with a median of $16.43. The interquartile range (the "middle" 50 percent or the 25th through 75th percentiles) was from $11.50 to $25.00.

The foregoing discussion of the NPHPRS-PHF data for 1978 suggests that many states had assigned functions that public health professionals consider to be primarily health-related to agencies other than the SHA. The reasons for this important trend, some additional instances

Table 3–6. Sources of Funds for LHD Public Health Expenditures in 44 States, Fiscal Year 1978[a]

Source of funds	Total LHD expenditures		SHA grants to LHDs		Additional expenditures of LHDs	
	Amount (in millions of dollars)	Percent of total	Amount (in millions of dollars)	Percent of total	Amount (in millions of dollars)	Percent of total
Total	$1,644.0	100.0	$693.3	100.0	$950.7	100.0
Federal	264.1	16.1	215.4	13.1	48.7	2.962287
State	358.4	21.8	353.5	21.5	4.9	0.298053
Local	837.4	50.9	77.9	4.7	759.5	46.19829
Fees, reimbursements and other[b]	184.1	11.2	46.5	2.8	137.6	8.369829

Source Association of State and Territorial Health Officials (1980, p. 71).

[a]This does not include the expenditures of all LHDs. For purposes of this table, the funds reported as "source unknown" ($447 million) were proportionately distributed to the other funding sources.

[b]This category is substantially underreported by the LHDs. See note 21 and discussion, p. 67.

of its manifestation, and its policy implications are discussed in the next two sections.

Issues and Historical Factors Influencing the Scope of Health Services Functions Assigned by States to Their Principal Health Agency

Dispersal of State Health Functions among Agencies other than the Principal Health Agency

At the beginning of this chapter, it was noted that the state's responsibilities for the protection of the public's health are much broader than those of the local government. There is, consequently, a wider range of functions that might appear in the list of programs run by any particular state health department than there would be for local health departments. This theoretically greater breadth of choice is in practice sharply constrained by the fact that the number of functions state health departments actually perform is generally but a part of all the health functions carried on by state governments, and the ones assigned to the health department vary markedly from state to state. The health department, or state health agency (SHA), has been and remains but one of many state agencies utilized for discharging the state's responsibilities for protecting the health of its residents. Responsibility and control are shared with other agencies.

Before 1950 That this has been so for a good many years is illustrated by the expenditure pattern for 1941. Table 3–7 shows the distribution by types of state agency of the average $1.90 per capita spent by the states for health services. The distribution of personnel, however, was quite different, with 11,269 of the 18,737 full-time health workers in state agencies being employed by the health department. The reasons for the discrepancy between the distribution of expenditures and that of personnel is that the work of supervising the state's public health system is much more personnel intensive than most other state functions, and many health functions in other agencies are not performed by persons whose training is in the health field, e.g., attorneys, engineers, clerks, and social workers.

Table 3–7. Distribution of Funds Spent by States for Health Services in 1941

Type of Service	Percent
Health department	18.5%
Special boards	25.0
Welfare department	21.3
Boards of control	16.0
All others	19.2
Total	100.0%

As early as 1950 a study conducted by the U.S. Public Health Service found that some sixty types of state agencies participated in carrying out health functions, with

the number of agencies performing health activities in a single state [ranging] from 10 to 32. . . . The variation among states in assignment of responsibility for health functions is due . . . to two main factors: Complexity of state governmental organization and extent of health services provided by the state. . . . Numerous other agencies are often responsible for a single activity within a state. As many as 13 separate agencies are engaged in accident prevention work in one state, while a total of 12 participate in some form of health education in another (USPHS, 1952).

And almost twenty years later in 1969, Hanlon wrote:

this complex and diffuse situation on the state level has not clarified appreciably since the survey was conducted. However, in every state without exception, some one agency is invested with primary responsibility for the *public health* [emphasis added] program. Usually this is a state department of public health, although in one instance, the state of Maine, public health is a subdivision of a department of welfare (1969).

Not only had "this complex and diffuse situation" not clarified "appreciably since the [U.S.P.H.S.] survey was conducted"; it continued to grow steadily murkier. After 1950 the frequency with which states assigned the administration of new health programs to agencies other than their principal state health agencies (SHAs) increased. This developing trend reached major proportions by the 1970s and received much attention from public health leaders and writers, culminating in the concerns expressed in the IOM Report of 1988. And well it should have, for it reflected some of the most important social and technical trends affecting the changing relationships between the newly evolving threats to the population's health and the states' organizational responses to the challenge.

As the quotation from the Public Health Service survey cited above implies, the states had already widely distributed their health functions among their operating departments by 1950 or earlier. The causes for this development reflect historical trends in politics, societal organization, and publicly held perceptions of governmental operations. Principal among those that played a part in determining (and that continue to influence) the departmental placement were:

1. The perception of the licensing and inspection function as primarily a police or general control function, even when health facilities and personnel are involved.
2. The perception that many direct curative health services run by governments are a charity for citizens who are at least medically indigent, rather than instruments for meeting a claimed right to a public service.
3. The fact that the introduction of many control functions antedated the 1870–1913 period during which permanent state boards and departments of health were established, so that these control functions were vested, by long-established tradition, in a special commission or board.

After 1950

TYPES OF CRITICISMS OF SHAS AND THEIR UNDERLYING IDEOLOGIES. The preceding three points have appeared in health service literature, but useful as they are in explaining the dispersal of health functions among state agencies already existing in the pre-1950 period, they do not adequately explain the accelerated growth of the practice of assigning *new* state health programs to agencies other than the health department in the years after 1960. The content of many of these new programs was such that they might reasonably have been expected to be assigned to the state health agency, and bypassing it in favor of other state government entities had a demoralizing effect on "the thoughtful public administrator since World War II," as Dr. Knutson, the incoming president of the APHA, noted in

1957. In addition to the portions of that address quoted in Chapter 2 he also remarked that

As he reviewed the new or growing public health problems, moreover, the public health administrator has observed that, in many instances, the programs dealing with them were not administered by the health department. In state after state the agencies that constructed new nursing homes, or abated water pollution, or promoted mental health were not part of the health department. To be sure, legislators are understandably inclined to create new agencies if only to make plain their high regard for the clientele of the new agency—crippled children, let us say, the handicapped, or perhaps the older people. But the legislators were not wholly responsible for the splintering of health functions and health responsibilities among a variety of agencies in state after state.

Too often a separate new agency, or commission, or authority was established when the legislators got the impression that the health department did not share their concern with a specific problem. On the other hand, advances in medicine and changed public attitudes have added medical components to programs located outside the health department. Examples of this are the expansion of medical rehabilitation activities in a program originally concerned primarily with vocational retraining, and the extension and broadening of the health component of the public assistance program.

In the face of this dispersion of health functions among a number of agencies, what then is the responsibility of the primary health agency? What are its obligations toward other agencies that have been given health functions to perform? *Again, and yet again, where are we going in public health?* [Emphasis added.]

More generally, the tendency to bypass the state health agency has been said to reflect dissatisfaction with the failures of state public health agencies to provide adequate protection against the newer types of environmental health hazards; to improve the delivery of medical care, primarily in the inner cities where access to care had sharply declined, but to also increase the availability of medical care for others who needed it; to help moderate the rising cost of medical care; and to bring some planned rationality to the wasteful chaos of the existing health services system.

The purported program failures have been variously ascribed to four main organizational deficiencies: an insufficiently adversarial pos-

Table 3–8. Schematic Presentation of the Types of Public Perceptions of SHA's Main Deficiency, the Ideological Basis of these Perceptions, and the Interest Groups Forming the Constituencies of the Perceptions

Organizational feature of SHA perceived as its main deficiency	Ideological basis for perception of main deficiency	Main interest groups forming the constituencies of the perceptions and ideologies
1. Insufficiently adversarial stance toward polluters (environment)	Aggressive confrontation of polluters leading to effective curbing of polluting practices is the most important criterion of agency operation	Environmental activists, technicians, others strongly interested in environmental issues, and some regulated large businesses
2. Management inefficiency (efficiency)	Managerial and economic efficiency is most important criterion of agency operations	Business and nonprofit organizations regulated by a program; many administrators, analysts, and planners working for a specialized regulatory agency
3. Technical inadequancy (effectiveness)	Effective outcomes constitute most important criterion of agency operation; advanced technology and skilled professionalism are the keystones to societal improvement	Professionals, technologists that are regulated by a program; many technicians working for specialized regulatory agencies
4. Lack of "holistic" approach to improving health; insensitivity to human needs (humanitarianism)	A recognition in practice of the multidimensional aspects of improivng health is the most important criterion of agency operation	Clients, their advocates, and professionals in social programs

ture toward organizations and individuals whose business activities damage the public's health, management inefficiency, technical inadequacy, and insensitivity to the "holistic" nature of human needs. For convenient reference we may label these concerns as *environment, efficiency, effectiveness,* and *humanitarianism* (see Table 3–8).

These four indictments originate in different systems of values with clashing priorities and are voiced by correspondingly different constituencies that are for the most part mutually antagonistic. The first criticism, asserting a lack of vigorous adversarialism, comes primarily from environmentalists who claim that the health departments are too much under the thumb of polluters, developers, and landlords who predict and sometimes threaten dire economic consequences to the community if "extremist" control measures are enforced. The efficiency criticism is typically rooted in a managerial and business ethic, while the effectiveness criticism is primarily voiced by those who see advanced technology and skilled professionalism as the keystones to society's improvement, including its health status. The insensitivity to human

needs complaint comes from social welfare protagonists who often claim that public health professionals are too one-sidedly concerned with the biomedical aspects of health threats and fail to appreciate the psychosocial determinants of ill health. Included in this criticism is an allegation that public health officials pay insufficient attention to personal health-enhancing behavior as a form of prevention. For the state health department as an institution to be accused of simultaneously having all these very different types of failings virtually guaranteed that it would have powerful detractors among all segments of the political spectrum and in many sectors of American life—government, business, consumer, environmental, social welfare activists, and professional and intellectual circles. Furthermore, this would be true whether the department's administration were under conservative or liberal leadership, although the primary source of opposition might vary with the current political situation.

Those for whom the most important criticism was the regulatory leniency of the health department toward polluters favored assigning the environmental control function to a specialized environmental control agency staffed mainly by experts in water quality, air quality, and the like. Persons who primarily blamed putative managerial inefficiency or professional technical inadequacy for the health departments' program failures were likely to press for various management and control functions being assigned to state agencies primarily staffed by practitioners or by general business-trained and -oriented managers or by scientific and technological professionals outside the health field. Those for whom the main criticism was a failure to respond to community needs in a humane and "people-oriented" manner generally pressed for assigning programs to departments of "resources development," human resources, or welfare.

The designation of a state agency to administer a health-related program could be a matter of state politics alone or could depend also on limitations written into federal law. If it was to be an agency essentially limited to intrastate functions, choices would likely be mainly decided in the state political arena. If it was to be a state conduit between a federal grant program and local health departments, and especially if it was to be the lead state agency for the federal program, both the federal and state political arenas were likely to see action in the course of the agency selection process. In the federal sphere, advocates of using the SHA may succeed in framing the law and regulations to provide that the single state agency in each state *shall* be the state health department, as they did in the original Hospital Construction and Survey Act (Hill-Burton) of 1946. Under this model the decision is made for the state by the provisions in the federal law, and obviously state politics does not enter into the choosing of the agency. But later federal legislation used another model specifying only that the state (governor or legislature) must choose *a* single agency, as in the case of the health planning acts. In that event political influences may enter at the federal level to frame the legislation in this optional model and then may subsequently also enter within any of the states to influence the actual choice of the agency. And a third model was used in at least one case, the Community Mental Health Center Construction and Retardation Act of 1963 (see Chapter 6), where the federal legislation point-

edly *prohibited* a particular type of state agency (the one that administers the state mental hospital), from being chosen to administer the new act in the state. This provision reflected a national political struggle between two camps of mental health advocates.

The choice of a single state agency to lead the administration of a national public health program within the state can thus be a deeply political process with the outcome reflecting the values and their advocates that are at work influencing state and federal policy development, including the required molding of public opinion. While much of the rhetoric is couched in purely logical argument that places blame on the state health department for being technically inadequate, managerially inefficient, or ineffective in implementing policy, and therefore inadequate to perform the tasks required by the proposed new program, actually there is evidence that various interest groups or constituencies seek the designation of another agency because they think it will enhance their leverage in influencing public policy development. Interest groups and constituencies like to have their "own" agencies. In the public health field the most important of these interest groups are of four broad kinds: the environmental conservationists, the business or professional organizations to be regulated by proposed programs, the representatives of and other advocates for clients of social programs, and the professional health planners, managers, and health systems experts (see Table 3–8).

INTEREST GROUPS AND CONSTITUENCIES AND THEIR CRITICISMS

Environmental conservationists. There is convincing evidence that the environmentalist constituency has favored the formation of special agencies. In this case, contributing strongly to the desire of the advocacy groups to have specialized agencies was an expressed perception that state health departments have too limited a view of their scope of function. The environmentalists wish to protect natural resources for the sake of the environment itself and not wait until direct threats to the public health become evident. In fact, the conservation of resources like wilderness areas is valued by environmental activists even if their alteration might not measurably affect the public's health.

The strongest elements of the environmentalist constituency are the voluntary environmental organizations like the Sierra Club and the more recently founded Conservation Foundation. One cannot say to what degree the resulting situation has been due to the influence of organized environmentalists, but Barry Rabe, whose study of state environmental management (1987) was previously cited in connection with local health departments, found that in 1983 only fifteen states used the "health departmental model" to manage their environmental protection activities. In nineteen states their function was given to an "environmental superagency" (one that operates air, water, and solid waste control programs and at least one conservation and development program) and in twelve states the "little EPA" model (a state agency approximately resembling the federal EPA) was used.

The environmentalists have also felt that the special environmental agency would be more adversarial in its relationships with polluters than the health agency could be (Rabe 1986, 1987), a perception that was largely based on the sharply more adversarial stance *enunciated* by such agencies toward polluters than by public health departments. But litigation by accused polluters and other factors have combined to produce an unclear record (Rabe, 1987). While a few states, all with specialized agencies (Rabe studied three), had developed a more "innovative" approach to pollution control, and no states with health department models did so, the actual outcomes were not impressive. The "revolving door" type of reasons discussed below very likely contributed to a cooperative rather than a true adversarial relation, but the research is not yet available on this question.

It is well to remember that state agencies are also constrained by economic considerations similar to those that produce the relative helplessness of local health departments in taking meaningful action against large corporate polluters noted in Chapter 2 (p. 93). Controlling the newer environmental threats means confronting industrial giants whose ability to influence state governments is very strong. It entails facing automobile, petrochemical, energy, trucking, and air transport industries. What is of interest here is the expectation that is said to have come to the fore in the 1960s and peaked in the 1970s,

that specialized environmental protection agencies would be more likely to be successful in curbing pollution than state (or, of course, local) health departments.

In fact, the primary thrust of the move to transfer the responsibility for the state government's environmental protection function from its health agency to a specialized agency has been regulatory relief. The concentration of these new agencies has been on simplifying the regulatory process for potential polluters.

Many states were determined in the late 1970s and early 1980s to make life easier for environmentally regulated constituencies. They devised a number of strategies to relieve the perceived excesses and burdens of the regulatory process. These were intended more to foster greater administrative efficiency and political acceptability than to provide superior protection or public health. Although these strategies did not necessarily weaken regulatory requirements, they did shift emphasis away from the substantive impact of regulatory programs and the consideration of integrated environmental management (Rabe, 1986, 44).

Thus, if future research and experience support Rabe's findings, it would seem that the preference of the regulated corporation for the special agency was based on a truer estimation of its self-interest than the environmentalists' preference for such agencies was of theirs.

It is interesting to note that the Institute of Medicine's report *The Future of Public Health* recommends that the states "bear the primary public sector responsibility for health" and that among its duties is the "assurance of appropriate organized statewide effort to develop personal, educational, and environmental health services . . ." (1988). The "appropriate organized statewide effort" is not designated, but one of the recommendations states:

The committee recommends that state and local health agencies strengthen their capacities for identification, understanding, and control of environmental problems as health hazards. The agencies cannot simply be advocates for the health aspects of environmental issues, but must have direct operational involvement (1988).

Regulated organizations. The politics of the second type of interest group, the one that is to be regulated by a proposed program, also calls for a separate agency. The members of this group fall into two subclasses: the professional practitioner organizations (e.g., the American Medical Association, the American Bar Association), and the regulated businesses. In the first subclass, perhaps the oldest and clearest examples in the health field are the state medical licensing boards, which nearly everywhere have been a more or less direct extension of the medical societies; and the hospital licensing bodies, which have been closely allied with the hospital associations. This source of pressure for health functions to be in separate agencies that are more easily controlled by the regulated group is of long standing, often largely because it predates establishment of state health departments and is primarily a byproduct of the growth of professionalism and its development of "old boy" networks.

The second subclass of regulated organizations driving this trend for "other agency" designation, especially since about 1950, includes the complex of powerful industrial, commercial, and financial enterprises that is involved in generating the "newer" and potentially more catastrophic environmental health threats attributable to the rapid growth and development of large-scale industry without sufficient attention to public health safeguards. The pressure for having a regulatory agency other than the state health department has been particularly insistent from this interest group. Many reasons for this strong preference have been advanced. For example, there is the question of better rapport between the personnel of the regulator and the regulated. The state regulatory agencies other than the SHAs have been more heavily staffed with engineers, accountants, economists, lawyers, and other personnel more typical of nonhealth regulating agencies, as well as chemists and statisticians who are specialists in environmental matters. The regulated large industries would be more likely to establish a better rapport with this type of regulatory agency than with one run by health-trained persons who look at health threats allegedly without due regard to the economic benefits brought by the processes that produce pollution as a side effect. This better rapport includes "revolving door" arrangements among the technical personnel of the regulators and the regulated described by numerous observers.[22]

When one hears it frequently reiterated that the reasons for choosing a department other than the state's principal health agency as the lead agency in a health protection program are the health agency's lack of technique or expertise in the field, or its lack of efficiency in its own internal management, two questions spring readily to mind. One is whether these generalizations may mostly be a rationale used to obscure large corporations' preferences for an agency that is more focused on the narrower technical aspects of environmental analysis, leading to fragmentation of regulatory efforts. Such an increased focus on technical considerations is often accompanied by a perceived greater appreciation on the part of regulating organizations for the economic benefits of processes that cause environmental deterioration. They might then be more inclined to look at side-effect damage as just another cost to be factored into the benefit/cost calculation and less likely to be "fanatical" about health threats, especially those that are forecast to emerge years after exposure.

The second question is to what degree specialists in various technological fields are led to prefer the specialized nonhealth agency because it brings them greater earnings and prestige than working for a general health agency.[23] Revolving-door policies are more easily implemented in the more technologically staffed nonhealth agencies and thereby tend to raise the earning levels of personnel in the specialized agencies over those prevailing in the state's principal health agency. This can be done directly by the revolving-door practice of offering stints of service in the regulated private corporation for employees of the regulating agency at higher than civil service salaries. It can also be done indirectly by forcing civil service scales to rise in non-SHA public agency because of the requirement for comparability with going "market" rates set by the regulated private industry for its own employees of similar training. The resulting greater financial rewards available in the "other" agency can then be expected to attract more qualified personnel, keep them longer, and contribute to making these agencies truly superior to health agencies in managerial and technical expertise.

Social program supporters. This group involves the beneficiaries of the program, their representatives, and their advocates. They strive to have a special agency whose fortunes, perhaps even whose very existence, will depend on expansion of benefits or greater attention paid to their interests. Such behavior has been well documented in empirical studies and is a widely accepted tenet of political science theory (Alford, 1975; Edelman, 1964). Examples at the national level include the symbiotic relationships between the veterans organizations, the Veterans Administration, and the congressional committees with whom they work; and those between farm organizations, the Department of Agriculture, and again, the congressional committees with whom they work. A particularly good example in the health field is the mental health lobby, which has been strong nationally and in many states, having been instrumental in getting the 1963 Mental Health Act passed (Connery, 1965) and in obtaining legislation aimed at changing the focus of mental health care from state mental hospitals to community mental health centers (see Gruenberg and Archer, 1979, and Chapter 6). There has also been a long history of such activities by children's advocates (getting MCH Title V funds to be administered by the Children's Bureau instead of the Public Health Service—see Chapter 2), welfare client organizations, and others. Many of them have distrusted public health officials, deeming them too wedded to "the medical model" instead of total personalized care and integration of clients into society. An extreme example is the psychiatrist Thomas Szasz, who thinks that public health officials are jailers and liberal witch hunters (1970). Most of the social program supporters, except possibly Dr. Szasz, prefer to have their programs located in specialized agencies such as mental health and a children's bureau.

Health planners and health systems experts. Many of the professional health planners in the period 1966–1980 were on the technical staffs of local and state health planning agencies, funded and supervised with major federal participation, under the provisions of the national health planning acts. Their experience with areawide, population-based health planning had been largely within the structure of these national acts, which concentrated on developing local areawide health planning agencies that almost everywhere were totally independent of the local health department. It was natural for many of them to prefer that there be a state specialized health planning agency staffed with persons like themselves, technical health planners. Technical health planning literature and practice in this period had been moving toward seeking solutions to the problems of health delivery in increased applications of generalized ("generic") managerial, model-making, and computing technology, which were generally subsumed under such terms as "cost benefit analysis" and "systems analysis."

Review of the State Health Department as Intermediary Between Local Public Health Agencies and the Federal Government

While there is insufficient research to warrant definitive statements about which factors were in truth the most influential in creating the trend toward choosing agencies other than the SHA as the single or lead agency for federal programs, the fact of the existence of the trend is undeniable. This will be discussed further in Chapter 4, but because it has been so important a component of the pattern of development of state health departments, and because the choice by a state of a lead agency for one of its health programs can affect the operation of the entire federal system, it is worth pausing to briefly review the evidence that corroborates its existence.

Most of the early federal acts appropriating grant money for public health (especially after the passage of the federal Social Security Act) *mandated* using the state's health department as the conduit and liaison between the federal government and local public health agencies. The original Titles V and VI of the 1935 Social Security Act, for example, required that the state health department be *the* agency for distributing monies granted under the provisions of these titles for use by local public health departments. Furthermore, the plan for the use of these funds and their distribution among local health departments was to be drawn up by the state health departments subject only to some general guidelines laid down by the Surgeon General of the United States Public Health Service. Eleven years later, when the Hill-Burton Act to aid hospital construction was passed in 1946, the state health department was again mandated as *the* single state agency to administer the distribution of the federal grant money within the states. Although not all of these early federal programs mandated use of the state health department as the state agency for every health grant distribution, the exceptions were special circumstances. The crippled children's services, grants, for example, consisted essentially of specialized, and often expensive, medical services and were therefore perceived as not constituting "public health" services. The state authority for crippled children's grants was, therefore, usually vested in agencies of the state such as departments of hospitals, welfare, or vocational rehabilitation. In general, however, use of the state health department was *mandated* by the early post-1935 legislation.

Beginning with the 1950s, federal legislation increasingly *permitted* the state health department to be bypassed in designating the state agency responsible for administering the distribution of federal funds to localities for health activities. Many states picked up their option and did not choose the state health department.

We recall, for example, that under the Environmental Protection Act, only nineteen of fifty-four SHAs having environmental health programs had been designated the "lead agency" for their state in 1978. Only seventeen SHAs operated air quality monitoring stations in that year; only nine SHAs had responsibility for controlling motor vehicle emissions; and only twenty-two were responsible for control of noise pollution. Under the Medicaid Act only nine SHAs were the designated state agencies for administering the program[24] although the SHAs had considerable experience with administering medical care for the poor. In 1978, for example, nearly all SHAs had programs of inpatient care (mostly chronic) that were either directly provided or paid for under contracts with providers, and some SHAs had programs of general ambulatory care. The amount of $800 million was spent by SHAs for inpatient care, of which 83 percent went to SHA-operated institutions, i.e., on direct provision of care.

Also by 1971–72, six states (Florida, Louisiana, Mississippi, New Jersey, North Carolina, and Pennsylvania) were using state agencies other than health departments to administer hospital and medical facilities construction programs (HEW, 1972), the original Hill-Burton proviso mandating choice of the SHA having been repealed by that time. Under the provisions of the 1974 Planning Act we recall that only thirty-six states had by 1978 designated the state health agency as their SHPDAS, the remaining twenty-one designating other agencies. Other examples could be cited, but these are among the main ones supporting the assertion that the bypassing of the state health department as chief administrator and federal-local liaison for new statewide health programs since 1950 is a fact, whatever one chooses to believe about its causes.

The bypassing has been particularly pointed in the case of health planning, because for many years a substantial body of opinion in the public health profession had advocated that areawide and state health planning be a function, perhaps *the* basic function[25] of state and local health departments. The portions of Dr. Knutson's APHA presidential address cited on pages 41 and 69 deal with the difficulties presented to public health department leadership stemming from lack of clear role definition. In the same address he also came to this conclusion:

The one role that public health officials are uniquely qualified to fill is that of maintaining a *total view of the varied health activities conducted in their jurisdictions* by all groups, public and private. They are especially fitted to maintain a broad professional interest in and concern for the public health as a totality. Certainly, public health practice includes the care of crippled children, the operation of mental hospitals, and the abatement of polluted air and water. Although these functions may be assigned to others, that does not mean that the primary public health agency should not maintain an active interest in and concern for them. Indeed, public health leaders should take the initiative in establishing working relationships with all programs having a health component. Only in this way can they determine their relationship to each other and to the needs of the community. [Emphasis added.]

In other words, health planning was the irreducible sine qua non of state health department functions. Yet, as I have noted, the Comprehensive Health Planning Act of 1966 specified only that *a* single state agency in each state be designated to administer federal grants to that state and a substantial number of states (twenty-three as of 1971–72) (USPHS, 1972) did not, in fact, choose to place this function in their health departments. Most of these other agencies were general program planning agencies, which are generally staffed by management technicians; and some of them were welfare or "human resources" agencies. With the advent of federally supported independent planning agencies at the local and often at the state level, the role of public health agencies in health planning became ambiguous. The 1968 APHA position statement on the role of state health departments (described on page 59, point 1) stressed this function, but with the compromise proviso that the health department's planning activities should "relate to the comprehensive health plan of the State," as opposed to flatly asserting that the state health department should draw up the plan and be *the* planning agency. But when this compromise was passed it was already two years after passage of the Comprehensive Health Planning Act of 1966, and many states had already chosen an agency other than the state health department as the principal state health planning agency under the act. The position apparently merely reflected a fact of life, for we recall that ten years later in 1978 some fifteen of the state health agencies that had not been designated as the SHPDAs were in fact providing planning services for the SHPDA.

Thus, although the 1968 APHA statement asserted that "The State's obligation to maintain a wholesome living environment devolves largely upon the State health department," the transformation of this professionally enunciated policy to de facto status was frustrated.

SUMMARY AND COMMENTS

The trend toward using specialized state agencies, largely staffed with specialized program personnel, rather than the principal state health agency to lead health programs has been gaining momentum since about 1950. Public health leadership has decried this trend, but it obviously has had wide support in the councils of political power, as its continuing implementation has demonstrated. The public policy question is whether this trend is a good direction for the nation to take—a continuation of the older

question about the role and functions appropriate for state public health departments. It reflects the fundamental public health problem of balancing the benefits of the increased productivity resulting from entrepreneurial activities against the adverse side effects of rapid development on social and physical environments.[26] Because the effects consist in large measure of threats to the public's health, an important way of evaluating whether and to what degree advances in production or commerce are or may be deleterious to mankind is measuring their actual and estimating their potential effects on health. If these are judged to be sufficiently serious to warrant giving their abatement a high priority, then this, it seems to me, is the main justification for the public health position that health services planning, regulation, and monitoring be assigned to the health agency.

It is, of course, seldom wise to make inviolate rules in such matters, but in general, assigning to narrowly specialized agencies the planning, regulation, and monitoring of programs that deal fundamentally with questions of the public health does tend to direct the focus toward the technical problems of measurement of environmental phenomena and control of industrial processes and away from the monitoring of the health effects themselves. There is evidence that this has been happening. For example, the very concentration and decision-making dominance of specialized technicians in specialized agencies has been one of the barriers to achieving cross-media integration in the important area of environmental protection. A principal aim of governmental reorganization to enhance environmental protection has been to improve the coordination of efforts to control the effects of designated toxic materials found in various media: water, air, solid wastes, and biota. But the work in specialized agencies tends to cluster around the media themselves: clean water, clean air, cleanup of toxic dumps. The pollutants, however, are more or less readily transmitted from one medium to another, and the formation of consolidated environmental agencies that was to have facilitated programmatic coordination has not materially done so (Rabe, 1986). In light of this situation, assumptions about the increased effectiveness of the specialized environmental agency over the better integrated and health-focused health department must be seen as at least questionable.

There scarcely seems to be any serious question, however, that if the state health agency is to recoup the leading position it once had—and indeed, to improve it from the modest role it played even at its peak—public health leadership and training will have to meet the valid criticisms of its shortcomings. The primary support for such a renewal will of course have to come from an awakened public appreciation of the importance of these agencies that will affect the "councils of political power." But it will also be incumbent upon the public health leadership to show the way by igniting public interest and leading the public's education. If the trend toward specialized agencies continues, two things are likely to happen. An unduly large share of the national resources put into environmental control will go into increased technology development and managerial improvement while a comparatively small amount will be allocated for inducing more environmentally conscious behavior and monitoring actual changes in health status and their environmental etiology. Similarly, an unduly large proportion of resources allocated for medical care for the poor is likely to be consumed in controlling (usually meaning reducing) eligibility and utilization compared with measuring health status and need for appropriate health services.

Public health professionals have taken increasingly stronger positions in favor of a state's total health service system being coordinated by and under the surveillance of its principal health agency, asserting that the assurance of a healthful environment is a state health department function, and favoring expansion of scope of authority and interest by that agency. But positions taken at conventions (privately enunciated policy) are not the same as actions taken by federal and state governments and their health departments (de facto public policy). The actual implementation of these advanced positions has been weak in the face of the state and federal governments' increasing tendency to assign authority over new (especially newer *type*) health programs to agencies other than the state health agency.

While this trend has largely been a response to the pressure of special constituencies accompanied by widespread apathy and lack of knowledge of public health issues on the part of the general public, other developments have also affected the move toward choice of specialized agencies to coordinate specified public health programs in many states. These had to do with the formation of specialized agencies within the federal government to carry out national public health programs (e.g., EPA, OSHA) and the models they provided for state agencies. The federal administrative organization of these programs often required using a lead agency within each cooperating state, and as has been noted, these were more often than not agencies other than the SHA. Perhaps it was only to be expected that the state lead agency would be organized in the image of its mother federal agency, but the reasons that have been discussed above for choosing the specialized agency—the influence of special interests and constituencies—continue to hold. In fact, they are also part of the explanation of why the *federal* agency was often set up as a relatively autonomous entity rather than as a part of the United States Public Health Service.

It is clear that from 1950 on, developments in the evolution of the scope of function of the state health department have been ever more inextricably intertwined with developments in federal legislation. With many of the health threats in the United States being increasingly viewed as at least nationwide in impact, their abatement was increasingly perceived as needing to be national in scope. Appropriations for newer health programs have at least since 1965 or so increasingly tilted toward a greater role for federal policy leadership in a reconfigured federal public health system. The relationships among the federal, state, and local health agencies has been changing under this reconfiguration. In particular, the state health department's role as a conduit for transmitting federal money to local public health departments and monitoring its use has been changing rapidly. Overall these changes have promoted the use of non-SHA agencies as lead agencies. And the Reagan administration's policy of attempting to transfer control and financing of government-sponsored personal services health programs to the states resulted in some cases in sharply cutting back government roles in health overall and in others in increasing the *relative* importance of the role of the state in the federal system. Treating these issues adequately requires turning next to a more detailed consideration of the role of the federal government in public health.

NOTES

1. Even today, the state health department carries on the functions of local public health work entirely without any local government public health departments in some states. These exceptional cases are discussed later in this chapter.

2. This date cannot be regarded as that of the first *permanent* state organization, for after the immediate problem abated in the port of New Orleans, the board lay quiescent for over forty years.

3. Although this chapter is titled "The State *Health* Department" rather than the "State *Board* of Health," the discussion of the origins of state public health agencies generally is in terms of the founding of boards of health. Most historical accounts I have consulted refer to the early formation of boards rather than departments and at the state level in the earlier years (1870–1915) it seems safe to presume that the health department, even if it consisted only of a very few full-time officials, became its administrative arm. In the last twenty-five years or so there has been a marked increase in the numbers of state health departments that operate without accompanying boards of health. This development has been regarded with concern by leading public health figures and is deplored in the IOM report of 1988.

4. See, for example, the APHA policy statements discussed in Chapter 2 and summarized in Table 2-4.

5. At the time of Mountin's report, nearly all the states were actually heavily involved in "mental hygiene," in the form of maintaining large censuses in state mental hospitals. The administration of these functions was generally lodged in state hospital departments or special departments of mental hospitals rather than in public health departments. The separation of mental health from "public health" functions still obtains, by and large. The seven states designated in the Mountin report are those in which the state public health department listed this as a function. As late as 1988, the IOM's *Future of Public Health* found that "the relationship between public health and mental health remains undeveloped [and] . . . the committee recommends that those engaged in knowledge development and policy planning in public health and in mental health, respectively, devote specific effort to strengthening linkages with the other field . . ." (IOM, 1988).

6. This is not a complete list; only the sixteen most frequently performed functions are shown here.

7. Other programs that were very infrequently encountered, such as "professional registration and licensure," appearing as state public health department functions in only three states, represent the type of program generally administered by a special licensing body of the state.

8. Now called the Public Health Foundation (PHF).

9. Not all SHAs are independent public health departments. As has been noted, many of them are parts of agencies encompassing more than the public health function. The SHA is the governmental unit, whatever it is called and wherever it is placed in the state government's organization plan, that performs the functions of a state *public health* department. The use of the generic term SHA instead of "state public health department" is analogous to the use of public health "units" in place of local public health departments described on page 29. It reflects similar developments in both cases, mainly the trend to merging public social and health services departments, but also the growing practice of having an overarching state department of health services of which a public health division is a part.

10. At this writing, annual data collected by the Public Health Foundation is available through 1990. The IOM report (1988) used PHF data mostly for the year 1984 (in its Appendix A). For the discussion of this section I use primarily the PHF data for 1978 because I find them and the accompanying analysis to have been in greater depth than those of later years. The trends drawn from the 1978 PHF annual data certainly apply to 1980, the closing year of the period covered by this book, but these trends have by and large continued into later years also. Of course, the influence of the budget cuts and grant blocking of the Reagan years are not shown. I refer to these briefly whenever I can in this chapter, but they are most fully discussed in Chapter 4.

11. The Census Bureau's reporting of state governments' finances gives $4.52 billion for state expenditures for 1978 for "health" (U.S. Bureau of the Census). This expenditure category excludes hospitals and other institutions so that the Census Bureau figure of $4.52 billion compares with the NPHPRS figure of $3.26 billion less $665 million for SHA-operated institutions, or $2.60 billion. While the discrepancy between $4.52 and $2.60 billion is undoubtedly due in some degree to various technical differences in the way the agencies reported similar items to the two data-collecting entities, the major difference most probably represents the underlying fact that the state is reporting its *total health expenditures* (excluding hospital operation) to the Census Bureau, including outlays for environmental and "general" health activities spent by state units other than the public health agency. On the other hand, the data given by the NPHPRS in Table 3-3 reports only the expenditures of the *State Health Agency*. The most

likely explanation of the substantial difference between the two figures is to take it as an indication of the degree to which many states have been using agencies other than their SHA for health functions, a phenomenon discussed later in this chapter as well as in Chapter 4.

12. The four functional areas (excluding SHA-operated institutions)—personal health, environmental health, health resources, and laboratory—are designated in the NPHPRS reports as program areas. Each contains a number of *programs* (or "program categories"), as shown in Table 3-2. A "program" is defined by NPHPRS as "a set of identifiable services organized to solve health-related problems or to meet specific health or health-related needs, provided to or on behalf of the public, by or under the direction of an organizational entity in a State Health Agency, and for which reasonably accurate estimates of expenditures can be made."

13. Total public health expenditures by state *and* local public health agencies in the United States in 1978 were $5.0 billion (U.S. Dept. of HEW, 1979, table 73); state health agencies spent 65 percent of this amount.

14. This is not to say that the role of state government in health activities did not grow, for it did. Here we are talking about the role of the direct organizational descendants of the original state public health departments only. The significance of this difference is discussed later, but it is helpful to keep it in mind here.

15. Perhaps mental health would also remain in the SHA bailiwick, but this area has a unique history and special issues. They are discussed in Chapter 6.

16. As previously noted, the data for 1978 are taken from [Association of State and Territorial Health Officials (1980)]. Intermittent portions of the text are at times directly reproduced without further attribution.

17. See Chapter 4 for a discussion of this act.

18. The nineteen states in which the SHA was the lead environmental protection agency in 1978 were Alabama, Arizona, Colorado, Hawaii, Indiana, Kansas, Louisiana, Maryland, Montana, New Hampshire, New Mexico, North Dakota, Oklahoma, South Carolina, Tennessee, Texas, Utah, Virginia, and West Virginia.

19. It will be noted that a state-operated local public health agency may not strictly meet the NPHPRS definition of an LHD. Such a local agency may not be at all "responsible to a substate governmental entity," but in practice usually has to work with it.

20. Delaware, District of Columbia, Rhode Island, South Dakota, Vermont, American Samoa, Guam, Northern Marianas Islands, Trust Territory, and the Virgin Islands.

21. In the distribution of sources of funds that were financing LHDs for forty-four states estimated by NPHPRS, the local non-SHA sources (fees, reimbursements, and other, Table 3–6) are "grossly understated" in the opinion of the estimators. The most serious underestimation included some metropolitan areas like Chicago, Reno, Las Vegas, Nashville, Knoxville, Memphis, and Chattanooga, which provided no estimate of these local non-SHA-funded expenditures.

22. Havighurst's discussion of his research in regulation of the air transport industry (1973) is particularly worth noting as an example. The "revolving door" refers to the easy back and forth passage of administrative and technical personnel between the payroll of the regulating agency and that of the regulated industry. It has often been pointed out, for example, that this flow is particularly free between the Pentagon and its military contractors. It is not necessary that there be any conspiracy or collusion. It is simply that the technical personnel come from the same schools, read the same literature, and conjointly get to view almost every aspect of the interests of the industry as synonymous with the public interest.

23. Specialist technicians are also likely to support the special agency approach on the basis of perceived superior "management efficiency/technical adequacy" grounds.

24. These were called Medicaid Single State Agencies (MSSAs). The Medicaid program is discussed in Chapter 10.

25. Reiterated in the 1988 IOM study. It should be noted, however, that although many states did not choose the SHA as their state health planning agency under the federal planning act, neither did they place the health planning function in a state *health planning* agency. This is further discussed in Chapter 15.

26. There is, of course, also the problem of balancing the activities that individuals wish to engage in because they find them enjoyable or because they make life easier for themselves against the undesirable effects that these activities have on other individuals. Control of such activities had been achieved reasonably well by "standard" public health efforts. The very much greater severity of the problems of the last half century is what I am principally addressing here.

4

The Public Health Role of the Federal Government

The development of the federal government's role in local and state public health services is conveniently considered in five identifiable periods:

1. From the founding of the republic until 1935: the period of minimal federal involvement.
2. From 1936 through 1945: the early period of major federal financial support. This support was directed primarily toward expanding the outreach and improving the staffing of state and local public health departments through public health grants. While this involved program enrichment, the programs added or expanded as a result of increased funding were confined mainly to long-standing functions.
3. From 1946 through 1968: the period of changing emphases in goals and methods of federal financial support. The purpose of these changes was to encourage increased health activities by health departments and nonprofit private agencies in specific, newer target areas and types of functions favored by the federal government.
4. From 1969 through 1980: the "New Federalism" program of the Nixon and Ford administrations and the relative quiescence of the Carter administration. This period was characterized by the reappearance of vigorous foreign trade competition, accelerating inflation, and their economic consequences, all of which had important repercussions on public health policy; a rising interest in environmental protection against the newer and larger-scale threats to health and safety as well as a renewed and growing public interest in personal health maintenance and disease prevention; attempts at retrenchment in government expenditures and early attempts by

Nixon and Ford to transfer control of government health programs from federal to state auspices and to combine federal appropriations for categorical programs into "block" grants; and the caution or indecision of the Carter administration in formulating definitive federal health policy.

5. After 1980, retrenchment and continuation of the major outlines of Nixon's "New Federalism" by the Reagan administration. The main features of this period that affected government public health policy were the continued sharpening of foreign business competition and American firms' stepped-up response to it, which included accelerating efforts to reduce health care costs; sharp cuts in federal taxes aimed at increasing business activity accompanied by a substantial relaxation of environmental protection regulation; a very large increase in military spending; and the enormous federal budget deficits that resulted from the combination of these policies and were a major factor contributing to the substantial reductions of federal expenditures for public health.

Although each of these periods will be separately considered in the discussion that follows, the major dividing points are the years 1935 and 1970. In 1935, the passage of the Social Security Act launched the United States government on a course leading toward the development of a social welfare state; and the year 1970 marks a fundamental change in the economy and accompanying politics of the United States that was to affect our public health and personal health care systems profoundly, reversing the direction of many policies followed during 1935–1970.

The fifth of these periods, the Reagan administration, will be treated only in passing here because it is not part of the main time period covered by this book.

THE NATIONAL GOVERNMENT'S ROLE IN STATE AND LOCAL PUBLIC HEALTH SERVICES: THE FEDERAL SYSTEM THROUGH 1935

Although public health services have been supervised or delivered by state and local public health departments, the pattern and nature of these services were in large part guided and to some degree determined by national government policy after 1935. Beginning slowly with Titles V and VI of the Social Security Act, federal grants-in-aid and the regulations accompanying them increasingly affected the direction of state and local policy so that by the end of World War II, federal policy direction had become dominant. The states supervised public health, set standards, and engaged only minimally in direct service delivery; localities delivered direct services; and the federal government helped meet much of the cost and set national policy. This made for an intricate federal system with intergovernmental relations among local, state, and national levels whose complexity lent itself to simplistic characterizations by critics and supporters alike. These characterizations often descended to the level of caricature during political campaigns. Critics, for example, often attributed the increasing role of the central government almost entirely to a relentless drive of faceless bureaucrats and megalomaniacal politicians for more power over the people. Supporters have often attributed the opposition to increasing centralization mainly to power-hungry forces within the states that were loath to give up control of their local fiefdoms. While there was some merit to both these assertions, they were far from the whole story. The relationships among federal, state and local governments with respect to public health policy formation and implementation were formed over time and reflected developments in the larger society. The purpose of much of the discussion that follows is to develop the background of events in the United States that foreshadowed and helped form the pattern of the rapid increase in federal involvement after 1935.

Although the role of the national government in the pre-1935 period was actually very small, it did influence subsequent relationships. Foremost among the pre-1935 factors that helped shape the post-1935 federal system were the provisions of the federal Constitution with respect to the relationship between the states and the national government. Article X of the Constitution states: "The powers not delegated to the United States by the Constitution [under Article I, Section VIII], nor prohibited by it to the States, are reserved to the States respectively, or to the people." Under this proviso the protection of the health of its people, as a general proposition, is implicitly reserved to the individual state under its police powers, since a health function per se is not explicitly assigned by the Constitution to Congress under the section that enumerates the explicit powers of Congress, as noted in Chapter 3. Nor was this power given to the president. Whenever Constitutional authorization was invoked to justify early federal action in public health matters that were not explicitly assigned to the federal government, one or both of two clauses of the Constitution were cited.

Under the first of these, Congress is given the power "to regulate commerce with foreign nations, and among the several States. . . ." This section was used to justify the earliest federal public health activities, which centered on control of communicable diseases at ports of entry, and somewhat later, included attempts to control communicable disease in interstate commerce. Under the second, Congress is empowered "to . . . provide for the . . . general welfare of the United States." This latter clause was the justification advanced by those who sought federal intervention in health problems in the interests of countrywide uniformity, equity, and efficiency (Grad, 1970).

Beginning in 1796, early federal legislation concentrated on attempting to control the introduction into the United States of communicable diseases such as malaria, yellow fever, and cholera. To this end, various laws were passed authorizing federal assistance for quarantine procedures at the major ports of entry. Because of the extreme sensitivity of the newly independent nation to the states' rights issue, the early laws, such as the act of 1796 relative to quarantine, merely *offered* federal cooperation to local and state quarantine authorities "in enforcing State and local quarantine relating to ships" (Mustard, 1945). This posture of offering assistance in enforcing state or local laws, rather than requiring compliance with federal laws, persisted in later work by the U.S. Public Health Service with states and localities with respect to communicable disease control. Until 1877 the quarantine function remained in the hands of state or local authorities with federal enforcement assistance available if requested by these authorities. The specific content of this assistance was limited to the use of federal power to prevent ships from entering ports where local quarantine authorities wanted them kept out. However, the number of serious epidemics, particularly of yellow fever and cholera, that ravaged different parts of the United States during the first seventy-five years of the 1800s kept public attention focused on this problem, and in 1878 the Marine Hospital Service, which had been established in 1798 to provide medical care for merchant seamen, was empowered to assist any state or community that *requested* its services by acting "as officers or agents of a *national quarantine system* [emphasis added]" (Mustard, 1945, 33).

From the time of its founding in 1872, the American Public Health Association had been urging the formation of a national department of health. In 1879 a National Board of Health with a four-year term of office was voted by Congress to "have charge of interstate and foreign quarantine," thereby repealing the power of quarantine granted to the Federal Marine Hospital Service only the year before. Serious dissension between the national board and various other public health bodies led to its becoming effectively defunct at the end of the mandated four years and to its abolition in 1893, with quarantine duties along with increased enforcement powers[1] restored to the Marine Hospital Service (Mustard, 1945, 54). A significant element of the dissension in public health officer circles was centered in the southern states, stemming from their opposition to the overriding of states' rights by empowerment of a federal agency; but it was also due to a difference of opinion over the relative merits of quarantine versus sanitation in controlling epidemics. It also became in part an organizational struggle between the National Board of Health members and their supporters and those in the Marine Hospital Service over which organization would be *the* national health agency.

Since the Marine Hospital Service had been doing quarantine at ports of entry when requested by local authorities, it was only to be expected that persons associated with that agency would favor it as the agency of choice for epidemic control. The National Board of Health, on the other hand, consisted primarily of people involved in local public health administration and the activities of the American Public Health Association. Their work experience and observation of conditions in the towns that were growing into cities led them to be more familiar with sanitation than with quarantine in seaports as means of controlling epidemics. Clearly the situation favored the selection of the Marine Hospital Service, which had already officially done port quarantine for one year and had for many years been operating out of medical facilities in all the major ports in connection with its duties of caring for sick merchant seamen. The National Board of Health people, on the other hand, because of their preference for sanitation over quarantine, could not have been enthuasiastic administrators in carrying out their charge to administer quarantine during the four years they were in office and empowered to do so.[2]

The 1893 restoration of the quarantine power to the Marine Hospital Service, augmented by the newly added legal sanction to *enforce* quarantine regulations without the necessity of obtaining local approval, was a significant step toward establishing a federal presence in health matters. Further, while states and localities could continue to pass their own quarantine laws, they now had to conform to federal law, and if state or local laws were nonexistent or inadequate, the United States government "might supersede them" (Mustard, 1945, 55). The 1893 act also empowered the federal government to purchase any existing local and state quarantine stations "if necessary to the United States." By 1921, the federal government had acquired ownership of and was operating all quarantine stations.

Congress also passed laws regulating interstate quarantine measures. These enforcement powers, too, were delegated to the National Board of Health in 1879, then to the Marine

Hospital Service in 1890 and were also strengthened in 1893. Thereafter, the public health aspects of the work of the Marine Hospital Service concerned itself with communicable disease control, both with respect to introduction of disease from abroad *and* its spread domestically among the states. As has been previously noted, it continued to use its domestic powers very cautiously, for the most part helping states with advice and personnel only when asked, despite the 1893 mandate to use enforcement.

Another aspect of the Marine Hospital Service's work in communicable disease control consisted of administering federal grants-in-aid to localities and lending personnel for demonstration projects in the various states, hoping thereby to encourage better local rural public health practice. But this was a relatively minor facet of its operations. Despite the change of name from the Marine Hospital Service to the United States Public Health and Marine Hospital Service in 1902, it was still concentrating mainly on medical care for seamen and other stipulated eligible persons, and on foreign quarantine. In 1912, however, its name was changed to the United States Public Health Service, and in 1913, when Congress started to appropriate funds for local demonstration and research in public health, a gradual broadening of perspective on the functions of the agency began. During the years 1914–1916 the service conducted a series of field studies in typhoid fever control with some sixteen states cooperating. These field investigations contained a large "demonstration" component, and from 1917 to 1934 annual amounts were appropriated by Congress for rural sanitation development by the U.S. Public Health Service Service. Mustard describes the importance of this development in these terms:

The work evolved from an undertaking concerned only with methods of control of typhoid fever to a demonstration of the effectiveness of reasonably adequate local rural health departments responsible for broad community health services . . . the effect of the program reached far beyond the local areas and even beyond the states in which the combined federal state-local activities were in progress (1945, 61).

These grants-in-aid required local fund matching to stimulate greater state and local appropriations for public health work and as an indicator of local interest in improving rural education.

Two other examples of federal stimulation of state and local public health work during the years 1915 through 1935 were grants for venereal disease control and for maternal and child hygiene. The impetus for the former program was the rapid increase in the incidence of venereal disease (now included in the term sexually transmitted diseases, STD[3]) in 1917 and the years immediately following, associated with the induction of large numbers of young men into the armed forces in World War I. Federal grants for venereal disease control began with the Chamberlain-Kahn Act of 1918, which allocated funds to the states according to population. Distribution of these grants was administered not by the U.S. Public Health Service alone, but by an interdepartmental Social Hygiene Board, and matching of federal funds by the states was required. The appropriations for this program eventually dwindled away, disappearing in 1926, but they left strengthened venereal disease control laws and programs in effect in many states.

Federal grants for maternal and child health began in 1921 with passage of the Sheppard-Towner Act. An interdepartmental federal Board of Maternity and Infant Hygiene was set up to help administer the act, but its powers were mostly advisory. Actual day-to-day administration of the act was assigned to the Children's Bureau, which had been established as part of the Department of Labor in 1912. The bureau had been conducting research and educational work on matters pertaining to the welfare of children and was a leading proponent of the 1921 legislation. Mustard (1945) wrote that "between 1922 and 1927 the Division of Maternal and Infant Hygiene carried on an aggressive and productive program." The act provided for allocation of the appropriated money among the states using a three-part formula that gave a constant sum outright to each state with no conditions attached, an additional constant sum to be matched by the state, and a third sum varying with the state's population. This last amount also required state matching. The program ended in 1929, following the discontinuance of federal funds.

The period up to 1935 saw the development

of public health both as a professional calling equipped to do effective battle against epidemic disease and as a government organizational form. As noted in Chapters 2 and 3, the public health scene by 1935 was one in which the organization of the delivery of services was principally local, with many of the large cities having impressive departments and boards. The states' public health agencies concentrated on standard setting, developing and monitoring of local services, and encouraging the formation of local departments in areas where none existed. They also provided local public health services directly via state "districts" in areas that needed the services but did not have a local department. The federal government, through an agency that became the United States Public Health Service in 1912, was performing quarantine services at the major ports and aiding some localities, in cooperation with the states, to improve their local sanitation services in rural areas. It also supervised interstate quarantine when asked to do so.

However, fundamental economic and social changes in United States society were creating strains on this arrangement. First, there was the inequality of tax resources among the states referred to in Chapters 2 and 3. If public health services were considered a public good, they could not be left to depend on the vagaries of state and local distribution of tax resources for their financing. To equalize the quality of these services across the nation, the use of federal tax collection according to ability to pay and the redistribution of tax revenues among the states according to public health need were advocated. It did not seem equitable for a child to be subjected to inadequately financed public health services merely because it was born in an economically undeveloped state, a state whose residents bought products largely manufactured by corporations headquartered in other states where they paid most of their local and state taxes. A second factor was that the responsibility for delivering local public health services (and many other social services like education) continued to rest with the states, which generally delegated them to the cities and localities. The main source of total tax collections in the United States, however, was moving from the local and state levels to the federal levels. While this trend did not become glaringly obvious until about 1945, the

growing disparity between service responsibility and available tax sources was already in evidence by the 1930s. It helped bring the question of the federal government returning some of its tax money to states and localities for local services increasingly to the fore as 1935 approached.

The federal aid provided by the demonstration grants for public health work was limited to rural public health, directed only to some of the states, and minimal in quantity. It was clearly insufficient to rectify the growing disparities. The Sheppard-Towner and Kahn-Chamberlain Acts had proved temporary. As part of the response to the upheaval created by the Great Depression of 1929, new legislation was passed giving the federal government more power to aid the states and localities. The most important of these laws, the Social Security Act of 1935, transformed the federal grants-in-aid for public health programs, increasing their size as well as altering and formalizing relationships among the three levels of government. Before turning to this legislation, it will be useful to consider some general questions relating to grants-in-aid and tax sharing among governmental units of different levels: local, state, and federal.

GRANTS-IN-AID AND TAX SHARING

Issues

An important aspect of the fiscal interrelationships among the three levels of American government with respect to the financing of health activities is the alignment of the service responsibilities of the respective levels with the tax revenues available to them. The disparity between the degree of responsibility for providing health services and the proportion of total tax revenues collected by the respective levels of government grew wider over time, reaching a peak between 1950 and 1960.

With the passing of time, local governmental responsibility for providing services[4] grew enormously while its share of the total taxes collected nationally by all governmental levels declined. Instead, the major portion of total taxes collected eventually went to the federal government, whose local service responsibilities were minimal compared with those of state and especially local governments. Furthermore, most of the national wealth and income was passing from being based on agriculture to being based on commerce and industry. Along with this transition, the center of gravity of the tax base shifted from rural real capital (agricultural land, buildings, livestock, and farm machinery) to urban-centered money income, money capital, industrial plant and machinery, and urban real estate capital. Taxes on money capital are not collected in the United States (unless one considers the special case of inheritance taxes), and taxes on money income are collected primarily by the federal government and secondarily, at a far lesser rate, by the state governments. Taxes on the value of real property have been local governments' principal source of tax revenue. As a consequence, although the proportion of the tax base available to the different governmental levels shifted in favor of the federal government, the responsibility for financing public health services (and other social services) continued to remain primarily with state and local governments. Many problems grew out of this "cultural lag."

In the early years of our nation's history, when the principal tax base was real estate and other real (mostly rural and semirural) property, and when probably over 90 percent[5] of the population was rural and semirural, residing on the land and making a living from it, it made sense for the local property tax to be the principal source of tax revenue nationally. Since the property tax was available to the states, and under state legislation and regulations to subdivisions of the states, the tax resources available to the states and their local subdivisions matched the larger share of the total governmental service and regulatory responsibilities that they held under the Constitution. And because property values were higher in more urbanized centers, local property taxes tended to be roughly proportionate to their greater needs for local services. But even in the towns and cities, such services were modest by modern standards. This was especially true before 1900 when the public health importance of good water and sewage systems was insufficiently recognized.

The federal government, on the other hand, was under the Constitution delegated relatively few functions—those involving principally the handling of foreign affairs, providing for national armed forces, and regulating commerce both with foreign governments and among the states. Except in time of war, these required modest resources in the early years. The conception of the Founding Fathers clearly seemed to be that the basic internal regulatory and administrative unit of government, as far as the individual citizen was concerned, was to be the individual state, with the federal government handling only those problems that involved all or at least several of the states. It was thus entirely appropriate that the federal government's revenues come mostly from various national excise taxes and tariffs. The main function of the tariffs was to protect the infant American industry, and the fact that they were also revenue producing was an added benefit—what economists call an "externality." And if the revenues yielded by these measures were modest, so were the funds needed by the national government to carry out the limited functions assigned to it by the Constitution.

As late as 1910, 54 percent of the population was still listed as rural and only 46 percent as urban. At some point between 1910 and 1920 the urban-rural balance in the population shifted from being predominantly rural to urban and remained so thereafter. By 1970, 73 percent of the population was urban (see Fig. 4–1). Concomitantly, and more importantly, the predominant way of making a living shifted from agriculture to nonagricultural pursuits during these same years. By 1980 the proportion of employed workers who worked on farms (including farm owners and family members) was only 3.4 percent, and the percentage of the population living on farms was only 3.2. This contrasts with 30.2 percent living on farms in 1920, 24.9 percent in 1930, and 8.7 percent only some thirty odd years ago in 1960 (U.S. Bureau of the Census, 1980, tables 103, 108, 634). (See Fig. 4–2.)

As the predominant basis of personal wealth and income, especially income, shifted markedly from ownership of real (especially agricultural) property and agricultural production to ownership of money capital and nonagricultural sources of income, the federal government sought to tap this rising money income source whenever it needed large amounts of tax revenue. During the Civil War, for example, Congress enacted its first income tax, which remained in effect from 1861 through 1871, with substantial collections during several of these

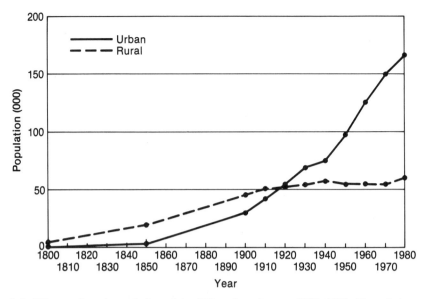

Fig. 4–1. Urban and rural population of the U.S., selected years, 1800–1980. *Note*: Only markers on lines represent actual data. *Source*: U.S. Bureau of the Census (1960, 1970).

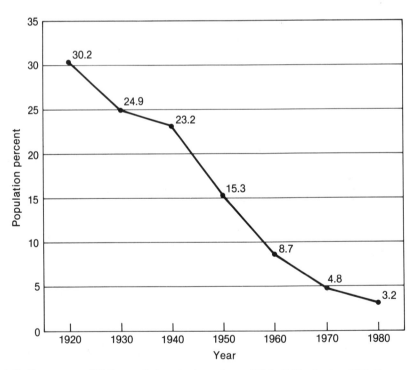

Fig. 4–2. Percentage of U.S. population that was farm, 1920–1980. *Source*: U.S. Bureau of the Census (1975; 1981, tables 703, 634, 118).

years; but this was seen as a temporary crisis situation. However, as more regulatory functions were assumed by the federal government after the Civil War to meet the requirements of an expanding American capitalism whose control centers were steadily amalgamating into ever larger units, and as military expenditures rose, the federal government's need for additional revenue grew and became permanent. Efforts were made to establish a national income tax as a permanent feature of our tax structure. An 1894 law reintroduced a federal income tax, but the law was struck down as unconstitutional by a five-to-four decision of the Supreme Court (*Pollock* vs. *Farmer's Loan and Trust Co.*). However, the Sixteenth Amendment to the Constitution, passed in 1913, explicitly permitted the federal government to levy an income tax, and thereafter it rapidly became the most important single source of tax revenue for the federal government and the main revenue generator of all the taxes levied in the United States. Income taxes accounted for 26 of the total 35 billion dollars (75 percent) of federal receipts by 1950, and 173 of 201 billion dollars (86 percent) in 1976. Customs revenues, which accounted for 84 percent of total revenue in 1800, 91 percent in 1850, and as much as 41 percent even as late

as 1900, had shrunk to an insignificant 1 percent by 1950.

The growing need of the federal government for additional tax revenues to support its expanding responsibilities was met from 1920 on by the newly sanctioned income tax, but the pressures for more services from state and local governments also multiplied as the nation's towns and cities grew. Yet the local source of tax revenue remained largely restricted to the real property tax base and did not keep up with expanding needs. Over time the percentage of total tax revenues collected by state and local governments fell compared with the percent collected by the federal government. In 1913, 71 percent was collected by the states and localities and 29 percent by the federal government. The federal percentage began to rise in 1940, and by 1950 the relative weights had been almost exactly reversed from the 1900–1940 pattern, with 69 percent of all taxes being collected by the federal government. Thus, by the time the country had reached the immediate post–World War II years, some 65 to 70 percent of total taxes was being collected by the federal government[6] (see Fig. 4–3).

The importance of the shift of the major tax base from real property to money income lay not

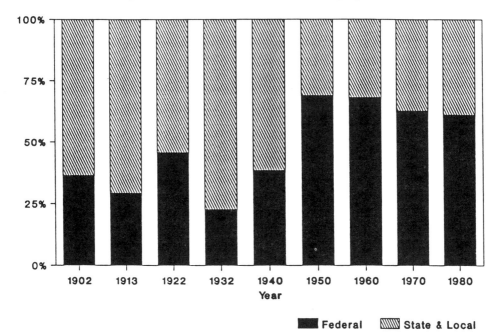

Fig. 4–3. Percentage distribution of total tax revenue by government level. *Source*: U.S. Bureau of the Census (1960; 1981, table 473).

only in the shifting of taxable resources from state and local to federal levels while responsibility for public health services remained largely state and local; the relative composition of the base of state and local tax revenues also became increasingly more money dependent. While the property tax was overwhelmingly the main tax revenue source through about 1935 and still provided more than 50 percent of total state and local tax revenues in 1940, by about 1950 and thereafter it yielded less than half of all state and local taxes. By 1980, 25 percent of all state and local tax revenues came from income taxes, 36 percent from sales taxes, and only 31 percent from property taxes (see Fig. 4–4). Thus, after about 1935, state and local tax revenues were becoming rapidly more dependent on taxable income and spending, and the geographical distribution of this money tax base was very uneven among the states and regions. Money income was concentrated in relatively few states. Those states containing industrial, "agri-business," commercial, and financial centers enjoyed high per capita incomes, while predominantly rural states with few or no centers of industry, com-

merce, and finance suffered from low per capita incomes. The available base for state and local taxation became ever more unevenly distributed, not only among states but also among localities within states. Furthermore, the need for health services from state and local government was often inversely related to the available tax base. Study after study of expenditures for public health services of the various states in the 1920s, 1930s, and 1940s revealed two important facts:

1. The amounts spent per capita were very uneven from state to state.
2. Often the states spending lower amounts per capita were making a greater proportional effort relative to their total tax base resources and income than were the more affluent states. Yet their per capita expenditures were deemed insufficient to provide minimally adequate public health services, often woefully so.[1]

Clearly, increasing local and state taxes could not equitably provide a nationally uniform level of public health services to match local needs because local taxable income was generally in-

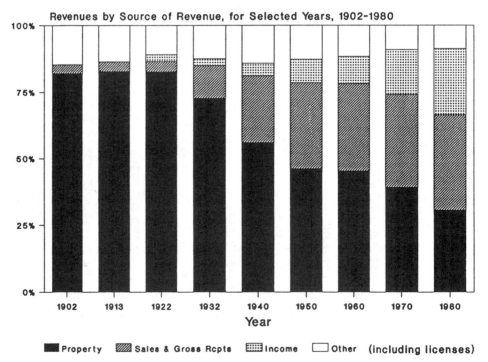

Fig. 4–4. Percentage distribution of state and local government revenues by source of revenue, for selected years, 1902–1980. *Source*: U.S. Bureau of the Census (1957, table 408; 1960; 1981, tables 468, 470, 473).

versely related to such needs, and despite the shifts in tax base to favor the federal level, the preponderant responsibilities of the states for providing public health and other social services were not correspondingly diminished. A solution to the problem boiled down to a choice between two alternatives or some combination of them. Either:

1. The responsibility for many health and other services could be directly transferred to the federal government by legislative, constitutional, or judicial action; or
2. The states could keep their responsibilities, but federal funds would be siphoned back from the federal treasury to the states to discharge these responsibilities.

The latter course was mainly followed, especially in the early years after 1935, but some shift of responsibility and control in the public health (and other) fields to the federal government also took place, corroborating the well-established maxim about control following the dollar.

Redistribution of Tax Revenues among the Different Levels of Government: Different Mechanisms and Their Implications

The redistribution of tax revenue among government levels is a process whereby a superior government, such as a state, collects taxes from persons living in its jurisdiction on one basis, such as ''ability to pay,'' and redistributes the proceeds on the basis of average community-wide need among units of lower levels of government, such as counties or cities. The allocative basis for distribution among these lower governmental units might be not only some measure of average need in a county or a city but also of compliance with the goals of the state in some respect. In the United States, redistribution of tax revenues takes place directly between the federal government and the states, between the states and localities, and between the federal government and localities. Federal tax revenue is also indirectly redistributed from the federal government to localities using the state government as intermediary.

Historically, two principal methods were used for sharing tax revenues between a superior gov-ernmental unit and its subdivisions: tax sharing[8] and grants-in-aid. The discussion here focuses almost entirely on federal grants-in-aid and considers only grant-in-aid plans in which the monies are all collected by the federal government from individuals across the nation under the general taxing power of the United States;[9] a portion of the revenues are returned by the federal government to the states or localities; and the amount redistributed as well as its method of allocation among states and localities is set by the terms of Congressional appropriation acts. Three major purposes of such grants-in-aid have been identified:

1. To assure the availability of sufficient funds to the lower government for carrying out, on at least minimally acceptable levels, specified health programs that it is federal policy to further.
2. To help restore the balance between Constitutionally delegated service responsibilities on the one hand and available tax resources on the other.
3. To equalize relative tax burdens among states and localities; that is, to enable state and local governments to achieve a uniform, minimally adequate level of health service with the same relative tax effort as measured by a ratio of tax rates to an indicator of ability to pay.
4. To stimulate state and local financial participation in programs deemed desirable by the federal government.

A number of methods have been used to allocate federal money among states and localities. These methods fall under two broad classifications, the formula grant and the project grant.

Formula Grants

Under this scheme, grants are distributed among lower levels of government, such as states,[10] according to a formula established by law. The bases for distribution among the states have been equal allocation, variable allocation, or a combination of the two.

1. *Equal allocation:* The same fixed amount is allocated to each state. This procedure has been used rather infrequently. When it was

utilized, it was generally only part of a larger overall formula that also included criteria for variable allocation of a portion of the appropriation among the states. The purpose of the same across-the-board grant was to guarantee that no state wound up with almost no money because of the way the formula for variable distribution might work out. The grants for maternal and child care provided by the Sheppard-Towner Act of 1921, for example, provided that each state receive a fixed $5,000 outright. Other parts of the formula provided additional variable amounts for each state, based on certain population characteristics within the state that indicated the degree of need for maternal and child health services.

2. *Variable allocation:* Under this method certain "need" characteristics of each state determine the percentage of the total national appropriation it receives. This type of grant allocation was the most common one for health purposes until about 1965 and continued to be widely used thereafter. It permits the appropriation to be distributed in a manner that helps equalize service availability and tax burdens throughout the nation. The most frequently used variables that enter into this type of allocation formula are the size of the program's target population, per capita income or other measures of financial need, and the severity of the existing problem of interest in the particular state, all indicating the degree of need for the program and the state's ability to pay for it. The "severity of the problem" variable was sometimes quantified by an indicator measuring the prevalence of a certain health condition, rather than the "size of the target population" criterion.

In addition to the distribution formulas, grants to the states often have also had stipulations about how the monies may be spent. Funds appropriated for health purposes are, of course, all restricted to health programs; but within this broad classification, formula grants have also been divided into general purpose, or block grants, and earmarked, or categorical grants, depending on the degree of restriction placed by the grantor on how they may be spent.

Block grants for public health may be used for broadly defined purposes without detailed specific program restrictions, such as grants to improve and expand local health department services. They have sometimes been designated as "general health grants." Categorical grants, on the other hand, may be spent by a local public health department only for a specific type of activity such as cancer control. It is important to note that what may seem to be an unrestricted or block grant at one level of administration would be viewed as a restricted or categorical grant at a higher level. For example, a general-purpose health grant to a local health department is an unearmarked block grant for that department, but it is categorically restricted from the point of view of the local government, which might perhaps like to use part of it on law enforcement. It should also be noted that in practice, what is legislated as a block grant may be administered with so many binding regulations and such narrowly interpreted oversight on the spending of the money that it is transformed de facto into a categorical grant substantially restricted to items favored by the granting agency.

Project Grants

As opposed to the formula grant, this type of grant was not generally given as a matter of course to all state governments according to an allocation formula but was distributed directly to selected qualified operating organizations for carrying out activities stipulated by the congressional authorization. The grantee could be a state or a general-purpose local government, but it could also be any other type of special-purpose governmental or nongovernmental organization deemed capable of carrying out a specific project that had been previously approved by the federal granting agency. It did not automatically accrue to any general-purpose governmental unit as a matter of entitlement.

Usually the grant award was made to an applicant in competition with several applicants each of which was generally required to provide evidence of competence to carry out the designated task. Its purpose was to directly carry out a federal program under federal oversight and was not essentially a systemic fiscal relationship between the federal and all state governments. This form of grant is especially well suited to furthering or demonstrating a particular type of activity or an experimental health care system. It is also well adapted to providing particular services to pinpointed areas or populations. It is, in general, ill suited for permanent equalization purposes among the states and indeed may work at cross-purposes with this aim, for under criteria used for awarding these grants, the bulk of the money may go to areas that have the best resources—special medical centers, for example—and therefore offer the best chances of achieving favorable outcomes. However, if lack of resources or other indicators of need are written into the criteria (as positive priorities) for awarding a project grant for service delivery, such as operating a local free clinic, it may then serve to help equalize the availability of health services among populations.

An objection to this form of grant, even if it does establish priorities for the neediest places, is precisely its lack of systemic institutionalization of federal-state relationships with all the states. It tends to be more time delimited than the formula grant, and the awards often go to only a few areas chosen for demonstration purposes. The necessity for continual renewal of the federal project grant makes such types of equalization assume a temporary and operationally unstable character, with the projects often being perceived as supported by ''soft money'' programs. The fact that these programs are instituted only in some, often a very few, places implies that they are temporary demonstration-type grants. These features have sometimes discouraged local public health and other public agencies from applying for them in the first place, especially in communities where there was little prospect that local resources could fund the project when the grant expired. Also, the reliance on applications for awarding grants often placed great importance on the local existence of, or the ability to buy, ''grantsmanship'' expertise in determining which areas were awarded grants. The availability of such expertise did not always correlate well with the suitability of the applicant for receiving a grant when measured by objective criteria.

In terms of the actual grant structure that developed, frequently used types of federal health grants may then be summarized under the following categories:

1. Formula general health grant: Distributed to the states by formula with no restriction on expenditure categories. The states redistributed most of these grants to local public health departments.
2. Formula categorical grant: Distributed to the states by formula with specific program restrictions on expenditure categories. The states also redistributed most of these grants to local public health departments.
3. Project grant: Awarded to applicants that were not necessarily general-purpose government bodies or government entities at all. Spending was restricted by a budget submitted with the application. The fact that project grants could be awarded to nongovernmental (non-profit) organizations proved to be a particularly important factor in the development of intergovernmental relations in public health.

THE NATIONAL GOVERNMENT'S ROLE IN STATE AND LOCAL PUBLIC HEALTH SERVICES: THE FEDERAL SYSTEM AFTER 1935

1936–1945 Period

It was previously noted that passage of the Social Security Act in 1935 heralded the beginning of a major program of grants-in-aid to the states for health purposes, and that the portions of the act affecting public health departments were Titles V (Section 1) and VI. These constitute the seminal legislation that set the pattern for later laws and their administration, which molded the national-state-local system of public health services for at least the next fifty years.

Title V Grants

The amount of 3.8 million dollars in federal grants was authorized to be appropriated under Title V to the states for ''promoting the health of mothers and children'' (Mustard, 1945). The funds were distributed by the Children's Bureau (then in the Department of Labor) to the state health departments to be used for supporting these services in state and local health departments. An additional 2.9 million dollars was appropriated for federal grants to the states, "enabling each State to extend and improve ... services for locating crippled children and for providing medical, surgical, corrective and other services and care. . . ." These funds were also distributed by the Children's Bureau[11] to state agencies, but these were generally not health departments. This grant of 6.7 million dollars authorized for fiscal year (FY) 1936 was renewed with increased amounts in the following years. The total amount actually appropriated by the federal government for both maternal and child care and crippled children's services grew from $1.9 million in FY 1936 to $87.3 million in FY 1966 (USDHEW, 1966–67)

Several features of the structure of these maternal and child health grants as they were originally legislated provide good examples of the structure of the grants-in-aid mechanisms. First, these grants were formula grants using a combination of several allocative methods. Each state received a flat allotment to ensure a floor to the grant for each state; an additional amount proportional to "the extent of the problem," using, in this case, the number of live births as the indicator; and a further amount inversely proportional to the financial need in each state. All of these, except the flat allotments, required matching by the state. Second, the states were required to give special emphasis to rural and economically distressed areas. Third, employees supported by Title V funds were required to be on a merit system,[12] and fourth, each state was required to submit a state plan for maternal and child health services and for services for crippled children. The plan was required to provide for financial participation by the state; to provide for the administration of the plan by the "state health agency" unless another state agency had previously been administering these services; and to have the state agency make reports as mandated by the administering federal agency.

The four provisions are worth noting for they were setting up a national program that was to develop into a public health services national network over the following years. The main features of the system would include: federal overall program delineation and major financing; state administration and mandatory matching of federal financing; local delivery of services, with the state having the option of mandating local

participation in the state's share of the financing; and statewide health planning for the program in conformance with federal guidelines.

While actual federal appropriations for maternal and child health and crippled children's services rose substantially between 1936 and 1966, the relative state and local contribution fell between 1954 and 1966. In 1954, the ratio of state and local funds to federal funds spent for maternal and child health was about 3½ to 1; in 1966 it was only just over 2 to 1. In the grants for crippled children's services, the same trend was in evidence, but it was not as marked. Clearly, federal funds were to an important degree displacing the state and local efforts rather than only augmenting them. Maintenance of state and local effort[13] was not fully attained.

Later amendments, mainly those passed in 1963 and in 1965 (as part of P.L. 89–97), provided for grants to state and local health agencies for comprehensive maternity care to high-risk mothers (Section 508) and for the development and delivery of high-quality, comprehensive health services to children and youth of school age or preschool age (Section 509). These only needed to be matched 25 percent by the recipient operating agency, which could be a public or an appropriate nonprofit, private agency. Amounts were subsequently also appropriated for research projects "relating to Maternal and Child Health and crippled children's services." In his book on public health administration, John Hanlon, a former U.S. Public Health Service Surgeon General, described the use of these funds in the following terms:

These funds have been used in the support of prenatal, postnatal, and well-child clinics, of demonstration of delivery and other services, and of public health nursing services for maternal and child care supervision. The [Children's] Bureau has played an important role in the promotion and development of divisions of maternal and child health in all of the State health departments (1969).

These expansions in federal support for maternal and child health activities by state and local health departments continued until 1981 when the grants were consolidated with six other programs into a Maternal and Child Health Services Block Grant. This was part of the reductions in social programs of the Reagan administration embodied in the Omnibus Budget Reconciliation Act of 1981, which will be discussed further at the end of this chapter.

Although not a part of the Title V legislation, it is important to direct attention again to the Supplemental Food Program for Women, Infants and Children (WIC), a nutrition program whose importance in local public health department operations was noted in Chapter 3. This program was established by federal legislation in 1972 but not implemented until 1974. Services are provided through state health departments and entail providing food supplements to pregnant, breastfeeding, and postpartum women as well as to children up to age five who are poor and nutritionally "at risk." Congress voted $900 million for the program in FY 1981 and $950 million for FY 1982.[14] The national program has been coordinated under the Department of Agriculture.

Title VI Grants

The purpose of this title of the Social Security Act of 1935 was to build up the state and local health departments across all their programs. The appropriated monies were administered by the United States Public Health Service (then in the Treasury Department). The original provisions of Title VI authorized $8.0 million in federal funds annually for the years 1936–1940 "[f]or the purpose of assisting States, counties, health districts, and other political subdivisions of the States in establishing and maintaining adequate public health services ..." (Mustard, 1945). In 1944 its provisions, with some changes, were transferred from the Social Security Act to Section 314 of the newly constituted Public Health Service Act. The $2.5 million amount actually appropriated in 1936 rose sharply in subsequent years to $9.5 million in 1940 and $65.0 million in 1965.

The original Social Security Act required these funds to be allocated among the states on the basis of a formula promulgated by the U.S. Surgeon General taking into account three factors: the state's population size, its economic status relative to other states, and the prevalence of special health problems in the state. Federal allotments required state matching except that funds allocated on the basis of economic status

were granted outright; apparently it was deemed illogical to attempt to rectify economic inequalities by including an additional economic burden on those states that could ill afford to match. Each state health department was required to file an acceptable plan with the Surgeon General indicating how the grant would be used by the state, and a report at the end of the year detailing how it had actually been used.

Several important aspects of the allocation and administration provisions of Title VI are particularly worth noting:

1. The federal funds were to be administered nationally by a federal general *health* agency. This contrasts with the child health funds of Title V, which were to be administered by the Children's Bureau of the Labor Department.
2. The method of allocating the grants-in-aid was partly a simple per capita redistribution of federal tax revenues and partly an attempt to equalize relative local and state tax burdens among the states and bring their public health service resources into conformity with their health needs. There was no constant dollar amount provided for each state as in the case of Title V funds.
3. The requirement of filing state plans and annual reports was a modest attempt at quality control and, again, at encouraging statewide *planning*. It established the pattern of a national system of public health services with basic directions largely determined by the federal government.
4. And, as in the case of Title V, the federal funds to be redistributed within the state went directly to a single state agency for administration and the agency was *mandated to be the state health department*.

In the years immediately following the passage of this law, the proportion of the total appropriation allocated according to the equalization and "special problem" factors in the distribution formula was increased and the proportion allocated on a strict population basis was reduced. For the three years 1936, 1941, and 1945, for example, the percentages allocated on a straightforward population basis were 57.4, 29.4, and 27.5, respectively. The fact that the equalization and "special problem" factors became relatively more important with the passage of time was an indication of attempts to better align public health programs with federal policy.

Some of these federal policy goals were articulated by the assistant Surgeon General, Joseph W. Mountin, in the Public Health Service report of 1946 (Mountin et al., 1947), discussed in Chapter 2. In the recommendations of this report, Mountin delineated desirable future directions in public health practice. The recommendations anticipated many of the problems subsequently encountered in federal-state-local governmental relationships with respect to public health programs and health services grants. Mountin's summary of the 1936–1946 period and the situation prevailing at the end of it (Mountin et al. (1947), 65–67) is so remarkably concise and prescient that it will amply repay reading in its entirety. Here I can only note that as early as 1946 he was recognizing and calling attention to the implications of several emerging trends that were to grow in importance as time went by: chronic and degenerative diseases would increasingly become the focus of public health problems; the relationships between preventive work and clinical practice would need to become closer; and the definition of public health would have to come to rest on a foundation of "applied sanitary and medical sciences combined with social organization"—implying the necessity for research on health service delivery as well as on biomedical questions. He also was very early in characterizing the aims of the tripartite "grant-in-aid mechanism"—what later came to be called "cooperative federalism"—as providing for local initiative and control, state technical guidance with some supplementary direct services, and federal resources for equalizing economic differences among the states and regions "and to perform studies and demonstrations which are essential for high quality of work and progressive development of programs."

A careful reading of these conclusions in the light of subsequent developments indicates that although Mountin was perhaps too sanguine about how completely acute infectious diseases would remain "fairly well under control,"[15] in many areas his forecasts were remarkably well borne out by events, proving in some cases to have been all too accurate. The years after his

report saw public health agencies wrestling with these problems, which are still largely unsolved. The move to augment the traditional and well-worn paths of communicable disease and sanitation control with functions to meet the changing health conditions, which Mountin foresaw as being so necessary, was not made with sufficient alacrity to satisfy either the general public or public health professionals, particularly the medical care experts. We recall Sanders's remarks to the effect that from 1950 until the year of his analysis in 1959, "there has been no growth in local health departments. . . ." The period 1936–1945 turned out to have been in many respects a honeymoon period between the public health departments and the federal health agencies during which the Public Health Service, the Children's Bureau and the ardent constituency grouped about it, and state and local public health leaders were thinking along similar lines, while federal funds kept lubricating the wheels with which the three levels of public health activities were meshing. After 1945 things began to change.

The 1946–1968 Period

With the passage of time, public health professionals, some members of Congress, and the Democratic administrations increasingly expressed concern that state and local health departments were being inordinately slow to enter the newer fields of health work. These were the fields indicated by Joseph Mountin, and identified by publicists, scholars, social advocates, and activists as belonging within the province of the local health department because of changing conditions. Principal among these new areas were the persistence of inadequate access to medical care, especially ambulatory care, for a large number of persons; the prevalence of unhealthy habits of personal living; and the newer types and increased magnitude of environmental health threats. Where they did enter these areas, public health departments were perceived to be insufficiently effective in developing programs required to meet the emerging or existing health problems, especially those for which solutions were becoming politically urgent. Attempts by the federal government to encourage greater attention to these special programs by local health departments led to increased use of the more narrowly targeted categorical formula grants as opposed to the general purpose formula grants (Kenadjian, 1966).

Growth of Categorical Formula Grants

The categorical public health grants were still formula grants with every state receiving an allotment and requiring state matching, usually on a dollar-for-dollar basis; they were intended primarily to promote emphasis on specific health activities that the federal government deemed nationally desirable rather than to support the locally formulated general public health budget, and thereby the priorities, of the local and state health departments. The first year in which the spending of any part of the Title VI formula health grants-in-aid was restricted to a given program (i.e., "earmarked") was 1939, the particular restriction in this case being to venereal disease control. In 1946, earmarking of a portion of the formula grants for tuberculosis control was initiated, and by 1965 there were categorical formula grants set aside for cancer control, the chronically ill and aged, dental health, heart disease control, mental health, radiological health, and water pollution control. From about 1950 onward, the federal health grant-in-aid structure increasingly reflected the efforts of the United States Public Health service to strengthen the incentives for state and local public health agencies to move more aggressively into areas of national health policy that were priorities of the federal government. The number of classes of categorically earmarked formula grants increased with the passing years, as did the proportion of the total appropriation for formula grants that were so earmarked, and by 1965, out of about $50 million in Title VI formula grants, only $10 million, or 20 percent of the total appropriation for formula grants, was left for "general health," with the rest restricted to specified categories of health problems (Zwick, 1967).

While the granting of funds on a line-by-line, earmarked basis was meant to push public health spending in desired directions, there are often undesirable side effects from this type of allotment, as budget analysts and administrators know only too well. A uniform national set of priorities may be generally desirable but not particularly applicable to the problems of some states and localities. If the line-item earmarking turns out to be inappropriate for the configuration of health problems in a particular state, then programs that are the most urgently needed may be starved while money lies unused or is frittered away because it is restricted to other and perhaps locally less relevant purposes. However, perhaps the most important basis for the recalcitrance of some state governments in energetically promoting programs for which federal funds had been earmarked was the existence of political antagonisms based on differences between the goals and values of many state office incumbents and those of federal officials.

Growth of Project Grants

We recall that federal project grants for rural sanitation projects had been made in very modest amounts prior to 1935. First legislated in 1916, they were continued during the years 1917–1934. After 1935, the first of the project grant programs to be administered by the U.S. Public Health Service was initiated in 1946 for venereal disease control and amounted to about $4 million per year (Mountin, Hankla, and Druzina, 69ff.) Between 1947 and 1959, the project grant program for venereal disease control remained unique. By 1959 the amount of these grants had decreased to an annual total of $2.4 million, while Public Health Service formula grants, by comparison, totaled approximately $30 million. But after 1960 project grant programs proliferated. A government analyst wrote:

The first half of the 1960s have been marked by a flood of new project grant programs. Grants for cancer demonstration projects began the trend in fiscal year 1960. Two years later, project grants for community health services, tuberculosis, and water pollution control appeared. In fiscal year 1963, three more similar programs were started—for vaccination assistance, neurological and sensory disease services, and migrant health. The next fiscal year was marked by the start of project grants for mental retardation planning. In fiscal year 1965, project grants were initiated to assist in planning of hospitals and other medical facilities and in conducting air pollution surveys, demonstration, and control programs. Thus, by the end of the five-year period, the Public Health Service was administering eleven health services project grant programs (Zwick, 1967).

The largest pre-1966 changes in grant composition took place during 1963–65. While formula (including both block and categorical) grants were 77 percent of the total $76 million in 1963, they were only 48 percent of the $105 million total granted in 1965. In the latter year the proportion of total grants-in-aid for project grants exceeded that for formula grants for the first time.

Project grants had two advantages over formula grants from the federal government's viewpoint during this period. First, they could save money, because grants could be awarded only to *some* selected sites instead of having to be spread over all states and all local health departments. Thus, an elected federal official could win points with a desired constituency by enunciating a bold new program, while actually awarding only a limited number of project grants that would not unduly exacerbate the fiscal problems of the federal government. Project grants lent themselves well to the political symbolic action without great cost described by Edelman (1964).

Second, it would be possible to award project grants only to applicants who really wanted to operate the program, thereby avoiding the continual wrestling with those unwilling health departments and their state or local governments that did not view some of the categorical formula grant programs with favor.

But perhaps the most important force pushing Congress toward greater use of project grants-in-aid was the political configuration of the country in these years. The large metropolitan centers, Congress, and the presidency, for most of these years, were generally liberal in politics and supported the public health policy being urged on the states and localities by the federal health agency. On the other hand, many state legislatures had been structured to represent the conservative rural sections of the state more heavily than their relative population sizes warranted. These states tended to be slow in moving toward assigning comprehensive health care and ecological control responsibilities to their state health departments. Circumstances in the large cities and their suburbs, on the other hand, had increasingly driven them toward demanding expansion of such activities. Spending by public agencies for increased services to the core cities

and the metropolitan suburbs was being promoted, especially in some of the more populous states, by a political alliance of metropolitan poor and ethnic minority groups, some labor unions, suburban liberal groups, and federal leadership, and opposed by many of the more conservative state legislatures and administrations. The implementation of the newer programs promoted by the federal government via formula categorical grants was being obstructed by the conflict between some large metropolitan centers and their state governments, and failing to prevail in the state capital, the urban and suburban dwellers could and did turn with growing frequency to Washington for aid in the form of direct project grants bypassing the state government entirely. Through sympathetic members of Congress and executives in the federal bureaucracy, the mayors, city and county councils, and citizen groups could work for legislation to establish project grant programs that would meet the needs of the metropolitan centers. If such programs already existed, the centers could lobby to have project grants awarded their areas. In times of a Democratically controlled Congress and federal executive, the activities of this coalition of urban and suburban forces with federal officials might be particularly effective. These factors were among those that led to the emergence of project grants as an increasingly important segment of the total federal grant picture in the 1960s.

In addition to the opposing views on project grants stemming from conflicting interests, differences in points of view also developed among public health administrators with respect to whether the project grants advanced the cause of optimizing statewide public health protection. Some state chief health officers felt that project grants given by Washington directly to applicants within a state served to undermine the state health authority in its efforts to plan for protecting the health of all the people throughout the entire state in a coordinated and efficient manner. An opposing view supported the idea of project grants directly from the federal government to local entities. Its proponents held that while federal grants, essentially unearmarked and granted only to the state health authority, might be desirable for a state with an aggressively active and forward-looking state health department, such a course would be quite inappropriate for states where this was not the case. Furthermore, they argued, direct federal project grants to the executors of a project were becoming increasingly necessary to meet interstate problems such as the "Ohio River Valley Sanitation Compact," which involved seven states in a joint effort to control pollution.[16]

Another implication of the consequences of the new emphasis on project grants also led to divided opinions about their desirability over formula grants. The project grants were in line with and thus encouraged a trend toward using the private sector on a contract basis to discharge health service duties presumed to be a responsibility of government. The formula grants were made exclusively to health departments with the expectation that these responsibilities would be carried out by public agencies responsible for protecting the health of entire health service jurisdiction, not just for the target populations of a project grant application. The appearance of a shift in emphasis from formula grants awarded to governments to project grants that could go to private entities was a harbinger of stronger moves in that direction yet to come.

Attempts to Realign the Public Health Grant System in 1966–1967

After some fifteen years of continued efforts by the federal government to encourage greater activity by state and local health departments in chronic disease control, pollution abatement, increasing access to medical care services, and similar programs, an attempt was made in 1966 to discontinue further efforts to accomplish these newer special goals via earmarked formula grants funneled through state governments. The "Comprehensive Health Planning and Public Health Service Amendments of 1966" (P.L. 89–749) and the related "Partnership for Health Amendments of 1967" (P.L. 90–174) abolished all categorical earmarking of formula grants (Cavanaugh, 1967). The intention of the legislation was that the federal government's efforts to direct the attention of local public health departments *and other agencies,* including nongovernmental ones, to its high-priority health service targets were thenceforth to be made solely through the use of the *project* grant. For-

mula grants for "general health" (i.e., to maintain standard services) would all be unearmarked.

The 1966 act authorized an amount of $62.5 million for a one-year program of block formula grants to states for comprehensive public health services. This compared with $50 million in formula grants for 1965, only $10 million of which had been for "general health" (i.e., unearmarked), and the rest earmarked for eight different categories. An amount of $62.5 million was also authorized for project grants that were to be available "to any public or nonprofit private agency, institution, or organization," in contrast to the general (formula) grants, which were to continue to be available only to "State health or mental health authorities." The 1966 act thus provided that for the time being both types of grants, the formula and the project, were to be continued with equal funding. The shift away from the overwhelming preponderance of block formula grants of 1936 was clearly evident in the provisions of the 1966 legislation and subsequent history of its implementation.

A major purpose of these 1966 and 1967 amendments to Section 314 (the successor to the old Title VI of the Social Security Act) of the Public Health Service Act was to entrench the project grant more deeply in the federal grant structure. It was hoped that decategorizing all the formula grants into block grants would remove the disintegrative effects on state and local areawide planning of categorical restrictions made in Washington, but the validity of the objections noted above to the disintegrative effects on statewide health planning by the project grants was also recognized by the framers of the legislation. To counteract the tendency of project grants to fragment the system of public health services within a state, the new law provided for grants for statewide comprehensive health planning. It also provided for grants to local health planning agencies to carry out local areawide comprehensive health planning.[17]

The 1966 Comprehensive Health Planning Act and Public Health Service Act, then, contained five major sections. The first three (establishing Section 314; A, B, and C) dealt with federal support for comprehensive health planning, and the last two (314 D and E) revised the public health grant structure as described above. In providing that the *general* formula grants replace all former categorical formula grants, Section 314D required them to be transmitted through the state health department, as before; but all plans for use of these funds now had to be approved by the statewide comprehensive health planning agency (Section 314A) as conforming to statewide plans developed by that agency. Section 314E, providing for project grants "for Health Services Development," required them to conform to the state plan of the state health planning agency also. The former project health grants were subsumed under this subsection. The appropriations for formula public health grants that were continued as block grants came to be known as "314D" monies after the section of the Public Health Act that provided for them, but in subsequent years appropriations for them dwindled to very small amounts. The subsequent atrophy of these funds indicated a retreat by the federal administrations from a policy of providing financial support to maintain and build the state and local public health department structure per se. This policy was replaced by one that called for the federal government to help fund only specific programs it wished to push and to increasingly regard the state and local health departments as field representatives of the national programs.

The following summarizes the situation after passage of the "Comprehensive Health Planning" legislation in 1966 and 1967:

Any local or state public or nonprofit private agency was eligible for project ("314E") grants for "health services development." These were required to conform to the State Comprehensive Health Plan and had to be approved by the State Comprehensive Health Planning Authority.

The state health department was to be the sole recipient of the general-purpose formula grants for public health services (Section 314D).

The State Comprehensive Health Planning Authority (called the "A" agency) was to be the recipient of the grants for doing statewide health planning (Section 314A), but this agency did *not* have to be the state health department. This was the earliest major national public health legislation that did not mandate

the state health department or its equivalent to be the single state agency as intermediary through which a national health program would be administered locally. The implications of this action are discussed more fully in Chapter 3.

That the choice of an alternative agency was not merely an infrequently used legal possibility is evidenced by the fact, noted previously, that as of March 1969 the state health department had been designated as the state Comprehensive Health Planning Authority in only twenty-two states; in the other states the planning agency was placed in the governor's office or in an interdepartmental commission, or some other mechanism was used (Health Insurance Council, 1969). (The designated agency was: the state health department in twenty-two states; the state health and welfare department in five states; in the office of the governor in nine states; and in a special commission in fourteen states and Puerto Rico.)[18]

The intended changes in grant-in-aid structure under this act may be characterized as involving three basic elements:

1. Abolition of categorical formula grants.
2. Reinforcement of the practice of health services grants going directly from the federal government to nongovernmental grantees through the increased emphasis on project grants.
3. An attempt to counterbalance the fragmentation of services exacerbated by project grants that bypass the state with increased support for local and state health planning.

Decline in Prestige and Influence of the Public Health Service

As has been noted, the attempt at a major recasting of the national public health law came partly in response to the mounting demands for improved access to at least minimally adequate medical care in underserved areas. This pressure emanated from some sectors of the public health profession, medical care organization scholars, activists, political leaders, and a substantial volume of writings appearing as popular books and in periodicals and newspapers. Interest also rose markedly during the 1960s in getting existing public health agencies to take a more active part in assuring that the nonpoor populations of their jurisdictions were being served by an effective and efficient system of health services; in improving safeguards against the intensifying threats to environmental safety; and in the continued proper maintenance of preventive community services of the more traditional type.

The efforts of the national public health agency, the United States Public Health Service (USPHS), to provide incentives to state and local agencies for innovative approaches to meeting these demands at the state and local levels via categorical and project grants were perceived as not sufficiently effective. The leaders and members of the Commissioned Corps of the United States Public Health Service did not create a strong public perception of their being wholeheartedly in the forefront of the drive for increased federal involvement in furthering publicly sponsored medical care services to at least the underserved poor. The perennial battles over the introduction of national health insurance were being waged with other troops in the front lines—largely medical care administrators, publicists, and scholars rather than leading federal public health professionals—so that when many of the new federal programs for improving access to medical care were passed, agencies other than the Public Health Service were assigned to administer them. The administration of Medicare was assigned to the Social Security Administration, the social insurance agency; Medicaid was assigned to Social and Rehabilitation Services, the welfare agency; and when federal attempts to provide greater access to ambulatory care were made by establishing community health centers (see Chapter 11), the program was placed under an independent agency in the office of the President, the Office of Economic Opportunity (OEO).

As one leading public health writer put it:

By the early 1960s there appeared to be substantial disenchantment and dissatisfaction on the part of the Administration toward the Commissioned Corps of the PHS. It was considered by many to be unwilling or unable to meet modern problems related to the administration and the delivery of health services. . . .

The status of the Commissioned Corps was not helped during the long battle over Medicare when it was believed that many members of the corps remained aloof. . . .

[O]ver the past few years, the existing organization of the PHS, with its limited number of career personnel and its traditional orientation, was overwhelmed and was bypassed. Health programs were developed at the Federal level outside of HEW, such as Head Start and Neighborhood Health Centers under the Office of Economic Opportunity, and Model Cities under Housing and Urban Development (Snoke, 1969).

The power of the Public Health Service and its chief were greatly curtailed within the Department of Health, Education and Welfare through a number of reorganizations that weakened the office of the Surgeon General. The status of that office and the role of the PHS remained in flux for a number of years, and the position was actually abolished under the reorganization of the Public Health Service in 1973 (see the next section). Despite the apparent intent of the 1966 legislation that appropriations for block formula grants to public health departments be about equal in total to the amount appropriated for project grants, Congress was unable to resist the importuning of the various advocates for specific programs. The appropriations for categorical public health programs continued to proliferate and grow in size, both openly and under the guise of project grants given to almost all health departments for these programs, while the unearmarked block 314D money that offered an opportunity for greater local flexibility in program planning continued to dwindle.

The termination of President Johnson's term of office in 1968 with his decision not to run for reelection marked the end of an era in federal health policy. After 1935, and more intensively after 1945, the cornerstone of this policy had been to exercise assertive federal leadership to create a more uniform, accessible, and comprehensive national health services system. In the public health area the main mechanism had been the federal grant structure, which distributed nationally collected taxes, mainly the income tax, to the states, localities, and nonprofit organizations to promote the federal objectives. These were increasing access to primary care, improving environmental protection, and decreasing inequality of health protection due to accident of geography or family resources. A formal mechanism was established to administer the implementation of these goals—the three-tiered federal system of the United States Public Health Service, state health agencies, and local public health departments. This system was expected to combine local initiative and policy input with national standards that worked toward uniform access to at least minimally adequate health services across the land.

The 1969–1980 Period

The Nixon Agenda

Enunciated federal health policy in the post-Johnson era was a proposed reversal of these trends by attempting to dismantle much of this three-tiered arrangement beginning with the federal grant system. There was to be a progressive shedding of federal responsibility for developing a uniform, cooperative, federal system of public health services and a transfer of these responsibilities to the states.

Following the election of Richard M. Nixon as president in 1968, the executive branch embarked on this policy of reversal with an announced new policy presented as a set of philosophical principles dubbed the "New Federalism" by the administration. It was summarized by President Nixon early in 1970 in the following manner: "after over a century and a half of power flowing from the people and from the local communities and from the States to Washington, D.C. let's get it back to the people and to the cities and to the States where it belongs"[19] (OMB, 1971).

The general thrust of the proposed implementation of this enunciated policy consisted of two main features:

1. Organizationally, federal granting programs were to be "streamlined" to simplify their administration and to facilitate the application process by according local governmental authorities and federal *regional* offices a greater degree of decision-making autonomy. There also was to be a major realignment of federal departments "to conform better to major purposes of government and to coordinate better the management of federal programs" (HEW, 1972).

The "streamlining" of federal machinery was a formulation with populist overtones. It was addressed to agencies and administrators, public and private, who sought federal grants for service programs. But its main political value lay in its appeal to entrepreneurial frustration with the intricacy of government procedures in granting permits for environmental impact clearances and similar regulatory impediments to rapid development. (See also note 21.)

2. Fiscally, there was an effort to revise the federal grants program to place increased emphasis on lump sums (block grants) to states and local governments and allow them to make their own decisions on how the monies should be spent. These lump sums were to be as global as possible; they were to be "lumped" for all purposes, not just health. Categorical grants,[20] including project grants for detailed programmatic purposes, were to be eliminated as far as possible. This proposed granting program was dubbed "revenue sharing," and all during the Nixon/Ford administrations, the term revenue sharing had this special meaning in public debates and discussions: global block grants to states, cities, and localities.

Whatever his ultimate intentions may have been, on the record President Nixon set out to carry out both parts of his enunciated policy, to simplify and improve the coordination of the federal machinery that deals with the public, and to consolidate as many of the state grants as possible into as few lump sums as feasible. There was no public statement of any intention to cut the overall total amount of grants—only to transfer the decision making about how they were to be spent to the state and localities.

The FAR Program To implement the first point of the "New Federalism," President Nixon in 1969 launched a three-year examination, the Federal Assistance Review (FAR), of all federal grant programs, and put into effect as many changes that would "streamline Federal assistance programs" as possible. Conducted by the Office of Management and Budget (OMB) and certain agencies of the "Domestic Council," made up of representatives of specified government agencies (1971), the announced three major objectives for implementing the goals of the "new federalism" were: "greater reliance on State and local governments in the operation and administration of Federal grant programs, decentralization of Federal programs from headquarters to regional offices, and increased interagency standardization of requirements and procedures for Federal grant programs" (HEW, 1972).[21]

The report issued at the conclusion of the program in 1972 claimed that the Department of Health, Education and Welfare (HEW) had benefited from measures taken to implement the FAR program findings, such as greater regional coordination among the field offices of the different federal granting agencies. The overall agency changes that the administration claimed to have brought about within HEW included:

1. Increased reliance on state and local governments, through HEW technical assistance in organizing local administration of health programs. This assistance was aided by the passage of the Intergovernmental Cooperation Act in 1970.
2. Improved management capability of state and local governments through the temporary exchange of personnel between the federal government and the states and localities, and federal assistance in developing management and evaluation skills for running federally funded programs. These were also provided for by the Intergovernmental Personnel Act of 1970.
3. Simplified funding of federal programs, establishing consistency in procedures, reducing government processing time and "cutting red tape." With the establishment of a Division of Consolidated Funding in HEW in March 1972, a project requiring funding from several sources in HEW could now be submitted as a single application, and if approved, would result in a single grant from this division, which would arrange for the grants to come from the various subdivisions of HEW.
4. Decentralization and regionalization of many HEW programs by transferring program and funding authority from national headquarters to regional offices. They were strengthened financially and by adding high-level super-

visory personnel capable of running the field offices with a great deal of autonomy. Compared with 1969 when "very few" programs were decentralized, by 1972, out of 318 grant programs, 199 were still "completely centralized," 49 "fully decentralized," and 70 programs "partially decentralized" (1972).[22]

Revenue Sharing I have briefly discussed the organizational change aspect of Nixon's New Federalism because it impinges on a number of themes that run through this book. The lack of technical competence as a source of the public health system's problems was emphasized, and an appeal was made to the country to rise up against the central government's voracious appetite for power over state and local institutions. An important transformation, however, soon took place in the original concept of simply making it easy for applicants to use the services available through grant programs. A principal focus of this goal became a concern with the ease of obtaining permits for commercial enterprises that had to meet environmental standards. Increasing the ease of application, in these cases, often involved an easing of environmental standards that became an important public health concern. This issue is further discussed later in this chapter.

The implementation of the second main point of the New Federalism, called for making a single, formula, block grant to state and (directly to) local governments the centerpiece of the federal granting program. As originally envisaged by the Nixon administration, this program was meant to comprise a "general" revenue-sharing portion and a "special" revenue-sharing portion. The general revenue sharing would be a single block grant almost entirely unencumbered by any categorical restrictions. The special revenue sharing would consist of a very few categorical grants, each earmarked for a single very broad category with no further earmarking within it. They would, in effect, be special block grants. The special revenue sharing, as presented in the 1974 federal budget, called for four special categorical grant programs covering the broad fields of urban community development, manpower training, education, and law enforcement. Note that there was to be no special health grant. States and localities were to have complete discretion on whether to use any of their general revenue-sharing block grant money for health purposes.

On October 20, 1972, *general* revenue sharing was enacted into law (P.L. 92–512) as the State and Local Fiscal Assistance Act of 1972. An amount of $30.2 billion was appropriated to the states and localities to be distributed over a five-year period beginning January 1, 1972. The money the states received was entirely unrestricted except that it could not be used as matching funds for other federal grants. The local government grants could be used only for "priority expenditures" that were "ordinary and necessary." Maintenance and operating expenses were limited to public safety, environmental protection, public transportation, *health*, recreation, libraries, social services for poor or aged, and financial administration. For the states, a "maintenance of effort" clause prohibited cut backs in their previous rate of aid to localities from state revenues. The previous federal grants for public health were seen by the administration to have been "folded in"[23] to the general revenue-sharing grant, except that a few categorical grant programs judged to be "effective" and nationally needed would be continued. The state and local governments were now free to spend what they thought appropriate on public health, and in some places general revenue funds were indeed used to help finance health services. In Alameda County, California, for example, a number of community health centers providing ambulatory care were financed out of these funds.

The state government kept one-third of the money and the remaining two-thirds was divided among its subgovernments using an intricate formula based on population, tax effort (related to personal income and indirectly adjusted for education expenditures[24]), and relative poverty. Thus, the method of using "need" factors for allocating national formula grants among the states established in 1935 was maintained and extended to local areas. No monies from federal revenue sharing could be used on any projects that discriminated on the basis of race, color, national origin, or sex.

Three of the four originally contemplated special revenue-sharing programs were subse-quently enacted: manpower, community development (housing), and law enforcement.

Two of these directly affected health services for the poor. One was the manpower program represented by the Comprehensive Employment and Training Act of 1973 (CETA), signed into law by President Nixon on December 28, 1973, which provided $1.65 billion over a period of five years for state and local governments. The other was the community development program in the form of the Housing and Community Development Act of 1974 passed in August 1973. Under the CETA legislation, many public hospitals, neighborhood health clinics, and local public health departments were able to employ poor persons, who would otherwise have been unemployed, to help relieve some of the chronic understaffing of these agencies. The Housing and Community Development Act superseded the previous urban development legislation, including the "Model Cities" program under which some neighborhood health centers were financed.

The general Revenue Sharing Act was extended in 1977 for five years through 1981, and again in 1981 for 1982 through 1986. Much of the special revenue sharing program was, however, severely cut in 1982 under the Reagan administration's retrenchment program. The entire revenue-sharing program was finally discontinued in 1986.

The revenue-sharing program was of substantial potential importance to state and local public health programs, for the block grants gave the states and localities increased power to reduce or augment public health programs in relation to other spending areas. This very fact aroused suspicion among President Nixon's political opponents. President Nixon's 1971 budget had called for discontinuing many of the categorical programs and cutting others substantially, thereby reinforcing the suspicions of many of his opponents about the real aim of his revenue-sharing program. It was feared by some that much of the terminology about local control and decentralization was a revival of the tactic of using the "states rights" philosophy to cover up an intent to subsequently reduce total outlays for federal social programs. This might be the underlying agenda, because the federal government might later find it easier to cut the total block grants than to cut the categorically specified programs.

Block grants for health, along with health planning support, was the concept of a "comprehensive health planning and services" law enacted by Congress in 1966. But when the Johnson Administration and later the Nixon Administration, began *chopping wholesale amounts off the block grants* [i.e., "314d" money] and some states began responding by eliminating health programs, categorical grant laws reappeared. The trend has been in that direction ever since Administration budgeteers had found it easier to trim a block grant than to cut back on a specifically labelled disease control program. (McGraw Hill, 1976, 151).

This quotation from a well-known Washington-based weekly newsletter on government developments in health legislation voiced the widespread perception that a federal administration stratagem for cutting or eliminating a categorical health program was first to "fold it in" to a block and then cut the block grant total. Whether this suspicion was well founded was never determined because of the truncation of President Nixon's second term in office in 1974. It remained for President Reagan to later turn these suspicious scenarios into actuality.

With such suspicions as a background, Congress, while going along with President Nixon's revenue-sharing proposals, opposed his proposed offsetting budget reductions that called for the elimination of appropriations for many ongoing categorical programs funded in past years. Thus what Congress was really proposing was to have both the revenue-sharing block grants and continuation of the categorical programs. Categorically defined health programs supported since 1966 continued to grow. Many members of Congress did not wish to reduce categorical appropriations, either by direct reduction or by "folding in" the categorical amounts into block grants, for programs targeted to diseases and classes of persons that had strong advocacy and lobbying constituencies.

Proposed Budget Reductions Although it seemed that cutting federal provision for health care services was indeed an underlying aim of the Nixon/Ford administrations, it should be noted that the programs specifically proposed for sharp reduction were mainly in the medical care (Medicaid) and mental health fields, because the largest money savings were available in these programs rather than in standard public health. The apparent primary aim was to cut federal costs. A more explicitly ideological war on particular public programs because of their content and for other general ideological reasons came later, under President Reagan. Nixon's avowed aim was to shift the center of gravity of decision making on how public health appropriations were spent from the national to state and local governments.[25] Therefore, the proposed cuts were not centered on the grants for public health. In addition to Medicaid, the reductions proposed by Nixon were mainly directed at programs whose budgets were relatively large. Those proposed for major cutting included Hill-Burton, Community Mental Health Centers, Regional Medical Programs, and the Public Health Service hospital system with allocations for health personnel education being cut in half. For the time being, at least, formula grants for state public health programs, on the other hand, were to be maintained at the previous year's level. Migrant health, maternal and child health, and family planning were to remain about the same, although the budget request was for maternal and child health Title V project grants to be "folded in" to general 314d public health department grants—an early but unsuccessful attempt at consolidating post-1966 categorical health grants into block grants.

In addition to the cuts being again proposed for the following year, the 1974 budget also proposed rescinding about $550 million that had been appropriated in 1973 that the administration had decided not to spend (i.e., had "impounded"). This impounding of already appropriated funds and later asking for the cancellation of their prior appropriation ("rescission") had become a bone of contention between the president and Congress, which subsequently revoked the power of presidents to impound appropriated funds. An apparent truce in the administration-Congress battle over the federally funded programs was declared when in June 1973 the president signed a bill into law (S.1136) extending expiring health programs for one year, and the proposed 1975 budget contained much more modest reductions of these programs than Nixon had asked for. The country was indeed operating under both general revenue-sharing and categorical health grant money, the latter appropriated at 1973 levels in 1974, and only modestly reduced for 1975.

Further contest between the Republican President Nixon and the Democratic Congress was cut short by Mr. Nixon's resignation on August 9, 1974, and the accession of Vice President Gerald Ford to the presidency. President Ford continued Nixon's health policies, in the main. The principal administration thrusts continued: attempts at overall reduction of health budgets and consolidation of appropriations for existing categorical programs into block formula health grants.

Many state and local officials might have welcomed the consolidations into block grants because of the greater discretion they allowed in how they could be spent, had they not involved reduction in total amounts for FY 1975, but given the fact of the overall reductions, they looked askance at them. The specific Ford proposals, for example, proposed cuts in Medicaid money. In addition, they objected to the "folding-in" being done all at once rather than gradually over a ten-year period (McGraw Hill, 1976). Not surprisingly then, the efforts of the Ford administration to convince state, county, and city officials of the benefits to them of health block grants were not successful. The Democratic Congress continued to oppose them, and the idea got nowhere because of lack of political support. Nevertheless, in his last State of the Union Address, President Ford unveiled a budget request for FY 1976 calling for consolidation of sixteen health programs, including a number of public health programs such as formula block public health grants (314d), immunization, rat control, lead-paint poisoning prevention, maternal and child health, state health grants, and family planning. Because the states were not required to match the federal block health grant funds in this budget proposal they would also have been free to reduce their own outlays for these programs. The proposal seemed clearly tied to a perspective of reducing health services unless the states spent more to make up for the federal reductions in the total block grant, and it

again got nowhere in Congress. In January of 1977 President Carter assumed office.

The Carter Administration

Although the Carter administration (1977–1980) discontinued the Ford attempts to put most public health categorical grants into a single block grant, the Carter budget for 1977–78 provided very little more for health services than the Ford budget had (McGraw Hill, 2/28/77). The Carter administration focused on three major public health goals: expansion of preventive and some treatment services for poor children; health promotion and disease prevention; and mental health services, especially community-based ones.

The measures suggested for expanding services for children were embodied in a proposal that came to be known as Comprehensive Health Assessment and Treatment for Poor Children (CHAP). It was intended to reach 1.8 million children in addition to the 12 million already eligible for such services through Medicaid. During 1977 CHAP bills were introduced both in the Senate and the House, and throughout the entire four years of President Carter's term this proposal was pushed in Congress, but it did not pass. A leading tactic used to defeat it was the attachment of an anti–abortion rights rider to it by legislators opposed to abortion, effectively splitting its congressional support.

The proposed health promotion and disease prevention program consisted of two parts. One was a number of stepped-up national campaigns to inform people about the importance to health of life style choices in such matters as smoking, eating, and exercise, and the issuance of documents outlining a public health campaign against the diseases that were now the leading causes of death and chronic morbidity. The other was a reorganization of the Communicable Disease Control section of the Public Health Service into the Centers for Disease Control (CDC). The two-part program was the centerpiece of Dr. Julius Richmond, the new Surgeon General of the Public Health Service.

We recall that under the Nixon-Ford administrations the role of Surgeon General had been reduced. After 1968 the position had at times been left unfilled, and a 1973 government reorganization had actually abolished it. In July 1977 the Carter administration reinstated the position and sought to restore its prestige by appointing Dr. Julius Richmond, a prominent physician widely known for his work with children, to the posts of USPHS Surgeon General and Assistant Secretary for Health of HEW.

Dr. Richmond's Public Health Goals for 1990 In two reports issued in 1979 and 1980 (HEW, 1979a & b) (DHHS, 1980), the importance of disease prevention and health promotion was carefully delineated and national "achievable" goals for 1990 were laid out. The introductory part of the first report described the orientation in this way:

In the modern era, there have been periodic surges of interest leading to major advances in prevention. The sanitary reforms of the latter half of the 19th century and the introduction of effective vaccines in the middle of the 20th century are two examples.
But during the 1950s and 1960s, concern with the treatment of chronic diseases and lack of knowledge about their causes resulted in a decline in emphasis on prevention.
Now, however, with the growing understanding of causes and risk factors for chronic diseases, the 1980s present new opportunities for major gains.
Prevention is an idea whose time has come. We have the scientific knowledge to begin to formulate recommendations for improved health. And, although the degenerative diseases differ from their infectious disease predecessors in having more—and more complex—causes, it is now clear that many are preventable (HEW, 1979).

The 1979 report presented justifications for allocating a greater portion of the health dollar to prevention, while the 1980 report identified the leading health problems facing the nation and set feasible improvement targets for fifteen priority areas.[26] Using extant reported research, the reports came to the conclusion that for the ten leading causes of death in 1976, 50 percent of deaths were due to unhealthy behavior or life style, 20 percent to environmental factors, 20 percent to human biological factors, and only 10 percent to inadequacies in the existing health care system. It seemed to follow clearly that changing unhealthy behavior was the key measure on which to concentrate in order to most effectively prevent or control disease, and much of the attention of the Public Health Service was subsequently directed to this activity, with oc-

cupational health and safety next in importance. However, other measures, such as immunizations, were also recommended for controlling specific health hazards.

The main organizational form adopted to implement the campaign was enhancement of the disease control agency of the federal government. This was effectuated in October 1980 with the reorganization that changed the Communicable Disease Center of the United States Public Health Service to the six Centers for Disease Control (CDC): the Center for Prevention Services, the Center for Environmental Health, the National Institute for Occupational Safety and Health, the Center for Health Promotion and Education, the Center for Professional Development and Training, and the Center for Disease Investigation and Diagnosis.

Thus was a campaign organized and energized to combat the newer threats to health in the classical fashion of past public health campaigns that had worked so well when the leading health threats were acute infectious diseases. There was the identification of health threats, determination of probable causes, the choice of measures to combat them based on the best scientific evidence available, and the choice of an organization to lead the campaign. But the proposed revitalization of the public health prevention campaign differed from the previous successful campaign in an important respect—the nature of the organizational form chosen to lead the battle. The earlier campaign had made the local public health department the center of the frontline battle, the field command post as it were, supported and backed up by federal and state money, state technical guidance and supervision, and overall federal program guidance. The new campaign proposed in the Surgeon General's reports made virtually no mention of what, if anything, would or even should be done to revitalize, rebuild, and restructure the national network of local departments to meet the challenge of the newer threats to health. Nor did it suggest any other changes or improvements that might be needed in the system of local provision of medical care, public or private.[27] The reorganization that brought forth the Centers for Disease Control implied reliance on developing a centralized, high-technology federal organization that would disseminate findings and propose activities, but with little indication of what sort of local agencies would be needed to disseminate anything effectively at the community level. Glaringly absent from the list of the names of the six centers were any that clearly indicated major responsibility for regular and systemic liaison, guidance, and contact with state and local health departments to solidify the federal *system*.

With this omission the report not only failed to face the problem of the role of the local general governments, the counties and cities, in implementing federal health policy with respect to the newer environmental programs; it also implied a lack of intent to involve and actively lead them in the campaign to control the ravages of the chronic and degenerative diseases. And it also implied an insufficient appreciation by the federal government of the necessity to maintain the basic six functions for controlling the incidence of acute infectious diseases and the local health departments' role in this ongoing task. Whatever the thinking was in deciding that the CDC reorganization was the best way to mount the new public health battle, it is undeniable that the proposed choice would be much less costly than a ten-year program, for example, to revitalize the national network of local health agencies along newly needed lines.

One may also reasonably question the definitive tone used in allocating the ''blame'' for the ten leading causes of death. The configuration of numerous and interacting risk factors in causing death from degenerative disease is still rather sketchily known. It therefore seems questionable to allocate only 10 percent of the blame to inadequacies in the medical care system, particularly if one believes that it is part of that system's mission to help change patients' unhealthy behavior. It is quite likely that the overly positive assertion of these percentages was influenced by the eagerness of the Carter (and subsequent) administrations to reduce the costs of medical care by restricting access. Underplaying the benefits of medical care makes curtailment of its services more palatable.[28]

Yet while one may question the particular choice of public service organization and exercise caution in accepting some of the assertions about the deep-rooted causes of mortality, the prevention program put forward by the Surgeon General still deserves to be regarded as a worthwhile contribution to modern public health administration thinking. Ever since Mountin's 1946 report, and even earlier, public health advocates had been calling for a realignment of public health priorities and functions toward preventing the onset and ameliorating the severity of the most prevalent serious diseases in the developed countries today—the chronic and degenerative. Dr. Richmond's reports advanced the formulation of such a program and laid the basis for continuing work along these lines.

On the other hand, although the admonitions of Joseph Mountin about the rising contribution of the chronic diseases to morbidity and mortality among the population were being heeded by Dr. Richmond's program, Dr. Mountin's statement that acute infectious diseases were ''*fairly well under control* [emphasis added] and the required protective measures can be put on a maintenance basis in most areas'' (see p. 209) was improperly interpreted, as it had been for many years. The history of the incidence and prevalence of acute infectious disease in the twentieth century belies the notion that because control of these diseases and their epidemics was relatively stabilized, local control measures could be sharply relaxed and resources for maintaining them safely reduced to very low levels. Yet this has been done again and again.

In the first place, all sorts of societal and biological changes bring forth renewed threats of epidemics of nominally ''old'' acute diseases. As two authorities on these diseases put it:

[P]athogenic agents evolve or mutate. This may be illustrated by the pandemic of influenza of World War I, by frequent emergence of new strains of viruses and bacteriae, the development of chemotherapeutic and antibiotic resistance, as with the gonococcus . . . there are continuing changes in the risk of disease transmission within various geographic, social, and age groups because of the changing patterns of transportation, food movement, travel and in particular changes in social behavior such as age at onset and patterns of sexual activity, patterns of marriage and breakup, public reaction to sexual behavior, etc. (Cutler and Arnold, 1988).

The pattern of federal public health policy has been to respond reactively by mobilizing the state and local public health departments to intensify the battle against a public health threat of exceptional virulence with specially enhanced grant-in-aid programs—and when the force of the threat subsided, severely curtailing the aid programs. The threat then often returned, albeit usually with reduced strength, fortunately. This pattern of lack of maintenance of local public health capacity during lulls in disease virulence is clearly shown in the history of the control of sexually transmitted diseases from World War I through the present (Cutler and Arnold, 1988).

Second, in addition to the continued existence of an underlying residue of cases of acute infectious disease that can spring forth as epidemics if surveillance and control measures are allowed to slacken, new acute infectious diseases do continue to appear. Such was the case with Legionnaires' disease, which made its appearance in 1976 in Philadelphia. But the most telling evidence of the continued threat from new acute infectious epidemic disease was not to appear until 1981, when the first cases of AIDS were detected in New York and Los Angeles. By 1988 some 47,000 cases had been diagnosed, and some 250,000–300,000 were projected to be diagnosed by 1991. For fiscal year 1988 alone, state-only expenditure for AIDS had reached some $156 million and PHS expenditures 790 million. Including all programs, about $1.9 billion was spent by state and federal governments in that year. It is reasonable to suppose that much of the initial confusion and hesitation in the response by the Reagan administration and many states was due not only to ideological factors, but also to the erosion of the professional and administrative structure of the national network of public health departments over the years after 1960. A similar pattern prevailed in the child immunization program, which showed sharp reductions in the percentage of children immunized against preventable serious childhood diseases. It is evident that the maintenance of a well-supported national network of local public health agencies monitored by state and federal public health agencies is an important national requirement if ''required protective measures'' are really to be put on a maintenance basis sufficient to keep acute infectious diseases ''fairly well under control.''

Perhaps it is unfair to construe the lack of attention in the Surgeon General's reports to development of the public health network as a fault of the policy adopted or the planning done,

given the short time that proved to be available to complete it. One term of four years is scarcely long enough. The new CDC was not organized until October 1980 and in November Ronald Reagan won the presidential election. In January he assumed office determined to dismantle as much of the federal health structure as possible. Yet one must also bear in mind the major advances toward the social welfare state made in the first terms of previous Democratic presidents (Roosevelt, Kennedy, Johnson) coming into office after Republican rule. It is fair to question whether President Carter was strongly dedicated to all the goals of the social welfare state that had been the hallmark of the Democratic Party's stance since 1930. How may we describe and characterize the public health goals of the Carter administration, and why was their implementation not more successful?

An Evaluation of the Carter Public Health Policy The Carter administration seemed to have difficulty determining its identity with respect to some aspects of social welfare policy, especially public health policy. Except for the eight year hiatus (1953–1960) of the Eisenhower presidency, the administrations from 1933 through 1968 were Democratic and pursued an enunciated and de facto policy of expanding federally supported and guided social welfare including a large expansion in health legislation (de jure health policy). The Nixon/Ford administrations enunciated and tried to implement a counter policy of federal disengagement from social welfare issues, and President Carter was expected by many adherents of the social welfare state concept to return the temporarily derailed social welfare train to the mainline Democratic tracks leading toward increased federal roles in public health protection, including greater access to medical care for needy populations.

But even if he had really wished to take this course, and it is doubtful that he did, Carter would have faced an uphill battle. The downward move of the United States economy in the late 1960s placed a restraining hand on continued expansion of social welfare programs. Europe, particularly West Germany, and Japan had returned to the status of economic competitors rather than being primarily pliant customers of the United States. The growing pressures of this competition on the United States economy intensified the perception that government cost cutting was a prime political requirement so that taxes and inflation could be reduced and the competitiveness of United States industry improved. These trends probably would have affected the administration's goals even if the White House incumbent were of the "mainstream," liberal, New Deal, Democratic lineage. But he was not; the mantle of that leadership was worn by Senator Edward Kennedy, for Carter did not have a history of congressional leadership against the Nixon assaults on the social welfare state as Kennedy did. Carter had been governor of Georgia and had won the presidential nomination as a relative unknown using unorthodox methods, and neither his advisers nor he had extensive experience with the national social welfare issues that had long held center stage in the concerns of Democratic administrations. He seemed on the one hand to perceive a need to cut health costs or at least reduce the rate of expansion of federal programs, and on the other hand to wish to be counted as a president who was continuing the Rooseveltian tradition of advancing social welfare programs, especially for the needy of society. The end product of these two conflicting pulls was an administration health services policy that was characterized by the attempt to appear compassionate but also, and first and foremost, fiscally prudent. He was perhaps the earliest major embodiment of what in the 1980s and 1990s was to be known as the "new Democrats."

Passage of truly comprehensive national health insurance, which would have lifted an albatross from the backs of local governments under pressure to provide a major volume of ambulatory general medical care in the face of depleted local funds, was put on the back burner, and a major federal shoring-up of state and local public health departments was never contemplated. Despite the Carter administration's declared support for public health, a substantial increase in expenditures for preventive and health promotion activities was not realized. In place of these measures, priorities for prevention, self care, and health maintenance were announced as policy. The only part of this enunciated policy that became de facto policy was the reorgani-

zation of the Center for Disease Control into the CDC centers, a relatively low-cost measure from which great improvements in health status were said to be expected.

The problems involved in strengthening and organizing state and local health agencies for effective implementation even of these enunciated priorities were largely ignored. It is unclear just what role, if any, the Carter administration envisioned for these entities. And the relative inattention to environmental protection activities compared with the proposed focus on changing personal health behavior was evident. All these reflected the general benign neglect by the Carter administration health policy toward maintaining and building the tripartite federal health system.

The Carter administration heavily promoted (i.e., emphatically "enunciated") a policy of federally supported health care for children that could be presented as a cautious opening wedge for national health insurance and which again was claimed to be a high-yield area in terms of cost/benefit ratio (see Chapter 10). Children's care was, on the whole, a relatively inexpensive component of general medical care, dealing as it does, largely in preventive measures, and the returns in terms of increased health in adult life might be expected to be relatively high; again, a prudent approach. But this enunciated policy did not become de facto policy; a major child health bill was never passed.

Finally, the Carter administration promoted organizational changes and increases in community mental health support that were claimed to hold promise for improved care. The passage of the Mental Health Systems Act (P.L. 96–398) in October 1980 was the culmination of administration efforts to improve the community mental health system, but it came just as the Carter administration was ending. The background and details of this issue are discussed in Chapter 6.

It appears that the central direction of the administration plan was to decrease the total outlay for health services, however. The increases for preventive, health promotion, and child health programs were to come from reductions in the more expensive federal medical care programs. Much, perhaps most, of President Carter's efforts in the medical care or "curative" health care field were directed to attempts to control costs in the Medicare and Medicaid programs, a record strongly reminiscent of the predecessor Nixon and Ford administrations.

In the context of the existing political climate featuring growing assaults on social programs, Carter's strong advocacy of disease prevention through personal health promotion and his neglect of national health insurance were seen by some as a one-sided overemphasis on personal responsibility for ill health. It was perceived by such persons as an attempt to "blame the victim" (Crawford, 1977) for his or her bad health, and thus divert attention from the prevailing lack of access to proper medical care and the administration's failure to grapple vigorously with polluters who were responsible for much if not most of the current burden of disease.

The administration positions were being articulated by Carter's Assistant Secretary for Health and Surgeon General (we recall that both positions were occupied by one person, Dr. Richmond). Supporting the administration position with respect to the relatively low importance of medical care as a determinant of population's health status were some writers, activists, and various public figures who argued that the most important determinants were indeed lifestyle and other forms of prevention.[29] Although the different authors in this camp did not all come to these views from the same direction, a number of basic themes run through their writings: access to modern medical care in developed countries, especially the United States, is a very small determinant of a population's health status; in fact, it even causes or exacerbates some illnesses ("iatrogenic" effects, see especially Illich, 1973); most illness is caused by personal behavior injurious to health and therefore changing such damaging behavior to health-enhancing behavior should be the fundamental aim of health services, especially public health programs.

This position was strongly opposed by others, including a number of liberal and labor figures. They did not argue that disease prevention through health-enhancing behavior was unimportant, but that for the present and for a long time to come, people will continue to get sick and when they do will need medical care. Poor people get sick more often and more seriously than others do (Hurley, 1971) and therefore need medical care more often, but they frequently do

not get it because they are socially and economically disadvantaged. Adherents of this position therefore distrusted voices that called for paying primary attention to inducing healthful behavior when the context in which it was presented implied a concomitant neglect of first assuring access to good medical care for all who need it. The access problem had to be solved, they argued, before real political support could be mustered behind personal prevention. Furthermore, liberals, labor, and some environmentalists took issue with the idea that most illness was now caused by individual failure to practice healthful behavior. It was due primarily, they asserted, to the effects of polluters and unhealthful working conditions (Epstein, 1976; Page and O'Brien, 1973; Brodeur, 1974) including the stress caused by unemployment. The controversy added to their distrust of those they perceived as one-sidedly concentrating on changing personal behavior.

Thus the Carter administration lost the support of medical care activists, of many environmental activists, and of many liberals and working people on the health question. He of course never had the support of conservatives, and his control of Congress eroded over the last two years of his term partially because of similar tactical approaches in areas other than health. Congress could come to no agreement on an appropriation bill for fiscal years 1980 and 1981, and the federal government existed entirely on continuing resolutions in these years.

It may fairly be said that funding support for public health did not increase substantially under Carter's stewardship despite his avowed commitment to expanding public health. In fact, considering inflation, it shrank. Carter's own budgets for FY 1980 and 1981 called for cuts in public health funds. The main contribution was the Surgeon General's leadership in beginning to define more specifically what a modern prevention program might look like. But the definition was not specific enough. The proposed new public health campaign did not include a plan or even an allusion to some sort of a national network of greatly strengthened state and local agencies to provide on-the-ground leadership throughout the land. Similarly, no plan for nationally enhancing environmental protection was presented. The failure to include this organizational structure in the plan allowed the proposal to stress prevention and health promotion to look relatively inexpensive on the budget and project an aura of prudence over Carter's public health policy. To have obtained funding resources for a nationwide network of agencies properly equipped to carry out the campaign would have required a level of political leadership that the administration lacked. Carter was too neoconservative for the mainline Democrats of the time and not conservative enough for the dominant Republicans. The lack of political support was reflected in the stalling of the advance toward health services for all during his incumbency.

The Reagan Administration's First Term

The Reagan administration took office in January of 1981 determined to slash all government social welfare programs to the greatest extent possible. In a new and more extreme form it was a resumption of the Nixon/Ford administration policy to reduce the outlays for these programs. The tactic of folding the categorical grants into block grants, cutting the total for the ''block,'' and turning the money over to the states for administration, unsuccessfully put forward under Ford, was reinstituted as de facto federal policy. Unlike the cuts Nixon had proposed, public health, rather than medical care, was now a primary target. This was foreshadowed by the composition of the Health Policy Task Force appointed to lay out policy for the incoming administration. It included representatives from the American Medical Association, American Hospital Association, American Dental Association, and the Pharmaceutical Manufacturers Association. There were none from the American Public Health Association. Most were practicing medical care providers and administrators, and social scientists with a strong leaning toward the use of conservative, neoclassical economic theory as the fundamental guide to health policy formation. There were no leaders of public health, either practitioners or theoreticians. The new president called for a severe cutback in federal support for public health, to be accomplished by discontinuing some programs, cutting appropriations for others, and folding as many as possible into ''blocks'' whose totals could be reduced without designating exactly which programs the state had to cut. Reagan originally hoped to consolidate all remaining federal money for public health given to the states into one block grant (later expanded to two).

The first major legislative achievement of the new administration was the Omnibus Budget Reconciliation Act of 1981 (OBRA), P.L. 97–35, passed on August 13, 1981. It was a global piece of legislation that contained in one bill both authorizations and appropriations through March 15, 1982, for a great many programs that had previously been separately considered. The result was that individual programs were given little or no detailed scrutiny and debate by Congress. The law was passed at the height of the new president's prestige and power and formed the basis for his actions on social programs for the remainder of his incumbency. It may be regarded as the administration's grand plan representing a planning document.

While the administration did not get its original budget request that twenty-six[30] programs be combined into two block grants for public health, it did succeed in getting twenty categorical programs combined into four block grants, with six programs remaining categorical. The block grants were set up as a new section of the Public Health Service Act, Title XIX.[31]

The authorization for the block grants was reduced some 21 percent from what it had been for the total individual programs folded into the respective blocks. After accounting for inflation, the actual reduction in resources was higher, coming to perhaps 30 percent. When one considers the simultaneous reduction in tax revenues available to states and localities because of the then-current (1982) recession and the state and local ''tax revolts'' of the late 1970s and early 1980s, it is clear that local and state public health services faced a severe financial shortfall bordering on crisis. An interesting commentary on the strong ideological component of the motivation for these reductions, over and above any cost-cutting aims, is provided by the folding in of the existing program for adolescent pregnancy into the Maternal and Child Health block grant, while a brand new categorical program called ''Adolescent Family Life'' was authorized at $30 million per year for three years. The folded-in adolescent program had permitted abortion as an optional service, if the grantee agency wanted to offer it, as well as freely dispensed information on contraception. The new Adolescent Family Life program restricted eligibility for grants to those centers that did not counsel or provide abortion and that stressed sexual abstinence as the principal method of preventing pregnancy.

During the formulation of the FY 1983 budget, political jockeying continued between the president and his supporters in Congress on one side and his opponents in Congress on the other. The president's budget proposals for 1983 called for a further reduction in federal grants for public health, to be accomplished by further folding in of remaining categorical grants into blocks and reducing their totals. In his State of the Union Address, the president also called for turning over the administration of forty-three federal programs, or the block grants containing them, entirely to the states by 1984 and giving them the choice of continuing or discontinuing them. Included in these were preventive health and health services block grant; alcohol, drug abuse, and mental health block grant; family planning; migrant health centers; black lung disease clinics; and the Women, Infants and Children (WIC) nutrition program (McGraw Hill, Feb. 1 1982). Family planning, migrant health centers, and black-lung clinics were to be added to the primary care block grants and WIC to the MCH block grant.[32] But the congressional atmosphere of a stampede to approve Reagan's proposals that prevailed during the 1982 budget considerations in 1981 had subsided considerably, and the request for further cuts met with substantial opposition in Congress. By the middle of 1982 Congress was attempting to write its own budget instead of merely waiting for the president's budget and largely approving it.

The Reagan program was seen as a basic reversal in federal policy with respect to the national cooperative system (Palmer and Sawhill, 1982, 10–11). The reversal applied to all three policy levels, de facto, de jure, and certainly enunciated. What were its essential features and implications for public health in the United States? First, it enunciated a call for an end to many federal grants to the states and especially localities for social programs, including public health services. During a transition period money would be given to the states for public health and ambulatory care services on a block grant basis with no categorical restrictions on how it was to be spent by program. Federal regulation was to be minimal. Second, direct federal health activities would be limited to a few programs, such as research, that were seen to be clearly national in character. Environmental protection activities would be sharply reduced. Third, federal income taxes would be substantially reduced so that persons would have more disposable income available and find it easier to vote more state or local taxes if they wanted particular public health programs.

Supporters of this program argued that the federal government had become too large and its influence too pervasive on state and local health activities (as well as other social program activities, of course). Local requirements and needs are not well determined in distant Washington and therefore decisions on priorities should be made locally. The amount of federal regulation that had developed had made most programs inefficient; they were top-heavy with administrative personnel and procedures and stifled innovation and operational efficiency. Many of the environmental and workplace protections were extreme and hurt the growth of the economy, a sine qua non for the nation's welfare. Furthermore, many programs had not achieved their purposes. The basic and almost the only solution to the problem of maintaining and improving the well-being of the American public was to give private industry unfettered liberty to expand the scope of its activities, including that of surveillance of health services. The mechanisms of the marketplace would see to it that industry served the American people in the best manner. Only if our private economy prospered would there be employment for all who can work, enabling people to pay for the personal and environmental health services they need and want. They will vote the local and state taxes to accomplish the public health objectives they perceive to be important to their local circumstances. Private philanthropy and minimal government "safety net" programs will provide needed services for that irreducible minimum number of persons who cannot earn enough to pay for them because of illness or old age and who are not able to provide for these contingencies through privately arranged insurance and pension plans. Not only will people be better provided for, but the services they receive will be better and more efficiently delivered because they will be subject to the rigors of the marketplace and to effective local control. The severity of environmental regulation will similarly be properly balanced with its effect on the local economy. In short, the federal role in health (and other social programs) had ballooned out of all due proportion because of the mistaken philosophy of "big government." The air must now be let of the balloon.

Opponents of the Reagan program included many who had personally lived through or studied the history of the development of the federal system of grants and environmental protections. Their opposition was based on their reading of the lessons to be drawn from the experience of that period. Many of them looked on in disbelief as attempts to dismantle this system continued under a rationale that assumed that the states and localities could do the job better without federal money or supervision. They argued that the history of the development of the American economy from a local to a regional and national one was inexorable, not the product of capricious ideology. Some of this development has been outlined in previous chapters, but we recall here that it led to a centralization of tax revenue in the federal government while the responsibility for public health services remained with the states and localities. This contradiction, in turn, led to ever-growing disparities between needs and available tax bases among states and among localities within states. A growing consensus in America had held that all persons, especially children and youth, should have equal or as nearly equal opportunity as possible to develop their potential (Tobin, 1981), regardless of the state or locality in which they happened to have been born or reared. To accomplish this had required either that programs be entirely federally run or that federal money be redistributed among states and localities according to measures of need.

Such opponents also pointed to the fact that the American corporate system was rapidly consolidating and centralizing its control into fewer and larger centers with ever wider geographic networks and more centralized command and

that therefore the governmental organization required to protect the public interest needed to respond with control over increasingly wider jurisdictions. In the public health field, for example, the emergence of many of the chronic and degenerative diseases as leading health threats pointed to nationwide causation and the need for nationwide prevention measures. Local agencies could not act effectively to control the activities of national and international combines. Returning environmental controls to the states, for example, could trigger a scramble among the states to offer the least environmental control possible in an effort to attract national industry to their states. Reaganism's opponents, for the most part, did not uniformly advocate complete control and administration from Washington. Rather the idea of most of them was to have as much local administration as possible, but with goals and aims coordinated on a national basis, which was the central idea informing the formation of the federal tri-partite "partnership" system in the first place.

Finally, critics argued, this system had grown in a typically "American" way, that is, pragmatically; it developed as a series of responses to problems that were empirically found to exist. The Reagan program, by contrast, was based on an abstract ultra-right ideology that had never been tried and consisted merely of a set of assertions stemming from theoretical assumptions about the functioning of a hypothetical construct called "the market," based on the simple early capitalism of Adam Smith's time. In other words, the growth of federal leadership in the health field was not instigated by a philosophical desire for "big government"; it was a measured response to the transition of the entrepreneurial organization to "big business."

An important part of the conflict involved the question of the relative roles of the federal government and those of the states in setting health policy and administering health programs. The opponents of the Reagan approach argued that too large a measure of state and local control cannot produce sufficient uniformity to provide equal opportunity for citizens across the country, not only because of state and local disparities in the resources-to-need ratio, but also because of differences in political outlook of the dominant groups in different places. An underlying enunciated goal of the Reagan program, on the other hand, was to enable the states and localities to use federal funds to support only those public health programs that their governing bodies found desirable.

A final question is: How was the Reagan "new federalism" actually implemented during the first term and what were its prospects? A major study found that by 1982 states and localities were reporting that the program had created great fiscal stress for them and that needed services had to be cut back (Palmer and Sawhill, 1982). However, a central tenet of the Reagan programs was that its sharp cuts in federal income taxes would make needed capital available to business for growth and thereby make additional tax revenues available to local and state governments to operate those programs transferred from the federal government that their citizenry favored. Large federal tax cuts did indeed take place, but the expected large increases in tax revenue did not materialize. The very large defense expenditures of the Reagan administration greatly exacerbated the federal deficit and an economic recession, stemming partly from government monetary policy, helped keep real interest rates high and reduce the states' income tax and sales tax revenues. This decreased their abilities even to continue past programs, not to speak of taking on additional expenditures for public health (and other) programs newly transferred with reduced federal contributions from federal sponsorship. Furthermore, many states passed "Proposition 13"-type laws strongly restricting local government taxes, especially local property taxes, the former mainstay of local public health services financing. The previously cited 1982 study by the Urban Institute stated:

Thus far the consequences of the 1981–1982 recession have far out-weighed the impact on individual or family income of the tax reduction, the defense build-up and the domestic budget cuts. By mid-1982 civilian employment and real hourly earnings were no higher than those they had been in 1980, and the unemployment rate had risen by more than two percentage points. After adjustment for inflation, median family income declined by 3.5 percent in 1981. And the incidence of poverty increased from 13.2 percent in 1980 to 14.0 percent in 1981, its highest level since 1967.

The recession also has severely restricted the ability of state and local governments to pay for current services (Palmer and Sawhill, 1982, 19–20).

The recession was mitigated in mid-1983 and during all of 1984. Although the recovery was not quite the boom that Reagan supporters characterized it, many parts of the economy did return to pre-1981 levels as increased defense expenditures percolated through the system. Furthermore, the relatively high interest rates and the large credit needs of the federal government to meet the huge budget deficits induced a flow of foreign investment to the United States. With this flow came a great appreciation of the United States dollar relative to foreign currency, helping foreign-made goods sell cheaply on the United States market and contributing to the maintenance of a relatively low rate of inflation, even after the economy climbed out of its depressed state back to the Carter administration levels. The combination of a rising economy, especially the fuller employment, and modest inflation helped local and especially state revenues. Many states began to show a surplus and were thereby able to reduce the effects of the Reagan cuts and local property tax reductions.[33]

The Reagan administration continued to demand federal program elimination and reduction and although the Democratic House resisted many of them, the resulting compromises all brought about further reductions in federally supported public health programs. The reelection of Reagan in 1984 by an overwhelming majority was followed by even more determined attempts to eliminate health programs as federal responsibilities.

DIRECT FEDERAL GOVERNMENT PUBLIC HEALTH ACTIVITIES: NATIONAL CONSUMER, ENVIRONMENTAL, AND WORKPLACE PROTECTION

This chapter has thus far been given over to a discussion of the federal role in developing and guiding the direction of the *federal* (i.e. "cooperative") system of state and local public health departments—which was de facto national government policy from 1935 until 1980. In addition to these public health activities carried out by the national network consisting of the states and localities with significant funding and guidance from the federal government, the latter has also been operating certain nationwide public health activities directly. In these activities policy formation and operational decisions are more explicitly centralized in the federal government. This section of the chapter is concerned with these directly operated federal public health programs.

There are many such programs; a reasonably complete list can be obtained by consulting Hanlon (1969) and Wilson and Neuhauser (1982). I deal here only with the food and drug regulation, environmental protection, and occupational health protection activities because they provide examples of public health functions that once could be carried out adequately by state and local health agencies, but in time were found to require direct federal administration to deal with the centralizing tendencies of the sectors of the American economy that these public health activities were required to regulate. While each of these direct national activities utilize state and sometimes local agencies to some degree, they have not developed into programs whose major activities are carried out via the federal-state-local general public health network described in Chapters 2 and 3 and in the preceding portion of this chapter. State agencies that participate in direct national programs as "lead agencies" with federal grants and supervision tend more often to be specialist agencies in environmental health, pharmaceutical safety regulation, or occupational health rather than the general state health agency. Therefore, even though intergovernmental arrangements do exist to perform these three types of functions, it clarifies matters to identify these public health activities separately as being carried out directly by the federal government in contrast to those previously discussed that have been administered under a federal partnership system of public health agencies.

The Food and Drug Administration

The main responsibilities of the Food and Drug Administration (FDA) are to monitor the purity, standard potency, and accurate labeling of substances that, in addition to food, include pharmaceuticals, drugs, cosmetics, and poisons. It is the principal consumer-protection agency of the federal government.

Local public health departments had for years been monitoring drinking water, milk and milk products, and other types of food sold in their jurisdictions for purity in terms of freedom from disease-causing microorganisms and chemicals. But the need for a national agency to assure the proper labeling of food and drugs was becoming evident toward the end of the 1800s. Again, the steady development of ever larger, more centralized, and more technologically advanced industries was making the control problem a national one. Not only were more foods and drugs being purchased and distributed nationally, but the ability to analyze the contents, safety, and potency of new food and especially new drug products required ever-increasing sophistication from laboratories and testing facilities. With the rise of the U.S. reform movement during the years 1890 through about 1915, much of the "muckraking" literature that protested the reckless manner in which American industry was developing was directed at the health-endangering impurities introduced into foods as part of processing procedures. The political activity around this issue culminated in the passage of the Food and Drug Act in 1906, during Theodore Roosevelt's presidency. The original legal justification for legislating federal authority to regulate food and drugs was the interstate nature of much of the commerce in these items. The act prohibited the manufacture and sale of impure or mislabeled food and was administered by the Bureau of Chemistry of the Department of Agriculture. In 1927 the Food, Drug and Insecticide Administration was established, replacing the Bureau of Chemistry in the Department of Agriculture, and in 1931 its name was simplified to the present one of the Food and Drug Administration. In 1940 it was transferred to the Federal Security Agency, but inspection of meat and poultry remained with the Department of Agriculture, a division of function that continues to complicate enforcement to the present day. When the Federal Security Agency was transferred to the newly formed Department of Health, Education and Welfare in 1953, the Food and Drug Administration went with it.

After 1906 more acts dealing with pure food and drugs were passed and given to the FDA (or its successor agencies) to administer. The scope of substances covered was constantly expanded, as was the scope of criteria to be monitored. Prominent among the foods specifically addressed were meats (including meat inspection until 1940), butter, canned foods, and seafood. The expanded criteria included the specification of correct weights, proper packaging, and correct specification of contents. The first formulation of the present form of the act was passed as the Federal Food, Drug and Cosmetic Act in 1938, and thereafter standards for both food and pharmaceuticals multiplied rapidly. With respect to pharmaceuticals, the law provided that the FDA must approve a New Drug Application (NDA) before the new drug could be marketed. The company had to report results of animal and human research to indicate the safety of the drug. A ''package insert'' giving complete information on the contents of the drug was required to accompany every container of the pharmaceutical sold. The FDA was to determine whether a drug could be sold over the counter (OTC) or only by prescription, and it regulated advertising for prescription drugs. (Over-the-counter drugs are regulated by the Federal Trade Commission.)

Major amendments were made to the law in 1962. These required that a drug must be demonstrated to be effective as well as safe to be approved. It established many ''human subjects'' protection measures for testing drugs on humans, leading to some complaints about the length of time needed to get approval for a new, effective drug. With the passage of the 1962 amendments requiring effectiveness as well as safety for new drug approval, some 2,500 prescription drugs that had been approved as safe between 1939 and 1962 were reevaluated for effectiveness by National Academy of Sciences/ National Research Council review panels, resulting in the withdrawal of a number of these drugs. (Over-the-counter drugs were separately reviewed by a similar review process.)

States also engage in food control activities, which they have sometimes placed in their agriculture departments (twenty-three states in 1973), sometimes in their departments of health (forty-three states in 1973), and sometimes in other departments (four states in 1973). In some states the function has been shared by more than one department, as it has been in the federal government (Hanlon, 1974). As has been noted, there is no formal federal-state-local network corresponding to that for other public health activities previously discussed.

There is also considerable state regulation of the pharmaceutical industry, but it is confined primarily to regulation of retail trade and wholesale distribution. Pharmacies are regulated with respect to the right to substitute a cheaper equivalent (''generic'') drug for that prescribed, and pharmacists must be state licensed. Thus, both in the case of food and of drugs, the federal government concerns itself mainly, but not exclusively, with conditions of manufacture and distribution, while states concern themselves mainly with conditions in retail establishments and wholesale distribution. This division of authority coincides broadly with the division of power among states and the federal government assigned by the Constitution because the distribution by manufacturers is generally interstate, and wholesale distribution to retailers and retail trade has been largely an intrastate concern.

The Environmental Protection Agency

The role of the federal government in environmental protection grew most rapidly during the years 1965–1973, spanning the administrations of two presidents, Johnson, and Nixon. It was noted in previous chapters that the steadily accelerating pace of environmental pollution and resource depletion was generating problems that were transcending the boundaries of local jurisdictions. They were steadily becoming regionwide, nationwide, and even worldwide problems, and were rarely amenable to a strictly local solution and often not even to a statewide solution. The heightened national awareness of the extent of the environmental degradation, aided by a growing organized environmental protection movement, led to the creation of a special federal agency for environmental protection, the EPA, in 1970. Many environmentalists, and their associations, as I have noted, were interested in preserving the natural environment for its own sake, not only for health reasons. They were also motivated by considerations of aesthetic, religious, and other feelings of humanity's oneness with nature and the general importance of the environment to pleasant living. The official governmental public health agencies had generally not allied themselves strongly with these forces because of the agencies' concentrated focus on immediate health threats. This contributed to the centering of federal environmental protection in specialized environmental agencies rather than in the broader spectrum general public health agencies.

Many federal Acts dealing with environmental health were passed in piecemeal fashion before 1970, beginning in about 1948. They concerned four main areas of control:

1. *Water pollution control* Under this caption are the 1948 and 1956 Water Pollution Control Acts, the 1965 Water Control Act, the 1966 Clean Water Restoration Act, and the 1970 Water Quality Improvement Act. These laws included such provisions as setting of standards; regulation of oil and vessel pollution by enforcement and information diffusion procedures such as conferences, hearings, and court action; *transfer of program control* from the U.S. Public Health Service to the federal Water Pollution Control Administration in 1965; and federal construction and improvement grants. The transfer of control from the national public health agency to a specialized technical agency located in the office of the president is of particular interest in the light of my previous discussions of the issues involved in choosing between a health agency and a specialized technical one for health-related environmental functions.

2. *Air pollution control* A number of fatal smog "epidemics" brought to national attention the health threat from air polluted by emissions from industrial plants and motor vehicles. Among these incidents were one occurring in the Meuse Valley of Belgium in 1930 in which thousands of people died from exposure to a mixture of industrial fumes and fog over four days; one in Donora, Pennsylvania, in 1948, in which 20 persons died and 14,000 became ill; the Poza Rica, Mexico, incident in 1950 in which 320 persons were hospitalized of whom 20 died; the Los Angeles smog of 1950; and the London "killer" smog of 1963 in which 700 persons died. The national legislation to mitigate air pollution included the first federal air pollution legislation passed in 1955; the 1963 Clean Air Act; the 1967 Clean Air Act and Amendments of 1967, which established nationwide clean air quality standards and set exhaust emission standards; and motor vehicle controls, enacted in 1968.

3. *Solid waste control* The 1965 Solid Waste Disposal Act and the 1970 Resources Recovery Act.

4. *Noise Control* The Noise Pollution and Abatement Act of 1970.

These laws were aimed largely at protecting the public's health against the environmental hazards, but they were broader in concept and geographic jurisdiction than the ordinances that local health departments had been enforcing for over a century. The national laws were directed at preserving the environment itself—the atmosphere, rivers, forests, plants and animals (biota)—even if the threats to the public's health were not immediate. Of course, abatement of all environmental damage that did pose immediate health threats were included in the aims of these overall environmental protection acts, and, as I have noted, the supportive constituency for these environmental acts was not identical with that of public health although there was overlap between the two.

The professionals who administered these acts were technically trained in controlling the environmental media: water, air, solid wastes, and biota (see Chapter 3). They worked mostly in agencies dedicated to these media-centered programs, and some environmental leaders had been deploring the media-centered approach of the legislation described above. They called for an integrated, cross-media approach to environmental protection. (See Rabe, 1986, 1987, for example.)

A Task Force on Environmental Health and Related Problems was convened in June 1967 after five two-day conferences during 1966–67 at which about 100 persons testified. Also, 100 experts had held informal meetings with the task force staff. Two actions resulted from this conference. One was a call for a White House conference on financing local government efforts at environmental action. The other was the issuance of recommendations, chief among which was a statement of ten goals, including restoration of air quality by controlling emissions into the air; mounting an effort to improve water quality, especially that of drinking water; improvement of waste disposal methods; careful monitoring of the effects on populations of environmental degradations; urban improvement; consumer protection; protection from radiation effects; and protection from occupational disease.

Some three years after this conference Congress passed the National Environmental Policy Act (NEPA) of 1970, which established "the environmental impact statement (EIS) as a fundamental tool for environmental regulation" (Rabe, 1986, 8) by federal agencies. The big policy question in this type of control centered on the implications of the choices that had to be made between protectiong health and the environment on the one hand, and creating impediments to the most economically efficient organization of industry on the other. These alternatives involved such choices as those between minimizing atomic radiation hazards versus promoting nuclear power, the health dangers of smoking versus the needs of the tobacco industry, and high farm yields versus the health dangers of using strong pesticides. The act also established a Council on Environmental Quality (CEQ) to oversee and coordinate all environmental efforts of the federal government" and urged all federal agencies to approach environmental protection in an interdisciplinary fashion (Rabe, 1986, 8). In December of the same year the Environmental Protection Agency was created by President Nixon to integrate the environmental activities of the federal government, including those under the earlier legislation previously described.[34]

The Occupational Safety and Health Act of 1970

A substantial part of the increased public consciousness about the new environmental threats dealt with health and safety in the workplace. We recall that one of the findings of the Mountin report of 1946 was that although the main effect of Social Security Act funds for public health had been to enrich existing types of programs rather than add new ones, one new program that had indeed been added by many state health departments during the period 1936–1946 was oc-

cupational safety. The issue had been strongly pressed by trade unions and brought to the fore by the operation of workers' compensation laws. Beginning with the 1950s the issues quickly became more complicated as the developing technology of the second industrial revolution introduced new hazards into the workplace whose effects were not easy to identify clearly and diseases whose causation could not easily be attributed to conditions of the workplace. Occupational *safety* dealt with avoiding injuries that were, for the most part, clearly attributable to the workplace. The new hazards were from occupational *health* hazards whose effects often only became evident years after exposure. It was increasingly being found that a "surprising" proportion of disease was occupationally caused.[35] The increased number of workplace accidents due to safety hazards was also becoming clearer as the reported injury rate in industry rose. The National Safety Council estimated 14,000 deaths due to accidents on the job and millions of disabling injuries for 1970. But the incidence of occupationally caused disease was much harder to identify. These occupational health hazards

typically include toxic and carcinogenic chemicals and dusts, often in combination with noise, heat, and other forms of stress. Other health hazards include physical and biological agents. The interaction of health hazards and the human organism can occur either through the senses, by absorption through the skin, by intake into the digestive tract via the mouth, or by inhalation into the lungs. [They can cause] respiratory disease, heart disease, cancer, neurological disorder, systemic poisoning or a shortening of life expectancy due to general physiological deterioration. The disease or sickness can be acute or chronic, can require a long latency period even if the original exposure is brief, and can be difficult or impossible to diagnose early or with certainty. . . .

Unlike safety hazards, the effects of health hazards may be slow, cumulative, irreversible, and complicated by nonoccupational factors . . . it is often difficult to perceive the severity or imminent danger contained in a brief exposure to a potential carcinogen that can take years to cause a tumor or death (Ashford, 1975).

The legislative response to the rising consciousness of these dangers was the Occupational Safety and Health Act (OSHAct) of 1970 (P.L. 91–596). It established the Occupational

Safety and Health Administration in the Department of Labor, the National Institute for Occupational Safety and Health (NIOSH) in the Department of Health, Education and Welfare, and a National Advisory Committee on Occupational Safety and Health (NACOSH).

The Occupational Safety and Health Administration (OSHA)

The law required nearly all employers to offer a place of employment "free from recognized hazards." All employers were required to comply with standards promulgated and enforced by OSHA, which was given "the authority to enter any workplace without advance notice and to propose penalties upon discovery of violations." Employees and their representatives were given the right to request an OSHA inspection anonymously and to accompany inspectors on their tour of inspection. States were permitted to operate their own programs if they could show them to be at least as effective as the national program. The law also established the Occupational Safety and Health Review Commission to rule on all enforcement actions of OSHA, with the decisions being court reviewable under certain circumstances.

The 1975 Ashford analysis of the effects of the OSHAct indicated that it had "had little measurable impact in reducing injuries and deaths, and the problems in the health area have become even more serious since 1970." The reasons for this slow progress were given as too few inspectors to monitor compliance; continuing opposition and noncompliance by employers; continuing emphasis on safety hazards and neglect of many serious health hazards; insufficiently severe penalties for infractions; difficulty in establishing an adequate data base; difficulty in establishing the levels of exposure that led to disease, especially if the result were long delayed; and the option for states to establish their own programs, thus diluting the effectiveness of the national system.

The appointment in 1977 of Dr. Eula Bingham as head of OSHA under the Carter administration provided the agency with a strong and knowledgeable administrator. She established a reputation for vigorous attempts to enforce the intent of the law in the face of continued opposition by employers, adversarial White House economists, and adverse court decisions that struck down some OSHA standards for toxic substances and carcinogens like benzene, on the grounds of inadequacy of knowledge about the levels of a particular substance that are necessary to cause disease. Despite these obstacles, a number of advances were made during these years, such as establishing standards for the hazardous agricultural pesticide DBCP (Last, 1980, 742) and some other substances.

Under the Reagan administration, cutbacks were made in the agencies' resources and activities. Thorne Auchter became head of OSHA, and his activities concentrated on attempting to repeal or stay the enforcement of standards.

The National Institute for Occupational Safety and Health (NIOSH)

NIOSH[36] was to be a research institute that would develop health and safety standards for the operating field agency, OSHA. It was to use its research resources "to publish a list of all known toxic substances and the concentrations at which these substances exhibit toxicity effects." Established within the Department of Health, Education, and Welfare, it was administratively part of the department's Center for Disease Control. NIOSH was designated as the main federal agency for research in the national effort to eliminate on-the-job hazards to the health and safety of America's workers; it was given the responsibility for identifying occupational safety and health hazards and for recommending changes in the regulations controlling them. It also was assigned obligations for training occupational health personnel. NIOSH not only fulfilled HEW's (later HHS's) research responsibilities under the Occupational Safety and Health Act, but also conducted the health program provided by the Federal Coal Mine Health and Safety Act of 1969 (P.L. 91–173). Its recommendations for new occupational safety and health standards were to be transmitted to the Department of Labor, which had the responsibility for setting, promulgating, and enforcing the standards. In the case of the federal Coal Mine Health and Safety Act, NIOSH was to recommend health standards to the Department of the Interior, which had the enforcement responsibilities under that law.

The institute's main research laboratories were established in Cincinnati, Ohio, where studies included not only the effects of exposure to existing general work environments and to hazardous substances used in the workplace, but also the psychological, motivational, and behavioral factors involved in occupational safety and health. Much of the institute's research focused on specific hazards; substances such as asbestos, beryllium, carbon monoxide, lead, and mercury, and conditions like noise, and heat stress. At NIOSH's Appalachian Center for Occupational Safety and Health in Morgantown, West Virginia, the research focus was on coal workers' pneumoconiosis, black-lung disease, and other occupational respiratory diseases. Thousands of coal miners were given X-ray and medical examinations as part of NIOSH's research on the incidence and prevalence of black-lung disease. Also located there was NIOSH's Testing and Certification Laboratory, which evaluates and certifies the performance of workers' personal safety equipment and instrumentation for measuring environmental contaminants. NIOSH's Western Area Occupational Health Laboratory, in Salt Lake City, has primarily studied the hazards of uranium mining and provided technical assistance to western states. This laboratory also provided chemical analyses and calibrated instruments for Department of Labor officers in the field, services also provided by the Cincinnati laboratories.

There has been a severe national shortage of occupational safety and health professionals. The Occupational Safety and Health Act required NIOSH to conduct "education programs to provide an adequate supply of qualified personnel to carry out the purposes of this Act. . . ." To do this, NIOSH has offered a spectrum of courses for upgrading the knowledge and skills of present occupational health practitioners. These short training courses, conducted at the Cincinnati laboratories and at other sites across the nation, helped to provide the qualified personnel needed to deal with the problems of occupational safety and health. NIOSH also has maintained staff in ten regional offices throughout the United States. These have been focal points for special surveys, evaluations of existing occupational hazards, and consultative services to the states.

Accidents

In 1978, accidents were the fourth leading cause of death, with a crude death rate of 48.4 per 100,000 persons, following deaths from diseases of the heart (334.3 rate), malignancies (181.9), and cerebral-vascular diseases (80.5) (U.S. Department of Commerce, 1981, table 113). About half the total death rate from accidents was due to motor vehicles (24.0); falls accounted for 6.3, drowning 2.7, industrial accidents 2.4, fire 2.8, accidental poisoning 2.2, and the remainder for 2.2. Injury and disability rates caused by accidents are very much higher, of course, than the death rates. In 1979, 69.1 million persons were injured, or 32.0 per 100.

A number of issues important to public health are highlighted by these figures. The death rate from industrial accidents of 2.4 per 100,000 represented some 5,200 deaths out of a total of 106,000 deaths (less than 5 percent) from accidents recorded for 1978. While this figure is certainly too high, it would seem that mortality from industrial accidents is not a leading cause of death overall, nor is it one of the more important contributors to the death rate from accidents. On the other hand, the crude death rate per 100,000 persons from malignancies was 181.9 in 1978 compared with 149.2 in 1960, a 22 percent increase. When adjusted for age the rate of increase is much smaller—the 125.8 age-adjusted death rate of 1960 increased to 133.8 in 1978, a rise of only 6 percent, but nonetheless a nontrivial one.[37] Many of the occupational *health* hazards are suspected to be carcinogenic in nature, and these figures may be more important indicators of the main workplace danger than the accident data are.

The most important cause of *death* from accidents is clearly related to motor vehicle accidents, but they are not the most important cause of *injury*. Of the 69.1 million persons injured in 1979, only 5.0 million (7.2 percent) injuries were due to motor vehicles whereas 24.7 million (35.8 percent) occurred at home, 12.0 million (17.4 percent) occurred at work, and 30.1 million (43.6 percent) in other locations. Thus home accidents constitute the greatest number of injuries, but motor vehicles are the leading cause of fatal injuries, and while workplace accidents accounted for only 5 percent of the deaths from accidents, they accounted for 17.4 percent of the injuries. A running battle between the federal government and the automobile manufacturers took place after about 1970 with respect to mandatory installation of automated or passive restraints in new automobiles. The battle was carried forward in the courts all through the Reagan incumbency despite the generally hostile attitude of his administration toward mandatory regulations.

Public Health Service to the American Indians

The United States Public Health Service has been providing sanitation and other community preventive services to American Indians through the Indian Health Service, an agency of the Department of Health and Human Services. These are discussed in Chapter 5 where the activities of the Indian Health Service are considered.

REORGANIZATIONS OF THE FEDERAL PUBLIC HEALTH AGENCY

In the discussions in Chapters 2, 3, and the preceding part of this chapter there have been intermittent references to reorganizations in federal government structure reflecting changes in programs, and sometimes policies, of different administrations affecting the public health structure. It may therefore be useful to briefly outline some of the principal reorganizations at this point.

The federal cabinet departments are each headed by a Secretary, appointed by the President with the advice and consent of the Senate. The first Secretaries appointed were for State, Treasury, and War. There are now fourteen cabinet departments. Until 1953 the United States government had no Departments or Secretaries of social welfare services; in particular, there were no Departments or Secretaries of health, education, or welfare, because such functions had long been envisioned as being relegated by the Constitution to the states under their police powers. When changing conditions resulted in

some health functions being assigned to the federal government, there was, consequently, no national cabinet department of health available in which to place the administration of health programs legislated by Congress. (The same was true of other social welfare programs.) The administration of these federal health functions was accordingly placed in other departments, the choice being determined by various historical happenstances that led Congressional sponsors of the health laws to feel that one or another existing agency was a logical place to put the new function. For example, the Public Health Service (and its antecedent agencies) was placed in the Treasury Department; the Children's Bureau, originally in the Labor Department; and the antecedent to the Food and Drug Administration in the Agriculture Department. In some cases, the politics of creating a new administrative agency were such that no existing cabinet department was deemed an appropriate home for it; then it was made a bureau or other subdivision within the Office of the President, as the group of administrative assistants to the President and their staffs was collectively called. The Social Security Board, created in 1935 to administer the Social Security Act, is an example of this type of arrangement.

During the years 1935 through 1939 of the Roosevelt New Deal period, a large number of social program agencies were created and some existing ones were expanded. The need for new cabinet departments dealing with social program areas was being advocated, and as an interim step the overall administration of a number of disparate social welfare programs was combined into a newly created Federal Security Agency (FSA) in 1939. Among the agencies included under the FSA authority were the Social Security Board and the United States Office of Education. The FSA was an "independent" agency—that is, it did not reside in any of the established cabinet departments—and it served as the umbrella agency for many federal social programs. In 1944 the United States Public Health Service was also transferred to the FSA from the Treasury Department, where it had resided since 1898 (when it was called the United States Marine Hospital Service). With this transfer, the section of the Social Security Act dealing with general public health grants (Title VI) was moved to the newly created Public Health Service Act, which was added to the United States Code (USC) to codify the health laws under a health title. Finally, in 1953 the cabinet department of Health, Education and Welfare (HEW) was formed, absorbing the entire independent FSA, the Children's Bureau from the Labor Department, and most remaining other agencies dealing with social welfare areas. Each of the three major subdivisions of the new department was almost a subdepartment with its own assistant secretary (one each for health, education, and welfare). In 1981 the education component of HEW was organized into a separate cabinet department of education and the remainder was renamed the Department of Health and Human Services (HHS), comprising the health and welfare ("human services") functions of the previous HEW in one cabinet department. Subsequently there was some advocacy for a separate department of health but this suggestion never materialized. The advocacy seems to have been coming from organized medicine. Figures 4–5 and 4–6 are visual representations of the organization of HEW modeled after one of the major organizations taken from Wilson and Newhauser (1982) which provides organizational charts that illustrate the changing structure of the federal cabinet department containing the health agencies after several significant reorganizations.

The reorganizations affected not only the high-level staffing of complete agencies, but also rearrangement of many of the offices, bureaus, divisions, and other subdivisions. Many of these also dealt with the federal government's medical care functions and are discussed in the chapters that follow. Principal among those involving public health functions were periodic rearrangements of the Public Health Service reflecting various contending views about the proper scope of function of the service.

SUMMARY AND COMMENTS: WHERE DO WE STAND?

Given the background and development of public health in the United States described here, what may be said about its future direction? Af-

ter almost fifty years of progress in one general direction, albeit with many minor zigs and zags, a reversal of "cooperative federalism" was attempted by the Nixon/Ford administrations and strongly pushed with some success in implementation by the Reagan administration. The direction established in 1935 for the support of state and local public health work was labeled inappropriate for today by the Reagan administration and reversal was its key word. The Urban Institute's study of the first two years of the "Reagan experiment" put it well:

The [Reagan] administration has endorsed a special interpretation of the federal government's past relations with the state-local and nonprofit sectors. This interpretation holds that the federal government has improperly supplanted—"usurped" is the term sometimes used—the roles of both lower levels of governmental and nonprofit organizations. . . . Viewing the federal government as in competition with other organized associations is a distinctly conservative perspective. It contrasts with the cooperative model of federal relations. The ties to the federal government that the president condemns were developed in the belief that they fostered a constructive partnership between Washington and the States and localities. . . . Eliminating this "cooperative federalism" is a fundamental and controversial element of the Reagan experiment (Palmer and Sawhill, 1982, 10).

Pursuing this notion a bit further, the opposing view to the Reagan "experiment" holds that there were compelling historical reasons why with respect to public health at least, local government should have been involved first, state government later, and federal government last. The reasons have become, if anything, more cogent over time, and attempts to devolve basic control of public health policy down to the localities and states are doomed to harmful failure. The main features of the long-run direction of government public health policy will be decided less by the ideologically based intent of politicians than by the imperatives of political, social, and economic developments in the United States and how they affect the public health. Because the assumptions on which the arguments for reversal are based run counter to the objective facts of this development, it is difficult to see how it can be continued indefinitely without grave damage to our society's well-being.

The United States economy continues to

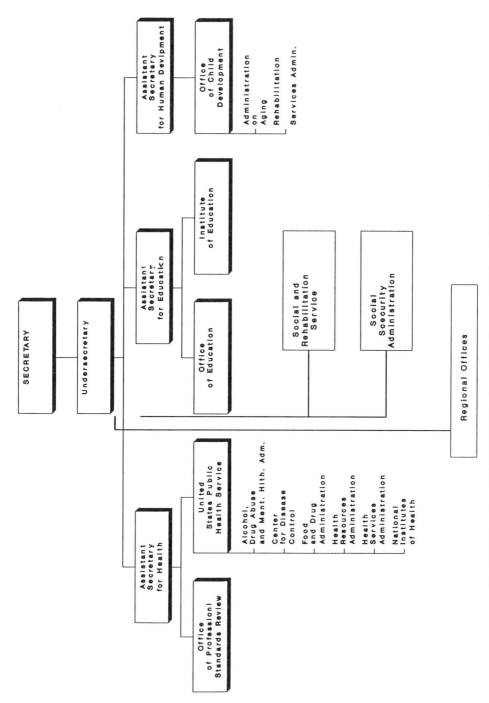

Fig. 4-5. Department of Health, Education and Welfare organization, 1976. *Note:* This is an abbreviated chart. There are additional entitites not shown. *Source:* Wilson and Neuhauser (1982).

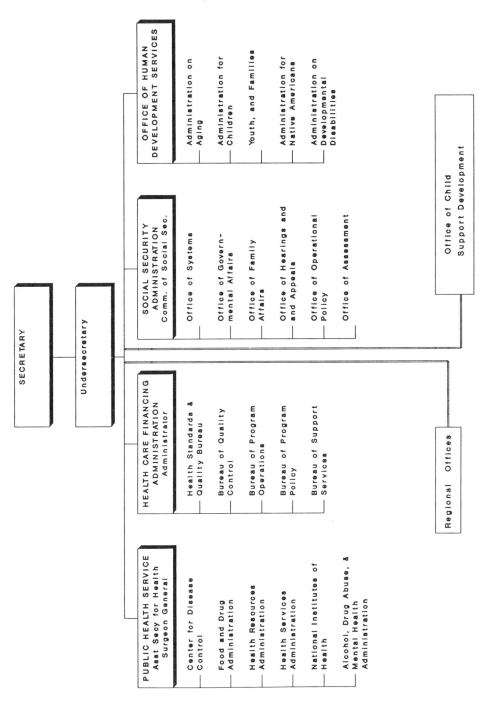

Fig. 4–6. Department of Health and Human Services organization, 1981. *Note:* This is an abbreviated chart. There are additional entitites not shown. *Source:* Wilson and Neuhauser (1982).

move ever more rapidly in the direction of using workplace processes that place additional stress on employees' health and materials that increasingly consist of man-made substances of unknown virulence and destructive power. The sociological results of the rapid organizational changes in the economy include such phenomena as increased occupational mobility of populations (both geographically and across changing occupations), increased introduction of new environmental health hazards that affect regions and even the entire country, and increased ravages upon body and psyche of stress and uncertainty. None of these are handled well by overly autonomous local and state efforts. The combination of national standard setting and financing with state and local service delivery and administration, a direction in which we had been moving, seems to be more than ever in consonance with the demands created by the incessant and rapid changes in our social structure responding to the constant changes in our economic structures. Health threats are increasingly national, and even international, in scope, with many of the environmental threats endangering the very future of the planet. International cooperation will be required to defend against them. It is difficult to see how anything but a strong national public health agency, with adequate authority to enforce decisions nationwide, will be able to represent the United States effectively in forging international agreements.

From the point of view of the content of public health services, one of the most important facts is the changed nature of the major threats to health—the chronic and degenerative diseases followed by accidents in transportation, the home, and the workplace. It may be that public health now stands with respect to the chronic and degenerative diseases where it stood with respect to acute infectious epidemic diseases in the mid-1850s. We are beginning to know something about the determinants or risk factors of these diseases. Certain preventive measures against them can therefore reasonably be advocated, but for such measures to be as effective against the chronic and degenerative diseases as public health measures became against acute infectious diseases, after 1915, considerably more epidemiological and biological research is needed. Given the nationwide nature of these

new health threats and some of the suspected environmental causes, it is reasonable to suppose that nothing less than strong federal coordination of a network of competent state and local health agencies can be successful in combatting them. We shall continue to need public health leaders who keep up with research and have the political and administrative ability to incorporate the worthwhile findings into well-supported public health practice. And we shall continue to need public health scholars and writers who can effectively transmit these findings to policy makers and the general public.

Experience has also made it clear that we have not rid ourselves of the appearance of new transmissible diseases. The experience with the occurrence of Legionnaires' disease, the Guillain-Barré syndrome, and especially the actual and impending menace of the AIDS epidemic all testify to the importance of maintaining a close check on evolving disease patterns. They also speak of the importance of keeping our epidemiological skills and resources intact and well supported. Whatever the answers to these questions may prove to be, one thing is certain: a challenging period lies ahead for future public health services administrators that will test the mettle of even the most talented and hard-working aspirants.

In addition to the community-wide services aspect of public health, the other important factor that underlies the question of governmental roles in health services in the United States is the provision of personal therapeutic medical services, which for brevity I shall henceforth call "medical care," following common usage. Many persons in the public health profession have long taken the position that the government's role is most appropriately concentrated almost exclusively on community-wide prevention measures, which are commonly referred to as "public health," a usage I have followed when the context is clear. I shall, however, continue to call these community-wide preventive services "standard public health" when greater precision is required. Others have vehemently asserted that medical care is simply a part of public health and should be vigorously regulated, and where necessary, operated by government. I shall discuss this fundamental question further at the end of Parts II and III, which deal with government and medical care, as well as in summary sections near the end of the book. In order to do this rationally it will first be necessary to discuss what the role of government has been in the provision of medical care and what the existing configuration of medical care provision is in the United States. This is done in Parts II and III.

NOTES

1. The Marine Hospital Service would thenceforth no longer need to obtain local approval to enforce quarantine in the seaports.

2. It is interesting to note that a similar experience with a national health board took place in Great Britain. It was established in 1848 under Edwin Chadwick's goading but was abolished in 1854. Apparently, the opposition to it also came from entrenched institutions, in this instance from the British local health authorities who did not wish to accede to the board's regulations (Rosen, 1958, 223).

3. While the diseases included in the old term "venereal disease," principally gonorrhea and syphilis, are included in the definition of sexually transmitted disease, the STDs include many more diseases. See Last, 1980, 257 ff. for a detailed modern treatment of the subject.

4. We are interested here in public health services, but this trend is observable with respect to many other governmental services that are generally provided locally, many of them also with state supervision and federal financial assistance.

5. The U.S. Bureau of the Census (1960, 9) indicates that 94.8 percent of the population was rural in 1790. This includes both rural nonfarm and rural farm, but until 1940 most of the rural population was farm-dwelling.

6. A decline in this percentage began only after 1960 as state and local services began to expand to meet the post–World War II population shifts and the increased demands occasioned by a period of economic well-being. By 1980 the federal percentage was down to 61, the trend was for states to use the income tax more than they had, and local property taxes were rising rapidly. Although property taxes rose, this source of tax revenue declined relatively as a source of state and local revenues as the use of sales and income taxes increased, despite the claims of the advocates of the local property tax "revolt" of the late 1970s. What was rising, in relative (that is, percentage of total) terms, is the state income tax as well as the state, and especially the local, sales tax (see Fig. 4–4). The main vulnerability of the property tax to being singled out for taxpayer revolt lay in its being a tax on capital instead of on earnings. This gave rise to many instances of persons owning relatively highly

taxed property on which they resided but unable to pay the taxes because their income had become low. As noted elsewhere, money capital ownership is not taxed per se. It is only subject to tax when it produces earnings—interest, dividends, and capital gains. The heavy reliance of local government on the unpopular personal property tax has long been an important barrier to achieving proper financing for local health services.

7. For example, the 1929 Ferrell, et al., study of health departments (cited in Chapters 2 and 3) found the configuration of the per capita state budgets in 1925 for public health work in relation to per capita income of 1926 to be such that New York state, with a per capita income of $1,250, had a per capita health appropriation of 11.6 cents, while Alabama, with a per capita income of $300, had a per capita health appropriation of 8.3 cents (see fig. 11 of Ferrell et al., 1929). That is, Alabama, with less than one-fourth the per capita income of New York, was spending almost two-thirds per capita of what New York was spending, and yet judging by the size of the per capita expenditure providing a less adequate set of health services.

8. I use the term here as it was commonly understood before about 1960 (see Mountin and Greve, 1949 for a discussion of this usage.) It should not be confused with the later term "revenue sharing" which described a program of what really were grants-in-aid.

9. That is, the revenue collected goes to the general fund of the United States to be appropriated by Congress for purposes it deems desirable. This is in contrast to special taxes in which the revenue goes into special trust funds earmarked for special purposes only.

10. For illustrative purposes I shall use the example of a federal appropriation that is to be allocated among the states, although these remarks apply to any similar relationship between any "superior" and "inferior" governments.

11. The Children's Bureau and its successor offices administering these grants went through a series of title changes and reorganizations. These reflected changes in policy dealing with the relationship of maternal and child health services to overall federal child protection policy. While a detailed consideration of the politics of the policy formation struggles underlying these changes would not be in keeping with the purposes of this book, it is important to be aware of their existence. A brief account of some of the reorganizations will at least give some feeling for their bewildering nature and frequency. In 1935 the Children's Bureau was located not in the Public Health Service, which was unaffiliated with any cabinet department, but in the cabinet Department of Labor, where it had been since its inception in 1912. In 1946, it was transferred to the non-Cabinet Federal Security Agency as a subsection of the Social Security Administration. It moved to the newly organized Department of Health, Education and Welfare (HEW)

when the latter absorbed the Federal Security Agency in 1953 and thereby became part of the first federal cabinet-level health agency. Within HEW, the Children's Bureau had a brief sojourn in the Social and Rehabilitation Services (SRS), followed by the public welfare and social services part of HEW, and finally in 1969 its health programs were put into the Health Services and Mental Health Administration (HSMHA) of the Public Health Service while its other social service programs went to the Office of Child Development, within which an entity named the "Children's Bureau" was retained. The administration of the Maternal and Child Health Grants was put under the Administration for Children, Youth and Families in the Office of Human Development Services in 1980. The Office of Human Development Services was placed in the cabinet Department of Health and Human Services, organized in 1980 when HEW was split into two cabinet departments, Health and Human Services (HHS) and Education. Wilson and Neuhauser (1985) present illuminating diagrams of federal government health organization (see also Figs. 4–5 and 4–6, and text pages 120–121).

12. The requirement of a civil service merit system for employees was a hallmark of APHA standards throughout the years. In recent years the disadvantages of this system have been dwelt on by various observers and officials. It has been claimed that it generates inefficiencies by making it difficult to discipline unproductive employees. There is undoubtedly some truth to these allegations, but their prevalence is not well documented. The fact is that the merit system is a deterrent to financially beleaguered departments discharging employees with substantial seniority and replacing them with lower-paid new workers, although in later years beginning in the mid-1970s, the so-called "contracting out" procedure was to be increasingly used to accomplish this aim even when it involved discharging tenured workers. In any case, a primary purpose of the advocates of a merit system for public health employees is to protect them from arbitrary reprisals for carrying out their monitoring and control functions. The Institute of Medicine (IOM) felt it necessary to note this fact in its 1988 report on public health and called for strengthening such protection (Institute of Medicine, 1988, 11).

13. In the lexicon of intergovernmental grants the term "maintenance of effort" refers to the state not diminishing its own contribution to a program in the face of federal increased contributions. In other words, the federal grants should be purely additive to the state's outlays before increases from federal grants.

14. See Pickett and Hanlon (1990), Chapter 22, passim for more information on this program.

15. Also, he seems not to have anticipated the exponential magnification of the environmental threats in later years even though he appreciated the need for extended research to develop "sanitary" sciences.

16. These differing views are exemplified in an exchange of views in 1965 between Hollis S. Ingraham, New York State Health Department Commissioner,

and Sewall Milliken and Marvin Strauss, executive director and research associate, respectively, of the Public Health Federation of Cincinnati, Ohio, who presented points of view opposed to that of Dr. Ingraham. These arguments are presented in some detail in Ingraham, 1965, which well repays reading.

17. These local agencies, in actuality, confined their work almost entirely to planning for the regulation of hospital bed resources in their jurisdictions. This aspect of these amendments thus became the most widely known feature of the 1966 act and led to its being generally called "The Comprehensive Health Planning Act of 1966."

18. Various tabulations differ slightly about the exact number because of differing interpretations as to whether certain public health units within state agencies with multiservice names are "really" health departments.

19. There is an amusing irony in this rhetoric. A policy that was later, under the Reagan administration, to culminte in an openly avowed single-minded effort to cut federal outlays for social programs, was initially presented as, in effect, one of returning "power to the people," a slogan then in vogue among Black Power and other protest and revolutionary movements.

20. Note that in this context the block health grants for health departments were categorical grants as far as the state and local governments were concerned, as described on page 90.

21. In his analysis of federal policy on environmental management, Barry Rabe refers to Nixon's "demonstrated belief that government should be organized around functions rather than programs and . . . his administration's efforts to coordinate programs in a number of policy areas" (1986, 10). He also notes that a reflection of this attitude existed in state governments (1986). A specific aim of reorganizations to promote such coordination was to move toward consolidated applications for permits and grants involving activities that needed clearance with respect to environmental impact. The FAR program moved along these lines generally. See Chapter 3, page 73.

22. It should be noted that this was the federal administration's "in-house" evaluation of the program's accomplishments. I am not aware of an independent study covering the same ground. We can only assume that this overview was in large measure accurate.

23. Folding a categorical grant into a block grant means adding the previous appropriation for the categorical program to the total block grant appropriation and eliminating the categorical identity of the original categorical grant.

24. The adjustment was calculated to *increase* the allotment to those substate governments (e.g., county, municipality, township) that spent *more* of their tax revenue for education.

25. Shifting spending decisions to states may be as much motivated by a subtle political calculus on the part of a federal administration as on any ideological

considerations about states rights, local autonomy, or grass-roots democracy. If the strategy is to reduce the total block grant in later years the administration will not have to specify which programs within the block will have to be reduced or even eliminated. The states will have to make that decision, and when the disappointed and enraged beneficiaries of the cut programs remonstrate against the reductions, it is the state or local governments that will bear the brunt of the anger. After all, it was not the federal government that will have made the decision to cut any particular program.

26. These were in the areas of high blood pressure control; family planning; pregnancy and infant health; immunization; sexually transmitted diseases; toxic agent control; occupational safety and health; accident prevention and injury control; fluoridation and dental health; surveillance and control of infectious diseases; smoking and health; misuse of alcohol and drugs; physical fitness and exercise; and control of stress and violent behavior (DHHS, 1980).

27. This point is discussed at greater length in Chapter 10 under "The Carter Administration."

28. See Crawford, 1977 for a critical literature review of this type of issue.

29. As noted previously, Robert Crawford (1977) lists many such writings (e.g., Illich, 1973; McKeown, 1971) and gives partial summaries of their views.

30. Different people writing about the folding-in process come up with differing counts of the number of programs involved. The differences are due to the various definitions of what constitutes a "program," but the resulting discrepancies among different accounts do not alter the general pattern described here.

31. Because many of the programs I have been talking about (e.g., Title V of the Social Security Act and Section 314d of the Public Health Service Act) and some that I shall be discussing later finally lost their individual budget identity through this act, I think the following description of how programs were folded in to form the block grants may be of interest:

a. Preventive Health and Health Services block grant. Programs folded in were: (1) rodent control; (2) fluoridation; (3) hypertension control; (4) health services and centers (rape crisis centers); (5) 314d money; (6) home health services; and (7) emergency services. The grants were distributed among the states according to a formula based on population and other factors deemed "appropriate" by the secretary of HHS. Despite the formula, each state now had to apply for these grants, a notable departure from previous practice in allocating formula grants among the states.

b. Alcohol Abuse, Drug Abuse, and Mental Health block grant. Programs folded in were: (a) Community Mental Health Centers Act; (2) Mental Health Systems Act; (3) Comprehensive Alcohol Abuse and Alcoholism Prevention, Treatment and Rehabilitation Act of 1970; and (4) Drug Abuse Prevention, Treatment, and Rehabilitation Act.

c. Primary Care block grant. This section consisted entirely of one program, the Community Health Cen-

ters. States could begin to take them over beginning with FY 1983.

d. Maternal and Child Health Services block grant (Title V of the original 1935 Social Security Act, as amended over the years). Programs folded in were: (1) maternal and child health and crippled children's services of Title V; (2) supplementary security income for disabled children used to provide rehabilitation services for blind and disabled children; (3) lead-based paint poisoning prevention; (4) genetic disease services; (5) sudden infant death syndrome; (6) hemophilia treatment; and (7) adolescent pregnancy services originally in the Health Services and Centers Amendment of 1978. The state health agency was mandated to be the administering agency, and the allocation formula for FY 1982 and 1983 was based on number of low-income children. Alternative bases for the allocation formula in the future were to be submitted to Congress by the secretary of HHS by June 1982. The states had to match $3 for every $4 of federal funds received.

The six HHS programs that were left as categorical grants were: (1) childhood immunization; (2) tuberculosis control; (3) family planning; (4) regional health centers; (5) venereal disease control; and (6) an amount equal to 15 percent of the total MCH grant that was to be set aside for use by HHS to fund projects of "regional or national significance" in training and research, genetic disease testing, counseling and information development, and for comprehensive hemophilia diagnostic and treatment centers. In addition, the Women, Infants, and Children (WIC) nutrition program of the Agriculture Department budget was also left categorical. Leaving six programs as categorical and dividing the remaining twenty into four instead of two block grants resulted from vigorous lobbying in Congress by advocates of the various programs.

32. See note 25 for further remarks on the political advantages to the federal administration of turning underfunded programs over to the states.

33. A few years later, in 1989–90, the states' fiscal status took a precipitous nose dive and by 1991 the revenue shortfalls in many states were extremely acute, with some states facing possible bankruptcy. The state reductions in support for health services have been heavy.

34. A 1986 study by Barry Rabe found that as of 1985 "EPA remains as devoted as ever to its separate statutes." (page 12)

35. Much of the material in this section is based on Ashford, 1975. Wherever quotations appear without citation in this section they are attributable to this source.

36. Much of this material is from HEW, NIOSH Fact Sheet.

37. The fact that the age-adjusted death rate increased by a lesser percentage than the crude rate implies that most of the percent increase was due to the population being more heavily weighted with older persons in 1978 than in 1960.

II

Direct Provision of Personal Health Care by Government in the United States

Government activities in the realm of "public health" services were examined in Part I. The scope of public health services was long a matter of dispute, with the debate becoming acrimonious at times. The main bone of contention has been the responsibility of government to assure access to personal health services, or medical care, for its citizens. Access to medical care comprises two elements: the *availability* of providers (the supply) and the *eligibility* for services. Here I speak only of perhaps the most important aspect of eligibility, the ability to pay the going price. Government policy to increase financial access to personal health care has been implemented in three ways:

1. Direct provision. Government provides care directly with its own personnel and facilities.
2. Private provider reimbursement. Government pays private providers or organizations to provide care for a specified population. Such payment may be direct fees to providers or grants to private organizations.
3. Tax incentives. Payments for health insurance premiums are wholly or partially exempted from taxation as are philanthropic contributions to health care organizations. There are also other exemptions, which will be discussed in the chapters that follow.

The most visible and commonly used arrangements for increasing access to medical care have involved direct provision and provider reimbursement for the care of special population groups. The tax incentive method has been used primarily to increase access for employed persons via indirect public subsidy of private health insurance premiums. The argument over the relative merits of public and private provision or assurance of medical care has centered almost entirely on the first two approaches, and the present discussion is confined to these. The stance taken on this question has varied across a wide spectrum between two polar positions. The advocates at one end of the spectrum, which I shall call the restrictive public health approach, hold that public health consists only of those community health activities that affect populations as groups—environmental controls, population disease monitoring, public education on health matters, immunization campaigns, and the like. In this view, all personal medical care belongs in the realm of privately provided medical care. If it is government policy to increase access for low-income persons to personal medical care, it should buy the services at market prices from private providers. If government cannot or will not purchase such services from private providers, an acceptable but distinctly less desirable alternative is to provide it directly to medically indigent populations, but under the aegis of a public charity or welfare department—not a public health department. In general, the appropriate relationship of government to the providers of medical care is, in this view, limited to regulating them, and then only insofar as it is necessary to protect the public against incompetent medical personnel or inadequate medical facilities.

The polar opposite of this position, which I shall call the comprehensive public health approach, holds that assuring the provision of all forms of needed health care is part of the overall responsibility of government for protecting the public's health. Public assurance of the provision of needed personal health care is in this view a public service rather than merely another private market commodity subject to government regulation. No capitalist country has adopted the pure form of direct government provision of all medical care in publicly owned facilities, although Great Britain has come closest to it. However, all developed capitalist countries (except the Union of South Africa) have at least implicitly recognized medical care as a right for all people by guaranteeing access to the preponderance of medical care services for all their residents. This guarantee has been met by a combination of services directly provided by government and government payment to private providers for medical care.

Because the advocates of the restrictive definition of public health placed so great an emphasis on personal medical services being privately provided, they preferred the private-provider payment method of government participation, for it did not require general use of government providers. Historical circumstances, however, led to many government programs of direct service, and the restrictive public health advocates were not entirely able to prevent their establishment. These services, although government provided, were nevertheless usually controlled by a nonhealth government agency. They were conceived as an extension of government functions other than health—poor relief, veterans' services, control of mental patients, part of the government's relations with Indians, or part of the maintenance of active-duty armed services and merchant marine personnel and their dependents. It was thus that many of the largest direct-service health programs of government could be defined or viewed not as public health but as public assistance, veterans' benefits, relationship with Indians, armed service operations, or confining mentally dangerous people.

Although the general tenor of the various attitudes expressed toward direct provision of health services was that it was for the most part an inappropriate function of government vis-à-vis the *general* population (Chapman and Talmadge, 1971; Sade, 1971), there was comparatively little opposition to its provision for certain special groups in the population. These subpopulations consisted of four major categories of persons:

1. Specially *deserving persons,* e.g., veterans, dependents of members of the armed forces, merchant seamen.
2. Persons with *special diseases* whose treatment was considered to lie in the public domain, e.g., mental illness, tuberculosis. The care of persons with these diseases was often seen to include isolation from the general population.
3. *Poor persons* carried as public charges under the police powers of the state. In this case it was appropriate to dole out medical care as other commodities such as food, housing, and clothing were doled out.
4. Other persons whose care was originally part of a total complex of *custodial responsibility* of the government for administrative or historical reasons, e.g., armed forces personnel, American Indians, prisoners.

These and other issues dealing with the past and continuing role of government in the direct provision of medical care, that is, providing personal health services using its own facilities and employing its own personnel, are developed in the three chapters of Part II.

Chapter 5 deals with federally operated direct services and treats the Veterans Administration health care system; the Public Health Service hospitals; and the Indian Health Services—all part of the direct services provided by the United State Public Health Services; and the medical care system of the armed forces. The United States Public Health Service Hospitals ceased operations in 1981, but they existed for 180 years and are a good example of a type of government-provided direct health service that was organized for a special group of persons but was discontinued when that group no longer needed special provisions for access to health care.

Chapter 6 deals with state directly operated personal health services. The main areas covered are the state mental hospital and state-sponsored community mental health services. Although the latter are not operated as direct government services, they grew out of the state mental hospital services and are therefore included in this chapter.

Chapter 7 addresses direct medical care services by local government. It covers local government provision for health care to the poor, with particular reference to the local public general hospital for the poor.

5

Federally Operated Medical Care Services

MEDICAL CARE FOR VETERANS

The medical care activities of the United States Veterans Administration (VA) constitute the most important segment of federally operated medical care services in terms of service load carried; indeed they provide a sizable portion of the total medical care delivered in the United States. In 1981, the VA was the largest centrally directed health care system in the nation. Its facilities included 172 medical centers, each with outpatient departments, 50 freestanding outpatient clinics, 95 nursing homes, and 16 domiciliaries. It directly ran a daily average of 82,000 operating hospital beds with an occupancy rate of 80.9 percent, as well as 8,700 nursing home beds and 8,400 domiciliary beds. On an average day there were 102,751 inpatients under care in the entire system (i.e., average daily census— see Table 5–1)—81,874 in VA facilities and 20,878 in other facilities. Of the 102,700 average daily inpatient census, 68,500 (66 percent) were patients in hospitals, 22,300 (22 percent) in nursing homes, and 11,900 (12 percent) were living in domiciliaries. An annual total of 1,360,000 inpatients were treated, 94 percent of them in VA facilities. There were 17,900,000 outpatient visits, 88 percent to VA facilities. The inpatient service in non-VA facilities was paid for under contract with the VA and the outpatient visits to non-VA providers were paid on a fee-for-service basis. The operating cost of this program in 1981 was $6,642.2 million[1] (VA, 1981, 9 and 130).

In 1980 approximately 9 percent of all hospital beds in the United States were under federal auspices; of these, about 70 percent were operated by the Veterans Administration. Thus 6 percent of all hospital beds in the United States

were operated by the VA, and total patient days in VA hospitals accounted for almost 6½ percent of the total hospital inpatient utilization for the country (Table 5–2). Virtually all the federal psychiatric beds were operated by the VA (approximately 25,000). These constituted about 29 percent of the VA hospital beds and 31 percent of the total 1981 year-end VA hospital census (VA, 1981).

Pre–World War II Background

After each war, the question of benefits to veterans was posed, with medical benefits being an important component of the demands raised by veterans ever since World War I. In each case, the definition of eligibility for benefits has been a central issue, with veterans' organizations generally seeking unlimited eligibility for all veterans, and opponents of this view advocating restriction of eligibility to those whose need for care resulted from service-connected injuries. Usually something in between these two alternatives prevailed. At different times, benefits have been granted under three different categories of entitlement, which in descending order of frequency of use have been: (1) for those with service-connected disability[2], (2) for special non-service-connected categories, e.g., age or presence of disease; and (3) solely on account of having been in the service. All three of these continue to serve as a framework for defining eligibility for VA medical services. During periods when all three have been in effect simultaneously, there has usually been a priority ordering of eligibility for service, with service-connected disability having the highest priority and "solely on account of having been in the service" the lowest. Often some types of

Table 5–1. Average Daily Census under VA Care[a] and Average Number of Operating Beds in VA Facilities: Selected Fiscal Years 1925–1981

| | Average Daily Census under VA Care (in thousands) | | | | Average Operating Beds in VA Facilities (in thousands) | | | |
| | | | | | | VA Hospitals | | |
Fiscal Year	Total Hospital Inpatients, Domiciliary Residents, and Nursing Bed Care Patients	Hospital Inpatients	Domiciliary Residents[b]	Nursing Bed Care Patients	All VA Facilities	Hospital Beds	Nursing Home Beds in VA Hospitals[c]	VA Domiciliaries
1981	102.7	68.5	11.9	22.3	99.2	82.1	8.7	8.4
1980	105.1	70.3	12.8	22.0	101.7	84.1	8.4	9.2
1979	106.8	72.0	13.7	21.1	105.5	87.7	8.4	9.4
1978	109.8	75.4	14.0	20.4	108.9	91.2	7.9	9.8
1977	111.2	77.7	14.2	19.3	109.9	92.4	7.6	9.9
1968	128.2	99.4	20.7	8.1	130.7	112.4	4.0	14.3
1963	137.8	112.6	25.2	c	137.2	120.3	—	16.9
1958	140.6	114.6	26.0	—	138.9	121.2	—	17.7
1953	129.5	104.5	25.0	—	126.8	109.0	—	17.8
1948	126.5	105.9	20.6	—	118.4	102.4	—	16.0
1947	116.8	98.2	18.6	—	111.9	96.5	—	15.4
1946	93.8	78.6	15.2	—	95.8	80.9	—	14.9
1945	81.5	68.3	13.2	—	87.2	73.8	—	13.4
1944	75.2	61.3	13.9	—	79.3	66.0	—	13.3
1940	79.2	56.3	22.9	—	74.9	56.4	—	18.5
1935	55.9	41.3	14.6	—	60.9	43.0	—	17.9
1930	n.a.	30.3	n.a.	—	n.a.	22.7	—	n.a.
1925	n.a.	26.6	n.a.	—	n.a.	20.7	—	n.a.

Source: (VA, 1981) for years 1935 and later; (Dillingham, 1952) for years before 1935.

[a]Includes veterans in VA facilities, non-VA hospitals, state homes, and community nursing homes.

[b]Includes residents who are also employees.

[c]Program was begun in 1965.

services have been available to all veterans and other types only to priority number 1 or 1 and 2 veterans.

Only since World War I has the medical care benefit as such been a particularly important component of the demands raised by veterans. Before then, economic assistance for veterans or their surviving dependents and provision of custodial residences were the all-important elements in government benefits. Cash pensions as well as domiciliary arrangements ("soldier's homes") were provided, with eligibility center-

Table 5–2. Number and Percent Distribution of Admissions, Number of Hospitals, and Average Number of Operating Beds—VA, Total Federal, and Total U.S., Fiscal Year 1980

	Number of Admissions (000)	ADC (000)	Number of Hospitals	Number of Beds (000)
Veterans administration[a]	1,183 (3.1%)	68 (6.4%)	172 (2.5%)	84 (6.2%)
Total federal[b]	2,044 (5.3%)	94 (8.9%)	359 (5.2%)	117 (8.6%)
Total U.S.[b]	38,892 (100.0%)	1,060 (100.0%)	6,965 (100.0%)	1,365 (100.0%)

Source: (VA, 1981).

[a]These statistics represent services in VA hospitals only (AHA, 1981).

[b]These data are for hospitals registered with the American Hospital Association.

ing on veterans who had been disabled as a direct result of military service and on families of soldiers who had lost their lives as a result of military service.

This traditional pattern goes back to the earliest colonial times.[3] As early as 1636 a law was passed in the Plymouth settlement providing for maintenance of soldiers disabled in battles with the Indians. The Virginia, Maryland, New York, and Rhode Island colonies had similar laws. In 1776 the Continental Congress provided for pensions to enlistees who were disabled as a consequence of their military service, and benefits to survivors of veterans of the American Revolution were still being paid as late as 1911.

The first Congress of the new nation passed a veterans' pension law in 1789, and in 1818 the administration of these pensions was transferred from Congress to the War Department, where it was administered by a special office called the Bureau of Pensions (after 1833, the Office of Pensions). With the organization of the Department of Interior in 1849, this function was again transferred, this time from the War Department to Interior, where it was administered by an agency once again called the Bureau of Pensions. Survivors of pensioners dating from the War of 1812 were still receiving benefit payments as late as 1946. These benefits were also extended to Union volunteers in the Civil War. In 1862 a formal pension system was established for disabled soldiers and for dependents of soldiers who died on active duty. To be eligible for a pension the soldier must have been disabled in the line of duty, that is, his disability must have been what was later called service-connected. The present motto of the Veterans Administration, which comes from President Lincoln's second inaugural address in 1865, reads: "to care for him who shall have borne the battle, and for his widow, and his orphan."

The first veterans' benefit that offered anything other than cash pensions was provided by the U.S. Naval Home, built in Philadelphia in 1811 as a domiciliary for "decrepit Naval officers, seamen and Marines." Because it was mainly a sheltered residence facility, any medical care offered was incidental to the provision of living facilities to the veterans. By 1860, however, a separate Philadephia Naval Hospital with

130 beds was built specifically to give medical care. In 1851 the U.S. Soldiers' Home for disabled and invalid soldiers (Army) had been built and was still operating in 1977 in Washington, D.C., as the U.S. Soldiers' and Airmen's Home.

The instituting of specifically identified medical benefits for veterans was materially advanced during the Civil War as a direct outcome of the recommendations of a Sanitary Commission appointed by the Secretary of War in 1861 to study medical and hospital conditions in the Union armies. Following one of its recommendations dealing with "needy and sick" discharged soldiers, temporary hospital or domiciliary care was provided at different locations to care for discharged soldiers until they were well enough to return home. In 1865 Congress established the National Home for Disabled Volunteer Soldiers, which later developed into a system of soldiers' homes. Many states also built soldiers' homes. All these homes provided complete domiciliary care, and because the soldiers had disabilities upon admission that generally became more severe as they aged, medical and hospital treatment was a part of the service provided without regard to "whether or not [the injuries or disease] were of service origin."

When World War I broke out in Europe in 1914, Congress created a Bureau of War Risk Insurance in the Treasury Department to insure U.S. ships and their cargoes against the risk of being sunk. Upon America's entering the war in 1917, Congress, as it had in the period of the Civil War, again revised and upgraded the system of veterans' benefits. The benefits under the 1917 law included disability compensation, voluntary low-cost life insurance for servicemen and veterans, financial support for the dependents of servicemen during their period of service, and vocational rehabilitation for the disabled. The administration of the three programs of financial payments—disability, life insurance, and dependents' support—was assigned to the Bureau of War Risk Insurance that had been established in 1914, while responsibility for administering vocational rehabilitation was not specified in the Act (Dillingham, 1952). In addition, the Public Health Service provided physical examinations to certify veterans for disability compensation or vocational training or for medical and hospital care, the latter offered under authority of previously established laws.

Shortly after the end of World War I in 1918, the Federal Board for Vocational Education was given responsibility for administering the vocational rehabilitation program, while in 1919 the responsibility for providing hospital and medical care was assigned to the Public Health Service. With the end of the war, the life insurance and dependents' allowances functions of the War Risk Bureau virtually disappeared and

determination of eligiblity for compensation, vocational rehabilitation and medical care and hospitalization became a major function. In the Public Health Service and the Federal Board for Vocational Education, veterans' services soon came to overshadow other activities (Dillingham, 1952, 13).

This was apparently perceived as an undesirable state of affairs, for it resulted in the appointment of a Presidential citizens' committee in 1921 to investigate the situation and propose a solution. Its recommendation that a single agency to handle all veterans' benefits be created led to legislation in 1921 (the Sweet Act) establishing the United States Veteran's Bureau. This agency took over the World War I veterans' benefits functions of the Bureau of War Risk Insurance for disability compensation, pensions, and life insurance, those of the Federal Board for Vocational Education for rehabilitation and training, and those of the Public Health Service for eligibility-certifying physical examinations and medical care for veterans. Under this law and the Executive Orders based on its authority, all veterans' hospitals then being operated by the U.S. Public Health Service for the care of World War I veterans were transferred to the Veterans' Bureau in 1922, and in 1923 forty-six U.S. Veterans' Bureau hospitals were in operation with the care of additional patients contracted out to other hospitals. Eligibility requirements for care in these hospitals were liberalized in 1924 to include veterans of other U.S. wars, to extend priorities for admission to medically indigent veterans for non–service-connected illness, and to cover care for non-service-connected illness for all other veterans, provided facilities were available.

The increased demand for service resulting from this liberalization of eligibility caused the Veteran's Bureau to embark on a long-term program of facility construction, and by 1932 there were fifty-six veterans' hospitals with 30,000 beds and ten veterans' homes (domiciliaries) with 20,000 beds. As late as 1930, however, veterans' benefits were still being administered by three different agencies: the Veteran's Bureau was administering a number of programs for veterans of World War I only as well as the medical program for veterans of all other wars, while the Bureau of Pensions of the Interior Department and the National Homes for Disabled Volunteer Soldiers were administering a number of programs only for veterans of wars other than World War I. The *Veterans Administration,*[4] established by Congress in 1930, consolidated the Bureau of Pensions, the National Homes for Disabled Volunteer Soldiers, and the United States Veterans' Bureau, each agency becoming a bureau in the VA with some rationalizing realignment of responsibilities. The new agency had three identifiable functions: paying compensation and pensions; supervising the provision of medical and rehabilitative services; and operating a system of residences for indigent and disabled veterans (domiciliaries). The Veterans Administration organization chart for 1977 clearly displayed the continuation of these three functions over the years. There were three departments in 1977: Medicine and Surgery, which was in charge of hospitals, outpatient clinics, nursing homes and domiciliaries; Veterans Benefits, which handled the regional offices and Veterans Assistance Centers for paying cash benefits, and a data management department.

The Great Depression brought a temporary hiatus in the trend of increasing veterans' benefits. In fact, retrenchment set in with all benefits previously voted to veterans of the Spanish-American and subsequent wars being rescinded in 1933. The President was empowered to grant benefits by executive order for a period of two years, and any other provisions would have to be newly legislated by Congress. The initial executive orders issued under this legislation provided for veterans' benefits that were sharply reduced from what they had been before 1933, including medical, hospital, and domiciliary services, but they were soon restored by legislation as well as by further executive orders. However, hospitalization for non-service-connected cases remained limited to the beds available in Veterans Administration hospitals. The use of contract beds in other government hospitals, such as Army, Navy, Public Health Service, and Interior Department, was restricted to service-connected cases, eliminating about one-fourth of all available beds. In addition, the veteran's cash pension was reduced while the veteran was in the hospital. These measures combined to reduce the patient load by about 23 percent.

This two-year period of Depression executive orders ended in 1935 with the advent of new legislation reestablishing a wide range of veterans' benefits. Hospitalization benefits were restored to all veterans of all wars and what was in essence the system of priorities for admission prevailing through at least 1980 was installed. The priorities for service eligibility in descending order of preference were: (1) medical care needs arising out of service-connected disabilities; (2) medical care not arising out of service-connected disabilities, provided the patient also had a service-connected disability and if a bed were available and; (3) all other cases, if the veteran swore he could not afford to pay for services needed and if a bed were available.

The agency settled down to care for existing veterans, whose numbers were expected to dwindle with time. As may be seen from Table 5–1, the number of hospital beds operated by the VA (and its predecessor agencies) rose from 20,700 in 1925 to 56,400 in 1940, and the total average daily number of veterans hospitalized under VA auspices (average daily census) rose from 26,600 to 56,300 during the same years. Then, in 1941, came America's entry into World War II.

We recall that implementation of the loosely defined entitlement to medical care under the War Risk Act of 1917 had been assigned to the Public Health Service, which proceeded to build a medical care system, and that this work was continued by the Veterans' Bureau after 1921. The emphasis was on providing an adequate quantity of facilities and services to meet a growing demand, and the quality of care was most often criticized in the 1920s in terms of lack of sufficient facilities. Veterans' organizations pressed for appropriations primarily for the construction of more facilities and liberalization of eligibility categories. However, the quality and economic efficiency of the care actually given were also criticized. A Senate investigation in 1923 revealed that about 40 percent of the inpatients

could be served equally well by dispensaries. However, as the men [patients] were unable to earn a living or to profit by rehabilitation training, they remained in the hospitals through the connivance of Bureau officials. . . . The medical service of the Bureau was inefficient, moreover, because it could not attract the better class of men [physicians] (Dillingham, 1952, 62, 63).

Over the next decade, the types of services available were steadily expanded to more nearly meet the special needs of veterans, and attempts were made to improve the technical quality of medical care by creating conditions calculated to attract better-qualified physicians.

In an attempt to place the medical service of the Bureau on a higher level a Medical Council was appointed in 1924. Council members were chosen from among men of important attainments in different fields of medical activity to advise the Bureau as to the best and most modern methods of diagnosis and treatment, hospital management, and other functions of the medical service. The Council recommended the establishment of a section of medical research in the medical service, the establishment of two diagnostic centers for the study of difficult cases, the establishment of an advisory council on nursing, and the establishment of an arrangement with the American College of Surgeons for a survey of Veterans' Bureau hospitals with a view to meeting the standards of that body. The recommendations were followed, and in addition a medical bulletin was published and such other steps as were possible were taken to make the medical service of the Bureau feel a closer connection with other medical circles.

The Bureau's campaign to improve medical service was a continuous one. In 1928, Director Hines proposed to establish points throughout the country where medical officers could be trained to meet the Bureau's particular problems and from which they could be assigned to facilities as needed. The policy was also established of assigning initially appointed medical personnel to veterans hospitals for the purpose of testing in practice their professional qualifications before they were assigned to definite duties and responsibilities. Postgraduate schools were established in Washington, D.C., and Palo Alto, California, for special training of Bureau doctors in the field of neuropsychiatry. Other similar courses and aids to medical personnel were used from time to time to improve further the medical service (Dillingham, 1952, 64).

Services and equipment that were introduced and more widely provided during these early years under the Veterans' Bureau were prosthetic appliances and supplies, dental care, and outpatient dispensary care.

The use of outpatient dispensaries by the Public Health Service prior to World War I led naturally to their use in the treatment of veterans as an alternative to the use of private physicians and dentists on a fee basis. The use of physicians and dentists prior to the establishment of the outpatient clinics proved to be inefficient, expensive, and subject to fraudulent practices; it was never possible to eliminate the use of private physicians completely, however, because there were many localities where the veteran was not close enough to a clinic to be able to make use of its facilities.

Shortly after the establishment of the Veterans' Bureau, experimentation with outpatient clinics and dispensaries led to the establishment of three types suited to the size and needs of the community to be served. . . . The highest number of dispensaries ever in operation at one time was 117 in 1922. The number of dispensaries in use varied with the reorganization of the Bureau. As more hospitals were constructed, dispensaries were transferred to the hospitals wherever this could be done without hampering operations (Dillingham, 1952, 66, 68).

Throughout the 1930s, the Veterans Administration, the successor to the Veterans' Bureau, continued to enlarge and improve training facilities and programs for its personnel. Training courses for physicians and other specialists were offered, short courses in general medicine and administrative procedure were given annually, and intensive orientation courses were offered for new physicians. Clinics and laboratories to be used in conjunction with specialties were organized, and special equipment for complicated procedures was installed (Dillingham, 1952, 110, 111).

It should be noted that these were all "in-house" training measures for the VA's own salaried staff. With the advent of World War II and the increased inroads made upon the VA's per-

sonnel to meet the demands of the armed forces (Dillingham, 1952, 114), concern was heightened after the 1943 action of Congress extending all veterans' benefits to World War II veterans and the potential enormous increase of the eligible population of veterans.

Post–World War II Expansion Through 1979

Voting veterans of World War II the same benefits as World War I veterans in 1943 increased the potential eligible population from approximately 5 million to about 20 million veterans. The Veterans Administration was already suffering a shortage of facilities and personnel during World War II because of the discharged new veterans requiring medical care coupled with the drain on personnel resulting from the call to military duty of many of the agency's medical and administration personnel, but the larger problem was the future shortage of resources anticipated with the end of the war (VA, 1977, 6). Faced with the threat of an expected huge potential increase in the use of VA facilities resulting from the fourfold increase in the number of eligible veterans, Congress passed legislation granting these rights and a program intended to greatly expand medical personnel and facilities to meet the expected rise in demand was instituted by the VA. This post–World War II expansion program had three main objectives: to increase the quantity and variety of facilities, programs, and personnel (resources); to increase the quantity of services delivered (utilization); and to improve the quality of care (quality). Each of these facets—resources, utilization, and quality—will be addressed separately.

Resources

Facilities The data in Table 5–1 document some aspects of the expansion in facilities during and after World War II. The number of hospital beds rose from 56,400 in 1940 to 121,200 in 1958 (the actual peak was 121,500, reached in 1960). After 1960 the number of hospital beds began a steady decline, and in 1981 the bed complement stood at 82,100.

The number of beds in domiciliary facilities

is largely a function of the aging of the veteran population. By 1940 there were 18,500 domiciliary beds, reflecting the aging of the World War I veterans. The deaths of World War I veterans were apparently offset by the aging of World War II veterans after 1950 so that the number of domiciliary beds for older veterans remained at about 17,000 thereafter. The sharp decrease in domiciliary beds after 1968 shown in the table did not represent a decline in the total number of beds for long-term care. Rather it signified a recognition that many of the veterans in the domiciliaries needed the more intensive level of care offered in nursing care beds. The program of nursing care beds, begun in 1965, soon came to include about half of the nonacute patients. The distribution of the types of facilities shifted toward stressing extended care more as compared with acute inpatient care.

Programs—Types of Services In addition to the nursing bed care program developed to accommodate the increasing number of veterans who were not well enough to manage with domiciliary care, which offered only supervised independent living, other special forms of health service were also instituted to keep pace with the changing health care needs stemming from the aging of the veteran population. This entailed adding new programs while retaining old ones at reduced levels of resource commitment, and the net result was an attempted widening in the *variety* of types of services.

The official 1981 annual report of the VA claimed that:

The VA now has developed a comprehensive, integrated, high quality program for long-term care for aging veterans, complemented by ambulatory and acute care. Nowhere else are all of these elements present for the appropriate care of aging patients.

Two examples of special extended are programs were cited:

The office of Geriatrics and Extended Care oversees a variety of programs, including VA nursing home care, community nursing home care, state home care (nursing home, domiciliary and hospitals), hospital-based home care, adult day care, [and] residential care. . . .

[*Hospital-based home care*] allows for early discharge of veterans with chronic illness to their own homes. . . . The family provides the necessary personal care under the coordinated supervision of a hospital-based multidisciplinary treatment team. . . . Thirty VA medical centers are providing hospital-based home care services. . . .

In FY 1981, 145,000 home vists were made. . . . Over 5,600 patients were treated, of whom about 20 percent were terminal cancer patients. . . .

[*The Residential Care Program* (formerly Personal Care Home Program)] provides residential care, including room, board, personal care, and general health care supervision to veterans who do not require hospital or nursing home care but who, because of health conditions, are not able to resume independent living and have no suitable family resources to provide the needed care. . . . Care is provided in private homes selected by the VA, at the veteran's own expense. Veterans receive monthly follow-up visits from VA social workers and other health care professionals, and are outpatients of the local VA facilities. An approximate average daily census of 12,500 was maintained in this program throughout FY 1981 (VA, 1981, 13–15).

It should be noted, however, that while the good quality of the nursing home program was corroborated by the the the NAS study (National Academy of Sciences, 1977), the statistics for the *hospital-based* home care and the *residential care* programs are not included in any of the agency's tables nor have we any other indication of their extent or quality. It would seem that these particular programs were in an early stage of development in 1981 and that the claim that "the VA now has developed a comprehensive, integrated high quality program of long-term care" should be approached with caution with respect to the newer type programs. But the trend and pressures that were producing such attempts and reports were inescapable.

Personnel There are no readily available data that show the post–World War II *quantitative* expansion of VA medical service personnel in a comprehensive manner on a year-to-year comparable basis. The main evidence of expansion derives from agency descriptions detailing the *qualitative* enrichment of medical personnel, (training, certification, and accreditation) which I treat separately below. Attempts to analyze the VA's progress in increasing the number of professional staff after World War II have been handicapped by the lack of comparability of the data of later years with that of the immediate postwar years, approximately 1945–1948, so that we do not have a really good base from which to start a comparison of postwar progress.

However, the agency's published data indicate that the inpatient staffing ratios per unit of service increased substantially over the years 1970–1981. On average, the full-time equivalent staff per inpatient (i.e., per daily average occupied bed) went from 1.28 to 2.13 during this period. However, for all community hospitals in the United States this ratio was 3.80 in 1980. In 1972 for all general hospitals in the United States the staff/(occupied bed) ratio had been 3.1 compared with 1.46 in VA hospitals indicating that the gap in 1981 had narrowed somewhat over 1972. But although the average staff per occupied bed increased over the ten years 1972–1981, the VA was not able to close the gap in staffing ratios between it and the community hospitals even after making a rough adjustment for the psychiatric load.[5]

Whether the low inpatient staffing ratios of the VA hospitals compared with all other community hospitals indicates inadequate numbers of staff remains a moot point, however. It has been asserted by some investigators that the VA acute beds held a substantial number of patients who did not require acute care. If this be true, then the VA may not have been understaffed for the care required by its case mix. A study of the Veterans Administration health care system in 1975 remarked:

The adequacy of staffing cannot be judged from staffing ratios alone. The patient-care requirements based on patient characteristics and treatment requirements can differ appreciably among hospitals.

There are no tested methods for determining the adequacy of physician staffing. On the basis of expert judgments made by the Committee's site visitors, it appears that the VA general hospitals quantitative staffing of physicians was considered adequate or better in 64% of the medical-service beds, 58% of the surgical-service beds, and 43% of the psychiatric service beds. In the psychiatric hospitals the quantity of physicians staffing was considered adequate in 59% of the medical beds, and 35% of the psychiatric beds. It is evident, however, that the adequacy of numbers is not closely correlated with the quality of care, as

judged by the same site visitors (National Academy of Sciences, 1977, 86, 100).

Utilization

Inpatient Services The average total daily hospital census under care (both in VA and non-VA facilities) rose from 56,300 patients in 1940 to a peak of 114,600 in 1958 and declined steadily thereafter (see Table 5–1). It was down to 68,500 by 1981. The total domiciliary census was also at its peak in 1958 with 26,000 residents, almost double the 13,900 level of 1944. Before 1965 the domiciliary census represented the entire nonhospital census, but in 1965 the program of nursing home care was started and thereafter one must add the domiciliary and nursing home (nursing bed care patients on Table 5–1) censuses to obtain the total nonhospital institutional census. In fact, after 1975 the nursing home patients outnumbered the domiciliary members, and if one takes the domiciliary and nursing bed occupants together, the combined census was in the neighborhood of 34,000 after 1976, almost two and a half times the 13,900 domiciliary census of 1944 and larger even than the prewar census of 22,900 (Table 5–1, Figs. 5–1 and 5–2). Thus, 84 percent of the total average daily institutional census was in acute hospitals in 1947 compared with only 66 percent in hospitals in 1981, when 22 percent was in nursing care beds and 12 percent in domiciliaries (Fig. 5–2).

The data in Table 5–3 illustrate another facet of the development of the VA census, the distribution of the total census paid for by the VA between the portion served in its own facilities and that served in state and community facilities. From that table we see that in 1981 the preponderance of the hospital census (66,400 out of 68,500 or 97 percent) was carried in VA hospitals. Although this percentage has been lower in some years after World War II (it was about 87 percent in 1947 and 1948) as the number of VA beds increased, most of the hospital census came to be carried in VA hospitals. The case with domiciliary care is markedly different. Some 30 percent of the census was always in state homes until about 1948, and thereafter the policy apparently was to increase that percent-

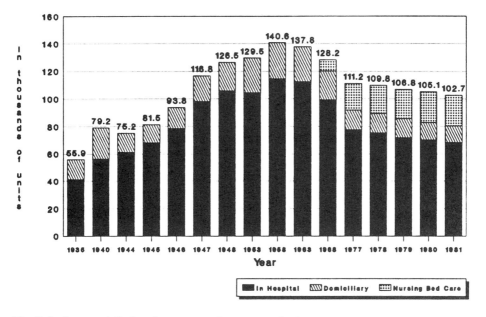

Fig. 5–1. Average daily inpatient census of veterans under VA care, totals and by type of facility, selected years. *Note*: Numbers above bars represent the total census cared for by the VA: In VA and in non-VA facilities. *Source*: Table 5–1.

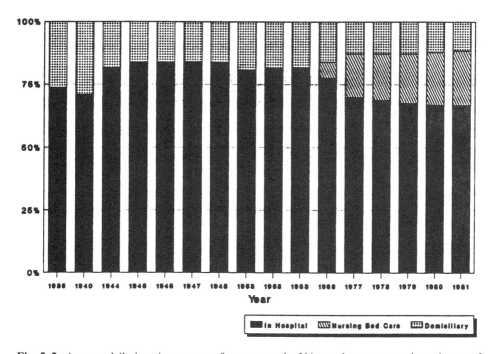

Fig. 5–2. Average daily inpatient census of veterans under VA care by percentage in each type of facility. *Source*: Table 5–1.

Table 5–3. Distribution of Average Daily Census Among VA Facilities and Non-VA Facilities by Hospital Inpatient Care, Domiciliary Members, and Nursing Home: for Selected Fiscal Years 1925–1981 (in thousands)

Fiscal Year	Hospitals				Domiciliaries			Nursing Homes			
	Total	VA Hospitals	Non-VA Hospitals	State Homes	Total	VA Domiciliaries	State Homes	Total	VA Hospitals	State Homes	Community Nursing Homes
1981	68.5	66.4	1.2	0.9	11.9	7.3	4.6	22.3	8.1	5.9	8.3
1980	70.3	68.2	1.2	0.9	12.8	7.9	4.9	22.0	7.9	5.6	8.5
1979	72.0	69.8	1.2	1.0	13.7	8.4	5.3	21.1	7.8	5.2	8.1
1978	75.4	73.0	1.4	1.0	14.0	8.7	5.2	20.4	7.5	4.9	8.0
1977	77.7	75.4	1.3	1.0	14.2	8.9	5.3	19.3	7.2	4.6	7.5
1968	99.4	97.4	2.0	[a]	20.7	13.2	7.5	8.1 [b]	3.5 [b]	1.8 [b]	2.8 [b]
1963	112.6	109.8	2.8	—	25.2	16.0	9.2	—	—	—	—
1958	114.6	111.6	3.0	—	26.0	16.7	9.3	—	—	—	—
1953	104.5	98.0	6.5	—	25.0	16.9	8.1	—	—	—	—
1948	105.9	92.9	13.0	—	20.6	14.4	6.2	—	—	—	—
1947	98.2	85.7	12.5	—	18.6	13.1	5.5	—	—	—	—
1946	78.6	71.5	7.1	—	15.2	10.5	4.6	—	—	—	—
1945	68.2	64.3	3.9	—	13.2	9.0	4.2	—	—	—	—
1944	61.3	58.3	3.0	—	13.9	9.4	4.4	—	—	—	—
1940	56.3	52.5	3.8	—	22.9	16.7	6.2	—	—	—	—
1935	41.3	39.0	2.3	—	14.6	10.4	4.2	—	—	—	—
1930	30.3	n.a.	n.a	—	n.a.	n.a.	n.a.	—	—	—	—
1925	26.6	n.a.	n.a.	—	n.a.	n.a.	n.a.	—	—	—	—

Sources: VA, 1981 for years 1935 and later; Dillingham, 1952 Table 4 for years before 1935.

n.a. = not available.

[a] Program was begun in 1970.

[b] Program was begun in 1965.

age, for in 1981 39 percent of the domiciliary census was in state homes that received grants from the VA to help pay for these veterans' care. The nursing home census has the lowest proportion housed in VA facilities, some 36 percent. About the same proportion, 37 percent, is carried by community nursing homes and the remaining 27 percent is accommodated in state nursing homes. Thus, 97 percent of the VA hospital census, 62 percent of its domiciliary census, and 36 percent of the nursing home census was being carried in the VA's own facilities in 1981. The rest was paid for by the VA, in whole or in part, and served in state and privately owned facilities. The data in Table 5–3 are displayed graphically in Figure 5–3, which shows the relative size of the census cared for in VA and non VA facilities for hospitals, domiciliaries and nursing homes.

CHARACTERISTICS OF INPATIENT CLIENTELE. In fiscal year 1981 almost 24 percent of the 82,079 hospital beds and about 31 percent of the average daily inpatient census were in the psychiatric diagnostic category. In a special analysis of a one-day census, about 53 percent were found to be World War II veterans, 15 percent Vietnam War veterans, and 12 percent Korean War veterans.

The average age of the hospitalized veteran had been holding steady, and in some years even declined slightly, during the years immediately before and after 1965. The aging of the veteran population from World War II and previous wars was being offset by the accretion of new young veterans from the Korean and Vietnam conflicts. In addition, some older veterans were turning to Medicare after 1965 as is implied by the approximately one-forth of the veterans who were over sixty-five and by decline of this age group both absolutely and relatively in VA hospital utilization. Although the use of Medicare, in some cases in conjunction with Medicaid, explains perhaps most of this decline, an additional cause was the expansion of the nursing home census for some patients who before 1965 would have been kept in a VA acute care hospital bed. This is discussed further below. What the data on the age distribution of all veterans as well as those using the VA hospitals illustrates pointedly is that the fifty-five-to-sixty-four age category steadily became the most important group.

Each year the percentage of total patients in this group was larger than the year before, and until 1977 the absolute number was also rising annually. After 1977, the numbers stabilized at about 22 or 23 thousand, but the relative percentage in this category continued to grow because of the drop in the other categories of census. This age group is the one whose members were past middle age, in whom health conditions associated with aging were beginning to come to the fore, but who were not eligible for Medicare.

ELIGIBILITY CRITERIA. Which veterans are to be eligible for what services has been a central political question throughout the development of all veterans' services; it has certainly been for health services. The central point of contention has been the appropriateness of treating non-service-connected conditions, especially for patients who had no service-connected disabilities. A National Academy of Science (NAS) study (1977) of VA health care considered "the extent to which the VA should be responsible for the health care of veterans without service-connected disabilities to be one of the three issues that it needed to explore," and an earlier study of some aspects of the VA medical program found that the American Medical Association (AMA) "has been consistently hostile in a political sense to the governmental provision of medical care to veterans with non-service-connected disability . . ." (Lewis, 1970).

The relative distribution of the inpatient census for 1981, by decreasing order of eligibility category on a sample census day, was found to be:

1. 15.9 percent were veterans receiving care for service-connected disabilities. These veterans were unconditionally eligible for VA care.
2. 13.5 percent were veterans with service-connected disabilities who were receiving care for non–service-connected disabilities and were not on pension rolls. These veterans were technically eligible for VA care only if a bed was available.
3. 25.9 percent were receiving care for non-service-connected disability but were on VA pension rolls, i.e., they were indigent. (Pensions were being awarded to indigent veter-

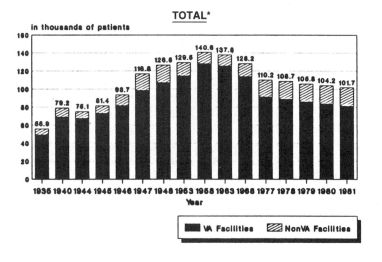

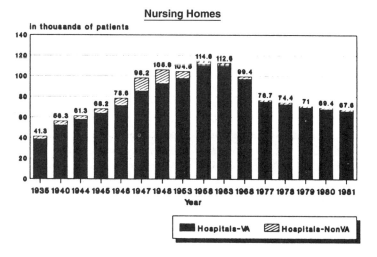

Fig. 5–3. Average daily census cared for in VA and non-VA facilities. *Note*: Numbers above bars represent combined census in VA and non-VA for total facilities, hospitals, nursing homes, and domicilliaries. *Source*: Table 5–3.

ans, and most pensioners were over sixty-five years of age.)

4. 44.2 percent were veterans without service-connected disabilities and were not receiving pensions. These veterans were technically eligible for VA care only if a bed were available, and they had to testify to inability to pay for hospitalization.

5. The remaining 0.4 percent were nonveterans.

Thus, 29.4 percent (categories 1 and 2, above) of the veterans on a typical census day in VA hospitals had a war-connected disability in 1981. Something over 70 percent had no service-con-

nected disability and most of these, 44.2 percent of the total census, were not receiving VA pensions and were largely under sixty-five years of age.

SUMMARY AND COMMENTS ON POSTWAR INCREASE IN INPATIENT USE. An increase in patient use did occur, but the flood of demand that had been feared did not materialize. The average occupancy of 81 percent that is shown for 1981 for total "hospital" beds is not very high for large hospitals with long average lengths of stay.[6] This indicates that there was not a large backlog of unmet demand due to lack of sufficient places, although local and regional short-

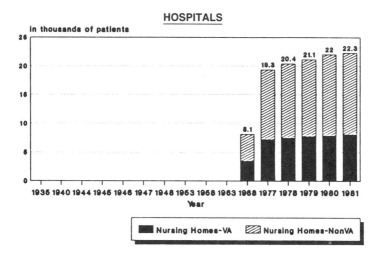

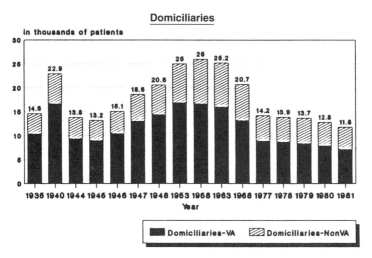

Fig. 5–3. *Continued*

ages as well as short-term shortages at any particular hospital from time to time cannot be ruled out. The reason for the comparatively moderate size of the post–World War II pressures on the veterans' hospitals was largely the postwar prosperity enjoyed by the United States, including low unemployment rates and the development of private health insurance during this period as an automatic fringe benefit of employment, especially for hospital benefits. The fact that Veterans Administration benefits covered only the veteran while private insurance often covered the entire family, as well as the widespread perception of the greater accessibility and desirability of private medicine, were undoubtedly

contributing factors to the privately insured veteran choosing not to use the VA services.

One would have thought that as World War II veterans grew older and sicker, they would have turned increasingly to the Veterans Administration facilities, and to some extent they did. The advent of Medicare, however, was undoubtedly a countervailing force to this expectation, especially for hospital care. In the case of poor veterans who were over sixty-five, Medicaid also provided alternative financing for their care. That this explanation is at least a reasonable one is shown by the use of extended care, a category of service that not only maintained its previous levels but exceeded them. Extended care is not well covered by private insurance or Medicare. Furthermore, the growing use of nursing home care and the declining use of domiciliary arrangements testifies to the aging and increasing morbidity among a large group of veterans, especially those of World War II. It also corroborates a well-known fact: nursing home care has been a particularly neglected sector for private health insurance and is very inadequately covered by Medicare. It is not all that surprising that veterans who might otherwise be well insured privately for acute care or be eligible for Medicare should turn to the VA for long-term care after having used private insurance and Medicare for acute care for many years.

Outpatient Services In the VA health care system, the outpatient services have historically been cast as an adjunct of the inpatient services rather than the usual arrangement in American medical practice, in which ambulatory services in the doctor's office are the main type of medical care, with inpatient services available as a backup service when needed. The previously cited NAS report (1977) noted that the VA clinics were for the most part located in the VA hospitals and that there were therefore too few locations at which ambulatory care could be conveniently obtained. Furthermore, the total outpatient capacity was too small for the need, especially for dental care.

Before August 1973, eligibility for the complete list of outpatient services available under VA auspices was limited to treatment for service-connected disabilities. Veterans with other classes of disabilities could obtain service for visits connected with prehospitalization and posthospitalization care only.[7] In 1973, eligibility for outpatient care was extended to veterans without service-connected disabilities, if such care were required to prevent hospitalization (P.L. 93–82). As a consequence, outpatient visits increased markedly after 1973. Faced with the evidence of the potential for a continuing sharp increase in the use of outpatient services following the 1973 liberalization of eligibility, Congress opted to restrain the rate of increase by a queuing system based on priorities rather than to expand resources to meet the expanded demand. The Veterans' Omnibus Health Care Act of 1976 (P.L. 94–581) established a six-category priority system and expressed the congressional intent that the VA limit its use of outside fee-for-service physicians as much as possible. But the NAS study had found in 1975 that "a large majority of veterans who use ambulatory services have no private physicians or other sources of care and are recurrent users of the outpatient and inpatient services of the VA. As currently set up, the ambulatory care programs in many VA facilities cannot provide comprehensive, continuous care of high quality." If the NAS assessment was correct, the restrictions imposed by the 1976 act curtailed services precisely in a service area most needed by veterans. The study was particularly critical of the organization and management of ambulatory care "in a substantial number of hospitals." (We recall that as of 1981 172 of the 226 VA outpatient clinics were located in hospitals and 50 were independent or satellite clinics.)

In 1979, P.L. 96–22 modestly expanded eligibility for dental care, which in 1981 alone brought 56,000 applications from veterans made newly eligible by this law. By 1981 outpatient services were being provided both by the VA staff and by private physicians and dentists who were reimbursed on a fee-for-service basis. Some of the ambulatory services now being provided were medical and dental care for service-connected disabilities and some other eligibles, the latter mainly involving prehospital and posthospital care; medical and dental care for veterans with service-connected disabilities who needed care for non-service-connected disabilities; and medical and dental care for other veterans on a priority waiting-list basis. Eligibility for dental care was more limited than for medical care and for examinations to determine medical eligibility for various aspects of the VA programs.

Eighty-eight percent of all outpatient visits were handled by VA staff in 1981. There was a sharp increase in visits between 1973 and 1976, when eligibility for outpatient care was first expanded, and a leveling off after 1976, when the restrictive priority queueing system was legislated.

The NAS study (1977) which included examination of VA internal records as well as site visits by the committee, noted that most VA dentistry, at least through 1975, was performed in conjunction with the inpatient services.[8]

CHAMPVA. In August 1973 a new medical program affecting veterans was enacted (P.L. 93–82) that provided some access for families of veterans. Known as Civilian Health and Medical Program of the VA (CHAMPVA), it provided for medical care for spouses and children of veterans who were totally and permanently disabled by service-connected conditions and for widows or widowers and children of veterans who had died from service-connected conditions. On January 1, 1980, surviving spouses or children of persons who died while on active duty were also made eligible for CHAMPVA, provided they were not eligible for Medicare or the Civilian Health and Medical Program of the Armed Forces (CHAMPUS), a similar program run for dependents of armed forces personnel. By the end of FY 1981, about 128,000 adults and 93,000 children, or 221,000 individuals enrolled in 137,000 family groups, were participating in the program. Interestingly enough, these benefits were to be provided primarily by private physicians and hospitals. VA hospitals were to be used only in cases for which these hospitals have a unique capability not available elsewhere, provided these unique facilities are not needed by a veteran. This program is administered by the Armed Forces CHAMPUS system, to be described later in this chapter. The program is an insurance-type operation and pays a percent of "reasonable charges" for outpatient services and for hospitalization. For outpatient services, there is an annual deductible per person with a maximum ceiling on cost sharing per family.

SUMMARY AND COMMENTS ON POSTWAR INCREASE IN OUTPATIENT USE. We have seen that the expected explosion in demand for acute impatient care did not materialize. Instead the main pressure was for more long-term care and for outpatient services. While the capacity for long-term care was expanded substantially to meet the growing demand, it would appear that a large measure of need and demand for ambulatory care remained unmet. The increased pressure for more ambulatory care was contained by maintaining and in some instances even increasing restrictions on eligibility.

Quality

In addition to expanding its resources quantitatively in anticipation of a post–World War II surge in demand, the VA also embarked on an ambitious program for improving the quality of its care. Much has been said about the elusive nature of medical care "quality" and how to measure it (Donabedian, 1966, 1969), (Brook), (Green), (Starfield), but the many aspects of this subject and the nuances associated with them cannot be entered into here. The following discussion of the post–World War II efforts of the Veterans Administration to improve quality of care will be based, for the most part, on the first of three widely accepted criteria—structure, process, and outcome—so cogently articulated in Donabedian's work (1966). It has been the main criterion implied by the VA efforts at quality enhancement and the only one of these three dimensions whose use has been reported in any detail. When using the "structure" criterion, one looks at aspects of the resources available for providing the requisite services, such as the qualifications and number of staff per patient and the appropriateness and quantitative adequacy of facilities and equipment. The assumption is that conformity to such structural criteria produces better medical practice ("process") and that the resulting better medical practice in turn results in improved health ("outcome"). Clearly, an appropriate quantity and professional mix of personnel is an integral part of judging proper quality with respect to personnel. Because the quantitative aspects of the quality criterion were discussed previously under "resource expansion," I shall concentrate here on the VA effort to increase the qualifications of its personnel and the quality of its facilities rather than their quantity, but some references to quantity will be unavoidable because the quality of personnel and facilities and their appropriate quantity are so inextricably intertwined in judging the overall quality of a medical care delivery system. Some reference to process and outcome evaluations will also be made but, as noted, reports on these appear sparsely, as is generaly the case in medical care literature, because they are more expensive and difficult both to carry out and to assess.

Under the leadership of General Bradley, who was appointed director of the Veterans Administration in 1945, plans were made to intensify efforts to improve the quality of the medical care available to all veterans by affiliating Veterans Administration hospitals with the medical education resources of the United States.

In 1946, the Department of Medicine and Surgery was established within the VA by congressional legislation (P.L. 79–293) to help effectuate General Bradley's plans. "This creation of a separate VA medical staff was intended to elevate the quality of the staff and the direction of the over-all medical program" (Lewis, 1970). It established a self-contained personnel system independent of the United States Civil Service Commission and provided for a physician Chief Medical Director to be appointed by the Administrator of Veterans Affairs. The act provided for the inauguration of a program of graduate training in association with medical schools that marked "a milestone in the progress of the Federal government in cooperation with civilian medicine." A "gentlemen's agreement" was entered into between the Veterans Administration and the deans of about 90 percent of the medical schools.

A 1950 article in the Journal of the American Medical Association stated:

The plan for affiliation with medical education forces envisaged the construction of new hospital facilities near the medical schools of the United States and the utilization of the faculties to aid in the programs of medical care and education. In such institutions the responsibility for hospital operations would be that of the Veterans Administration and the responsibility for the quality of the medical care would be accepted to a large degree by the medical schools.

In addition, the program would develop a situation whereby the Veterans' Administration would enlist as many high caliber medical practitioners as possible on full-time duty. The professional services of the medical colleges have been utilized by the appointment of consultants for actual service in the program of medical care. These consultants supervise the professional work, carry on the teaching program and make their services available in any other way deemed necessary by the full-time members of the staff. There has been appointed a large group of attending physicians and surgeons who, in general, are younger men but who do active service in the medical and surgical wards with residents working full time under their direction. Each affiliated veterans' hospital under this plan is operated by what is known as the Deans Committee, and today such institutions are referred to as 'Deans Committee hospitals.'

In these situations all consultants and attending men are recommended for appointment by the Deans Committee and the appointments made by the Veterans Administration. Thus, there has been developed a tremendous group of part-time, high-grade medical talent throughout the United States in the capacity of consultants and attending men, whose appointment have been recommended in every instance by Deans Committees of the various medical schools and who are utilized in addition to the gradually enlarging, full-time staffs in the various installations ... (Kracke, 1950).

It should be noted, however, that while some 90 percent of the medical schools were associated with VA hospitals by 1959, approximately half of the VA hospitals were not associated with medical schools because of their geographic location away from them. As of that year, 72 medical schools and 93 hospitals were participating in this program. In October 1959, George E. Armstrong, a physician, speaking for the Special Medical Advisory Group to the Veterans Administration, wrote:

In presenting this report as a spokesmen for the Special Medical Advisory Group, I am pleased to call attention to the tremendous contribution which American Medicine has made, and continues to make, to the total VA program. In this cooperative effort there has been an ever-increasing degree of understanding between practicing physicians and VA staffs' general acceptance of mutual obligations toward veteran patients, and, finally, a feeling of national pride in our democratic system which provides excellent medical care for the men and women who have earned their eligibility through service to the country (1959).

Dr. Armstrong then proceeds to describe the contribution of the VA to medical education, largely in terms of training facilities provided by the VA hospitals. There is ample evidence of the early perception by representatives of organized medicine, the VA, and the medical colleges that the contribution of the VA medical system to the professional training system in "American medicine" had been substantial and that the AMA committee concerned with medical education supported the move. However, a nonphysician student of the development of the VA medical program, B. J. Lewis, wrote in 1965 that the AMA had consistently opposed extension of VA medical services to non-service-connected disabilities. "American medicine has taken a dim view of the steady expansion of veterans' hospitals because this expansion obviously accommodates increasingly non-service-connected patient loads" (1970). Thus while the AMA Council on Medical Education and Hospitals of the American Medical Association supported the affiliation agreements as deepening the quality of care, the AMA's position on the VA services opposed the expansion of its volume. That this opposition did not prevent such an expansion is quite evident from the previous descriptions of post–World War II trends in changing numbers of facilities and use.

By the end of 1967, almost 12 percent (3,754) of the nation's medical residents, as well as a substantial portion of other medical personnel, were being trained in VA institutions. The VA had also become a major resource for schools of nursing and various allied health training programs, and VA personnel were holding faculty appointments in academic institutions of medicine, dentistry, and other health professions. By 1971, 82 medical schools had Deans Committees operating within their programs, and the number of participating VA hospitals was 96; by 1981, 132 out of 172 VA hospitals as well as 40 outpatient clinics were affiliated with 100 medical schools. In addition, a substantial number of these institutions also had affiliation agreements with schools of dentistry and with some other types of health professions training programs.

In 1981 the number of faculty appointments of VA staff totaled 9,259, including 7,232 physicians, 407 dentists, and 1,620 other staff. The 7,500 full-time medical residency positions supported by the VA in 1981 represented about a sixth of the nation's total number of medical residents in training.[9] About 40 percent of United States trainees in all medical specialties other than internal medicine, obstetrics/gynecology, and pediatrics were doing at least part of their training at the VA. About 27 percent of all fully approved general-practice programs in this country were at sixty-nine facilities of the VA. A large number of allied health professionals also were training at the VA.

While the training facilities have often been praised as excellent in both scope and quality from an educational point of view, occasional newspaper accounts reported poor care and dissatisfied patients (*Los Angeles Times,* 1970, 1972). The overall quality of care rendered to patients was not publicly assessed in a systematic fashion, however, until the previously cited 1977 study of the National Academy of Sciences (NAS). The NAS study was able to assess quality of care not by "structure" criteria alone but also by some "process" measures because of VA cooperation in granting access to site visits and to the use of survey questionnaires and interviews. In a few instances "outcome" measures, such as postoperative complications and patient satisfaction, were also available. It was found that access to needed care, with the exception of dental care, was rarely denied veterans. About 4 percent of the veterans responding to a questionnaire stated that they felt they could not obtain needed dental care. By contrast, only 1 percent complained that they could not obtain needed medical, surgical, or psychiatric services. It should be noted, however, that 1 percent still represents 300,000 veterans and "can easily explain the volume of complaints received by the VA and the Congress" (1977, 33). The NAS study included the following observations with respect to quality of care:[10]

1. The medical school affiliation program was found on balance to be beneficial to all parties concerned. "The quality of care furnished to the nation's veterans has improved, and the educational enterprise has been promoted." This opinion was based entirely on the affiliation between VA hospitals and medical schools; relationships with other professional schools (dental, nursing, pharmacy, social work, and others) were not studied because of constraints on time and resources. However, the VA does not depend to the same degree on its affiliation relationship with other professional schools to actually supply its nonphysician hospital staff as it does for its physician staff. Therefore, the study concentration on medical school affiliation was not as arbitrarily one-sided as it may seem at first glance.

2. The VA was a regular source of care for about 3 million of the 30 million living veterans. This core of frequent users consisted typically of low-income or socially isolated persons; only 17 percent of those under sixty-five had health insurance and only 30 percent had service-connected disabilities. There was "excessive reliance" on hospital care, and ambulatory services were inadequate, especially for those with non-service-connected disabilities. "Outpatient-care facilities are—for the most part—in the 171 hospitals and are therefore relatively sparse. The capacity to provide outpatient care in VA facilities appears to be insufficient in relation to current and potential demand. . . . The VA system is organized and its resources allocated primarily to supply inpatient hospital services." As a result outpatient services were found to be inadequately staffed, operating with inadequate facilities, and not well managed or organized. The report noted the broadening of eligibility for outpatient services in 1973, but instead of expanding outpatient service capacity in anticipation of increased demand, Congress in 1976 directed the VA to keep use within the confines of existing capacity by using eligibility priorities.

3. The overall quality of acute medical care was rated as outstanding in five hospitals, adequate in thirteen hospitals and inadequate in three hospitals by the team of site visitors to the twenty-one sample general hospitals. The quality of acute medical care was inadequate in five of the six psychiatric hospitals visited. Of the discharged patients responding to the questionnaire, more than 50 percent rated their physician and nurse care as excellent; 5 percent rated it poor.

4. Surgical care depended heavily on residents. Full-time VA surgeons performed few operations. Residents performed 79 percent of all operations and 69 percent of all the operations they performed were not supervised by a staff surgeon, either full- or part-time. Despite most operations being done by residents, adverse outcomes as measured by complication rates and surgical mortality were not higher than was to be expected in average hospitals. However, in the ten psychiatric hospitals that were visited the crude mortality rate was excessive, with the number of operations performed being too small to expect surgical proficiency.

The agency's data giving the numbers of health care personnel by certain categories of professionals clearly indicate that a smaller proportion of the physicians were full-time (60 percent in 1981) compared with nurses (90 percent). This largely reflects the fact that much of the physician staffing depended on VA relationships with medical schools. Building these medical school/VA relationships was stressed after World War II rather than concentrating on expanding the numbers of senior full-time inhouse staff. The account of the attempt to improve professional staffing technical quality to meet expected postwar demand centered therefore on the measures taken to implement medical school relationships.

5. Psychiatric care was evaluated as being of lesser quality overall than medical and surgical services. "In general, the Committee concluded, on the basis of comments by expert consultants, that substantial inadequacies in both quantity and quality of professional psychiatric staff—both psychiatrists and nurses—exist in many VA facilities." The report also noted that antipsychotic drugs were often administered in place of psychotherapy, such drugs often being administered "at variance with the VA's own policies and guidelines," and that "Relatively small numbers of the alcoholic-patient population appear to be receiving comprehensive care and rehabilitation services."

6. Rehabilitation medicine was, on the whole, adjudged a strong point of the VA medical systems. All VA hospitals had rehabilitation-bed sections. The resources were average or above average in 71 percent of the sample of 23 VA hospitals that were visited. None of the programs, however, were as good as two outstanding non-VA centers that were visited.

7. The VA was found to have met only a small fraction of the substantial needs of veterans for a broad range of dental care in 1975. Although this was largely due to severe eligibility constraints on dental care access, even those veterans eligible for dental care were receiving inadequate care due to insufficient service capacity, at least part of which resulted from a failure to adopt modern methods of service delivery.

8. A considerable portion of the inpatient census listed as "acute care" in official VA sta-

tistics was defined by the study as being nonacute in nature and being more properly classified
as needing "intermediate care"—somewhere
between nursing home and acute care.

The report indicated the presence of cost inefficiencies stemming from the inappropriate
use of acute beds and the installation and maintenance of underused expensive equipment and
programs. "The VA has installed many expensive specialized medical facilities that, in many
hospitals, are used at rates far below their capacity. Furthermore, in many communities in
which VA hospitals have underutilized services,
there are community hospitals offering the same
services and the community facilities also are
frequently utilized at rates well below their capacity."

The nursing home care was generally judged
to be very good compared with good quality
non-VA nursing homes. The intermediate care
units were judged to give less adequate care bordering on being quite poor. This was attributed
primarily to the understaffing of the intermediate
care units compared with the nursing homes.
"The quality of care in community nursing
homes in which veterans are placed on contract
is generally inferior to that in the VA nursing-
home-care units" even though the community
nursing homes with which the VA contracts

"represent a superior quality of care within the
community." In brief, the findings were that the
nonacute care provided by the VA, especially
the nursing home care, was superior to most of
the long-term care provided outside the VA. In
spite of this, the care was adjudged "generally
not excellent." This was thought to be because
"very few institutions either in the VA or in the
country at large are doing well in meeting the
needs of geriatric patients."

9. The domiciliary program was found to be
residential rather than rehabilitative. The care
was adequate but "austere" with few amenities.
The clients ("members") were "disaffiliated"
from society and infirm.

10. The major overall recommendation of the
committee was that "*VA policies and programs
should be designed to permit the VA system ultimately to be phased into the general delivery
of health service in communities across the
country.* [Emphasis in the original.]

Unit Costs

Table 5–4 displays the unit costs of various
types of health care in VA facilities and the adjusted[11] expenses per inpatient day of nonfederal
short-term general hospitals. The VA cost of inpatient care per inpatient day has clearly been

Table 5–4. Unit Cost (dollars) of Care in VA Facilities and National Averages: Selected Fiscal Years

	1965	1969	1974	1979	1980	1981
			Veterans Administration			
Inpatient day		34.17	65.08	133.82	154.00	168.36
Medical		42.66	68.02	139.44	159.10	175.1
Surgical			89.74	179.25	208.65	228.38
Psychiatric		22.58	46.45	95.87	111.03	119.62
Outpatient visit			56.29	61.60	64.09	
Domiciliary day		7.77	13.89	25.65	29.39	32.04
Nursing home day		15.69	35.83	65.65	75.40	81.72
			Nationwide averages			
Adjusted expenses per inpatient day in nonfederal short-term general hospitals*	40.56	64.26	113.21	215.75	244.44	

Average annual percent increase in cost per patient day—1980 over 1969	
VA per inpatient day	15.0 percent
All nonfederal short-term general hospitals per adjusted patient day	12.9 percent

Source: VA for VA data; AHA, 1981 for national hospital data.

*Said by the AHA to represent cost of inpatient care only.

much lower than the average for all nonfederal hospitals. One is not sure just what to make of this in light of the NAS assertion that a substantial fraction of the VA acute beds were occupied by patients who required and were receiving care that was much less intensive than acute medical care and that many required only domiciliary care. The NAS study made a big point of this, claiming that the system of resource allocation used by the VA budgeting system impelled administrators to classify the largest possible number of beds as acute and that the patient census conducted by the study found "that about half the patients in acute medical beds, one-third of the patients in surgical beds, and well over half the patients in psychiatric beds do not require—and are not receiving—the acute care services associated with these types of beds" (National Academy of Sciences, 1977). The NAS study implied strongly that the VA system was actually not cost efficient for two reasons: it had too many extended-care patients in acute beds, and it was not sufficiently aggressive in carrying out the congressional mandate to share expensive equipment and facilities with non-VA hospitals in the area wherever feasible. A study of comparative costs between VA hospitals and non-VA hospitals, adjusting for differences in case mix, has yet to been done, so the arguments of the NAS study committee and others that the VA may be expensive, given the type of cases it handles, stand as hypotheses but the raw data show the VA to be less expensive.

Another way to look at measures of the relative cost efficiency of the VA medical services is to look at rates of increase over time of total national health expenditures and compare them with rates of increase in VA expenditures. Using this approach, the NAS study found that national health expenditures increased by 71.2 percent from 1970 to 1975 and VA expenditures by 100 percent in the same period. The data in Table 5–5 indicate that if one takes a longer span of time that includes some years after the NAS report came out, the results are rather different. Between 1969 and 1981 national health expenditures increased 337 percent and VA expenditures by 327 percent (lines 6 and 7). Per capita expenditures similarly increased at a somewhat lower rate for the VA than for the nation as a whole. The annualized average rate of increase in total expenditures was about 13 percent per year for both. Furthermore, the percentage of national expenditures for health attributable to the VA remained between 2.3 and 2.5 for all years shown (line 3). Thus it is clear that whatever

Table 5–5. Total VA Health Expenditures Compared with National Health Expenditures

	1965	1969	1974	1979	1980	1981
Expenditures **Years as indicated: Fiscal Calendar for National and VA**						
1. National total health expenditures (millions of dollars)	41,700	65,600	116,400	215,000	249,000	286,600
Per capital	211	318	535	938	1,075	1,225
2. VA total health expenditures (millions of dollars)		1,554.0	2,950.6	5,448.0	6,157.8	6,642.1
Per capita		58	101	181	201	221
3. VA total as % of national total		2.37	2.50	2.53	2.47	2.32
		Percent increase over previously specified year				
Total expenditure:						
4. National		57.3	77.48	84.7	15.88	15.1
5. VA			89.9	84.6	7.9	

Changes in Expenditures over Time
(Total & average annual percent increase 1981 over 1969)

	Total	Annualized average
6. National Total	336.9	13.07
Per capita	285.2	
7. VA Total	327.4	12.87
Per capita	282.8	

Source: VA for VA data; Health Care Financing Administration, Sept. 1982, for national health expenditure data.

discrepancies in costliness there are between the VA and other health care systems, these discrepancies were not widening over these twelve years and fail to indicate that the VA was any more costly than the average of other health care systems. The raw figures seem to indicate that it is less costly, but as noted, strongly asserting this conclusion seems unjustified without comparative studies controlling for case mix. For the same reason the supposition that the VA would be found to be more costly than other hospitals remains only a supposition.

The Vietnam Veteran

Thus, the most comprehensive of the publicly circulated reviews of VA medical care during the core period encompassed by this book judged the large expansion in veterans' health services that took place after World War II to have included substantial improvement in quality, over and above that implied by the increase in quantity of resources alone. Most of the measures to increase the intrinsic quality of the care itself were centered on acute inpatient medicine and the principal method was medical school affiliation. However, during the years 1960–1975 a new problem was developing for the VA medical services, the entry of Vietnam veterans into the veteran population. By 1974 almost a fourth of all veterans were Vietnam veterans and in 1981 they constituted over 30 percent of the total. By the latter year the average age of all veterans was 48.0 years; for Vietnam veterans it was 34.3. In 1969 the average age for all veterans had been 44.3 and for Vietnam veterans, 26.2. While the World War II veteran continued to dominate the inpatient census, the Vietnam veteran component jumped from 11 percent in 1972 to 15 percent in 1981 (VA, 1981). When one adds part of the "between Korean conflict and Vietnam era" component, many of whom may also be Vietnam veterans, the growing extent of the patient load that consisted of the Vietnam veteran was even larger. The Vietnam veteran was different from veterans of previous periods, particularly those of World Wars I and II. These differences created problems for the VA's administration, including its administration of medical services.

One main difference manifested itself in the psychological problems emanating from the public opposition to the Vietnam war, in sharp contrast to the patriotic fervor and public support for World War II. The Vietnam veteran was reported to suffer from a feeling of having sacrificed for a cause that many Americans condemned as brutal murder of an underdeveloped people. Psychiatric problems, many attributed to this feeling, arose among Vietnam veterans at an earlier age than did the psychiatric problems of World War II veterans, which were viewed as largely due to the onset of psychiatric senility and other ailments associated with aging. An article in the *New York Times* in 1970 (reprinted in VA (1972)) put it in this fashion:

There were no victory parades, no brass bands, no cheering crowds when [the Vietnam veteran] ... came marching home from Vietnam. . . .

Most of the . . . veterans of the Vietnam war . . . have slipped quietly back into society. . . .

They seldom make news. Hardly anyone calls them heroes. They return one by one—not by regiment or division as their older brothers did from the Korean war or their fathers from World War II or their grandfathers from World War I. . . .

He is a silent veteran—perhaps the nation's first— and he is on his way to becoming the nation's first forgotten veteran.

A second difference lay in the social and ethnic composition of the Vietnam veteran population. In World War II the United States draft cut across most classes of Americans. In the Vietnam war, exemptions from the draft of college students and other more advantaged segments of the population were widespread. Consequently, Vietnam veterans came disproportionately from low-income and ethnic minority population groups. National concern grew over the problems of Vietnam veterans in obtaining proper medical and psychological help if they needed them; it was evidenced in the press, in Congress, and by the VA itself. A reflection of this concern is the special identification of Vietnam veterans in many of the VA statistics and the issuance of publications like *The Vietnam Veteran in Contemporary Society,* which in 1972 published a collection of articles written by social scientists and psychotherapists on the Vietnam veteran. In this collection, Dr.

Cecil P. Peck, a VA psychologist, describes the special nature of the Vietnam veteran's problems.

The Vietnam veteran is unique in that he has fought in a highly complex war which is interlocked with unprecedented social, educational, economic, political and cultural changes of the last twenty years that have had a profound influence on his human values, the intellectual and emotional aspects of his life style, and the personal conflicts . . . over meaningfulness and meaninglessness of life in our society have had a shaping impact. [As a consequence] . . . Vietnam patients are characteristically more rebellious, demanding and confrontational in contrast to more passivity, politeness, passive aggressiveness and reservation of WWII and Korean veterans (VA, 1972).

There were situations reported describing the conflict in the VA medical facilities between the young "new style" Vietnam veteran and the traditional older veteran. Accusations were made that the veterans' associations were dominated by the older veterans and did not defend the interests of the Vietnam veteran. For example, a writer, Jim Castelli, remarked in the *Catholic World* in 1971:

Some have suggested that the more traditional groups are more interested in protecting their lobbying position and their older members than in helping the younger veterans. Many patients and staff complain that many older veterans are needlessly occupying beds that are needed by younger men, using the VA system as a hotel. Even pro-war veterans have used drugs, wear long-hair, have 'loose morals' by the standards of World War II veterans, and in general are still different enough to represent a threat to these generally conservative groups. Many leaders of the older veterans groups have been active in trying to secure help for wounded GIs, but it appears that the power of the older organizations is rapidly becoming a thing of the past; they will have no new blood, having lost it in the rice paddies of Vietnam (VA, 1972).

A third factor that was new in the Vietnam veteran was the greater prevalence of severely disabled veterans among them. This resulted in large part from the newer and better emergency measures being used at the front. "One out of ten soldiers wounded today would have died of the same wound in any previous war; while quick evacuation methods and medical advances are keeping these men alive, doctors are faced with wounds of degree of severity that they have never had to cope with before in such numbers" (VA, 1972).

All in all, it would appear that during the early 1970s, at least, the younger Vietnam veterans were apparently not being easily assimilated into the VA care system, which had been treating largely older and chronically ill veterans. What the long-term influence of the Vietnam veteran upon VA operation and policy would be was not clear. These veterans continued to organize and to confront VA authorites in areas where they deemed the service inadequate. They made up 30 percent of the veteran population in 1981 and as the World War II and Korean veterans grew steadily fewer, they became an ever larger proportion of the VA population. This trend continued and their average age of thirty-four years in 1981 also continued to increase with time. It is rather likely, however, that those aging Vietnam veterans who entered normal civilian life upon their return will not prove to be much different as patients when they seek care than other previous veterans, except for the general differences due to the "generation gap" in the United States population at large.

That the problem had not gone away or begun to abate by 1980, however, was evidenced by the continuing frequent appearance of newspaper stories about Vietnam veterans, many of the stories dealing with the VA. In 1981 the VA annual report described a just completed study by the Center for Policy Research entitled "Legacies of Vietnam; Comparative Adjustment of Veterans and Their Peers." The VA cited the need for this study as stemming from "limited research findings, general consensus of experts, professional staff of VA medical centers and considerable direct feedback from Vietnam era veterans, their families and from other concerned groups of citizens that approximately 20 percent of Vietnam era veterans are continuing to have readjustment problems" (VA, 1981).

Summary

The Veterans Administration directly runs a comprehensive medical service for which, as of 1981, 30 million veterans,[12] or about 13 percent of the U.S. population, were eligible, in varying degree. For inpatient services, eligibility has been open to virtually all veterans requiring only the deposition of medical indigency for non–service-connected cases. Access to ambulatory services has been more restricted. The staff-per-occupied-bed ratios increased from 1970 to 1981 but were still far below those in nonfederal community hospitals nationally. This may reflect a less intensive case mix in the VA hospitals, and until this is carefully studied the adequacy of the staffing is not clear. About 3 million veterans were found to use VA facilities as their main source of health care in 1975. This rose to 4 million in 1991.

The post World War II anticipated degree of increased demand for the post–World War II period did not materialize. The increase was modest, with the demand being partially damped by the Medicare and Medicaid programs and the growth of private health insurance. The most substantial increase in demand was for nursing home care, for which private insurance and Medicare provided skimpily.

The VA medical services were provided at a ''structural'' level of quality that was approved by mainstream medicine and without any charge. A major study of the system as it was in 1975 judged it to be of quite good quality in terms of structure and process for its inpatient services but lacking adequate access in its ambulatory services, especially dental care. The extended-care services were not as good as they might be but better than the average non-VA-provided services, especially with respect to nursing homes. The psychiatric services were found to be the poorest of the inpatient services. Affiliation with medical schools and other health-professional training centers introduced a large component of the academic medicine milieu. Vietnam veterans brought with them a set of problems that many observers and experts called ''new,'' and which in 1981 were still in the process of resolution. Among the effects that seemed to be developing were new forms of veterans organization and more openly adversarial relationships between Vietnam veterans and the VA.

Despite the fact that the provision of dental care had been singled out as one of the medical services needing the most upgrading, the first major Reagan budget embodied in the Omnibus Reconciliation Act of 1981 (P.L. 97–35) curtailed outpatient dental treatment for veterans with non-service-connected dental conditions. The Reagan administration consistently attempted to reduce the appropriations for the VA medical services despite the campaign of the same administration to reverse the public perception of the Vietnam war as a mistaken venture. The details of this battle lie beyond the period covered by this book, which ends with year end 1981, but at the time of this writing (1991) the efforts to reduce the appropriations substantially have not been successful.

Some Policy Implications

The VA health care system is one of the clearest examples of government-sponsored, directly provided, health care set up in the United States for special populations, a central feature of the prevailing pattern of our national health care system. The dominant U.S. model has been that medical care is something one purchases in an entrepreneurial, albeit not really competitive, private market. Government supplying such care directly is a departure from the norm that must be justified as being for special persons and under special conditions. When the antecedent of the present government medical care system for veterans was first instituted in the early 1920s, there were insufficient hospital beds for veterans and there were no government programs like Medicare and Medicaid to help pay for the care of indigent people, including veterans. Since 1946, the Hill-Burton program (see Chapter 12) has produced what some believe to be a surfeit of acute hospital beds, and Medicare and Medicaid have, since 1965, helped pay for the care of elderly and of poor persons. To some analysts this has signaled a need for phasing out the VA program and integrating it into the general health care system. Prominent among such advocates was the Committee on Health Care Resources in the Veterans Administration, which formulated the report of the NAS (1977) cited rather extensively in this chapter. The committee's recommendations on ''phasing in'' the VA system were based on the assumptions that national health insurance ''in some form'' was imminent and that the veteran population will continue to age. Under these assumptions, it was argued that a separate system would be largely redundant in the near future since everyone would have access to the "mainstream" of community care. Because it was considered likely that early versions of national health insurance would emphasize acute care and underplay extended care, the committee saw a more protracted need for providing extended care and ambulatory care by the VA and urged a move away from what it perceived to be an overemphasis on acute hospital facilities and care arrangements.

There can be no reasonable argument with the central idea lying at the core of the committee's position that overlapping systems of care, each with a specially designated set of eligibles for the same service, is socially disintegrative and economically inefficient. If a national system of comprehensive health care were established that is universally accessible, that is, one that provides a true "mainstream" used by the overwhelming preponderance of the population, many[13] of the various systems for special eligibles should then be phased into the mainstream as rapidly as possible. In fact, if such a system had existed earlier, much of the VA medical system as well as most of the other special systems for special populations would very likely not have developed at all. But the ineluctable fact is that we do not have a comprehensive, universal national health care system, and no one can say with any assurance when we are likely to have one. Because of this, the care the VA is providing continues to serve millions of people who would otherwise have great difficulty in obtaining it. Furthermore, this care is claimed as a right, not as a patronizingly bestowed privilege or charity, and it is generally of better quality than is otherwise available to the low-income and poor persons and the long-term patients who are now the principal regular VA users. It is all well and good to remark that a neighboring private facility offers a service that the VA provides and can physically accommodate the VA load because both the VA and non-VA facility each now have this service underutilized. But statistics that are or could be collected on such places would not fully indicate how willing the other facility would be to take *all* VA patients, and how willing they would be and for what price they would agree to do so in years to come, after the VA facility was closed. The non-VA

facility may be ready to contract for an acceptable price now, but what if costs rise, federal budgets fall, and the contractor asks a price in the future the government will not pay?

This is not a fanciful scenario. It has happened with a number of programs, as we shall have occasion to see in later chapters, especially in the deinstitutionalization program for mental health care described in Chapter 6. This problem of cutting a program that is offering needed services because there is a better way to do it before the "better way" is established and funded runs through the history of our health (and other) service programs. First cutting a program with perceived problems to replace it with a better one, and then failing to follow through on replacing it has been a practice often used to reduce needed services. Other instances of the use of this policy are discussed in subsequent parts of this chapter as well as in later chapters.

DIRECT MEDICAL CARE SERVICES OF THE U.S. PUBLIC HEALTH SERVICE

The Public Health Service Hospitals

For many years the Veterans Administration has been the main medical care operation run by the federal government that provides direct services, but the U.S. Public Health Service represents the earliest entry of the federal government into direct provision of medical care via its original predecessor agency, the Marine Hospital Service. Although the Public Health Service hospitals were discontinued in the 1980s, their history spanning almost two hundred years illuminates an important aspect of public policy on government provision of medical care—its restriction of eligibility to special groups. We have seen that the Veterans Administration medical programs arose from the public perception that veterans were specially deserving of such care. Presumably this attitude was tied to the necessity to guarantee a continued positive feeling toward wartime service in the armed forces. The direct medical services of the United States Public Health Service (USPHS or PHS) had a similar origin except that the beneficiaries of special eligibility were persons who served in a civilian service deemed essential to the growth of United States commerce—the American merchant ships, collectively called the merchant marine.

The Marine Hospital Service Act of 1798 authorized the establishment of marine hospitals to care for American merchant seamen in several ports of the United States and provided for the deduction of twenty cents per month from each seaman's monthly wages to help finance the hospitals. Deficiencies in revenue were made up from general tax revenues. Harry Mustard, in his rather detailed analysis of the attitudes of the Congressmen of 1798 who voted for this bill (Mustard, 1945, 50), indicates that the legislators did not really have health insurance in mind, but in point of fact the act itself was an example of compulsory health insurance. It established a noncharity service available to all merchant seamen despite some of the debate in opposition to the bill centering on the assertion that demonstrably indigent seamen should be cared for by charity and the others could pay for themselves.

This act marked the beginning of the trend by government in the United States to provide medical care for select groups of people. In this case, not only was the merchant fleet deemed essential to United States prosperity, but the defined group also comprised persons who, because of their occupations, were often not officially residents of the locality in which they found themselves when they became ill and thus were not eligible for locally provided charity care. Their problem was seen by Mustard in 1945 as similar to that of the migratory worker of his day who fell prey to tuberculosis and was not eligible for state medical care. (It remains a continuing problem for the migratory worker of recent years, one which the federal program for migratory health centers was meant to abate. This is discussed in Chapter 11.)

The amount deducted from seamen's wages was raised to forty cents per month in 1870, and later a flat tonnage tax paid by the shippers became the sole source of user contribution and the deduction from seamen's wages was discontinued. The tonnage tax, too, was eliminated after 1905, and all financing for the marine hospitals thereafter came from general tax funds appropriated for this purpose.

Originally, the program was organized to operate "through local contracts for medical and hospital service." This system apparently did not work satisfactorily. Many of the difficulties encountered under the Marine Service Act arose in connection with the lack of a centralized administration and the consequent lack of uniformity of standards among the different hospitals. Each hospital operated under the authority of the customs collector of the port in which the hospital was situated and the customs collector worked for the state in which the port was located. As a result, conditions and standards varied among hospitals not only because of differences in conditions at the various ports but also because of the precarious tenure of the position of customs collector, which was a political spoils-system appointment. Hospitals could be built with federal funds, but even these were usually operated through local contracts. The initial practice of having the president of the United States appoint surgeons to the marine hospitals was soon abandoned and these appointments became one of the perquisites of the position of customer collector.

The act of 1870 that raised collections from seamen to forty cents per month also called for "nationalized supervision, under medical auspices," and a national supervising surgeon was appointed. This act, according to Mustard, created a national service "from an administrative standpoint." The first supervising surgeon under the new act, Dr. John M. Woodworth, proved to be a strong leader, and perhaps reflecting his military background, "he organized the new corps and its procedures along military lines," instituted entrance examinations for the service and tenure of office. In 1889 this organization came to be called the U.S. Public Health Service "Commissioned Corps" and in 1890 an act of Congress formalized its quasi-military status with the members of the corps being given commissions and uniforms.

In 1902 the name of the Marine Hospital Service was changed to the Public Health and Marine Hospital Service, and its organization was further formalized under the direction of a Surgeon General. In 1912 the name was changed again to the present one, the United States Public Health Service. By then the agency was operating in three areas:

1. The "public health" areas discussed in earlier sections of Part I, primarily in quarantine work;
2. The public health hospitals, as the Marine Hospitals were now called; and
3. The research area, to be discussed in Chapter 14.

In 1939 the U.S. Public Health Service was finally transferred out of the Treasury Department, where it had anomalously been lodged for 141 years as a consequence of its origins being tied to customs collections, and placed in the newly created Federal Security Agency. In 1953 it was transferred to the newly created Department of Health, Education and Welfare (HEW), which absorbed the parent Federal Security Agency. A total picture of the Public Health Service requires including a discussion of the National Institutes of Health, to be covered in Chapter 14; here I discuss only the later course of the public health hospitals and other medical care services and facilities that were or are operated directly by the U.S. Public Health Service.

By 1943 the Public Health Service hospitals were all under central administration and medical direction. As Mustard noted: "The system of indirect and contract medical service, at first entirely localized, had become strongly centralized. Except in minor instances, part-time physicians have given place to full-time medical officers employed on a career basis, though consultation staff (part-time private physicians) are maintained" (1945). There were by then twenty-six Marine Hospitals with 6,500 beds, all approved by the American Hospital Association. The system was supported from general tax revenues, and the merchant seamen had come to constitute but a small proportion of the eligible and actual users. Eligibility had been extended to include Coast Guard personnel and dependents, Coast and Geodetic Survey (now the National Oceanic and Atmospheric Administration) personnel and dependents, Public Health Service officers and employees, Army, Navy and Marine Corps, and a number of other government employees. It provided 2.5 million patient days and 3.1 million outpatient visits per annum.

This development is not only of historical interest in demonstrating how government medical care came to be extended as a right to special groups; it may also hold lessons for future policy on national insurance and on choice of delivery systems to be used by government medical care programs. A Mustard points out, one could conclude either "that locally autonomous and noncentrally directed medical services have proven themselves impracticable; or, with a different approach and attitude, it might be concluded that the tendency of the Federal Government, in operating a medical service, is to supplant local independence with centrally directed bureaucratic control. . . ."[14] However, Mustard himself supplies ample evidence of the poor quality and economic inefficiency of the local contracted-out system before it became a centrally controlled, federally operated system as a result of the changes begun in 1870. Even though much of the evidence comes from the writings of Dr. Woodworth whom we recall as the first supervising surgeon appointed in 1870, and therefore may perhaps be self-serving, much of his critique is probably true because it is corroborated by the reports of other subsequent supervising surgeons and by Congressional and the Secretary of the Navy's remarks. Dr. Woodworth wrote "that in the beginning things did not go well . . . and complaints and criticisms arose." He reported that there were instances of incompetence or malfeasance in the building of hospitals. Others reported that the care "in many instances farmed out through second parties, was not satisfactory to its recipients"; that hospitals being used were totally inadequate; that the physicians were either not good ones or paid more attention to their private practice than to the agency service; and, as noted, that appointment of medical officers had become a "perquisite of the collector of customs." In 1822, many seamen had protested to Congress about the unavailability of service. The location and building of hospitals became a political pork barrel with sites being purchased and never built on and hospitals being built, never occupied, and then "sold for a song." Parenthetically, it should be noted that similar problems were later to evidence themselves repeatedly in the contracting out of medical care for special populations by other government programs.

With the growth in private and some government health insurance and welfare programs after World War II, there was a steady decline in inpatient use of Public Health Service hospitals. While outpatient use also fell from the 1943 wartime high, it declined relatively less. The use of ambulatory services increased moderately during the 1960s and 1970s as a result of a particular effort to serve special groups of underserved people at some of the hospitals.

In 1970, there were still 37,000 hospital admissions, 1.7 million clinic visits, and 74,000 visits to contract physicians (HEW, 1970). In addition, a considerable program of postgraduate medical education and training was run at these hospitals. There were 244 residents and interns in training during 1970. Eligibility for service had been further expanded, and among the eligible now were American seamen, officers, and enlisted men of the U.S. Coast Guard and their dependents, military personnel and their dependents, federal employees who were injured or became ill while on work assignments, and special community groups whose medical care was provided for under contract.

But by 1976 (HEW, 1977) there were only nine Public Health Service hospitals left, comprising eight general hospitals and the National Hospital for Hansen's disease (Leprosy) at Carville, Louisiana. [In 1948 there were twenty-four hospitals (Wilson and Neuhauser, 1985)]. The service was also operating twenty-six outpatient clinics and contracting with private physicians to provide health services in areas with no PHS facilities. But utilization figures continued to show steady declines. The merchant seamen were by now members of powerful unions and had good private insurance and the location of the hospitals at waterfront sites were not appropriate for building a large general clientele among the poor.

With the decline in utilization and in numbers of hospitals, questions began to be persistently raised in federal administration circles as well as in Congress about the continued need for these hospitals. This was particularly true of conservative presidents and legislators. The services were shifting increasingly to ambulatory care, and the involvement of a number of the hospitals in providing care for special groups of disadvantaged persons probably helped to polarize the supporting and opposing factors in govern-

ment. The Nixon administration tried to divest the federal government of these hospitals, including an attempt to eliminate them from the 1974 budget, but Congress prevented this move. President Ford in his 1977 budget again proposed closing the eight remaining general Public Health Service general hospitals. It was pointed out that at least five of the hospitals were in areas—Galveston, Seattle, Baltimore, Boston, and San Francisco—with an excess of hospital beds for community needs. The Carter administration did not ask for federal divestment of these hospitals, but in June 1981, during the early months of the Reagan administration, while both the House and the Senate were debating bills to eliminate the PHS hospitals, the General Accounting Office released a study asserting that the PHS hospitals were providing free care to noneligible patients, failing to collect from third-party payers, and lacking control over contracting procedures (McGraw Hill, June 22, 1981). In the new conservative political environment this was effective in strengthening the sentiment for removing the hospitals from federal ownership.

President Reagan finally succeeded in obtaining legislation to divest the federal government of these hospitals in the Omnibus Reconciliation Act of 1981 (P.L. 97–35), passed in August 1981, which provided that existing Public Health Service hospitals be either transferred to state, local, or nonprofit auspices or simply closed in short order. The right to medical service from the Pubilc Health Service for specified groups was to be discontinued, and all of this was to be accomplished not later than September 30, 1982. By the end of October 1982, The New Orleans Public Health Service hospital had been taken over by the state of Louisiana; those in San Francisco and Norfolk, Virginia, by the Defense Department, who "mothballed" their inpatient facilities and turned them into strictly ambulatory facilities; a religious order was taking over the Nassau Bay, Texas, hospital; and the remaining four—Seattle, Boston, Baltimore, and Staten Island—which the Reagan administration had planned to close—were the subject of negotiation for transfer to local control.

Another important direct-service activity of the Public Health Service began to supply physicians and other medical personnel to medically underserved areas in 1972. These personnel were part of the National Health Service Corps (NHSC) which had been established by the Emergency Personnel Act of 1970 (P.L. 91–623) for the purpose of staffing areas that had an insufficient supply of medical personnel. The Corps was administered by the PHS and some of its physicians had been allowed to become part of the PHS Commissioned Corps. Most of them, however, after serving a stint in the underserved area to repay their medical scholarship money, went on to private practice or to work in other public institutions. This program is discussed in greater detail in Chapter 13 on government roles in development of health personnel.

The Indian Health Services

As of 1987 the Indian Health Service (IHS) was directly operating or funding operation by Indian tribes of 51 hospitals, 439 health centers and stations, and 265 others types of ambulatory health service units. It also contracted with private physicians, dentists, and other health professionals and hospitals for care for American Indians entitled to IHS services, including approximately 1,074,000 Indians and Alaskan natives residing in the United States in 1988. Of these, 97 percent resided in states in which the Indian Health Service had responsibilities (HEW, 1978, 1979; U.S. Department of Health, 1988). In 1980 it employed 620 physicians in addition to nurses and other supporting medical personnel.

The direct services of the IHS were divided into seventy-eight local administrative units in 1988. Most of these so-called "service units" were based on a single federal reservation and were located in or around a hospital or health center. The service units were grouped into larger central administrative units making up twelve area (regional) offices. In addition some programs were operated by tribes, and a few served Indians in urban centers.

Data published by the Indian Health Service on the health status of American Indians indicate substantial strides made since 1955, when the Public Health Service took over the Indian Health Service. Even with these improvements, however, the health status of American Indians in many important respects remains worse than the average of other Americans. This will be discussed in greater detail after an overview of the background to the present situation.[15]

Before the Introduction of Public Health Service Supervision in 1955

The founding fathers of the United States and the federal Constitution ostensibly envisaged a future in which the original thirteen states would negotiate with the Indian tribes as equal nations. The early treaties provided for assistance to the Indian tribes for education of their children, and some of these assistance funds were spent on health services (Cohen, 1941, 192). A law of 1802 effectively put whatever health care Indians would get from the United States under the supervision of the War Department, where it was assigned to an office of the Superintendent of Indian Trade in 1806. As the very title of the office implied, health care for the Indians would be part of the commercial trading between the United States and the Indian nations. Consequently, since the medical care was delivered by U.S. Army medical officers on an ad hoc basis as emergencies arose, only Indians living in the vicinity of military posts received any care at all. Much of the care was aimed at controlling the spread of communicable diseases among the Indians, largely out of fear that these would spread to the white community through trade contacts (HEW, 1957). It is ironic that a number of these diseases were introduced by the Europeans in the first place and that they were particularly deadly to Indians because they had very low natural immunity to these "foreign" diseases. Smallpox was a particularly virulent affliction, with an epidemic in 1838 killing 17,200 Indians in the Northwest alone (HEW, 1957).

During her first twenty-five years or so, the new nation's official Indian policy was at least ostensibly directed at preserving the territorial and national integrity of the Indians, but de facto policy, that is, actual performance, contradicted the enunciated official position. The two main aspects of the actual policy consisted of attempts to homogenize the Indian culture by inducing Indians to become more like Europeans, on the one hand, and to remove them from their lands if these lay in the path of white settlers on the other. These two policies, guided United States actions toward the Indians in the early years, and may be characterized as the integrationist policy versus the appropriationist policy. Those favoring integration thought it would eventually result in Indians being thoroughly integrated into the mainstream of American life, with many of them retaining parts of their former tribal lands as individual holdings while some would join the mainstream of Americans in cities and towns. They hoped to hold back the assault by settlers on Indian lands to permit the Indians' assimilation to evolve under protective federal legislation which would include provisions for educational and social services required to help further this assimilation. Most subsequent fluctuations in federal government policy toward the Indians reflected the struggle between the integrationists, who identified themselves as protectors of Indian rights, and those who moved to appropriate Indian lands as rapidly as possible. In later years, organizations of the Indians themselves entered this struggle, with some Indian voices calling for integration and others for a "nationalist" solution—retention of tribal lands with emphasis on developing the tribes as truly self-governing nations. This viewpoint abjured the integrationist solution. Federal Indian health services policy largely reflected these developments in U.S. government–Indian relations.

An early manifestation of the first aspect of federal Indian policy, homogenization, was embodied in an 1819 law authorizing annual amounts of $10,000 to establish a system of Indian education that would introduce "among them the habits and acts of civilization . . . for the purpose of providing against further decline and final extinction of the Indian tribes, adjoining the frontier settlements of the United States. . . . " (Tuler, 1973). The money was given to missionary societies who ran these programs and is referred to by one historian as "the civilization fund" (Tuler, 1973). Some of these monies were used for health services because the missionary groups were supporting medical programs among the Indians (HEW, 1957). Whatever beneficial effects may have been achieved by the integrationists' "civilization" program were more than undone by the appropriationists' relocation policy, which was also being carried out by the United States government. During the

period immediately after 1800, settlers widely violated rights guaranteed the Indians by treaties with the United States government, and Indian resistance to further incursion on their lands grew (Tuler, 1973). Some of the resistance escalated into open warfare between Indians and the U.S. Army.

The relocation or removal policy involved a large resettlement of Indian tribes in the name of " 'preservation and civilization' of the aborigines" (Tuler, 1973). Many tribes occupying eastern portions of the United States were moved west of the Mississippi to new locations during the years 1812 through the 1840s and was accomplished largely by treaty. The fact that tribes that were relocated included those who had adapted best to the "civilizing" program of the Bureau of Indian Affairs[16] (in fact five of them came to be known as the "five civilized tribes") strongly suggests that the removal was done mainly to seize Indian land. The wish to preserve tribal integrity from the corrupting influence of proximity to white settlement, a goal that was advanced by some "humanitarians" of that period, was clearly not a serious priority of the perpetrators of the forced migration. During this period of great suffering caused by the uprooting of entire peoples from their homelands and transported elsewhere, only oblique provision was made for the care of the health problems that developed among the transported Indians. There were appropriations for transportation, resettlement, and welfare services for the displaced Indians, but since these were allotted in lump sums to contractors who undertook to effect the moves, little of the intended services trickled down to the Indians. Additionally, a little money was allotted to missionary and other voluntary groups to provide some auxiliary services to the displaced persons (Foreman, 1953). In 1832, for example, Congress appropriated $12,000 for vaccinating Indians against smallpox.

In 1832, a treaty with the Winnebago Indians (Iowa and Michigan) provided that the federal government provide medical care for a period of twenty-seven years as part of the payment for the Indian cession of land. This was the first such explicit assumption by the federal government of the obligation to provide medical care to the Indians. The provision expressly stated that a physician be provided at each of two specified places at a stipulated annual salary. At least twenty-four subsequent treaties included provisions for medical care (HEW, 1957). Between 1855 and 1868 one finds listed fifteen treaties that provided for physicians and hospitals (Cohen, 1941). Although many of these provisos restricted the provision of medical care to a limited time period, the policy of extending the services beyond the original expiration date was adopted under what has been called "gratuity appropriations" (HEW, 1957). In 1849, with the creation of the Department of Interior, the Bureau of Indian Affairs (BIA) was moved from the War Department to the new department and with it went the responsibility for providing health services to the Indians. For the first time these services were under civilian rather than under military supervision. However, the quality of the medical care provided continued to be questionable.

After the end of the Civil War in 1865, the pace of westward expansion by white settlers accelerated, and the Indians west of the Mississippi were forced onto islands of land that were called Indian reservations, the years 1870 to 1876 coming to be known as the "reservation years." In 1871 all further formal treaty making with the Indians was discontinued (Tyler, 1973). BIA agents administered United States government policy inside the reservation, while outside the reservation the Army was "harrying those that resisted being confined within reservation boundaries." All during the period 1850–1900, federal policy was gradually but effectively changing the status of the Indians from even being nominally regarded as members of independent nations to be negotiated with to being wards of the U.S. government. This was especially true of the Indians on reservations, where rations of food and clothing were made available in lieu of the treaty privilege of hunting in "customary places."

Until the close of the Civil War the United States dealt with Indian tribes largely as individual self-governing units. Internal practices under tribal government had been left almost entirely to Indian leaders, and to local Indian custom. But after 1865, with its rapid westward movement of settlers and the impounding of Indians in reservations . . . the Indians were soon virtually surrounded by their conquerors and newly appointed rulers. The old way under Indian leadership was gradually disappearing. The Indian agent was the new taskmaster bringing a multitude of new programs foreign to Indian ideas of the proper role of man in his society. . . .

Indian leaders could see that further struggle was useless. Their economic base gradually disappeared. There was no longer a source of power adequate to a successful resistance. The tribe and its leaders had lost their political autonomy. Unable to maintain their own government, they became communities administered from Washington. The administrative structure was the Bureau of Indian Affairs. The local representative was the agent or superintendent given the administrative responsibility to look after the welfare of the Indians in relations with non-Indians, to maintain the resources of the reservation and to encourage "civilizing" influences. . . . A major trend that we observe running through much of the legislation of this period was a tendency to further minimize the functions of tribal leaders and tribal institutions and to continually strengthen the position of the Government representative and his subordinates, and to improve effectiveness of their programs to break down traditional patterns within the Indian communities. . . . [T]he loss of the local political autonomy traditionally maintained by Indian tribes came with or shortly after, the commencement of reservation life (Tyler, 1973).

This trend was accelerated with the completion of the transcontinental railroad in 1869 and the disappearance of the buffalo herds, the staple of the Plains Indians' economy.

The introduction of the reservation system as the predominant mode of Indian living brought with it an increase and formalization of federal programs for social services including health services. As has been noted, the practice of including government health care as a federal obligation had already been introduced by the provisos of many treaties during the treaty period of about 1830–1870 and these established precedents for a federal policy of a separate health care system for Indians. After 1870, congressional appropriations for "education and other purposes" became regularized, with "other purposes" usually including health care. The sum of $140,000 was appropriated in 1870, and by 1887 this had risen to $1,226,415. Most of the money went to establish and operate schools, and whatever expenditures were made for health care were generally in connection with the educational program. For example an Indian Service hospital was established in 1882 at the Carlisle Indian School, an off-reservation boarding school. By 1888 there were two more. Some schools were operated by the BIA (163 in 1887) and others by private agencies, "usually missionary societies" (64 in 1887) (Tyler, 1973).

In 1873, a special Division of Education and Medicine was organized in the Bureau of Indian Affairs. During the life of this division through 1877, its charge included centralizing and coordinating the system of Indian medical services (HEW, 1957; Cohen 1942). Upon discontinuance of the medical section of this division in 1877, medical care for Indians was entirely in the hands of physicians working for Indian schools or Indian agency offices until 1909, when a medical supervisor was appointed for the Educational Division of the BIA. The Indian health program became a regular part of the BIA in 1911, soon after the appointment of the medical supervisor.

Although half the Indian reservations had physicians in 1874, they were not required to be medical college graduates until 1878. The quality of care was generally quite low:

at no time during the 19th century were there nearly enough doctors to meet overall needs. Available Bureau doctors generally had such heavy caseloads that they could do little more than issue pills and some reservations still had no medical service at all. This, of course, hardly excuses the Pine Ridge Agency physician who in 1898 practiced medicine for 10,000 Sioux and Cheyennes by dispensing medicine upon the most cursory examinations made through a hole in the office wall (HEW, 1957).

One historian judges that "These doctors did some good work under discouraging financial, administrative and living conditions sometimes largely under the compulsion of the missionary spirit than characteristic of the medical profession" (HEW, 1957). It was not until 1891 that the personnel of the Bureau of Indian Affairs, including physicians, were placed under the civil service and required to pass professional competency examinations.

During the period of 1870–1900 there were major obstacles to the BIA's efforts in addition to inadequate funding. Considerable resistance to using even the existing meager governmental health services existed among Indians stemming both from the culturally based distrust of white medicine and the fears of competition on the part of traditional Indian healers.

States took almost no part in providing public health services to the Indians residing within their boundaries because first, few state health departments had been organized before 1900; second, the care of Indians had long been considered the responsibility of the federal government; and finally, the states had no legal power over the reservations, including that of taxation or enforcement of sanitary ordinances. Administration of public health therefore fell to the federal government, and in addition to the construction of some hospitals and infirmaries for Indians between 1880 and 1900,[17] promoting preventive health measures was a developing Indian Bureau policy. A BIA paper of 1889 outlining the duties of BIA physicians included visiting Indian houses and imparting health education; sanitary inspection of the school and Indian agency buildings; and visiting Indian schools to give health education. Field workers who were the predecessors of public health nurses were appointed in 1891. They made home vists and provided health instruction and emergency nursing. But these services, too, could not have been very intensive with only twenty-one field workers on staff by 1900.

An "alarming prevalence" of tuberculosis and trachoma was uncovered on reservations by a number of health and sanitary surveys, and in 1911 $40,000 in federal funds were appropriated for more general services to provide for care and prevention of contagious and infectious disease among the Indians (HEW, 1957). President Taft in a special message in 1912 asked Congress for a $253,000 appropriation for health service to the Indians. This message coming from so high a source was the first of many to follow from officials, commissions, committees of Congress and other sources, outlining the very poor state of Indian health. An excerpt from Taft's message appearing in the Congressional Record of August 10, 1912 and quoted in Tyler (1973) follows:

In many parts of the Indian country infant mortality, tuberculosis and disastrous diseases generally prevail to an extent exceeded only in some of the most insanitary of our white rural districts and in the worst slums of our large cities. The death rate of the Indian country is 35 per thousand as compared with 15 per thousand—the average death rate of the United States as a whole. . . . Last year, of 42,000 Indians examined for disease, over 16 percent of them had trachoma, a contagious disease of the eye, frequently resulting in blindness, and so easily spread that it threatens both the Indian communities and all their white neighbors. . . . Of the 40,000 Indians examined, 6,000 had tuberculosis. . . . Few Indian homes anywhere have proper sanitary conditions, and in most instances the bad conditions of their domestic surroundings is almost beyond belief.

As guardians of the welfare of the Indians, it is our immediate duty to give the race a fair chance for an unmaimed birth, healthy childhood, and a physically efficient maturity. [18] The most vigorous campaign ever waged against diseases among the Indians is now under way. It began in 1909. Prior to that time little attention had been given to the hygiene and health of the Indians. In some reservations, equal in area to a State, there were not more than two physicians, frequently only one. In 1909 tens of thousands of Indians were substantially without any chance to reach a doctor.

With this additional appropriation, if granted by Congress, it is believed that the tide can be turned, that the danger of infection among Indians themselves and to the several millions of white persons now living as neighbors to them can be greatly reduced, and genuine cooperation with local State boards of health now already under way can be adequately provided for.

In 1913 the Public Health Service conducted a survey of Indian health, focusing on trachoma and tuberculosis. The 1911 appropriation of $40,000 for Indian health services was increased in subsequent years until by 1918 it had reached $350,000; by 1955, it had grown to $17.8 million. The 1911 figure of $40,000 was the first earmarked specifically for general health services to Indians. Before then Indian health activities were financed out of miscellaneous funds, and for many years disbursements from "miscellaneous" funds continued to augment the specific appropriations. During the U.S. involvement in World War I and for some years thereafter, BIA services, including health services, declined, but in 1924 a special Division of Health was established in the BIA and thereafter the health service program grew. A major reorganization of the Indian Health Service in 1926 included the appointment of District Medical Directors (HEW, 1957).

During the period 1924–1932 there was much public discussion of the inadequacy of services given to and the living conditions prevailing among reservation Indians. In 1926, the Secretary of the Interior requested a private research group to study the workings of the BIA. Funded by John D. Rockefeller, Jr., this group submitted a report of its findings, "The Problem of Indian Administration," which came to be known as the Miriam report after its editor, Lewis Miriam. It asserted that more and better doctors were needed and recommended that there be clinics on all reservations, more emphasis on disease prevention, instruction in hygiene, collection of reliable statistics, and closer cooperation with state and local agencies (Tyler 1973).[19] Following the Miriam report, Congress passed an act to allow state government employees to enter Indian lands for sanitary inspections, surveys, and quarantine supervision. Some states delegated this responsibility to the local BIA health service office. The recommendations of the Report also led to closer liaison with the Public Health Service in improving personnel, facilities, and the collection and tabulation of vital statistics. An effort was also made to improve health education by teaching personal hygiene and disease prevention (Tyler, 1973) (public health nurses had already been added to BIA staffs in 1924).

The accession of Franklin Delano Roosevelt to the presidency in 1932 while the country was in the trough of the Great Depression had a marked effect on the development of federal Indian health service policy. Two main legislative developments embodied much of the changes. One comprised the Johnson-O'Malley and the Indian Reorganization Acts of 1934 [P.L. 73–383] and the other was the Social Security Act of 1935. It was after the passage of these three laws that the full import of the 1924 act giving all Indians United States citizenship became manifest. Under the U.S. Constitution, every United States citizen is also a citizen of the state wherein he or she resides, and now because of the 1924 law, Social Security Act benefits, both public health and income security, applied to Indians. Furthermore, the Johnson-O'Malley Act of 1934 specifically provided for federal-state cooperation in Indian affairs, allowing the Secretary of the Interior to enter into contracts with states, territories, and private institutions "for the education, medical attention, agricultural assistance, and social welfare, including relief of distress of Indians in each state or territory through the qualified agencies of each state or territory.'' The intent of the Act was to work toward Indians receiving services through the same local facilities as those used by other citizens rather than through special federal ones for Indians, with the federal government contracting with state authorities to implement this change. In 1936 the Johnson-O'Malley Act was amended to enable such contracts to be negotiated directly with local governments as well as with other public or private organizations. A leading barrier to fuller implementation of this Act was its perceived intent of shifting much of the federal responsibilities for Indian services to the states, and a belief that the depression was hardly the propitious time for state governments to take on additional financial responsibilities (Tyler, 1973).

The Indian Reorganization Act of 1934 (also known as the Wheeler-Howard Act) was directed at reversing the trend of 1887–1933 toward the breaking up of tribal governments and instead provided for strengthening tribal self-government (Tyler, 1973). Although the Wheeler-Howard Reorganization Act would have led one to expect that the health services would rapidly become more tribally controlled and operated after 1934, a serious attempt to do this on a wide scale would not be made until 1975. There was only partial implementation of the Act despite the efforts of the incumbent Commissioner of the BIA, John Collier (see below).

By 1937 considerable improvement in Indian living conditions was noted. In the health field, new hospitals had been built, there were ''improved medical resources, a new attack on trachoma that by 1939 saw vast improvement of treatment and by 1943 a virtual end to consideration of this disease as a major problem[20] . . . and enlargement of cooperation with other government agencies such as . . . the Public Health Service'' (Tyler, 1973). Despite the Johnson-O'Malley Act provisions seeking to transfer the site of a substantial amount of health services provision to ''mainstream'' (i.e., off-reservation) locations and despite bitter opposition in some quarters to the reorganization program, much of the development of the Indian health services during the Reorganization Act period, 1934–1945, was in facilities on the reservations

with growing tribal input into their development (a nationalist direction).

This period coincided with the tenure of John Collier as BIA commissioner (1933–1945). He was strongly identified with the nationalist approach of moving toward developing tribal autonomy and culture. Toward the end of Collier's term in office, beginning with about 1940, prointegrationist opposition by some Congressional figures and groups to the aims of the Indian Reorganization Act began to surface more strongly (Tyler, 1973). One form of this opposition became known as ''termination'' sentiment and called for discontinuing special provisions for Indians as soon as possible. Some expressions of this sentiment even called for abolition of the BIA. The advocates of rapid termination claimed that assimilation of the American Indian into American mainstream life would end an already decreasing paternalism and that they were thus proposing an accelerated version of the integrationist approach as against Collier's nationalist approach. The opponents of rapid termination argued that termination, in the context of existing reality, was nothing more than another move to usurp the Indian's land and resources, because he was ill prepared for assimilation and also because termination involved discontinuing the federal government's obligations under the Indian treaties. It was therefore, in reality, another appropriationist gambit in disguise.

During World War II some 65,000 Indians left the reservations to serve in the armed forces or work in war industries. The cultural influence of the war on Indian thought and life was profound. Indians returned with mixed perceptions of their futures. Some wanted to resume their roles on the Indian reservation while others wanted to join the world of the non-Indian (Tyler, 1973). Among the younger Indians especially, the war produced a deepening of the cleavage between integrationist and nationalist outlooks and the corresponding views toward the desirability of compensated termination as against federal support for developing the tribal government. With rising land values, some Indians wanted a return to the policy of parceling out the tribal lands as individual holdings to its members so that they could cultivate them as independent entrepreneurs or even sell them.

The controversy over the future direction of federal Indian policy accordingly took on a crucial added dimension after 1945. While participants in past debates had often largely been confined to non-Indian legislators and public figures, many of whom were lifelong advocates of justice for Indians as they saw it, the voice of the Indians themselves had now become more powerful, and Indian organizations played a very important part in the debate over policy. Some favored compensated termination, whereas others were opposed to assimilation. They also opposed increased federal paternalism toward reservation Indians and called for greater self-rule but with a continuance of federal support based on old treaty obligations rather than any idea of "civilizing" the Indian.

Thus, the opposing positions of integration versus self-rule were being espoused both in Congress and by Indian organizations, but the accelerated integration ("termination") idea prevailed in Congress after World War II. The 1945 law it passed set up an Indian Claims Commission empowered to adjudicate claims by Indian tribes against the United States government. The settlement of treaty claims could lay the basis for renouncing future federal obligations. Another important element in the preparation for termination was the establishment of service sources for Indians that would be independent of federal government management.

Beginning with 1948 a special job placement program was established by the BIA. At first it was only for Navajos and there were offices in Denver, Salt Lake City, and Los Angeles. Later, offices were also opened in Oklahoma, New Mexico, California, Arizona, Utah, and Colorado. In 1951 a Field Relocation Office was opened in Chicago, and the placement offices for Navajos in Los Angeles, Salt Lake City, and Denver were converted to Field Relocation Offices that served all tribes in those areas. The numbers of Indians using these offices to relocate from the reservation into mainstream America grew from year to year (Tyler, 1973). Also in 1951, the Bureau of Indian Affairs stated as program objectives "step-by-step transfer of Bureau functions to the Indians themselves or to appropriate agencies of State or Federal Government" (Tyler, 1973). In the area of health services the continued movement of Congress after

1945 toward termination featured efforts to establish local and autonomous sources for medical care and preventive services for Indians especially in urban areas.

The two opposing sets of pressures, one toward accelerated "termination" of the reservation and integration of the Indian into the mainstream of American life and the other toward greater autonomy and self-rule for the Indians that remained living in tribes on reservations were both reflected in the development of the Indian health services over time. From 1909 until World War II these services had been steadily built up as special services for Indians operated by the medical arm of the BIA. Despite a number of improvements made in these services, some of which have been previously mentioned, the numbers of health personnel in the Indian health services remained far below satisfactory levels until 1950, when passage of the national doctor-dentist draft law permitted physicians and dentists to discharge their military service obligations by serving in the Public Health Service. The number of physicians and dentists assigned to the Indian health service then quadrupled (HEW, 1957). In addition, up until 1940 hospital construction had been growing, and the previously mentioned health services development had increased the number of public health nurses and the programs for preventive care.

The integration trends began to be reflected in health service policy from about 1940 on, with a gradual shift toward the use of local community resources with the BIA closing more than thirty of its hospitals and sanitoria in seventeen states. By 1955, the Bureau had contracted out Indian health care to sixty-five general community hospitals, seventeen tuberculosis hospitals, and five mental hospitals. This de facto policy of closing Indian health facilities whenever suitable facilities were available, at first slowly put into practice after 1940, was officially enunciated as policy in 1952. In 1940, eighty-one hospitals with 4,253 beds (excluding Alaska) were being operated by the BIA. By 1955 the corresponding numbers were forty-eight hospitals with 2,804 beds (HEW, 1957). As against these reductions, the average daily Indian census in contract hospitals rose from 323 in 1950 to 936 in 1955[21] (HEW, 1957). In addition, during the period 1940–1955 (especially after 1945), the BIA issued regulations restricting eligibility for federally sponsored health care to certain classes of Indians generally based on percentage of pure-bloodedness, belonging to a recognized tribe, or being a descendant of a reservation Indian. The imposition of cost sharing was attempted in some cases but was not widely practiced.

The idea of transition to autonomous tribal governance had been conceived as a gradual process by John Collier in his twelve years of administering the Indian Reconstruction Act. While the ultimate aim was complete tribal autonomy, the interim measures were to include a three-pronged program of decentralization: decentralizing the BIA's functions to other agencies in the federal government that were better specialized to carry them out; decentralizing services to local, state, and county governments (also the aim of the Johnson-O'Malley Act); and finally decentralizing tribal governance to tribal councils. Part of these ideas continued as federal de facto policy in the health field after Collier left in 1945. The main decentralizing action in the health services area was taken in 1955, when the health services of the BIA were transferred to the Public Health Service (P.L. 83–869, passed August 5, 1954). "Fifty nine hospitals and other physical facilities plus about 25 percent of the total personnel of the BIA that had been assigned to the Indian health programs were involved in this transfer" (Tyler, 1973). Thus, the first of the three aspects of the decentralization program as it applied to health services, transfer of the specialized health services within the BIA to a specialized health agency, was implemented ten years after Collier had resigned his post. With this transfer, the Indian Health Service under the Public Health Service became the agency supervising federally sponsored health services for Indians.

Under Public Health Service Supervision, 1955 and After

In a 1957 report by the United States Public Health Service (PHS), the transfer was said to represent "an attempt to plan the program on a firmer administrative foundation for future development" (HEW, 1957). The report notes that such a transfer had been considered in 1919 and

in the 1930s and that from 1949 on, the Association of State and Territorial Health Officers, the American Public Health Association, the Association on American Indian Affairs, and others supported this move. Yet the 1955 transfer was not made without controversy. Some opposed it on the grounds that it was unwise to separate health programs from the complex of other programs being administered on the reservations by the BIA. Others, like the Oklahoma Indian tribes, feared a reduction in medical and hospital benefits. The arguments favoring the transfer were that it would help ease the staffing problems of the Indian health programs because the PHS could better attract health professionals; there would be direct medical provision of the program, which would be delivered from "nonprofessional" supervision; a public health agency was likelier to focus more sharply on the public health problems of the Indian than would an agency whose primary function was resource management; the PHS might obtain more adequate appropriations for Indian health; it would eliminate duplication in Federal health activities between the BIA and the PHS; and it would promote state and local cooperation because of the already existing federal-state-local connections in the system of grants for public health work administered by the PHS. All these assertions were advanced as factors likely to improve Indian health services and hopefully also Indian health status.

Some termination forces were among those favoring the transfer, seeing in it a step toward achieving their goal because it would help diminish the role of the special agency that administered the reservations, the Bureau of Indian Affairs. Termination advocates also saw contracting out of health services to some public, but mostly private, contractors as a transition toward termination, and the trend toward contracting for services with non-Indian Health Service agencies continued at an accelerated pace. Legislation passed in 1957 empowered the Public Health Service to assist communities with the construction of health facilities that would aid in the construction of those community hospitals that were expected to materially serve Indians (HEW, 1957). The transfer of the health services out of the BIA was not confined to health issues but was part of a general disengagement policy by the BIA of transferring its functions to other agencies and jurisdictions,[22] a policy being followed by Congress with particular vigor during the Eisenhower administration (1953–1960) as preparation for termination. When the Congressional enthusiasm for rapid termination of reservations cooled as the 1960s approached, federal health policy toward Indians changed its emphasis accordingly.

The push of the Eisenhower administration for termination was halted after the election of John F. Kennedy as President in 1960. The new administration adopted a policy of self-determination rather than one of single-minded concentration on rapid termination (Tyler, 1973). Self-determination was a policy of choice, allowing and encouraging Indians to choose from among at least three options: continuing and strengthening the autonomous tribal community and remaining on the reservation with continuing federal support based on the agreements negotiated in the original treaties; giving aliquot parts of the tribal lands to individual Indians who would continue to cultivate or otherwise use or dispose of them as individual owners; and leaving the reservation after receiving some form of "release" payment in settlement of treaty obligations to take up life in city and town. These options may be characterized respectively as tribal self-rule or autonomy, termination via individual land distribution, and termination via cash buyout.

That the option of self-rule along with continuing aid was a real one may be inferred from the publication by a 1961 task force of the Secretary of Interior of *A Program for Indian Citizens* calling for greater emphasis on development of human and natural resources on reservations and recommending the use of competent technical consultants, not restricted to BIA personnel, to help in this development, with loans and loan guarantees available to finance this assistance. Money for such financing was subsequently appropriated by explicitly including Indians in general acts to help depressed areas, such as the Area Redevelopment Act of 1961 (P.L. 87–27], and the Economic Opportunity Act establishing the Office of Economic Opportunity (OEO) in 1964. The Manpower Development Training Act of 1962 specifically included Indians among its beneficiaries. The OEO programs were particularly active among Indians in helping them organize their own economic and service activities on reservations (Tyler, 1973).

In a special message to Congress on "The Forgotton American" in 1968, President Johnson called for an end to discussion of tribal termination as the only or main solution and explicitly reaffirmed the Kennedy Administration's de facto support for the policy of self-determination or free choice between remaining on the reservation or moving into the mainstream of American life in either a rural or urban setting (Tyler, 1973). In the same year, the new policy calling for enhanced federal efforts to help develop the tribal services and resources of the Indians choosing to remain on reservations as well as improving Indian welfare and conditions in preparation for eventual termination for those Indians who preferred it was incorporated into a Senate concurrent resolution. It expressed the "sense of Congress" as being in support of the policy of promoting self-development and self-determination.

The self-determination policy was also reaffirmed by President Nixon in a special message to Congress in 1970, and his Commissioner of Indian Affairs (Louis R. Bruce) stated that government policy was handing "the right and the authority to Indian communities and tribes to take part in the planning and operation of activities that touch their daily lives" (Tyler, 1973). At the same time, a congressional committee noted in 1971 that 40 percent of the country's Indian population was living off the reservation, and after 1972 the activities of the BIA in helping Indians living off the reservations, mostly in cities and towns, increased. A program of vocational training and placement services was continued and intensified for Indians choosing to live in towns and cities.

The policy of self-determination avowed in 1960 and reaffirmed in 1968 and 1972, and the guarantee of continued services, both on and off the reservation, promised in 1960, were embodied in two important laws enacted during the mid-1970s. The first of these, the Indian Self-Determination Act (P.L. 93–638), passed in January 1975, permitted tribes the option of operating the Indian Health Service (IHS) programs in their communities themselves and provided for skilled assistance in improving the technical capability of the tribes to do so. The activities that might be managed by tribes were described by the IHS in 1978 as "broad, ranging from the provision of outreach services in the community, to the planning, construction, staffing and operation of health care facilities" (HEW, 1978).

The second of these two major acts was the Indian Health Care Improvement Act (P.L. 94–437), passed in 1976 during the Carter administration. It authorized higher Congressional appropriations for a seven-year period, beginning with fiscal year 1978, to expand health services and resources such as building and renovating health care facilities, increasing the number of Indian homes with safe drinking water and sanitary disposal facilities, and increasing the number of Indian health professionals in Indian communities by establishing health professions scholarships, health professions preparatory scholarships, and other health personnel training programs for Indians.

It also authorized programs for Indian urban organizations seeking to improve access to health services by Indians living in cities.

Standard Public Health Services

The particularly urgent need for the type of basic preventive services offered by the local public health department described in Chapter 2 has been and remains particularly urgent on Indian reservations. It demands special treatment here. For a long time these services were skimpily available. The BIA did not provide services comparable to those provided by the better local health departments, and for a long time the state and local health departments themselves did not have jurisdiction over the reservations. After 1955 the situation changed markedly for the better although these services never reached national average levels in the reservations. In the following sections the earlier background of this situation is sketched, but the situation after 1955 is the main focus. The previously cited description of Indian health services (HEW, 1957) excellently summarizes the background of the federal government's role in providing such services and is the basis for much of the following discussion.

Sanitation and Hygiene. The need to improve sanitation and health education has been long recognized as a serious problem in Indian health services. The following excerpts from the 1957 survey report of the Department of HEW (pp. 92–94) summarizes the background well:

The Public Health Service survey of 1913 (USPHS, 1913) carried out by order of Congress, has been described as the "first comprehensive survey of infectious diseases" among the Indians [Mountin and Townsend, 1936]. Besides revealing great prevalence of trachoma ..., tuberculosis (much more than among whites), and certain other communicable diseases, the survey made a variety of suggestions for improving Indian health. The most urgent need in the opinion of the Public Health Service was for better sanitary conditions. . . . In its capacity as health authority for the whole United States, the Service recognized in sick Indians a threat to the health not only of other Indians but also of the general population: "The control of communicable diseases among Indians and the prevention of their spread to other races is . . . indicated as a public health measure" (1913, p. 70). . . . The Public Health Service survey of 1936 (Mountin and Townsend), conducted at the direction of the Surgeon General of the Public Health Service, above all urged improved sanitation, health education, and other preventive health services. . . .

Improvement of water supply, waste disposal, and other sanitary facilities on Indian reservations occurred gradually, although as late as 1936 sanitation was described as "the most neglected element in the general health program" (Mountin and Townsend, p. 41). Prior to the late 1920s, sanitation efforts did not extend beyond occasional cleanup campaigns and physicians' inspections of homes, schools, and agencies. Beginning in 1927, the Public Health Service Sanitary Engineering Corps assisted the Bureau of Indian Affairs in surveying water and sewer systems and investigating other basic sanitary problems. However, the Corps usually restricted its work to Bureau installations such as schools, hospitals, and agency headquarters. Sanitary services provided from the 1930s under contracts with State and local health departments resembled those of the Public Health Service in being confined mainly to Bureau installations. To improve basic sanitation in individual homes as well as at Bureau installations, the Indian Bureau, beginning in 1950, obtained the services of a full-time Public Health Service sanitary engineer as supervisor, increased its sanitary staffs at major field offices, started a training course for Indian sanitarian aides, and launched reservation-wide sanitary surveys on a large scale.

Systematic attempts to raise the level of personal hygiene among Indians began as early as 1910, although progress toward an effective health education program was made slowly thereafter. Among the devices used in the early years to promote healthful living habits were pamphlets, illustrated lectures, and motion pictures. In 1924, the Indian Bureau obtained the help of the American Red Cross and American Child Health Association in designing health courses for Indian schools. Another step forward in the organization of health education for Indians was the appointment in 1934 of a supervisor of health education, to work under the joint auspices of the health and education units of the Indian Bureau. In general, low standards of living on the reservations retarded progress in health education. As one observer said, "The Indian still gets along very peaceably with flies" (U.S. Congress, 1931). Various Indian customs and medical practices introduced special complications, as in the case of the tuberculous mother accustomed to chewing food for her baby. . . .

The first Hoover Commission's Committee on Indian Affairs, also found in 1948 "that immediate need existed for more vigorous preventive health work" (HEW, 1957).

The continuing urgency of the need for improvement in public health environmental protection services for Indians was acknowledged by the passage of the Indian Sanitation Facilities Construction Act of 1959 (P.L. 96–121). Under the terms of this act the IHS constructed sanitation facilities for Indian communities. The services performed covered a wide range of environmental controls, including occupational health and safety and "environmental impact-type" evaluations for proposed tribal enterprises. In addition, special environmental service workers called environmental health aides or technicians were to be trained to perform many of these functions. Cooperation with local housing programs also helped improve sanitation.

While the existence of such activities was reported by the Public Health Service, it is evident that they were not provided in sufficient quantity to make them widespread among most of the Indian population. In 1978 HEW reported that "many families still lack basic facilities and are subject to the serious health hazards associated with such environmental deficiencies." Some of the effects of this law on Indian health services after 1975 are discussed further in the "Summary and Issues" section below.

Dental Services. Dental health among Indians has been persistently poor, with utilization of services far below the amount judged to be required. IHS data indicate the estimated shortfall in services as late as 1981 as still about 70 percent; that is, only about 30 percent of services estimated to be required by the IHS were given. The percentages of required services provided are somewhat higher for children and young persons but do not exceed 42 percent for the twenty-five to thirty-four age group. There has been an actual decline since 1976, when the overall percentage of required services provided was 41 percent (HEW, 1978). However, by 1980 the number of dental services provided had increased tenfold since the year of the transfer to the Public Health Service, 1955.

Maternal and Infant Health Infant mortality is often used as a surrogate indicator of a population's health status and by a further extension as a surrogate for the efficacy of that population's health care. The infant mortality rate of the American Indian has always been higher than that of the total United States population. It was 2.4 times as high as the United States rate in 1955 and 1.5 times as high as that of racial minority groups.[23] The 62.7 mortality rate (per 1,000 live births) of 1955 had declined to 14.6 by 1979, but it still was 1.1 times the 13.1 of the total population. (It had, however, fallen below the 19.8 of all other minorities.) There does not appear to have been a clear-cut increase in the rate of decline since the passage of the Self-determination and Health Improvement Act of 1975–76. Maternal deaths declined from 82.6 per 100,000 live births in 1958 (2.2 times the overall U.S. rate) to 15.7 (1.2 times the overall U.S. rate) in 1975 (HEW, 1978; U.S. Department of Health, 1988).

Summary and Issues

The Indian Health Service reflects the history of the changes in Indian policy of the United States government, which itself is a reflection of the economic and social development of the United States as it affected Indians. Beginning with an early policy of negotiating treaties with Indian tribes regarded as independent nations, the policy changed to appropriating Indian lands and confining the Indians to reservations on sites chosen by the United States government. The reservation Indians became wards of the federal government, which provided services and governed them with some participation of tribal councils. Health services were provided by the federal government. In the twentieth century, federal policy turned increasingly toward disengaging the national government from its obligations to reservation Indians. One part of this policy was to promote the provision of services to Indians on the reservations by local and state governments, a policy particularly applicable to health services. A concomitant of this approach was to encourage contracting for health services rather than expanding federally operated Indian health facilities and services. Another aspect of the policy was to encourage greater self-government by the tribal councils with continued federal funding assistance, an approach strongly pressed by John Collier. A third facet of the policy was to attempt to liquidate the reservation itself by giving lump-sum payments to Indians in settlement of all claims to reservation privileges as well as encouraging off-reservation settlement and employment of Indians. Basically, these different policies represent two different approaches: assimilationist and nationalist. In practice the most recent health services policy has been to permit Indians to opt for continuing on the reservation or to leave it and join the mainstream of American life as ordinary citizens. There has been available a further option for reservation Indians of continuing to receive services from the Indian Health Service or to choose to operate an autonomous tribal health system. For those leaving the reservation there have been, depending on the circumstances, lump-sum payments and off-reservation Indian health centers. As of 1980 the Indian Health Service was still directly operating most of the health services itself, contracting with some private and public providers for others, and some tribal organizations were operating their own facilities.[24] This reflects a legacy of the development of these services on reservations, many of which are isolated, sparsely settled, and far from adequate general health services. It also stems from the history of resistance of state and local governments to taking responsibility for the health care of Indians living in their jurisdictions. Increasingly the personnel of the Indian Health Service have been of Indian descent, re-

flecting the policies started by the 1934 Reorganization Act and the administration of the BIA under John Collier. The highest-ranking professionals, physicians and dentists, however, were always and still are overwhelmingly non-Indian.

The use of contracts with private groups for services reflects, again, both the inability of the PHS to always recruit the required personnel to provide the service directly and the aim of termination, which had always had adherents in Congress but became dominant policy in the 1950s, when preparations were being made to remove all direct services from the reservations. This policy was reflected in the Indian Health Facilities Act of 1957, which authorized the Indian Health Service to contribute to the construction costs of community hospitals wherever it was judged that this would supply hospital care to Indians more efficiently than providing it in PHS facilities. The extent of these contract services grew from 14.7 percent of all hospital admissions in 1955 to 28.1 percent in 1976.

The actual percentage of patient days in contract hospitals was less than their percentage of admissions, which implies that the length of stay of IHS clients in contract hospitals was less than that of Indians served in IHS facilities. This in turn suggests that the Indian patients served by the community contract hospitals were less sick and less chronically ill than those in the IHS facility.[25] This pattern has been observed in many cases when government health facilities contract some of their patients out to private ones. A number of tribes availed themselves of the opportunity provided by the 1975 Self-Determination Act to engage health planning and management consultants who helped guide them in establishing tribe-operated systems of health care, but a relatively small portion of total services to Indians have been handled by tribes.

After the transfer of Indian health services to the PHS in 1955, there is evidence of major improvement in the quantity of health resources available to and used by Indians and some improvement in health status. This may be taken to reflect ths increase in access as well as the better training of personnel. The number of IHS physicians per 100,000 target population rose from 57 in 1956 to 105 in 1976, and while the number per capita in 1956 was 39 percent of the general United States rate, in 1976 it had risen to 57 percent of the general number per capita. Similar improvements appear in some health status indicators, the most impressive being the infant death rate, which went from 62.5 per 1,000 live births in 1955 to 18.2 in 1975. However, even in 1975 it was still above the 16.1 for the entire U.S. This improvement may be partly due to the fact that in 1955 88.2 percent of Indian births were in hospitals while in 1975 this had grown to 98.1 percent (HEW, 1978).

The age-adjusted overall annual death rate for Indians averaged about 1,020.0 per 100,000 during 1949–53 (HEW, 1957), and by 1975 it was down to 824.8. Again, however, it was still 1.3 times the 630.4 rate for the United States as a whole. While the major causes of death are not much different in priority order from the overall U.S. order of importance, some individual rates are much higher. The data show motor vehicle death rates to be 4.4 times higher than those of the United States, and the rate from cirrhosis of the liver, a disease linked to chronic alcoholism, is high on the list. Tuberculosis, with a rate 8.3 times as high as the U.S. overall, is especially flagrant. The trend in tuberculosis cases is distinctly down, with a sharp reduction in tuberculosis hospitalizations. New active cases per 100,000 population fell from 758.1 in 1955 to 69.4 in 1976, although again the U.S. rate of 48.0 in 1976 was much lower than that of Indians. These causes are related to the substandard living conditions that still prevail in poor areas. The change in some health indicators has been distinctly negative. The age-adjusted death rate from suicides among Indians was 17.0 in 1959 and 26.0 in 1975, more than twice the overall population rate; homicide rates went from 9.1 to 10.5; and the average number of decayed, missing, and filled teeth among persons five to nineteen year of age went from 4.00 in 1957 to 5.97 in 1976.

The advent of Medicare, and especially Medicaid, in 1965 took some of the pressure off the push to expand special Indian health clinics in urban areas. The future shape of Indian health services clearly depends on the course of the Indian mode of community organization. If reservations flourish and become a relatively permanent feature of Indian life, the services on many of them will probably be increasingly Indian controlled and operated. If assimilated ur-

banization becomes the prevailing mode of Indian life, then it would seem that special health services for Indians would be at most a transitional phenomenon. The two factors in American life that will probably affect the future of Indian health services most are the state of the economy, in particular the job market, and the passage of comprehensive national health insurance.

The evolution of Indian health services, embedded as it is in the evolution of Indian health policy, is of particular interest as a microcosm of the evolution of health systems in response to social and political circumstances. It presents another aspect of the United States pattern of providing special subsystems for special populations in the absence of an overriding comprehensive system.

MEDICAL CARE ACTIVITIES OF THE ARMED FORCES

Background and Overview

Other examples of a comprehensive medical service operated by the federal government for specially defined population groups are those of the armed forces: the Army, Navy, and Air Force. One of the main differences between the health services of the armed forces and those of the Veterans Administration stems from differing missions. The VA services are directed toward maintaining the health of a civilian population as it ages over time, so that long-term care is an integral part of its mission. Furthermore, the VA is especially responsible for providing all needed care to veterans with service-connected disabilities. Care of chronic conditions, psychiatric care, and long-term maintenance and rehabilitative care are again indicated.

In contrast, the armed forces health care system is in the first instance charged with the medical aspects of maintaining the combat readiness of the armed forces. Whatever long-term and chronic care the services provide is mainly for the dependents of active-duty personnel and for retired personnel and their survivors, who remain eligible for the armed forces medical services. In the words of an internally conducted study: ''The mission of the Military Health

Service System is to provide the health services necessary to support and maintain all military forces in fulfilling their approved missions, to create and maintain morale in the uniformed Services by providing a comprehensive and high-quality uniform program of health services for members and other eligible beneficiaries, and to be responsive to missions directed by the Executive Branch of the Government'' (U.S. Department of Defense, 1975).

On its face, this statement implies that care for long-term needs and chronic disabilities is peripheral to the concerns of the Military Health Service System (MHSS). However, because retired personnel and their dependents and survivors do remain eligible for health services, for whatever reasons, the growing fraction of the service load that they constitute presents an increasing challenge to the MHSS to provide services for long-range and chronic disability. In 1975 active-duty personnel and their dependents were estimated to constitute 58 percent of the beneficiary population of the Military Health Services System and retired personnel and their dependents 38 percent. In 1955, the corresponding proportions had been active-duty and dependents, 89 percent, and retired, 9 percent. In 1975 they had been estimated to be 52 percent active duty and 43 percent retired by 1990, ''on the assumption that no war occurs between 1975 and 1990.''[26] The estimated age and sex distribution of the beneficiaries of the Military Health Service System in 1975 and 1990 is shown in Table 5–6. The proportion of beneficiaries fifty-five years of age and older was expected to rise

from 10.3 percent in 1975 to 19.2 percent in 1990. But even these percentages underestimate the proportion of the actual workload of military medical facilities that consists of nonactive personnel, because they are based on total eligibles and not on actual users. An Army study found that in 1953 22 percent of the overall workload of Army Continental United States (CONUS) hospitals was attributable to dependents, and in 1963 this figure was 44 percent (see page 179).

Notwithstanding the formal merger of the three departments into a single Department of Defense (DOD) in 1947, the Military Health Services continue to comprise three substantially autonomous segments—those of the Army, the Navy and the Air Force. There are both similarities and differences in the way the three are organized. Each provides health services both within the boundaries of the continental United States and to troops stationed abroad or aboard ships.[27] The organization of services is further differentiated into one portion that provides services under a separately organized, medically focused authority (''command'') and another that provides services to combat units and is under the authority or command of the regional military commander. The discussion will address the CONUS medically commanded services almost exclusively because they have a wider impact on the complex of health services operated by government within the United States health care system and are therefore more germane to the purposes of this book. Furthermore, in peacetime the CONUS medical command services have constituted

Table 5–6. Estimated Age and Sex Distribution of Military Health Care Sysem Eligible CONUS Population for 1975 and 1990

Age	Male (percent)		Female (percent)		Total (percent)	
	1975	1990	1975	1990	1975	1990
0–4	26.4	24.1	28.3	24.9	27.3	24.5
15–22	27.8	26.2	21.1	19.5	24.6	22.9
23–44	24.8	21.4	26.9	23.2	25.8	22.3
45–54	11.2	9.5	12.9	12.7	11.9	11.1
55–64	6.9	9.9	6.8	10.5	6.8	10.2
65+	2.9	8.8	4.1	9.2	3.5	9.0
TOTAL	100.0	100.0	100.0	100.0	100.0	100.0
0–54	90.2	81.3	89.1	80.3	89.7	80.8
55+	9.8	18.7	10.0	19.7	10.3	19.2
Number (in thousands)	4,091	4,463	3,737	4,239	7,828	8,703

Source: U.S. Department of Defense, 1975.

overwhelmingly the most important segment of the armed forces health services provided. In 1975, 69 percent of the total active-duty physician force was directly involved in military medical care delivery in the continental United States, most of them serving in the medical commands.[28]

The Department of Defense is a cabinet department; that is, the Secretary of Defense is a member of the President's cabinet.[29] The DOD was established de facto in 1947 and reorganized under its present name in 1949. Under the Secretary of Defense are three Departments—Army, Navy and Air Force—each with its own secretary. Each of the three departments has its own medical services ("military medical departments"), although increasingly attempts have being made to coordinate them into "tri-service" organizations. These military medical departments provide "environmental, preventive, diagnostic, therapeutic, and authorized restorative and rehabilitative patient care and ancillary support services" (U.S. Department of Defense, 1975).

In 1975 the Military Health Service System (MHSS) had 6,929 physicians in the United States (5,442 in direct patient care and 1,487 in preventive medicine, research, and various administrative capacities) and was sponsoring 2,834 interns and residents (2,599 in military and 234 in civilian facilities). In total there were 9,763 military physicians in the United States. An additional 1,901 physicians were serving outside the United States (U.S. Department of Defense, 1975).

The Army medical service was first established as the Hospital Department of the Revolutionary Army in 1775, and in 1818 Congress authorized a Surgeon General and a medical service as a permanent part of the Army. With every war, the medical service of the Army was reorganized. Additional reorganizations also took place between wars. Most of the Army hospitals currently in operation in the United States were established after 1900, particularly during the two World Wars (Hamilton, 1961).

As of December 1975, the health services provided by the Army Medical Department consisted of those provided by the Health Services Command (HSC), headed by a Surgeon General,

and those provided under the authority of the Forces Command. (The HSC is the previously described medically centered authority and the Forces Command the operational combat centered authority.) In 1975 the Health Services Command was in charge of thirty-three areawide health systems in the United States and eight medical centers. Each of the regions generally had a hospital and satellite health facilities. The medical centers were sophisticated referral and teaching hospitals that supported the areawide systems with specialized, i.e., secondary and tertiary care. The Forces Command consisted of combat units, and the medical services within them operated under the authority of the military commanders. They provided field medical units, such as mobile hospitals, as well as medical personnel who provided first aid and primary care within the combat units. The number of medical personnel within the United States Forces Command is very small during peacetime but expands rapidly in wartime, partly by transfers of personnel from the Health Service Command (HSC). All overseas medical services are under the command of combat commanders, although liaison is maintained with the Surgeon General of the HSC. As has been previously noted, the domestic, medically oriented services under the Health Service Command are the focus of this chapter. In addition to the direct services provided, the Health Services Command supervised programs for training medical personnel and for enhancing the recruitment potential of the military medical departments. It operated an Academy of Health Sciences for specialized training, ranging from basic medical training for enlisted personnel to postgraduate specialty training and also operated a division whose responsibility is medical research, development, testing, and evaluation. (See "Professional Education and Training Activities," below, for a more complete description of these activities by the Armed Forces health service system.)

In 1974, the Army Health Service Command had an average daily inpatient census of 6,800 and 46,000 daily clinic visits; it provided 9,800 clinic treatments daily in the United States (Surgeon General of the U.S. Army, 1974). A total of 16,000 medical department officers were employed worldwide, broken down into six categories: medical, dental, veterinary, medical service army nurse, and army medical specialist.

The personnel of the Medical Service Corps represented many administrative and certain ancillary and scientific fields, including audiology, podiatry, social work, and hospital administration. The Medical Specialist Corps is composed of dietitians and physical and occupational therapists. The service capability of the regular Army medical personnel is enhanced by a number of medical residents, interns, and medical students who train in Armed Forces medical facilities. In 1974, some 240 interns and residents were accepted to train at Army facilities and about 300 medical students served clerkships.

The Department of the Navy had a smaller but similar program. Like the Army, the Navy also had a bifurcated organization for health services. One branch, known as the shore establishment, covered the shore-based services and was analogous to the Health Services Command of the army. The other, the "operating forces," served the combat forces afloat and was analogous to the medical units of the forces. The Navy's shore establishment and its educational and training system were under the command of the navy Surgeon General, and the operating forces had medical units that were under the authority of the combat commanders. The bifurcation was slightly different from that of the army in that the shore-based health services commanded by the navy Surgeon General were worldwide, whereas the Health Services Command of the Army Surgeon General was essentially limited to continental United States territory. The shore-based health service system was called the Bureau of Medicine and Surgery (BuMED) and consisted of a network of regional subsystems, similar to those in the Army, each with a hospital or medical center and branch dispensaries. BuMED also operated a network of training schools and programs similar to those of the Army. As of 1975 it was operating eight training schools, a Medical Training Institute, a graduate dental school, a School of Health Administration, and a number of other institutes. In October 1982 BuMED was reorganized and redesignated as the headquarters of the Naval Medical Command. In December 1979 the active-duty

personnel and their dependents constituted 51 percent of the beneficiaries, and the average daily census in CONUS facilities was about 70 percent active-duty personnel and their dependents despite their being only 51 percent of the eligible population (U.S. Department of the Navy, 1978, 1979).

The Department of the Air Force has had no separate, quasi-autonomous medical command analogous to the Army's Health Services Command or the Navy's Medical Command. In 1975 all medical activities were subordinated to the military commanders of some of the fifteen major commands, such as the Strategic Air Command or the Military Airlift Command. The Surgeon General was a staff advisor to the Secretary of the Air Force and Air Force Chief of Staff rather than a line operations chief. Within the United States, the Air Force health services were operated in a system of six regions, each with a tertiary care hospital known as an Area Medical Center. Primary care was provided by small base hospitals and clinics. Of the fifteen major "commands," three were charged with operating medical training facilities and programs. In 1975 the organizations operated by these three commands were the School of Health Care Services of the Air Force Training Command, the School of Aerospace Medicine of the Air Force Systems Command, and the Air Force Institute of Technology, which was part of the Air University.

In addition to the programs of the three major military service departments, the Department of Defense developed overall departmental services—"tri-service" programs. As of 1975 there were eight such joint medical activities supporting the direct care system. The Army was given the "lead" responsibility; that is, it was appointed the executive agent, for six of the joint activities, and the Navy and Air Force each were assigned one. These functions included programs of pathology, epidemiology, vector control, data analysis of operations, and library.

All members of the uniformed services on active duty or retired, as well as their dependents and survivors, are entitled to service in any of the Military Health Services System (MHSS) installations. The uniformed services include the commissioned personnel of the U.S. Public Health Service, the commissioned corps of the

U.S. National Oceanic and Atmospheric Administration (formerly the Coast and Geodetic Survey), and the U.S. Coast Guard (U.S. Department of Defense, 1977). Whenever the members of one service are cared for in the facilities of another, an interchange of payments takes place. Table 5–7 shows the utilization of the "direct" medical services by type of beneficiary for 1984.

In 1974 the worldwide Armed Forces medical system had "approximately 190 hospitals and 120 free-standing clinics providing direct care, with payment for supplementary civilian care made through the Civilian Health and Medical Program of the Uniformed Services (CHAMPUS)" (U.S. Department of Defense, 1975). In 1984 the military health care system included "more than 160 hospitals and 300 clinics, supported by over 150,000 military and civilian personnel (Congressional Budget Office, 1984). Like other statistics comparing the status of DOD medical services over the last ten or fifteen years, these indicate a decline in inpatient facilities and a concomitant increase in outpatient facilities, reflecting the shift from inpatient to outpatient sites of much of the medical service in recent years generally.

Medical Care Insurance for Dependents (CHAMPUS)

In addition to these direct medical services, dependents of uniformed services personnel are also eligible to receive care at civilian facilities under an insurance program that began in 1943 with the Emergency Maternal and Infant Child Care Program (EMIC). EMIC was a war emergency measure that provided maternity and infant care benefits to the wives of servicemen on active duty and ended in 1946. It "was the first legislative step taken to provide other than 'space available' care to nonactive duty beneficiaries" and was succeeded by the Dependents' Medical Care Program Act of 1956 (military Medicare). The impetus for this law came from the overcrowding of military medical facilities during the Korean war and the fact that it was estimated that 40 percent of the dependents of active-duty personnel were located too far from military medical facilities to use them conveniently (U.S. Department of Defense, 1975). It provided for limited medical and dental care from civilian sources at government expense for wives and children of servicemen. The Act also established formal priorities for eligibility for direct-care services and instituted direct-care inpatient charges for active-duty officers as well as for retired personnel. It gave the the Secretary of Defense authority to limit the situations under which dependents could choose to use private-sector providers when Armed Forces facilities were accessible; set cost sharing ("fair charges") for inpatient care for all beneficiaries other than active duty and retired members; and imposed minimal charges for outpatient care. The intent of limiting use of outside providers

Table 5–7. Direct Medical Services: Distribution of Beneficiaries, Ambulatory Visits, and Hospital Days in the Continental United States by Category of Beneficiary, Fiscal Year 1984 (In Percent, Totals in Thousands).

Category	Beneficiaries	Beneficiaries in Catchment Areas[a]	Ambulatory Visits	Hospital Days
Active-duty personnel	20	24	28	39
Dependents of active-duty personnel[b]	27	32	41	27
Enlisted[c]		23	31	22
Officer[c]		9	10	5
Retirees and their dependents[b]	51	42	28	29
Enlisted[c]		30	21	20
Officer[c]		12	7	9
Survivors[b]	2	2	3	5
Enlisted[c]		1.5	2	4.5
Officer[c]		0.5	1	0.5
Totals	8,340	6,500	38,000	4,700

Source: Congressional Budget Office, 1984.

[a]Catchments are defined as the area in a roughly forty-mile radius around a hospital.

[b]Distribution among groups from the Department of Defense Resource Analysis and Planning (RAPS) model.

[c]Distribution between enlisted and officers within catgories from Department of Defense Health Use Survey.

in cases where adequate military medical facilities were readily available was to make the insurance system supplementary to the direct service system and to discourage considering it as an alternative system. The MHSS regarded services obtained from outside providers as more expensive for the Armed Forces than the cost of the same services provided directly by its own providers—a cogent consideration in view of the rise in the number of eligible dependents from 2,772,800 in 1956 to 3,960,000 in 1966.

Until 1966 the major portion of this program consisted of obstetrical care, but legislation passed in 1966 (P.L. 89–614) added additional classes of individuals entitled to use this service and also enlarged the scope of available benefits. Dependents of retired personnel and survivors of certain deceased military personnel were made eligible for the outpatient benefits, and these benefits were expanded to include routine ambulatory care and a special program of medical care for handicapped dependents of active-duty personnel. However, this legislation also further amplified the powers of the Secretary of Defense to restrict access to outside providers in areas considered to be adequately served by military facilities. This expansion resulted in expenditures of $170 million in 1968 compared with $75 million spent in 1966. By 1969 there were about 6.2 million potential participants in this service, which was named the Civilian Health and Medical Program of the Uniformed Services (CHAMPUS). A total of 1.3 million claims were processed in that year, representing approximately 593,000 beneficiaries.

CHAMPUS is a health insurance program that pays "for medically necessary services and supplies required in the diagnosis and treatment of illness or injury, including maternity care" (U.S. Department of Defense, 1977). It may be used by all persons eligible for the health services of the MHSS except for active-duty personnel and includes coverage for care in civilian hospitals, by civilian physicians and "other authorized individual professional providers," ambulance service, prescription drugs and "authorized" medical supplies, and rental of durable equipment. Considerable cost sharing is required "to encourage use of the Uniformed Services direct medical system" (U.S. Department of Defense, 1977). As of 1984 dependents of active-duty personnel, for example, were subject to annual deductibles for outpatient services ($50 per person with a $100 limit per family) and a 20 percent coinsurance for all expenditures exceeding the deductible. They were also paying $6.80 per day toward their inpatient costs (with a minimum of $25 per stay).[30] Retirees and their dependents and survivors were paying 25 percent of all expenses (Congressional Budget Office, 1984). As of 1984, many military dependents and retirees also had supplementary private health insurance to help them cover the required cost sharing, especially the coinsurance, which could become quite large with catastrophic illness. More than half the military retirees were buying this supplementary protection. In addition, many military families had private health insurance because a family member was working at a civilian job that provided health insurance.

As noted, the eligible military dependent does not have a completely free choice of using the military services or availing him- or herself of CHAMPUS to pay civilian providers, because the program is meant to be supplementary to the direct-service system, and both the laws and regulations prohibit payments by CHAMPUS for specified services available in accessible MHSS facilities. For example, in FY 1977, legislation specifically prohibited payment for nonemergency care to providers for services that were available in an MHSS facility within a forty-mile radius of the patient's residence. The methods of paying providers are similar to those of Blue Cross and Blue Shield and will be discussed in Part III, where health insurance issues are treated.

Professional Education and Training Activities

During the World War II period and much of the Vietnam War, the Army, along with the other two military departments, was able to draft physicians. To help the Armed Services obtain a proper mix and supply of physicians, legislation was passed instituting a training program called the Armed Forces Physicians' Appointment and Residency Cooperation Program, which came to be known as the Berry Plan. In fiscal year 1969, 5,781 medical school graduates participated in the Berry Plan, of which 2,928, or just over half, were allocated to the Army. Under this plan an intern in training could obtain financial support and have his or her draft obligations deferred until completion of training. Upon completion of internship training, military service could be deferred further in order to undergo residency training if the proposed training were in a specialty needed by the Army. In return, the participants in this program were obligated to serve a stipulated time in the military in the specialty for which they were being trained. (Again, this arrangement applied to the three military services.)

In 1973 the physician draft was discontinued and with it the Berry Plan. There had also been an early commissioning program to help recruit armed services physicians that was also discontinued. The successor to these discontinued recruiting incentive programs was the U.S. Army Health Professions Scholarship Program, established by P.L. 92–426, enacted in September 1972. Under this act, students in the health professions could get grants to support their education and training in return for service obligations. A "large number of grants . . . substantial in size and scope" were made available to "every student or potential student of medicine, osteopathy, dentistry, veterinary medicine, optometry, podiatry, or clinical psychology at the doctoral level" (Surgeon General of the U.S Army, 1974). Students were commissioned as officers in the U.S. Army Reserve and served about one and one half months at full pay during each year of training in professionally oriented active duty. Despite the designation of "U.S. Army" in the title of the act, all three services participated in the program. By June 1974, some 1,350 students were participating in the Army portion of the program alone.

The same 1972 act also authorized the establishment of a military services and health sciences (including medicine) school—the Uniformed Services University of the Health Sciences. Its mission was to train career military health professionals, and it was part of the Department of Defense serving all three services. The school is on the site of the National Naval Medical Center in Bethesda, Maryland. Graduates were required to serve at least seven years after graduation, not counting time spent in in-

ternship and residency programs. The first class was graduated in May 1980, the twenty-five men and four women graduates receiving captains' commissions as well as medical degrees. As of 1980, the total enrollment was 329 students.

There had been Congressional "opposition of budget makers in several administrations" (McGraw Hill, 1980) but backers were successful in obtaining support for the school from some members of Congress. A particularly strong attack on the continued existence of the school was launched under the Reagan administration when in August 1982 the Director of the Office of Management and Budget, David Stockman, attempted to delete the authorization for funding the school from the 1982 budget. By that time two classes had already graduated and this effort was also thwarted by backers of the school in Congress. It is interesting to note that the National Commission for Health Certifying Agencies reported in 1982 that the Department of Defense had in that year provided more government support for health profession education than did the Department of Health and Human Services.

An Institute of Medicine study found that it may be unnecessary for the Air Force and Navy to maintain their graduate medical education programs at existing levels but that the Army was still understaffed and should receive an increased allocation of personnel from the health professionals scholarship program. The Institute of Medicine suggestions were based on its perception that a sufficient number of physicians in the country could be recruited, as indicated by the ample staffing of the Air Force and Navy medical programs.

Costs

The Department of Defense and the Armed Services committees of Congress have been expressing a mounting interest in the cost efficiency of the Military Health Services System. The main questions that have come to the fore at different times were the costliness of the direct services compared with comparable civilian medical facilities, the relative costliness of using CHAMPUS compared with direct services, and the possible cost savings of using alternative health services and management systems. An early study, done in 1965 by the Army's Office of the Surgeon General, "A Study Comparing Utilization, Staffing and Cost Trends in Civilian and CONUS Army Hospitals" for the years 1953–1963, covered the period after the Korean war had ended and before American involvement in Vietnam had reached the point of producing large numbers of casualties. The proportion of the medical workload consisting of dependents had increased until it represented 44 percent of the overall workload in 1963, compared with 22 percent in 1953. It was, therefore, a period during which the function of the Army medical services more nearly approached that of maintaining the health of a civilian population and in which heavy inroads were not being made into CONUS staffing by the requirements of combat medicine. The main focus of this study was the first of the questions mentioned above, which asks how the cost of direct military medical services compares with comparable civilian-sponsored services. The 1965 investigation was confined to inpatient hospital services. After adjusting personnel, costs, and operating statistics to account for differences in medical practice necessitated by differences in patient case mix and conditions of army life (see quotation from the study cited below), the study concluded that "Army hospitals are found to have lower staffing ratios and patient day costs than comparable civilian non-Federal short-term (NFST) hospitals. This superior cost effectiveness despite the high standard of care is due to the nature of the Army hospital and its method of operation." The study found that in 1957 the CONUS hospitals used 24 graduate nurses per 100 beds occupied compared with 56 in NFST hospitals. Total personnel per 100 beds occupied in 1963 was 168 and 235, respectively. The CONUS hospitals were on average larger than the civilian ones, averaging 261 beds as opposed to 123 beds for NFST, and the proportion of CONUS hospitals having certain adjunct services was higher for almost every type of adjunct. Ninety-three percent of the CONUS hospitals were accredited compared with 64 percent of the NFST group.

A study made jointly by three government agencies[31] in 1975 covered the entire DOD—not just the Army—and addressed a number of the questions of interest with respect to costliness. It found that average annual cost per beneficiary

in FY 1974 was $270 ($449 for active-duty and $228 for non-active-duty personnel). This compared with the $464 per capita spent nationally for personal health care in CY 1974 (Health Care Finance Administration). Of course, the health risk mix of the eligible armed forces population was undoubtedly still considerably lower than that of the general population despite the growing proportion of retirees, but the study also showed that payment for similar care to civilian providers via CHAMPUS was higher than for care provided by the Military Health Service System. Moreover, using Kaiser or Blue Cross for non-active-duty personnel would have been more expensive than direct care (U.S. Department of Defense, 1975). While the premiums for Kaiser (California) and Blue Cross were each lower than the overall per capita cost of the DOD health system in CONUS, they were higher than the per capita cost of taking care of non-active-duty personnel in the existing system of direct care plus CHAMPUS. It was the cost of the active-duty personnel that raised the overall per capita direct cost figure. As noted above, the 1965 Army study described above had asserted that since the cost of direct inpatient services to active-duty personnel was not adjusted for the extra lengths of stay due to "conditions of army life," it was not clear whether the cost of inpatient care in MHSS was actually higher than in comparable civilian facilities, other things being equal.

The analysis in the study argued:

In the Army the multi-bed barracks is the soldier's home. This has a direct bearing upon both frequency and duration of hospitalization. . . . The barracks area is an unsuitable place for a sick soldier, since privacy is lacking and there is no one to administer to his needs. Also, commanders generally object to a non-effective soldier remaining in the barracks because of his potential effect not only on the health but on the morale of troops, particularly when the unit is roused at three o'clock in the morning for a training exercise. Thus, many soldiers who as civilians would be cared for at home with or without the supervision of a physician must be hospitalized in the Army. For the same reason, patients who in civilian life might be released for limited care or convalescence at home must remain under hospital jurisdiction until ready to return to duty. . . .

By their very nature, Army hospitals operate in a different manner from civilian hospitals in many respects. The Army hospital is the focal point for the provision of total medicine to the post population served. It is not only self-sufficient in the provision of hospital care but provides full clinic service for both inpatients and outpatients and, where necessary, dispensary care and sick call at outlying points throughout the post. It provides various preventive medicine services, including medical examinations, immunizations, inspections of units and facilities, accident prevention, and a health nursing program encompassing home visits, school nursing, and many other forms of extra-hospital nursing care. It is the hospital, the doctor's office, the pharmacy, the public health center, the medical laboratory, the dental clinic, and the dental laboratory all combined. In addition, its military staff, which includes nearly all professional and a large portion of the supporting personnel, is supervised by the hospital and is housed and fed on hospital grounds. As in civilian hospitals, the larger Army hospitals have the added mission of conducting internship and residency training and clinical research. However, unlike civilian hospitals, the military personnel in the Army facility must participate in certain military training and perform a variety of military duties.

Perhaps because of these difficulties in making valid comparisons for active-duty personnel, the major thrust of subsequent studies on the feasibility of cost savings were directed at the non-active-duty personnel health service eligibles—dependents and retirees.

The 1975 joint agency study also conducted "satisfaction" surveys of military personnel and dependents and found that dependents generally expressed a strongly positive opinion of military health care, as did those using civilian care, but when asked to compare the two, by a small margin they thought civilian care to be better.[32] The aspects of civilian care that were found to be inferior were its expensiveness and difficulty of obtaining emergency out-of-hours care. Military care was found to be less desirable than civilian care with respect to waiting time and patient-physician relationships.

Later investigations estimated potential savings from changing the proportion of dependents using CHAMPUS as well as the use of civilian contractors to provide care for CONUS non-active-duty personnel. The DOD also made efforts to increase use of ambulatory in place of inpatient care along the lines of recent cost containment trends in civilian health services, and a General Accounting Office (GAO) report in May 1985 concluded that the Defense Depart-

ment should make greater use of outpatient surgery. In a survey of 635 inpatient cases at six military hospitals, the GAO found that 65 percent of the cases could have been handled in outpatient settings (McGraw Hill, 1985).

Cost containment has been the central rationale put forth for the continued interest in alternative health care systems for non-active-duty personnel. In October 1980, the Department of Defense asked for legislative authority to proceed with an HMO project for Champus eligibles (McGraw Hill, 1980) and by 1982, two experimental HMO projects run by CHAMPUS were in operation, one in Portland, Oregon, and the other in Minneapolis-St. Paul, Minnesota (U.S. Senate, 1982). Another experimental pilot project for saving money in the CHAMPUS program through the use of outside civilian contractors to process and pay CHAMPUS claims had already been in effect for a number of years when in 1981 the General Accounting Office found that the program had "resulted in poor service to military facilities" and that the contractors "have rushed through approvals that should not have been made" (McGraw Hill, 1980). A definitive study of the efficacy of using outside contractors to perform this function remains to be done, but available data seem to find it wanting. In a move to place greater emphasis on ambulatory care, the 20 percent coinsurance required of CHAMPUS beneficiaries was changed to a $25 per visit flat copayment for services in ambulatory surgery facilities effective October 1, 1980.

Although the main changes in medical care organization being considered were those involving increased use of nonphysician personnel such as clinical psychologists, optometrists, and nurse midwives (U.S. Senate, 1982) a study by the Congressional Budget Office (CBO) in 1984 also looked at two immediate ways of saving money for the DOD medical system: increasing cost sharing for all but active duty personnel and increased collections from private health insurers for dependents who have such coverage. For the longer term the report investigated prospective reimbursement and "closed enrollment" (HMOs and similar arrangements). Savings from introducing such changes were estimated for Congress. The report derived estimates showing that military families spent much less for health care than did civilian families in similar economic strata (see Table 5–8). That the pressures of increasing medical costs were affecting the CHAMPUS system was demonstrated by the appearance of Defense Department health officials before the Defense Appropriations Subcommittee in June of 1982 to ask for an additional $100 million appropriation. The CHAMPUS costs were projected at $966 million for 1982 compared with about $570 million in 1975. A White House Working Group on Health Policy and Economics under the Reagan Administration completed a report in early 1985 for the president that included recommendations for cutting costs for DOD health services by requiring that hospitals participating in CHAMPUS accept the federal prospective payment system based on DRGs for CHAMPUS reimbursement. Other recommendations were that the DOD be empowered to collect from private insurers, to use private insurance plans including HMOs, and increase both deductibles and coinsurance (McGraw Hill, 1985).

A departure from the cost-containing direction of the recent changes was a 1977 law (P.L. 96–173) that explicitly guaranteed that all retired veterans with service-connected disabilities could use CHAMPUS, even though they have VA medical care eligibility. Before this law, army personnel who retired early because of physical disability were expected to use the VA and not the military system.

Quality of Care

With all the attention to cost reduction that has been paid by Congressional committees and the Department of Defense, remarkably little emphasis has been placed on maintaining quality of care. The assessment of quality of medical care and the process of maintaining it at a high level—quality assurance—is a difficult problem even for experts in the field. The main dimensions of quality—the technical quality of the medical procedures, the accessibility of appropriate services, and the degree of patient satisfaction—are difficult to measure. Even when measurements are made, there still remains the problem of establishing proper boundaries for characterizing the poor, the good, and the excellent among programs and practices. Although on balance, the skimpy evidence supports a hypothesis that there has been some deterioration in the quality of Armed Forces medical care, particularly for nonactive personnel, along all these three dimensions of quality, there has not been a sufficiently thoroughgoing study of this question. The evidence is sporadic, sparse, and often anecdotal, with little indication of how deep or widespread the deterioration may be.

For example, there has been an increase in medical malpractice suits. (Nonactive personnel have been permitted to sue while active personnel have not, although Senator James Sasser of Tennessee introduced a bill in 1985 to permit

Table 5–8. Average Spending on Medical Care by Families of Active and Retired Military Personnel and Hypothetical Urban Families of Four (In 1984 Dollars)

| | Average Out-of-Pocket Expenses[a] | Private Health Insurance | | Total Average Spending | Annual Budget for Urban Family of Four with Comparable Incomes |
		Percent Covered	Average Premium[a]		
Active-duty					
Enlisted	225	13	480	285	1,865[b]
Officer	160	13	430	215	1,955[c]
Retired					
Enlisted	530	52	590	835	1,875[d]
Officer	720	67	610	1,120	1,955[c]
Survivors					
Enlisted	260	39	275	365	1,865[b]
Officer	175	62	375	410	1,865[b]

Source: Congressional Budget Office, 1984.

[a]Figures were originally reported in 1978 dollars. Prices of medical services rose 64.4 percent between 1978 and 1983 and are projected to increase another 7.4 percent by 1984. Accordingly, CBO multiplied reported figures by 1.77.

[b]Lower-income living standard according to Bureau of Labor Statistics: $17,050 in1984 dollars.

[c]Higher-income living standard of $42,350.

[d]Intermediate-income living standard of $28,270.

malpractice suits by active-duty uniformed personnel.) And increasingly the news media have reported evidence of lapses in medical care quality in the MHSS. On July 29, 1988, the Los Angeles Public Television Station reported that medical audits within the Defense Department found the quality of care of Madigan Army Hospital in Takoma, Washington, to be questionable. Also, nonactive personnel users when interviewed complained of interminably long waits for ambulatory services. On the same program, Dr. William Mayer, the Assistant Secretary of Defense for Health Affairs, announced that a panel of civilian physicians would oversee medical quality in the military health system. From time to time reports of similar problems have appeared in the print media.

Thus, the federal policy toward the Military Health Services System in the latter half of the 1970s and during the 1980s has in many ways mirrored federal policy with respect to civilian medical services. The emphasis has been on cost containment, with quality assurance being almost entirely overlooked at first and later instituted slowly and very modestly in response to adverse public exposure and medical malpractice suits. The cost-containment measures proposed have taken the standard civilian forms: more cost sharing for all but active-duty personnel, better collections from private insurers, and use of alternative delivery systems that control utilization. It should be noted that such measures as the greater use of cost sharing and better collections from private health insurers were not designed to reduce the nation's total health care cost but only those of the federal government.

In a sense it seems surprising that measures aimed at reducing health care utilization and increasing the cost to military families should be discussed in budget hearings and government documents. After all, the Reagan policy had been to reduce social programs and cut taxes while amply funding the military services. That military medical services, especially those to all but active-service personnel, should have come under a cost-cutting scrutiny justified by language used to reduce civilian program spending while highly controversial and costly weapon systems were unswervingly supported seems puzzling. It is particularly difficult to understand when one considers that the entire budget for

DOD medical care was about $5 billion in 1984 and of this only about $1 billion, the CHAMPUS share, came under serious cost-cutting discussion. The total budget outlays of the Department of Defense for fiscal year 1984 was $227 billion (U.S. Bureau of the Census, 1987).

Summary and Comments

The Department of Defense spent $5 billion on medical services in fiscal 1984. With this expenditure it was supplying full medical services to 2.1 million active-duty personnel, about 1 million reserves when on active duty, and 7 million people not on active duty (Congressional Budget Office, 1984). There were 8,340,000 beneficiaries in the continental United States, of which 1,670,000, or 20 percent, were active-duty personnel. The majority were their dependents and retirees and their dependents. Thus 4 percent of the population was eligible for direct services under this system, and about 22 percent of these were also eligible for DOD-subsidized care in the private sector under the CHAMPUS program because they were non-active-duty personnel who lived more than forty miles from a DOD health facility. The direct system provided 38 million ambulatory visits and 4.8 million hospital days. The military health services system is therefore a small but not negligible part of the United States health service system.

Over time considerable interest has been evinced in how this subsystem compares with the rest of the United States health services system with respect to cost efficiency and medical quality. Although comparisons with the civilian medical system must be scrutinized with care, not only for the reasons already given, but also because most of them were made by interested parties, the presumptive evidence seems to be that a comprehensive service providing care to a target population has been run by the Armed Services at a cost at least as low as that of the private sector. Unless a war intervenes to expand the active-duty population, the CONUS beneficiary population may be expected to grow older steadily, with almost a fifth being fifty-five years or older by 1990. This may move the CONUS services toward increasingly offering more long-term and chronic care and would progressively make them resemble civilian-type services because the beneficiaries will not only be older but they will be civilians—retirees and their dependents and survivors—who in 1975 were expected to constitute 43 percent of the eligible MHSS population by 1990. If a universal, comprehensive, national medical care insurance system is established in the United States, it is likely that the problem of providing care for the MHSS beneficiaries who now use CONUS off-base facilities would be greatly simplified. This is especially true of the aging retirees and their dependents.

The largest unanswered question is the quality of care provided in the CONUS system. The Armed Forces issues little public information about its medical system. Perhaps good and comprehensive analyses of quality of care sit in internal archives, but on the basis of available material there seem to have been no such studies of the system as a whole. The DOD has not embarked on a program of affiliation with civilian medical schools or commissioned many outside studies as the Veterans Administration has, but the basic missions of the two agencies are fundamentally different and this may have been undesirable and perhaps impossible. Like other direct-service programs run by the federal government for special population, its average level of quality and cost must be considered to compare favorably with the general open-market system as a whole. It may be true that the quality of services provided by the best upper percentiles of the general open-market system surpass the average quality available in the MHSS, but if universal access and egalitarian considerations are principal criteria of system quality, the very fact that all its eligibles can get the services they need from recognized types of facilities and practitioners places the MHSS ahead of the general open-market system where millions of persons have little or no access to any medical care.

NOTES

1. Unit costs are discussed on page 151.
2. That is for veterans who need medical care because of a disability directly attributable to their military service.
3. Except where otherwise noted, most of the facts in this early history appearing on page 135 come from VA, 1977.

4. Originally it was the Veterans' Administration, but the use of the apostrophe fell into disuse except in certain legal documents.
5. If adjustments are made for the difference in handling outpatient staff statistics in VA and AHA data, this ratio for all community hospitals still comes to about 3.4 for 1981, which does not materially alter the conclusions. For all psychiatric hospitals the ratio was 2.17 (AHA, 1981). Since the psychiatric bed census was about 30 percent of the 1981 total average daily census in VA hospitals, one would expect the staffing to be about 3.3 per occupied bed if the VA were staffed on the national average pattern.
6. The overall length of stay averaged 27.3 days in 1981 (VA, 1981). There is some difficulty in using overall average stay to characterize VA hospitals in comparison with other acute general hospitals in the United States because of the previously noted inclusion of long psychiatric stays not found in the average community hospital. Thus for 1981 the VA statistics give the average stay for "psychotic" patients as 88.4 days, for "other psychiatric" as 30.3 days, and for medical and surgical as 20.2 days. The psychotic component accounted for 27 percent of the total days, the other psychiatric for 15 percent, and medical and surgical for 57 percent. Hospitals with a large proportion of long stays are statistically expected to be able to operate with higher occupancy rates than those with predominantly acute short stay cases, and an occupancy rate of 81 percent does not, in these circumstances, represent overtaxed facilities.
7. This is the principal reason for my characterizing the outpatient services as having been historically an adjunct of the inpatient services rather than the other way around.
8. For the years 1971–1975, and using VA supplied data, the study tabulated the number of dental visits by inpatient and outpatient categories. Inpatient visits outnumbered outpatient visits by about two to one (NAS, 1977).
9. Most of these data continue to be from VA, 1981, and some statements are reproduced verbatim without attribution.
10. Based on findings of site visits to a sample of twenty-one general VA hospitals, studying the medical records of a sample of patients in fourteen of the twenty-one sample hospitals, and responses to a questionnaire sent to patients eight weeks after discharge.
11. The hospital expenditures reported to the AHA for inclusion in its annual compilation of hospital statistics include outpatient costs. The formula used to arrive at "adjusted" expenses is claimed by the AHA to result in only the cost of inpatient care being represented by the adjusted figure. In the AHA's words the procedure is exactly equal to the removal from total expenses of that part incurred for outpatient care (AHA, 1981).
12. In March 1989 the VA acquired cabinet status as the Department of Veterans Affairs. The *Los Angeles Times* of January 26, 1991, reported that there were then 27 million veterans and that the VA med-

ical system had 172 medical centers, 233 outpatient clinics, 119 nursing homes, 12,000 physicians, 60,000 nurses, and served 4 million veterans a year.

13. I use this qualifier because even a national health insurance system is unlikely for a long time after its establishment to provide adequate resources for nonacute care, psychiatric care, and other services that are of special importance to the present clients of special programs like the VA medical system.

14. All these direct quotations are from Mustard, 1945, unless otherwise noted.

15. I am indebted for a portion of this background material to leads supplied by the papers of some of my students, especially James A. Morrisey, Ph.D.

16. In 1824 the office of the superintendent of Indian trade in the War Department was replaced by the Bureau of Indian Affairs (BIA), and after 1832 it was headed by a Commissioner of Indian Affairs.

17. By 1900 there were "five hospitals and infirmaries in existence . . . [that] served Indian boarding school students almost exclusively; it was not until later than the Bureau [of Indian Affairs] built any number of general reservation hospitals" (HEW, 1957)

18. One cannot help being struck by the startling resemblance of this 1912 presidential rhetoric to current formulations about the health conditions of the poor.

19. With respect to this last point, it is important to note that in 1924 Congress had granted American citizenship to all those Indians who had hitherto not been citizens. This later enabled the federal government to increase its pressure on states to make their services, including health services, more accessible to the Indians residing in their respective jurisdictions.

20. The virtual eradication of trachoma as a serious problem at Indian schools and reservations resulted not only from better attention to prevention but also to the discovery in 1938 by Dr. Fred Loe of the Indian medical service that sulfanilamide quickly cured or arrested the disease (HEW, 1957).

21. All data from this source (HEW, 1957) excludes Alaska, which joined the Union in 1959. Other data, even for years before 1959, taken from HEW, 1978, include Alaska. Hence, data for years 1955 and earlier that are quoted from these two sources will show higher figures for HEW, 1978 source.

22. For example, a similar type of transfer of the BIA's agricultural extension program to the U.S. Department of Agriculture took place shortly after the health services transfer, and P.L. 280, making the Indians of five states subject to the criminal and civil jurisdiction of those states, had already been passed in 1953.

23. "Indian" includes Alaska "native." Racial minority groups includes all "other than white."

24. For example, for hospital admissions: 71.9

percent were to IHS facilities, 27.0 percent to contracted facilities, and 1.2 percent to tribal facilities. For outpatient visits the corresponding percentages were: 82.6 percent, 7.1 percent, and 10.3 (U.S. Dept. of HHS: *Indian Health Service Chart Series Book*, Tables 5.5 and 5.12).

25. For example, in 1976 the average length of stay in contract hospitals was 5.3 days while in IHS hospitals it was 6.3, so that only 24.4 percent of the patient days in 1976 were in contract hospitals, despite their having 28.2 percent of the admissions.

26. In 1979, the active proportion for the navy department was already down to 51 percent (U.S. Department of the Navy, 1978, 1979), and in 1984 for the total Department of Defense (DOD) the proportion of active-duty personnel and their dependents was down to 47 percent. They used 69 percent of the direct service (that is, service provided in DOD medical facilities) ambulatory visits and 66 percent of the direct-service hospital days, however. The disparity between beneficiary composition and utilization percentages reflects the greater use of "outside" civilian medical services by non-active-duty beneficiaries (retirees and their dependents) under the armed forces medical insurance system, CHAMPUS, described below.

27. This description applies to the conditions prevailing in 1975, when a major study of the system was made (U.S. Department of Defense, 1975). Wherever more recent data are used their sources are identified.

28. It should be noted that the term "CONUS" excludes Hawaii and Alaska and is thus not fully comparable to the term "United States—domestic." However, most of the available statistics are arranged in this manner, and the CONUS data are sufficiently representative to fully illustrate the importance and nature of the domestic segment of the medical services.

29. The president's cabinet originally consisted of the secretaries of State, the Treasury, and War in 1789. In 1981 it comprised the heads of twelve executive departments: State, the Treasury, Defense, Justice, the Interior, Agriculture, Commerce, Labor, Health and Human Services, Education, Housing and Urban Development, and Transportation.

30. There were numerous modulating provisos in the regulations; the amounts quoted here were typical ones and are meant only to give an idea of their magnitude.

31. The Departments of Defense and HEW and the Office of Management and Budget.

32. The percentage found to be satisfied with their overall care in a national study of civilian care, however, was 91 percent compared with the 78–84 percent found in two states by the study of users of military health care, not a small margin of difference.

State-Operated Medical Care Services

NONFEDERAL GOVERNMENT SERVICES: INTRODUCTION

Aside from public health preventive services clinics, the main health services directly operated by state and local governments have been public hospitals. For many years state, county, district, and municipal hospitals have borne a significant part of the medical care burden of the United States. They still do, although in some specialty sectors their proportionate share has decreased in recent years. These hospitals range over a wide gamut of service types and populations served, so that any generalization about them will contain notable and significant exceptions, but profiles of "typical" state hospitals and local public general hospitals are sufficiently applicable to be useful. This chapter will deal with the state hospital and Chapter 7 will address the local public general hospital.

Most federal direct medical care is provided to well-delineated target populations for whose health federal agencies have clearly established responsibilities: veterans, armed services personnel, Indians, federal prison inmates, and before 1982, clients of the United State Public Health Service's hospitals and clinics. As noted in the preceding chapters, these populations have been legally entitled to a complete spectrum of health care by national legislation, extending in some cases to the family of the primary beneficiary. Essentially, the singling out of these populations as deserving of a special system of medical care has been based on a concept of an implicit or explicit contractual relationship between them and the federal government. In the case of those who have served or are serving in the armed forces, this right is part of the implicit contract between the federal government acting as surrogate for a grateful society and members

of the uniformed services, whether drafted or volunteer. It has been understood for many years that medical care, both during and after active service, will be provided by special programs (quite apart from battlefield medical care). In other cases, the provision of services is part of a broader obligation to the target populations perceived to be conferred on the federal government by history or circumstance: guardianship in the case of prisons, treaty obligations in the case of the Indian, and national economic interest in the case of the Marine (Public Health Service) hospitals. The underlying notion for most of these programs has been that the beneficiary populations have a *right* to their services because they have earned them or because the federal government is otherwise obligated to provide them.

The state and local hospitals, on the other hand, were usually established simply to fill gaps in our general system of medical care. They typically have served populations who were medically indigent or whose illness was perceived to pose a threat to the health and well-being of the community at large, or both. The provision of medical care for these populations has consequently been regarded either as a public charity, and therefore a *privilege* conferred upon the unfortunate by a moral and compassionate society, or as a public health function in the nature of a quarantine measure for the protection of society. The eligibility of medically indigent persons has been based on prevailing notions of public charity or equity, and while the concept of equity has at times been widely regarded as including a *right* to needed medical care, for all, this idea has never gained sufficient political support to have become the de facto policy of the United States government. The local public general hospital has been the main provider of direct general medical care for the indigent. The state hospital has been the main provider of care and often the place for forcible confinement of long-term patients whose condition, such as tuberculosis or mental illness, was perceived to make them unable to function in their community, or whose presence was considered to endanger the rest of the population. Appropriate alternatives in the form of community-based, preventive and on-going non-crisis care for these conditions have rarely been accessible in sufficient quantity to the populations using these hospitals, especially for psychiatric patients, although attempts to improve these have been made since World War II. A major part of this chapter is concerned with these attempts.

THE STATE HOSPITAL

There were 468 state hospitals "registered"[1] by the American Hospital Association (AHA) in fiscal year 1980 (see Table 6–1), constituting 6.7 percent of all United States hospitals and 18 percent of all government hospitals. Of these, 170, or 36 percent, were short-term, and the remaining 64 percent were long-term.[2] But most re-

vealing of the nature of the inpatient load carried by the state hospitals is the distribution of beds and average daily census. The total average daily census in state hospitals for fiscal year 1980 was 196,100, of which 168,900 (86 percent) was long-term. State hospitals furnished 18.5 percent of all patient days[3] but handled only 3.3 percent of all the admissions, testifying to the long average stay in most state hospitals. Nongovernmental hospitals, by contrast, handled almost 75 percent of all the admissions but only 59 percent of the total average daily census, reflecting the fact that 97 percent of the nongovernmental hospital census was short-term.

Looking further into the distribution of inpatient service load by type of medical service, we see in Table 6–1 that 81 percent of the beds and 83 percent of the average daily census of state hospitals were psychiatric. Indeed, 80 percent of both psychiatric beds and of the total average daily psychiatric inpatient census in the United States were in state hospitals.

The average daily census in nonfederal tuberculosis (and other respiratory disease) hospitals has virtually disappeared, having decreased from some 62,000 in 1950 to 11,000 in 1971 to about 1,000 in 1980. About 87 percent of these patients, 873, were in eight state tuberculosis

Table 6–1. Selected Operating Statistics of State-Controlled Hospitals by Service Type—Fiscal Year 1980

Service Type[a]	Hospitals		Beds[b]		Average daily census		Admissions	
	Number	Percent of total state	Number (in thousands)	Percent of total state	Number (in thousands)	Percent of total state	Number (in thousands)	Percent of total state
Short-term	170	36.4	36.4	15.6	27.2	13.9	960.4	74.81
Psychiatric	28	6	6.4	2.7	5.3	2.7	58.2	4.53
Tuberculosis	0	0	0	0	0	0	0	0.00
General	129	27.6	28.2	12.1	20.7	10.6	872.4	67.95
Other	13	2.8	1.8	0.8	1.2	0.6	29.8	2.32
Long-Term	298	63.7	197.4	84.4	168.9	86.2	323.4	25.19
Psychiatric	248	53	182.4	78	156.9	80	298.4	23.24
Tuberculosis	8	1.7	1.3	0.6	0.9	0.5	6.3	0.49
General	2	0.4	0.3	0.1	0.2	0.1	1.6	0.12
Other	40	8.6	13.4	5.7	10.9	5.6	17.1	1.33
Total state	468	100.1	233.8	100	196.1	100.1	1283.8	100.00
Total U.S.[c]	6965	6.7	1364.8	17.1	1059.8	18.5	38892.3	3.3

Source: AHA, 1981.

[a]Hospitals are classified by the American Hospital Association by the type of service provided to the majority of patients. Psychiatric includes care for the mentally retarded and treatment of alcoholism and other chemical dependencies. Tuberculosis includes other respiratory diseases. General includes medical and surgical. Other includes all other specialty services, such as obstetrics and gynecology; rehabilitation; orthopedic; chronic disease; and eye, ear, nose and throat.

[b]Number of beds set up and staffed for use.

[c]Percentages represent percent total state is of total U.S.

hospitals. There were 11 nonfederal tuberculosis hospitals in all in 1980; in 1950 there had been 398.

In 1980 the average size of the state hospital was about[4] 500 beds (but 662 for long-term hospitals and 735 for long-term psychiatric) compared with 327 for federal and 115 for local hospitals. The average nongovernmental, not-for-profit hospital had 204 beds. In 1969 the average state hospital had had 1,110 beds. We are justified, therefore, in characterizing the typical state hospital of 1980 as a large hospital, primarily composed of long-term beds, and with an inpatient census of persons who are mostly medically indigent due to psychiatric illnesses requiring long periods of hospitalization.

In the 1980 regional distribution of nonfederal psychiatric beds, of which about 88 percent were state controlled, most of the state psychiatric hospitals were east of the Mississippi, with Atlantic and East North Central States predominating in total numbers of hospitals, and the Atlantic and New England States having the most psychiatric beds per population (AHA, 1981; U.S. Department of Commerce, 1981). The early establishment of the state institution as a mental institution in the east is perhaps the most important reason for this distribution. Control over state hospitals was variously vested in departments of health, welfare, boards of charity, or in special hospital boards or commissions.

Some 44 university hospitals in 1975 were state-owned and -controlled in conjunction with state university medical schools. These hospitals comprised most of the beds and census of those state-sponsored hospitals that are classified under short-term "general" beds and census.[5] They had about 23,000 beds, served an average daily census of 17,000 persons, and delivered 348,000 outpatient visits (Hospital Research and Education Trust, 1978). Since these teaching institutions tend to be large (averaging 527 beds in 1975), they contribute to the large average size of the state hospital. If state hospitals are considered excluding these general teaching hospitals, the percentages of patient services that are long-term and that are psychiatric are even higher than those cited above.

Although tuberculosis hospitals constituted a larger component of state and local bed care

prior to the last two decades than they do today, even then state facilities never dominated nonfederal government tuberculosis inpatient care as they did psychiatric care. In 1971, for example, while state hospitals carried 86 percent of the psychiatric census and local psychiatric public hospitals accommodated only 3 percent, the tuberculosis census was distributed 71 percent to state hospitals and 26 percent to local governmental hospital. However, the census in the state hospitals providing primarily tuberculosis and other respiratory disease care was less than 2 percent of the total state hospital census even in 1971 and by 1980 had become negligible. Most tuberculosis (and other respiratory diseases) came to be treated in general hospitals. By 1980 there were about 2,800 tuberculosis beds in general hospitals (1,658 in federal and 1,165 in nonfederal) compared with 1,300 beds in tuberculosis hospitals.

THE STATES AND INPATIENT MENTAL HEALTH SERVICES

In terms of medical care expenditures for direct inpatient care, the data over the years clearly identify the big problem facing the states as having been psychiatric services. As late as 1975 a report of the GAO found that "[d]espite reductions in their institutional populations, State mental health and retardation agencies have had to devote the bulk of their resources to institutional care" (U.S. General Accounting Office, 1977). A total of $11.0 billion was spent by the states in 1980 for "direct expenditure" on all state hospitals (U.S. Bureau of the Census, 1980). This was 4 percent of the total $258 billion spent by states and one-fourth of all their expenditures for social services and income maintenance. It was almost double the $6.5 billion spent by states on public health activities. Two-thirds, or $6.7 billion of the $11.0 billion spent on state hospitals, was for state mental institutions. Although the states operated in 1980 with an overall surplus of about $19 billion (revenue of $277 billion and expenditures of $258 billion), state hospitals operated with a deficit of $7.5 billion ($11.0 billion in expenditures, partially offset by collection of $3.5 billion in patient charges). While the revenue from patient collections is not broken down by psychiatric and other hospitals, we may be sure that very little of it came fron long-term psychiatric patients. A sample survey by the National Institute of Mental Health (NIMH) in 1975 found[6] that one-third of the admissions constituted "free" patients and the other main sources of payment paid only a part of the cost or charges, either because of the low-income classes included in the "personal pay" category or because of the skimpy coverage of long-term psychiatric reimbursement by public and private insurers.[7] A study by the NIMH on the cost of mental illness had found that in 1971, fully 75 percent of the cost of operating the state mental hospitals was borne by the states (1975). Thus, state inpatient psychiatric care constitutes a large portion of the state-provided direct hospital care financed from state general tax funds. Moreover, in earlier years, going back to 1950, operation of the state psychiatric hospital constituted an even larger proportion of state expenses than it does today.

Owing to its origin as a place to forcibly stow away persons considered deranged, it has typically been understaffed and overcrowded, and treatment of its residents has very often been custodial, characterized by forcible restraint rather than therapy.

In the face of seriously inadequate resources, the dual mission of the state mental hospital, to alleviate the patient's condition and to keep him or her institutionalized, out of harm's way, usually was replaced by the single goal of restraint. The fact tht most patients ("inmates," as they were revealingly called) were poor contributed to this treatment by public authorities.

The first State asylum for the mentally ill in the United States was opened in 1773 [at Williamsburg, Virginia] and from that time the public came to accept isolation of mentally ill persons in large hospitals as the proper way of dealing with metnal illness. And despite the ever-increasing number of people afflicted and the steady advance of potentially useful medical knowledge, the public reliance on custodial isolation endured well into the twentieth century (Connery, 1965).

Although there were periods during which treatment became an important part of the state men-

tal hospital's services, forcible restraint without treatment continued to be widespread. Consequently, the state mental hospital has been the traditional "snake pit" in the public mind, a perception perpetuated by widely read articles and books, including the expository, investigative, advocacy, and fiction genres. (See, for example, Kesey, 1962; Elwood and Hoagberg, 1970).

Efforts to alleviate this situation were made periodically all throughout the 1800s under the leadership of reformers like Dorothea L. Dix and Horace Mann. In 1880 the National Association for the Protection of the Insane and the Prevention of Insanity was organized to help focus attention on the cruelties within the asylums. This organization soon dissolved, but by 1908 the mental hygiene movement in the United States began to make organizational strides forward. Perhaps the leading intellectual impetus given to this movement at that time came from the autobiography of Clifford W. Beers, *A Mind That Found Itself,* in which he detailed his experiences with incarceration in mental institutions and in 1909 the National Committee for Mental Hygiene was organized. While this organization and some individuals worked tirelessly to alleviate conditions in mental hospitals, only very modest gains were made as long as mental patients could be categorically labeled violent and therefore perceived as dangerous by their attendants. This justification was used to keep them under physical restraint for a large part of the time. The obstacles against which the mental hygiene protagnosists fought all those years to ameliorate conditions in mental hospitals inculcated in many of these advocates a deep and abiding antipathy to the institution of the state psychiatric hospital, an emotion that was to become an important factor in post–World War II developments in the mental health movement. When the National Association for Mental Health was formed in 1950 with the same sort of membership that had made up the National Committee for Mental Hygiene in 1909, the newer organization was strongly imbued with a desire to phase out the state mental hospital and replace it with a community-based mental health service system.

Would-be reformers of the treatment of the mentally ill had not always pressed for closing institutions. For many years they pressed for enlarging the number of such facilities and radically altering their treatment of patients. In the 1700s and 1800s the mentally ill had frequently been indiscriminately intermingled with the general class of "paupers" in abominable poorhouses. The initial campaign to separate those who were mentally ill into asylums[8] was motivated by the intention to substitute care, whether ameliorative, curative, or rehabilitative, for the harsh prisonlike conditions of the poorhouse. The initial concept of the asylum was that of a place of refuge and sanctuary,[9] but as the asylums also came to be associated with repressive restraints and little treatment, the reformers began to talk of mental *hospitals* as a better alternative for the mentally ill.

Some asylum directors as far back as the late 1700s had attempted to transform their institutions from custodial facilities based on forcible restraint into places of treatment and healing— that is, to transform them from madhouses into hospitals. One pioneer in this movement, Philippe Pinel, a physician in charge of two "madhouses" in Paris, Bicêtre and Salpêtrière, replaced chains with "moral treatment," seeking to meet the personal needs of patients and to "arouse their dormant faculties for self-care." Similar work was done by Quakers in England under the leadership of William Tuke, who established the York Retreat, where no restraints were used and all patients were treated only with kindness, "plain talk," and "honest efforts to understand and diminish their distress." A few years later, in the early 1800s, similar efforts were made in the United States, where mental hospitals using the principles of "moral treatment" were established by physicians and social reformers. Two such hospitals were the Hartford Retreat and the McClean Hospital, where "patients of independent means were seen daily by the superintending physician (Gruenberg and Archer, 1979). These were private hospitals for patients who could afford them, however, as the expression "patients of independent means" implies.

The early establishment of such institutions as state hospitals—twenty-eight of the then existing thirty-three states established such hospitals in the first half of the 1800s—was seen by many as an advance in the treatment of the mentally ill and is referred to by some as the first psychiatric revolution. This "revolution" attempted to extend moral treatment to the public mental hospital. During the second half of the 1800s the principle that the mentally ill were "wards of the State" promoted by Dorothea Dix and Horace Mann attained wide currency. To implement this precept, it was recommended that state *hospitals* dedicated to "moral treatment" be established. There the mentally ill could be treated humanely instead of being kept restrained in jails, poorhouses, and madhouses, or auctioned off to the lowest bidder for providing room and board. As I have noted, the term "asylum" had by this time become a term of opprobrium; in fact, it was more commonly termed a "madhouse." The hospital, by contrast, was increasingly perceived as the locus of scientific medicine, and science was riding high in public esteem toward the close of the 1800s when all things deemed to be based on science were highly regarded. "[M]edical superintendents were projecting 100 percent cure rates in these institutions and by 1900, 100 new State institutions were built" (Rose, 1979). However, as this principle of accommodating the mentally ill in scientific, treatment-oriented mental hospitals became established in more states, the large number of patients that entered them made mass institutions of them again. The results were that

even the best managed hospitals did not long continue to function as the small, rural, therapeutic retreats that Dix and Mann had envisioned. New asylums were built as older ones overflowed, and the demand for accommodation always seemed to exceed capacity. As chronic cases accumulated and new admissions rose, overcrowding led to a deterioration in the standards of care . . . moral treatment precepts were forgotten and patients' behavior was controlled with physical restraints and seclusion (Gruenberg and Archer, 1979).

Post–World War II efforts to alter this situation were encouraged both by the advent of new psychoactive drugs that altered violent behavior and by strong federal interest, which reached a peak during the Kennedy administration. Some attempts were made to improve the professional component of inpatient services, both qualitatively and quantitatively. Much more prominent, however, was the attempt to establish statewide networks of local community mental health facilities that would emphasize ambulatory care, preventive care, and postdischarge follow-up care. Because it was widely assumed that community-based mental health services would be much less costly than hospital-based ones, the community mental health facilities were expected not only to help the patients but also relieve state budgets by reducing the patient size of the large psychiatric hospitals.

THE STATES AND COMMUNITY MENTAL HEALTH SERVICES

The Federal Mental Health Acts

The National Mental Health Act of 1946 established a Division of Mental Hygiene in the U.S Public Health Service; in 1949 this division became the National Institute of Mental Health (NIMH). The act provided for federal grants to public and private institutions as well as to certain classes of private individuals for research on mental health topics. Public and other non-profit organizations could also receive grants for training, demonstration, and instruction in the field of mental health. With respect to support for mental health services, the 1946 law provided for formula grants to the states allocated on the basis of population size, extent of the mental health problem, and financial need for the development of state mental health services. Public Health Service personnel could be assigned under this act directly to the states and localities to provide technical assistance. The major orientation of Congressional purpose with respect to services may be found in a report of the Senate Committee on Education and Labor, which stated that: "Mental outpatient clinics, conveniently located and offering facilities for early diagnosis and treatment, give every promise of being the most effective means at our disposal for combatting mental disease" (U.S. General Accounting Office, 1977). The money provided for funding *services* was largely for staffing *outpatient* clinics "so persons could be released from institutions and continue to receive mental health care in communities" (U.S.

General Accounting Office, 1977). Connery further clarified this aim:

It is important to recognize that the Federal aid authorized by the Act was not intended to subsidize the operating costs of mental hospitals. Instead, the objective of the legislation was to stimulate a new form of community mental health activity. The desirability of treating mental illness in the patient's normal environment rather than in a mental hospital had been recognized . . . [and] the 1946 Act sought to provide . . . services through a network of outpatient psychiatric clinics.

At the time the Act was passed the problem was that "less than 20 percent of the number of outpatient clinics required . . . are available, and these are concentrated largely in cities having more than 150,000 population and are devoted almost exclusively to child care." The House subcommittee reported that "the nation should have as a minimum one all-purpose psychiatric outpatient clinic for each 100,000 of the population." . . . Testifying before the Senate subcommittee, Dr. Felix[10] stated: "The initial goal is the establishment of 100 clinics during the first full year of the operation of the program proposed in this bill. These would be set up in the areas of the greatest need, based on one clinic for 500,000 population." Congress recognized that most mental hospitals were equipped to provide treatment only for the chronically ill, and even that treatment primarily consisted of custodial care. For that reason, the funds authorized under the Act were not intended to "be used to finance routine bed care in mental hospitals but should be devoted in large measure to further development of existing and new techniques of preventive and treatment methods as well as to training of much-needed personnel" (1965).

Each state was required to designate a "mental health authority" to administer the distribution of the federal mental health grants within the state. This State Mental Health Authority (SMHA) was to be "the State health authority," with the exception of states that had certain pre-existing arrangements. In reporting on the bill, the House committee stated very unambiguously that the mental health authority was not to be a state agency "whose activities in the mental health field are restricted to jurisdiction over mental institutions and their patients." Thus it was clearly the purpose of the act to expand as well as to improve the quality of the mental health services available outside the inpatient facilities of the state mental hospitals. The strong antipathy to supporting almost any care in a state mental hospital was clearly evident.

It is useful to recall the discussion in Chapter 3 on the use of the state health department as a conduit for federal grants to be used for local health services. We note here that the state health ''authority'' was mandated to be the lead agency for handling the federal community mental health funds with the exception of some states. It should also be noted that this act initiated a program intended to develop into locally initiated and controlled mental health services focused on a mental health ''center,'' a term that was to be more carefully defined in later legislation. It was not made clear what was to become of the state mental hospitals, but there were strong indications that many in the mental health movement would have been only too happy to see their demise. The foundations were laid for a dual mental health system consisting of long-term care provided in state mental hospitals predominantly supported by state funds on the one hand, and on the other ambulatory and short-term crisis care, including short stays in acute short-term psychiatric sections of acute general hospitals, provided in local communities and partially supported by federal funds augmented in varying degrees by local and state funds.[11]

After almost ten years of operations under the 1946 Mental Health Act, a Joint Commission on Mental Illness and Health was organized in 1955 under the leadership of the American Psychiatric Association and members of the Council on Mental Health of the American Medical Association to study the needs for mental health care, the modes of treatment of mental illness that were likely to be most effective, and to make recommendations to Congress for action. Financed principally by $1,250,000 appropriated by Congress under the Mental Health Study Act of 1955, the Joint Commission, which ultimately listed thirty-six participating organizations and forty-five individuals as members, issued a report in 1960, *Action for Mental Health*. It recommended the establishment of community-based programs for the mentally ill that would provide expanded outpatient services for prevention and crisis intervention and intensive inpatient treatment for acute mental illness; help improve care in mental hospitals and reduce their size; and provide for community-based aftercare, intermediate care, and rehabilitation services. The Joint Commission also urged a greater federal role in helping state and local governments pay for mental health costs.

The objective of modern treatment of persons with major mental illness is to enable the patient to maintain himself in the community in a normal manner. To do so it is necessary (1) to save the patient from the debilitating effects of institutionalization as much as possible, (2) if the patient requires hospitalization, to return him to home and community life as soon as possible, and (3) thereafter to maintain him in the community as long as possible[12].

Thus, the report recommended continuing and enlarging the efforts to expand community-based treatment made under the 1946 act and developing treatment networks featuring coordination of mental hospitals and community-based services.

Shortly thereafter in 1962, a President's Panel on Mental Retardation issued a substantially parallel report dealing with treatment for mental retardation. Entitled *A Proposed Program for National Action to Combat Mental Retardation*, its main recommendations called for grants to support a program to help the mentally retarded that was similar in many respects to the 1960 recommendations on mental health. The grants would be project grants to state institutions for the retarded to improve services and to hasten the return of residents to local communities where comprehensive program of community-based services would be expanded through federal-state-local cooperative efforts.

[The] report of the Joint Commission on Mental Illness and Health of 1960 led to the ''bold new mental health program'' proposed by John F. Kennedy in a message to Congress in 1963.

The President's message had the revolutionary aim of shifting ''the focus of treatment of the mentally ill from State mental hospitals into community health centers.'' Accepting in principle the objectives of the President's program, Congress passed the *Mental Retardation* Facilities and Community *Mental Health* Centers Construction Act of 1963 [P.L. 88–164]. Thus the means were considered to have been provided [for moving] . . . toward a shift from the warehousing of patients in ''houses of horror'' to treatment in the patient's own community (Connery, 1965). [Emphasis added.]

The Act authorized funds for the construction of community-based mental health centers and facilities for the retarded. The share of the total cost provided by the federal government was 66 percent, with the remainder to come from local or state sources (Ozarin and Feldman, 1971).

It is worth noting that the act combined in one law the provisions for aiding two target populations that were not identical, although there was considerable overlap. This overlap often appeared even greater than it actually was because of misdiagnosis. The retarded and the mentally ill groups had differing needs. The retarded person typically mainly required a protected training and work environment and perhaps also special education and a protected living milieu. The mentally ill, while also frequently requiring specially protected living environments, also needed psychiatric therapy, including drugs in many cases. Reflecting such differences, the supporting constituencies of the two groups were not the same and did not see the problems of their clientele in the same way. The two programs were administered by separate offices in the DHEW, and later renewals of and amendments to the original legislation increasingly treated the two programs in separate acts. This culminated in the Developmental Disabilities Services and Facilities Construction Amendments of 1970, which defined a separate program for the "developmentally disabled" that provided formula grants to the states for services and construction. The mentally retarded program was thenceforth administered as part of the developmentally disabled program under the Developmental Disabilities Office in the offices of Assistant Secretary for Human Development of HEW, while the Community Mental Health Center program continued to be administered under the NIMH in the Office of Assistant Secretary for Health, also in HEW. After 1970, legislation concerning the mentally retarded was often included in legislation dealing with the more inclusive category "developmentally disabled."[13] I shall place much more emphasis in the subsequent discussion on the CMHC than the Developmental Disabilities program, because the former is more directly related to the states' mental hospitals and is more generally (but by no means unanimously) regarded as a health problem with its treatment more akin to medical care than is care of the retarded. Some material on the mental retardation program is

provided because there are similarities between the two programs as well as differences that are instructive to note.

Provisions of the original 1963 act, and of the companion piece of legislation that specifically authorized funds in the 1963 HEW budgets for grants to states for mental health services planning, required each state to demarcate geographic catchment areas and rank them in declining order of need for services. An estimated $4.2 million was disbursed to the states by the National Institute of Mental Health to help finance the work of laying out thest catchment areas for mental health services. Each mental health center was to serve 75,000–200,000 persons, and the minimal types of services a mental health center had to provide to be eligible for federal support were spelled out.[14]

A mental health center did not have to be a single building or group of contiguous buildings in which all the required services were provided. Inpatient acute services, for example, could be provided by arrangement with an appropriate general hospital in the community, and outpatient services could be provided at variously located clinic sites.

The recommendation of the Joint Commission in 1960 that federal aid include funds for upgrading the services in state mental hospitals went unheeded in the act itself. The House Committee on Interstate and Foreign Commerce in its report on the proposed legislation stated that it had purposely chosen to ignore providing funds for state mental hospitals because "a choice has to be made between developing community resources or improving State mental hospitals and that it had chosen the former because new methods of treatment were being developed, the mentally ill were capable of rehabilitation, and there was less inclination to reject and isolate the sufferers" (U.S. General Accounting Office, 1977). Thus it appeared that the advocates of substituting community-based mental health services for mental-hospital-based services had won out as far as the content of the 1946 and especially the 1963 legislation was concerned. It is clear that what was envisioned in the 1963 act was a substitution of one for the other rather than the development of a coordinated system between state mental hospitals and community-based mental health services, with the mental hospital playing an important and perhaps even a central role in the partnership.[15]

The NIMH had, in fact, already initiated a grant program in 1963 to improve services in mental hospitals, to develop more cooperative relationships between hospitals and existing community programs, and to establish precare and aftercare programs, which it claims succeeded in "moving a large number of hospital patients to communities" (U.S. General Accounting Office, 1977). Apparently this activity did not continue for very long, or was of insufficient scope, or was allowed to lapse, because two NIMH task forces or special committees reporting in 1970 and 1971 reported poor coordination between state mental hospitals and community mental health programs in providing proper placement for discharged patients. Much of the situation was clearly attributable to a lack of facilities in the community, but some seems to have been caused by insufficient coordination of resources. Thus the 1963 act solidified the tendencies of the 1946 act to stress community mental health at the expense of state inpatient mental hospital care. The new federal system channelled virtually all federal funds to the community centers and left the mental hospitals to be solely a state responsibility. The funds granted to state mental hospitals noted above were relatively small.

The early experience with the original 1963 act was that acceptable applications for grants to construct new Community Mental Health Centers (CMHCs) came in very slowly, at a rate below the objectives set for the program. The main difficulty seemed to be that the act provided funds for construction only; operating funds were to be raised either by the localities, states, or private organizations, and many states and communities felt that they would not have the resources to underwrite the operating costs of these centers after they were built. This was especially true in the areas that needed them most. The Mental Retardation Facilities and Community Mental Health Centers Construction Act Amendments of 1965 filled this gap by providing Federal funding for staffing new community mental health centers. The grants would cover 75 percent of the staffing cost in the first fifteen months of operation and declining percentages subsequently, down to a low of 30 percent. After

fifty-one months, no further federal staffing money would be available. By that time the localities, sponsoring private organizations, and the states were to have arranged to provide for the full cost of operating the centers. (Similar staffing funds for community facilities for the retarded was not provided until 1967.)

Two other mental health expense items that were not granted federal support by the original 1963 legislation were also provided for in 1965: help in defraying the living and support services costs of patients discharged from mental hospitals to live in the community and some help to the states for improving service in state mental hospitals for patients who needed to remain there.

In addition to the particularly strong necessity for staffing grants to CMHCs in low-income areas, it was also found that the financial strain of meeting the requirement that all five mandatory "essential elements" of service be available immediately upon opening was impeding the development of centers. These requirements had been modified by 1971 to allow temporary exceptions permitting new centers to open and operate for the first eighteen months with only three of the mandatory five services in place (see note 14). In some states, a State Community Mental Health Act provided a substantial portion of the local operating costs. For example, in California and Pennsylvania, state matching of federal funds was authorized up to 90 percent.

By June 30, 1971, 452 centers had been funded, with 300 being operational. Nearly three-fourths of these centers included short-term psychiatric beds in general hospitals, with about half the grantees being public and half private agencies (Ozarin and Feldman, 1971). By 1973, 400 were operational, 36 of them in California, by far the largest number in any state. The Community Mental Health Centers Act of 1970 liberalized the 1965 provisions for help to low-income areas by extending federal staffing support to cover an eight-year period, providing specially high ratios of construction costs, and raising staffing support ratios to start at 90 percent and end with 70 percent for the last three years, in these areas. High federal funding participation levels were also authorized for services to alcoholics, narcotics users, and children. The 1974 federal budget of the Nixon administration proposed discontinuance of further federal grants for construction of additional mental health centers, but the struggle with Congress (described in Chap. 4) resulted in restoration of this item. In 1980 there were 691 federally funded community health centers (Redick, Witkin, Bethel, & Manderssheid, 1985).

Effect of the Community Mental Health Centers Act on the State Mental Hospitals and the States' Finances

Patient censuses in state mental hospitals had begun to decline even before the passage of the 1963 act. The national average daily census fell steadily after 1955, the year when it reached its peak of 558,900. It had dropped to about 132,000 by 1980 and 115,000 by 1985 (Sunshine et al., 1990). That the drop in census of the state mental hospitals represented a shift in locus of treatment for mental illness rather than an absolute drop in incidence of mental illness "episodes" is shown by the data in Table 6–2 and Figure 6–1, which depict the change in the relative distribution of the locus of mental health therapy between inpatient and outpatient sites during the years 1955–1986. Table 6–2 lists the significant changes that occurred over this period.

1. The total number of episodes of care[16] had increased almost four and one-half times (from 1.7 million in 1955 to 6.4 million in 1981). Part of this increase was due to population increase, as the episode rate per 100,000 population increased less than threefold (from 1,028 to 2,810). The number of patient-care episodes in outpatient psychiatric services, however, increased more than nine times. NIMH publications point to the increase in episodes (which include readmissions) as evidence of the increase in the active quality of therapy achieved under the program over the years. The notion of active therapy is particularly pertinent for persons suffering from chronic mental illness that fluctuates between periods of remission and bouts of illness. The aim is to allow the patient to live in the least restrictive environment in which he or she can manage but to have appropriate impatient care available at

all times in case of a recurrence. Many NIMH statistics have been couched in terms of "patient movement."

2. Patient-care episodes in inpatient services, which accounted for over three-quarters of the total episodes in 1955, made up only 27 percent of the total in 1981. Outpatient mental health services, on the other hand, accounted for the largest proportion of patient care episodes—69 percent in 1981 compared with only 23 percent in 1955.

3. The number of patient-care episodes in nonfederal *general* hospital inpatient psychiatric units rose two and a half times from 1955 to 1981. This is considered to be a good trend because psychiatric care in nonfederal community hospitals is assumed to generally consist of active, relatively short term therapy.

4. Inpatient episodes in state (and county) mental hospitals, which accounted for almost half of the patient care episodes in 1955, accounted for only 8 percent of the yearly episodes in 1981.

5. By 1977, federally assisted community mental health centers were handling 38 percent of all outpatient episodes, and half of the increase in outpatient episodes from 1965 to 1977 was accounted for by the Community Mental Health Centers. After 1980, this category of statistics was discontinued by NIMH[17] and most of the services given in these centers are included in the new typology under "multiservice mental health organizations." In 1986, 53 percent of the total outpatient episodes were served by these organizations (Redick et al., 1990).

It is clear, therefore, that use of mental health therapeutic services greatly increased between 1955 and 1981, and that even before the proliferation of the federally Assisted Community Mental Health Centers the increase already was all in outpatient services and *acute* inpatient care in general hospitals. The effect of the activities of the mental health movement's advocacy and the funds of the 1946 Mental Health Act were already apparent by 1965. The further effects of the 1963 act became evident after 1965 when the trend toward outpatient community-based service, especially in the community mental health centers, accelerated, as did the decline in the census of state mental hospitals. The year-end census of psychiatric patients in the *general acute* hospital also continued to increase after 1965. Thus, the data unequivocally support the fact that, as a result of postwar legislation, deinstitutionalization of psychotherapeutic treatment from the state mental hospital occurred during these years. Some of it may have represented patients actually transferred to outpatient treatment and some to psychiatric inpatient services in acute hospitals, but how much cannot be confidently inferred from these data. Given the lack of a well-developed system for tracking discharges from state mental hospitals over these years, we do not know definitively how much of the increased ambulatory and acute hospital inpatient use consisted of former state mental hospital patients.[18] Nor do we know explicitly what proportion of the increased ambulatory use of community mental health centers served to prevent state mental hospital episodes.

Another factor in reducing both the percent occupancy and the year-end census in state mental hospitals was the Hill-Burton hospital construction program, initiated in 1946. This federal program granted money for hospital construction, and "by mid-1965, 19,295 beds had been added to mental hospitals; and another 10,020 beds for psychiatric patients had been added to general hospitals" (Connery, 1965). The latter helped to promote the trend toward an increased number of psychiatric hospitalizations being handled by general hospitals, but most of this effect was already observed before the effects of the Community Mental Health Act could take hold. (Inpatient episodes in nonfederal general hospitals increased by 95 percent from 1955 to 1965; they increased only 30 percent between 1965 and 1981. See Table 6–2). Also contributing to these trends were special demonstration grants by NIMH to encourage this development.

The failure to include any substantial help for state mental hospitals in the 1963 act had been defended by some on the grounds that the community mental health centers would reduce the burden on state inpatient psychiatric services, thereby creating savings for the state. These savings could then be applied to upgrading the services for the remaining irreducible core of patients who really needed inpatient services, or, at the state's option, they might be applied to

help fund the operating expenditures of the community mental health centers within the state. Also, the voluntary participation of many of the states, especially some of the large ones like California and Pennsylvania (p. 193) in financing operating costs and other forms of support for the Federally Assisted Community Mental Health Centers was partially based on expectation of such savings. But many states soon found themselves faced with surprisingly steep rises in community mental health expenditures as well as accelerating outlays for mental hospital care. Containing costs of mental health services became an increasingly pressing problem for state governments. The federal government was funding the operation of the community mental health centers in large part but the burden of funding the mental hospitals continued to fall largely on the states alone. Furthermore, hospitalization of persons with serious mental illness has always appeared more politically urgent than supporting ambulatory care for many persons seen as only "neurotic." The outcome was a foregone conclusion. All mental health care was inadequately funded by the states, and what support there was went preponderantly for state mental hospital care.

A study sponsored by the NIMH, *The Cost of Mental Illness—1971* (1975), estimated that $13.5 billion was spent "due to" mental illness in 1971. Of this, $9.5 billion was for "direct care."[19] Almost one-fourth (22.7 percent) of all direct-care expenditures was represented by the $2.2 billion spent on state and county mental hospitals. This compares with only $928 million spent on services in community mental health centers. Most important, 75 percent of the cost of mental hospital operation was borne by the state (and, in the case of a few county mental hospitals, some local) governments. It is true that financing care in state mental hospitals was assisted by the Medicare and Medicaid programs, enacted in 1965, which provided some reimbursement for patients in mental hospitals and nursing homes (see Chapter 10), but in 1971 the federal government, principally through Medicaid, paid for only 10.5 percent of the cost of state and county mental hospitals; self-pay and insurance payments, including private insurance and Medicare, met only 14.6 percent of the cost. This last figure clearly indicates how

Table 6–2. Number, Percent Distribution, and Rate per 100,000 Population of Inpatient, Outpatient, and Partial-care episodes in Mental Health Organizations, Selected Years, 1955–1986[a]

Year	Total episodes, all mental health organizations	Inpatient Care Episodes, by Type of Organization								Total outpatient care episodes[d,e]	Total partial care episodes[d,f]
		Total	State and county mental hospitals	Private psychiatric hospitals	VA medical centers	Nonfederal general hospitals with separate psychiatric services	Federally funded community mental health centers (CMHCs)	RTCs[b] for emotionally disturbed children	Multiservice mental health organizations[c]		
						Number of episodes (in thousands)					
1986	7,460.9	2,055.7	445.2	258.3	203.9	883.1	(g)	47.2	218.0	5,041.1	364.1
1983	6,926.1	1,900.3	499.2	180.8	170.5	820.0	(g)	32.5	197.3	4,718.0	307.8
1981	6,400.8	1,720.4	499.2	176.5	205.6	676.9	(g)	34.4	127.8	4,441.1	239.3
1977	6,639.2	1,846.1	574.2	150.7	217.5	571.7	269.0	33.5	29.5	4,576.4	216.7
1975	6,648.5	1,817.1	599.0	137.0	214.3	565.7	246.9	28.3	25.9	4,618.3	213.1
1971	4,190.9	1,755.8	745.3	98.0	176.8	542.6	130.1	28.6	34.4	2,316.8	118.3
1969	3,682.4	1,710.3	767.1	102.5	186.9	535.5	65.0	21.3	32.0	1,894.5	77.6
1965	2,636.4	1,565.4	804.9	125.4	115.8	519.3	—	—	—	1,071.0	—
1955	1,675.3	1,296.3	818.8	123.2	88.4	265.9	—	—	—	379.0	—
						Percent distribution of episodes					
1986	100.0	27.6	6.0	3.5	2.7	11.8	(g)	0.6	2.9	67.6	4.9
1983	100.0	27.4	7.2	2.6	2.5	11.8	(g)	0.5	2.8	68.1	4.5
1981	100.0	26.9	7.8	2.8	3.2	10.6	(g)	0.5	2.0	69.4	3.7
1977	100.0	27.8	8.6	2.3	3.3	8.6	4.1	0.5	0.4	68.9	3.3
1975	100.0	27.3	9.0	2.1	3.2	8/5	3.7	0.4	0.4	69.5	3.2
1971	100.0	41.9	17.8	2.3	4.2	12.9	3.1	0.7	0.8	55.3	2.8
1969	100.0	46.4	20.8	2.8	5.1	14.5	1.8	0.6	0.9	51.4	2.1

Year										
1965	100.0	59.4	30.5	4.8	4.4	19.7	—	—	—	40.6	—
1955	100.0	77.4	48.9	7.4	5.3	5.3	15.9	—	—	22.6	—

Number of episodes per 100,000 civilian population

Year										
1986	3,117	859	186	108	85	369	—	20	91	2,106	152
1983	2,952	799	198	78	73	351	—	14	85	2,021	132
1981	2,810	754	219	77	90	297	—	15	56	1,951	105
1977	3,079	857	266	70	101	265	125	16	14	2,122	100
1975	3,145	859	283	65	101	268	117	13	12	2,185	101
1971	2,053	861	365	48	87	266	64	14	17	1,134	58
1969	1,853	861	386	52	94	269	33	11	16	953	39
1965	1,375	816	420	65	60	271	—	—	—	559	—
1955	1,028	795	502	76	54	163	—	—	—	233	—

Source: Adapted from Redick, et al., 1990. Further detail on the definitions given in the Notes below are available in the Appendix of the same reference.

aSee note 16.

bResidential treatment center for disturbed children.

cA mental health organization that provides two or more types of services. In 1986, 86 percent of the episodes in this category were outpatient and are included only in the outpatient total on this table. See also note g below.

dExcludes episodes in VA programs for comparability with earlier years.

eIn 1986 total outpatient episodes were distributed as follows: multiservice mental health organizations, 53 percent; nonfederal general hospital psychiatric service, 17 percent; psychiatric outpatient clinics, 14 percent and the remaining 16 percent was distributed among four other categories.

f"A planned program of mental health treatment services generally provided to groups" in sessions of 3 or more hours.

gWhen the CMHC federal grants were converted to block grants in 1981 the mental health centers supported under the community health centers act were reclassified in NMHI records. The preponderance was thenceforth classified as multiservice mental health organizations and the rest were added to other classifications of mental health organizations.

(—)Data not reported.

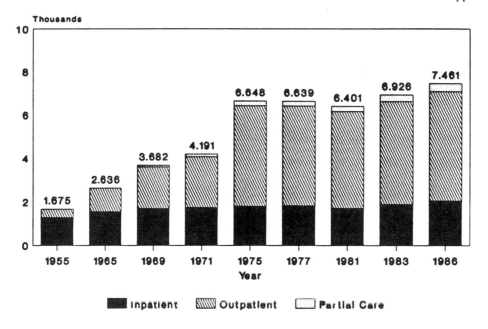

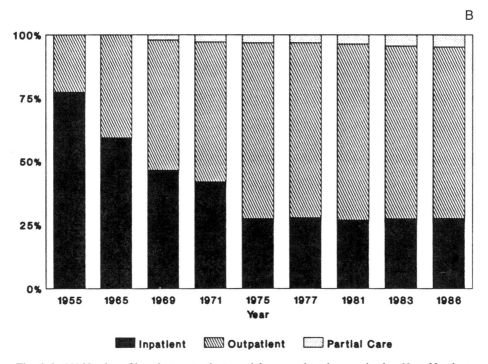

Fig. 6–1. (A) Number of inpatient, outpatient, partial care, and total care episodes. *Note*: Numbers on top represent total episodes (in millions). (B) Percentage distribution of inpatient, outpatient, and partial care. *Source*: Table 6–2.

198

small a percentage of the total cost of operating state mental hospitals was met by self-pay, privately insured, and Medicare patients combined.[20]

Looking at Table 6–3, we see that the operating expenses of state mental hospitals rose steadily between 1967 and 1977. If we adjust for inflation they rose more slowly and erratically, but they still increased 16 percent in constant 1967 dollars over these years[21]. However, during this period the year-end census dropped from 438,600 to 177,800, so that the average daily cost per patient, adjusted for inflation, rose more than threefold—from $8.84 per day in 1967 to $27.90 in 1977. Thus, the annual expenditures for operating state mental hospitals did not diminish in current or constant dollars, while the average inflation-adjusted amount spent per patient per day rose sharply with the overwhelmingly preponderant portion of the financial burden still being borne by the states. Furthermore, when one adds the states' share of the costs of the Community Mental Health Centers program, the states' share of the costs of Medicaid payments to nursing homes, and their contributions to other community programs, it is most likely that the states were paying more for mental health than they had before the implementation of deinstitutionalization, even after adjusting for inflation. It should be noted, however, that the steady rise in the real average daily

outlay per resident patient is consistent with the hypothesis that the care of the remaining inpatients has been improving.

However, some studies of possible "savings" from deinstitutionalization, cited in U.S. General Accounting Office, 1977 and Rose, 1979, were estimating that net savings of between $20,800 and $39,400 per person over ten years could be achieved by states for each patient served in community-based facilities, as opposed to state mental hospital care. These studies concluded that much of this estimated saving was not in total lower costs of care but due to *cost shifting* to the federal government. Formulations of this type only helped to whet the appetite of fiscally harried state officials for massive, and perhaps some indiscriminate, deinstitutionalization. Community-based treatment was stressed as more economical, and possible problems with it were ignored. For example, community-based facilities may not be adequate for many mental patients; *good* community facilities are not really cheap; and relying on cost shifting to the federal government may be poor long-term strategy. The ultimate questions therefore remained unanswered: How many and what kind of patients belonged in the mental hospital, and were there many such persons in the community who should be in hospitals? How many patients discharged from mental hospitals as needing only community-

Table 6–3. Maintenance[a] Expenditures and Daily Maintenance Expenditures per Resident Patient in State and County Mental Hospitals in Current and Constant Dollars: 1967–1977 and 1986

Fiscal year	Price deflator[b]	Maintenance expenditures			
		Annual amount		Daily per resident patient	
		Current dollars	Constant dollars		
		(in millions)		Current dollars	Constant dollars
1967	100.0	1,415	1,415	8.84	8.84
1968	106.1	1,578	1,487	10.47	9.87
1969	113.4	1,739	1,534	12.59	11.10
1970	120.6	1,890	1,567	14.89	12.35
1971	128.4	2,036	1,586	17.59	13.70
1972	132.5	2,146	1,620	20.68	15.61
1973	137.7	2,326	1,689	25.20	18.30
1974	150.5	2,479	1,647	30.86	20.50
1975	168.6	2,641	1,566	37.54	22.27
1976	184.7	3,141	1,701	43.55	23.58
1977	202.4	3,329	1,645	56.47	27.90
1986	433.5	6,326	1,459	155.25	35.81

Source: HEW, various issues (445, various cases): For 1986, NIMH, 1979.

[a]Maintenance expenditures are total expenditures less capital expenditures.

[b]Medical care component of the consumer price index, 1967=100.

based care were receiving such care? What kind of persons were the Community Mental Health Centers serving?

The Deinstitutionalization Program[22]

The Development of the Program

When the Mental Retardation Facilities and Community Mental Health Centers Construction Act was passed in 1963, the proposed Community Mental Health Centers were envisioned as the instrumentality for meeting the needs of discharged state mental hospital patients as well as those of future mentally disabled persons, many of whom would be spared the experience of a protracted stay in the mental hospital altogether. These centers would meet mental health needs through ambulatory therapy with social work supervision and monitoring of residents' living conditions in community facilities such as foster homes, apartments, halfway houses, and small group residences. Acute recurrences would be treated by crisis intervention centers with hospitalization available in the psychiatric services of short-term acute-care hospitals or in partial (day- or night-only) hospitalization facilities. If relapses requiring periods of longer-term care occurred, the CMHC would work in concert with the state mental hospital to arrange an appropriate mental hospital stay of as short a duration as possible. The initiation of the program would be federally sponsored, with state participation in varying degrees.

As the program developed, it soon became clear that many, perhaps most, of the discharged patients needed both financial support and help with making their living arrangements (''social support services'') if they were to be in a position to benefit from the therapeutic mental health services of the CMHC. Furthermore, a good many discharged patients needed little more than financial and social-service support, their degree of mental illness being slight or even nonexistent. This was especially true of persons who were found to be mentally retarded but who had been misdiagnosed as mentally ill, leading to a growing awareness of policymakers that the mental health program and the mental retardation program would need to be separately considered. In recognition of these factors a number

of federal laws were passed designed to provide such support for discharged patients and to differentiate the mental health from the mental retardation program. In addition, some of these acts provided limited financial help to states to care for some of their mental hospital patients in alternative facilities in the hope that this would release state money for financing improvements in community-based mental health services. This type of financial aid was not always legislated as amendments to the mental health center legislation but often appeared as sections of laws on various other subjects, as is frequently the case in United Stated federal legislative policy formation. In order to see more clearly what provisions for financial and social services were made for the mentally ill (and mentally retarded), it is necessary to pull together those that became part of the Community Mental Health Center Act by amendment and those that were passed as part of other legislation. They included:

1. Portions of the Medicare and Medicaid programs[23] enacted in 1965. Medicare, which provided federally sponsored health insurance for persons over sixty-five, provided for inpatient coverage for the elderly mentally ill in general acute hospitals on the same basis as any other illness. A limited number of inpatient days and outpatient visits in mental hospitals were also covered. Medicaid was a federally initiated and supervised program that paid for the medical care of certain classes of poor persons. Its financing was shared by the federal government and the states, and it was administered by the individual states under federally promulgated guidelines and regulations. Medicaid covered mental health care for nonelderly eligible poor persons, but only in *general* hospitals, both for inpatient and outpatient care, as well as for eligible elderly persons in mental hospitals. Although this latter benefit was optional with the states, in 1975 forty-two States included these services in their Medicaid programs. Thus the Medicare and Medicaid laws provided for inpatient mental hospital benefits for some of the mentally ill, hoping

to encourage States to discharge [from the mental hospital] the elderly who with *financial assistance and support services* [emphasis added] were able to care for themselves in the community. It was intended that the Federal assistance for the institutionalized mentally ill would enable the States to shift their funds to developing alternatives to care in mental hospitals and to improve the care provided in such facilities to help persons return to communities (Rose, 1979).

It is particularly important to note that the Medicaid program became a principal source of financing long-term care in nursing homes, because these institutions were where many persons discharged from state mental institutions landed. The Medicaid Act was laced with requirements intended to make states use the newly freed-up state funds both to improve inpatient care for those patients needing a continued stay in the mental hospital and to develop the community mental health system. For example, it was required that each inpatient have his or her continuing need for remaining in the mental hospital evaluated periodically; that mental health and welfare agencies actively work to develop and use alternatives to inpatient care; and that "maintenance of effort" be demonstrated by the states—that is, that the states use the funds freed up by the new federal funds for additional mental health services and not as substitute financing for the same services that they had been financing with their own funds.

2. In 1965, federal grants were voted to the states for state-operated and -supported schools for the handicapped, including those in public institutions for the mentally disabled. These grants helped to support the public institutions for the mentally retarded. It was hoped that this would discourage the practice of placing them in the mental hospital.

3. The 1965 amendments to the Vocational Rehabilitation Act provided for construction of community residences for retarded persons receiving vocational rehabilitation services in workshops that developed job skills.

4. The Comprehensive Health Planning and Public Health Services Amendments of 1966 required that at least 15 percent of the "314d" state formula grant money be used for community mental health services (not for mental hospitals). (The 1967 amendments to the 1966 act lowered the percentage required to be used for community mental health to 10.5 percent beginning with 1969.) (See Chapter 4).

5. In 1967, the act was amended to authorize special grants for initial staffing of community mental retardation facilities over a period of fifty-one months, and in 1968 the Vocational Rehabilitation Act was amended to provide project grants earmarked for rehabilitating the mentally retarded.

6. The 1972 amendments to the Social Security Act created a new category of institution eligible for reimbursement under Medicaid—the intermediate-care facility (ICF). Its purpose was to provide financial and social support services for persons needing inpatient care but not requiring intensive skilled nursing care. Public institutions for the mentally retarded were made eligible for reimbursement under this category but institutions specializing in care of the mentally ill were excluded (for persons under sixty-five). This was a further instance of the developing federal policy that perceived the mentally retarded program as essentially not being medically oriented while the mental health program was.

7. The Housing and Urban Development Act of 1970 required the Department of Housing and Urban Development (HUD) to encourage the development of residential settings specially designed for elderly and handicapped persons who could maintain independent (noninstitutional) living if provided such special setting and some support services.

8. For some time before 1975 the federal government had been reimbursing 75 percent of the states' costs for providing social services to the four[24] categories of persons eligible for federal "welfare" (i.e., cash assistance). This was provided under Titles IVA and VI of the Social Security Act[25] and was intended to help needy persons "attain or retain capability for self-support, self-care, and reduced dependency in the community and to remain in or return to communities" (U.S. General Accounting Office, 1977). Since many retarded (and the other developmentally) disabled persons were eligible for "welfare" cash assistance under the "disabled" welfare category, these titles were used by the states to help provide social support services as well as financial assistance for discharges of state mental hospitals and for persons who could avoid going to a state institution altogether as long as an appropriate type of shel-

tered living was available. Services included day care, arranging for and supervising foster care, protective services, services in halfway houses, and activity centers. These two Social Security Act titles were replaced in 1975 by a weaker Title XX, which allowed states greater freedom to relax the requirements on the standards for social service providers as well as to restrict eligibility to clients below specified income limits. Despite this lowering of standards, the appurtenant regulations clearly indicated that Title XX was intended to further deinstitutionalization. The services were to be directed toward achieving one of its five specified goals, "preventing or reducing inappropriate institutional care by providing community-based care, home care, or other less intensive care." Another of its goals, "securing referral or admission for institutional care when other care is not appropriate or providing services to individuals in institutions" (U.S. General Accounting Office, 1977) was scarcely addressed, but it is noteworthy that while Title XX still plainly identified noninstitutional care as the modality of choice, it now also recognized that for some persons institutional care was the appropriate modality and called for upgrading the social services provided to persons in institutions as well as in the community.

9. The Health Services and Nurse Training Act of 1975 (P.L. 94–63) amended the Community Mental Health Centers Act further by requiring federally funded centers to provide, in addition to the first five required services, screening, follow-up care, and transitional services in order to strengthen the implementation of the deinstitutionalization program.

Progress in bettering the care of the mentally disabled was also aided by a series of court decisions[26] in the 1970s establishing the proposition that mentally disabled persons had a constitutional right to treatment in the least restrictive setting necessary and that minimal standards of living conditions must be maintained for the mentally disabled, including avoidance of overcrowding. These decisions helped pave the way for advocacy groups, including branches of the federal legal aid program, to use the courts for obtaining more humane and therapeutically active treatment in the state mental hospitals and better conditions in

institutions for the mentally retarded as well as better and more adequate community-based facilities for caring for patients who did not need to remain in other institutions.

By 1975 then, federal legislative policy was directed toward encouraging states to improve both their noninstitutional and institutional care for the mentally disabled, to sharpen their discriminating power for placing them in the most appropriate setting, and to develop a coordinated system of state institutions and community-based services that referred persons back and forth as needed. In this formulation, evidenced further in other legislation discussed below, we see the beginnings of a modification of the single-minded deinstitutionalization spirit that informed the original 1963 act and the early years of its administration. In those years the idea was often put forth that almost anything was better than a state mental hospital (or a state institution for the retarded) and that it might be a reasonable goal to close them all down as rapidly as possible. Portions of President Kennedy's message to Congress in 1963 on the CMHCs implied this by suggesting that the state mental institutions could, if improved, at best "perform a valuable transitional role" (Gruenberg and Archer, 1979). The emergency federal policy, modified largely because of the experience with implementing the program, was that both long-term institutional and other kinds of care were needed. These objectives implied a good follow-up system that kept track of individuals and their progress and that made plans for their future care, keeping clients' needs in mind and meshing them with the appropriate and available services. Other acts, also passed in 1975[27], further advanced this goal by requiring that states receiving grants plan and work toward eliminating inappropriate placement of mentally disabled persons in institutions, improving institutional services for those who needed them, and ensuring the availability of appropriate community services.

Thus, a panoply of Federal programs was brought into existence incrementally to aid in properly implementing deinstitutionalization and to steer it in the direction of providing community-based services only for those clients for whom they were appropriate rather than encouraging an overly precipitous and indiscriminate emptying of the state institutions. Although it largely financed these programs and drew up their regulations, the federal government attempted to have the states, principally through the state mental health authorities, coordinate and monitor the local operation of the programs. A problem that developed with the administration of the programs was that responsibility for them was lodged in different federal agencies, some of which were even in different cabinet departments. Getting so many more or less disparate government entities to work as a coordinated system for providing coordinated care to the mentally disabled was a formidable task. By 1975 coordination of services had been only poorly accomplished (U.S. General Accounting Office, 1977), reflecting the difficulties encountered in attempting to change course from one that originally promoted the establishment of two independent systems—the state mental hospitals and the community mental health centers—to one that would promote integration of the two into a single coordinated system.

In the political battle over the direction to be taken by the original act, the protagonists of the two systems saw themselves as ideological adversaries. The CMHC advocates, particularly, would have nothing to do with the state mental hospitals, which they viewed as abominations and barriers to progress in mental health care. Transforming the goal from creating a fragmented dual system to creating a coordinated one came about slowly through a series of patches applied incrementally as weak spots surfaced. Each patch was an attempt to correct one or more of the remaining weaknesses that came to light in the deinstitutionalization program, but some of these attempts at repair produced new problems.

Prominent among these was the nursing home care made available by Medicaid (see points 1 and 6, above). The change in distribution of mentally ill persons in selected long-term institutions during the first few years of operation under the 1963 Mental Health Act, shown in Table 6–4, is illuminating. In 1969, there were 852,000 persons with mental disorders residing in long-term facilities, a 7 percent increase over the 1963 census count of 794,000. However, the state (and county) mental hospital census had dropped from 505,000 to 370,000, a 27 percent

reduction, while the main increase was in the census of nursing home residents, which in 1963 had held 28 percent of the patients but in 1969 accounted for fully 50 percent of them. In contrast, in 1963 64 percent of the long-term mental patients were in state mental hospitals but by 1969 only 44 percent were. The drop of 35,000 in the number of patients in state hospitals was more than compensated for by an increase of 146,000 in the census of nursing homes. Thus, at least in the early days of the CMHC program, the deinstitutionalization from the state mental hospital seems to have been largely to the nursing home, that is, from one long-term institution to another; the total number of residents in all long-term facilities did not fall.

There were strong financial incentives for the states to discharge mental hospital patients to nursing homes even if some of them they should have remained in the mental hospital. In the mental hospital the state usually paid the entire cost; in the nursing home the federal government contributed from 50 to about 80 percent of the cost under Medicaid. But nursing homes were not suitable places for many discharged patients. Nearly all the activities and quality standards were based on patients whose main disability was physical; mentally retarded patients, especially, did not need a medically oriented setting so much as they needed social support services, special education, and training. As noted in point 6, above, the 1972 amendments to the Social Security Act tried to patch up this weak spot in the deinstitutionalization program by making the mentally disabled eligible for federal payments in ICFs, homes with minimal medical orientation. The intent presumably was for persons in ICFs who needed mental health services to have access to them through a CMHC. The incentive for states to move patients from the state mental hospital to the ICF, where the federal government would participate in paying for their stays, remained. It was an incentive to close mental hospitals or otherwise discharge patients who needed long-term intensive mental health care to the minimal-care ICFs where at best the often inadequate therapy offered by a CMHC would be available.

A General Accounting Office report of 1977 found that by 1975 it was still true that many persons released from mental hospitals (and in-

Table 6-4. Number and Percent Distribution of Patients with Mental Disorders in Selected Long-term Institutions by Age, 1963 and 1969

Institutions	Number (in thousands)						Percent					
	1963			1969			1963			1969		
	Under 65	65+	Total	Under 65	65+	Total	Under 65	65+	Total	Under 65	65+	Total
State & county mental hospitals	356	149	505	259	111	370	81.3	41.9	63.6	71.8	22.7	43.5
Private mental hospitals	7	3	10	9	2	11	1.6	0.9	1.3	2.4	0.5	1.3
VA hospitals	41	16	57	34	10	44	9.3	4.5	7.1	9.4	2.0	5.1
Nursing homes	34	188	222	59	368	427	7.8	52.7	28.0	16.4	74.8	50.1
Total	438	356	794	361	491	852	100.0	100.0	100.0	100.0	100.0	100.0

Source: Redick, R. W. Patterns in Use of Nursing Homes by the Aged Mentally Ill, Dept. of HEW, Public Health Service, Alcohol, Drug Abuse, and Mental Health Administration, National Institute of Mental Health, Rockville, 1974, Table 2.

stitutions for the retarded) were being placed in nursing homes. While the GAO found that full information on the number of mentally disabled persons in nursing homes who were released from public institutions was lacking, available evidence suggested that "substantial numbers" were being placed in nursing homes and that apparently more mentally ill persons were in nursing homes than in public mental hospitals, as had been the case in 1969 (as shown in Table 6–4). The GAO noted that:

According to National Institute of Mental Health (NIMH) estimates, nursing homes are the largest single place of care for the mentally ill. They represent 29.3 percent, or $4.2 billion, of the estimated total direct care costs for the mentally ill of $14.5 billion in 1974. In contrast, State, county and other public mental hospitals accounted for 22.8 percent of the total direct care costs.

In addition, nursing homes housed about 2,350, or 26 percent, of the more than 9,000 mentally retarded persons released from 115 public institutions in 1974 . . . (1977).

Although it was a weakness of this report that it did not contain more detail on whether the mentally ill persons in the nursing homes in 1975 were under the therapeutic care of CMCHs,[28] still, transfer to nursing homes was not what had been meant by the deinstitutionalization advocates when they had called for discharge into the community. They had envisioned the discharged persons living alone, with families, or in small residential centers, not living in nursing homes, many very large and generally "without provision being made for needed services."

Although considerable controversy arose over the quality of the care in nursing facilities for mentally disabled patients, some other alternatives to long-term hospitalization came under even stronger criticism. Developments in California illustrate a set of problems that arose in connection with one of these—the board and care home. Critics cited it as yet another result of overly precipitous discharge of patients from state mental hospitals to inadequately funded local programs. Many of these patients were placed in privately owned board and care homes. The care in these homes was reimbursed by the state but monitored by the counties. Their adequacy was hotly debated among public officials,

with most articles being sharply critical and presented as exposés (Los Angeles Times, May 13, 1972). Between 1965 and 1972, as the state mental hospital census in California dropped from 30,000 to 8,000, newspaper features stories described appalling conditions in these board and care homes. In this period two state mental hospitals were closed, two partially closed, and two were expected to close shortly.[29] One writer stated in 1972:

There is still a lack of effective alternatives to hospitalization, and many who are kept out of hospitals get *no* service. . . . Patients are entering the revolving doors between the community and the hospitals faster and faster. It is often difficult to see what the patients get from this. There is far too little evidence to date that keeping people out of hospitals *without* providing alternative services is free enough of disadvantage to justify it (Schwartz, 1972).

Controversy over whether "deinstitutionalization" of patients from mental hospitals was too rapid went on for many years with mental health professionals, publicists, political activists, government officials, and consumer groups lined up on one or another side of the issue. Most of the writings and speeches argued that deinstitutionalization had been too drastic and therefore on the whole harmful to the cause of mental health. Many contended that the main motive was to save money for the states rather than to serve the well-being of the patients. The inadequacy of the federal financial commitment to the operation of community mental health, many cities alleged, virtually preordained that the deinstitutionalization programs would have serious shortcomings. Writing in January 1971, Raymond M. Glasscote, Chief of the Joint Information Service of the American Psychiatric Association and the National Association for Mental Health, after noting the positive accomplishments of the 1963 act, such as the declining state hospital census, mental health centers brought closer to poor people, the use of "new" social modalities of treatment in some centers, and the development of new categories of psychiatric therapeutic personnel, went on to conclude:

Clinically, the picture is promising. Financially, it is not. The Federal contribution—only about $350 million over a six-year period—is, in aggregate, considerably smaller than the annual budget of the New York Department of Mental Hygiene. The prospects for the future are dismal.

The inadequate federal contribution to the cost of operating the Community Mental Health Centers stemmed from the orientation of the original act toward construction, with only partial contributions toward operations limited to the first few years after opening. In 1971 federal grants to the 295 federally funded Community Mental Health Centers totaled $103 million, which was only 34 percent of the centers' total income; state funds contributed $87 million, or 29 percent; and local government contributed $26 million, or 9 percent. Most, but not all, of the $103 million federal funds, $83 million, was for staffing (NIMH, August 1973).

Two years after the 1977 General Accounting Office (GAO) report to Congress of its investigation into the progress of the deinstitutionalization policy, the journal *Milbank Memorial Fund Quarterly/Health and Society* published a special issue devoted to arguments on the pros and cons of the deinstitutionalization. All the articles agreed that sufficient provision for community-based services for patients discharged from state mental hospitals (and state institutions for the retarded) had not been made. There was less agreement over the causes and extent of these inadequacies, as well as what remedies were appropriate.

Appraising the Outcomes of Deinstitutionalization

By 1977 it was evident that much had been done since 1963 to deinstitutionalize patients from state mental hospitals and institutions for the retarded. This included efforts to encourage construction of appropriate community mental health facilities and to provide living income and social services support. It was also evident that what had been done was not enough and had been put in place by a crazy quilt of patchwork legislation. How should the program be evaluated? Had it been, on the whole, successful, or should it more appropriately be judged a failure? Were its shortcomings due merely to lack of resources and administrative coordination, or were they symptomatic of basic misconceptions upon

which the program was based? Not surprisingly, the answers to these questions were seen differently by persons with different viewpoints about what mental health services should do and whom they should serve.

Three different views on deinstitutionalization are discernible in articles appearing in the special issue of the Milbank Journal (1979, no. 4). The first, that of G. J. Clarke (1979), and by far the most commonly expressed view in the professional literature of the day, was that the aims and principles of the deinstitutionalization program implied by the 1963 Community Mental Health Centers Act were correct. The relatively isolated state long-term mental hospital was no place to treat anybody and it was time to replace it by a network of community-based services. The program's weaknesses lay only in the implementation, which provided insufficient followup and coordination placement of discharged patients and inadequate aftercare. It followed that the remedy was to improve implementation by providing better coordination and more community resources.

A contrasting and less widespread view, presented by Gruening and Archer (1979), was that the deinstitutionalization process envisioned by the 1963 act was fundamentally wrong in concept. A national program should have as its first priority caring for the seriously mentally ill. Discharge to the community should be done under the aegis of a mental health therapy team of the state mental hospital. The proposed remedies for the existing programs entailed increased support for improving the professional services in the state mental hospitals and for constructing and operating a system of community aftercare facilities supervised by the hospital mental health therapeutic teams.

A third view, put forth by Rose (1979), and also less widely held than Clarke's, agreed with Gruening and Archer that the basic concept of deinstitutionalization embodied in the 1963 act was incorrect but for different, and in a certain sense diametrically opposed, reasons than those given by the improve-the-mental-hospital advocates. This view held that most of the care, whether in the mental hospital or community-based, was premised on the mistaken concept of mental disability as being essentially a disease to be treated under a "medical model." As long as this erroneous concept underlay the organization of the system, the central question was not whether mental health care should be carried out in the more restrictive mental hospital or the sorry environments to which many deinstitutionalized persons were relegated. Rose proposed no alternative system of services to remedy the weaknesses of the existing system. Instead, he called for recognition of the general principle that much mental disability is socially caused rather than the result of a fundamental internal failure of the individual.

The proponents of each of these views asserted that the observed events provided empirical support for the correctness of their views. Defenders of deinstitutionalization characterized the changes as improvements and pointed to the data on implementation as evidence of the mounting successes of deinstitutionalization. They argued that only further enhancement of resources for community living was necessary or desirable and that ''The central question . . . today is no longer *whether* to deinstitutionalize but *how*. . . . Too many critics of the deinstitutionalization movement have failed to offer any better alternatives'' (Clarke, 1979).

Among the opposing viewpoints, the anti–medical model advocates represented by the S. M. Rose article asserted that based on experience with the program, the overly rapid rate of discharge from the mental hospitals was essentially an ''abandonment of organizational responsibility, as well as of patients'' and judged the empirical outcomes of deinstitutionalization a failure (1979). Rose argued that while the early advocates of deinstitutionalization had been motivated by the lamentable conditions prevailing in most state mental hospitals, with their custodial warehousing of patients and little or no active treatment, the main factor motivating the states had been their grasp of ''a political and economic measure designed primarily to sustain near-bankrupt state governments and to establish the basis for transferring funds from public services to the private sector'' (1979). He pointed to the resulting disposition of discharged patients, as has been discussed previously: relatively few went to CMHCs; support services were not coordinated with the needs of discharged patients; a preponderance went to inappropriately organized nursing homes; and

some went to inadequate board and care programs. It was charged that inappropriately placed patients were kept pacified with psychoactive drugs, which was not much better, if at all, than drugging them in the mental hospital. Neither system provided adequate, active therapy. Furthermore, many of the residences used to house patients were run by the private sector, and many instances of gross abuse, neglect, and exploitation of residents were reported. ''The abuse, leading to state investigations and federal congressional hearings, has become so widespread that it has paralleled the general medical abuse of Medicaid and Medicare programs, but without many of the useful services delivered.'' This line of criticism laid the blame for the inadequacies of deinstitutionalization both on the insufficient resources provided, and more important, on the faulty conception of providing the care along medical-model lines (1979).

The other opposing viewpoint, the improve-the-mental-hospital position, focused on the charge that the deinstitutionalization program had been particularly harmful to patients with serious mental illness. Gruenberg and Archer argued that the treatment of the seriously ill patient constituted its most shameful failure (1979). The one-sided concentration of government money spent on improving mental health care resources in the community and in training psychiatrists for private office practice[30] had wrongfully neglected the mental hospital. Community-based therapy, they asserted, focused on relatively mild mental illness; the seriously ill needed the mental hospital. They contrasted the program experience of the deinstitutionalization program in the United States with some forward-looking, hospital-based programs in Britain as well as in the United States.

In Britain, the directors of three mental hospitals (D. MacMillan, T. P. Reas, and G. Bell) had introduced new measures for treating their patients, and their reports of the favorable results with these approaches had begun to reach the United States in the early postwar years. Their reports were investigated by Dr. Robert C. Hunt, ''who had years of experience working in New York State mental hospital.'' His favorable report was followed by a visit from a committee of American mental hospital directors who were also favorably impressed with what they saw.

They reported that all patients were admitted to these three hospitals only on a voluntary basis, were not under restraints, and stayed in the hospital during periods of crisis that were alternated with long-term stays in the community. The same clinical team that supervised the patient's care in the hospitals took responsibility for his or her care in the community.

Gruenberg and Archer further reported that "By the early 1960s many state hospitals in the United States were operating as open hospitals and some were providing comprehensive services to most of their patients in the community. This movement toward *state-hospital-based community care* for the mentally ill had little connection with the rapidly proliferating *community-based mental health services,* which rarely served people with severe mental disorders who often needed inpatient care" (1979). One of the better known of these reorganizations of state mental hospital services was carried out by Dr. Hunt himself in Dutchess County, New York. Gruenberg and Archer assert that careful evaluations of the Dutchess County program showed its real promise of being able to create a system that transferred patients to the community appropriately, that is, only after proper arrangements for aftercare had been made. The system did not "abandon" responsibility for the care of the seriously mentally ill[31] (1979).

The Mental Health Systems Act of 1980

Thus, by the time President Carter took office in 1977, the content of proposed legislation as well as academic and professional writing had implicitly acknowledged the pertinence of some of the arguments of Hunt, Gruenberg, and others (Gruenberg and Archer, 1979; Bennett, 1979) about the need to improve services for the severely mentally ill in psychiatric institutions. It was also recognized by some that while the improvement of the mental health care system should include paying major attention to the seriously mentally ill, the best way to approach the task was not by turning it into a question of choosing between "hospital care *or* community care when, in fact, both are needed at different times and in different circumstances and must always complement each other" (Bennett, 1979)—an importance element of the British ex-

perimental model described previously. These considerations, taken together with the observed inadequacy of follow-up and support in existing aftercare arrangements, led to an increased emphasis on making the mental health services a better-coordinated system.

But the federal government's attempts to improve the coordination of the care of mental patients was not based on the British notion that the mental hospital would, as a matter of course, be the coordinating agent. Instead, it sought to assign this role to one of a number of different community agencies. There was no apparent support for the idea that it ever, let along generally, should be the state mental hospital. The theme of the NIMH was to weld existing services into Community Support Systems (CSS) under a federally supported Community Support Program (CSP), again a federal "partnership" system. By January 1978 the NIMH had contracted with sixteen states to work on building Community Support Systems, either by formulating strategies for their development over time or actually instituting pilot CSS organizations in short order. "The purpose of these pilot programs was to fix responsibility at Federal, State, and local levels for meeting the full range of needs of the *seriously* mentally ill in the community" [emphasis added]. Each local CSS was designated as a "core service agency"[32] with case managers responsible for maintaining continuous contact with each client "regardless of how many other agencies are involved" (Child Welfare League or America). States with such pilot projects were urged to try to use HUD funds to provide housing alternatives for deinstitutionalized mental patients.

A President's Commission on Mental Health, appointed by President Carter in early 1977, reported in April 1978 that after considering the work of the 32 task panels and 450 volunteers used to help it assess the nation's mental health needs, it was recommending that the CMHC program be recodified and amended to stress coordinated service systems as well as community supports in addition to ongoing support of mental health research and services. Yet while the commission recommended closing only "large" mental hospitals, its report continued to reflect the longstanding dominant trend in the mental health movement to pay scant attention to improving state mental hospitals compared with enhancing community programs.

The activity in the mental health field during the Carter administration culminated in the passage of the Mental Health Systems Act (P.L. 96–398), signed into law by President Carter on October 7, 1980. It incorporated many of the recommendations of his President's Commission on Mental Health. The provisions of the act indicated that the administration intended to stick by the commitment to developing the community mental health system as the core of the mental health care delivery system with some adjustments called for by the empirical experience with it. Chief among these were to stress a coordinated system of services and to give greater attention to seriously ill persons. The main provisions, for our present purposes, were to continue providing operating support grants to newly established public or nonprofit private community mental health centers for eight-year periods on a declining percentage basis (starting with 90 percent and going down to 30 percent in poverty areas and going from 80 percent down to 25 percent in other areas). Grants were also instituted for services to chronically mentally ill persons, with one of the eligibility requirements being that the applicant undertake to provide a case manager; assure coordination of mental health services; and assure related support services. These grants were intended primarily either for State Mental Health Authorities (SMHA) or CMHCs. Other nonprofit entities could receive grants only under exceptional circumstances. State Mental Health Authorities were required to achieve appropriate placement of all mentally disabled persons in the least restrictive *appropriate* setting within five years. The remonstrances of those who had called for instituting a better system of care for the seriously mentally ill that would be centered on the state mental hospital apparently again went largely unheeded. Whatever coordination was anticipated from the effects of this bill was clearly to be based in the community organizations.

The Reagan Administration

One month after this act became law, Ronald Reagan won the presidential election, assuming office in January 1981. The entire mental health program became a target for cuts, and the entire public mental health community was thrown on the defensive. Efforts by mental health advocates to improve the care of the mentally disabled were replaced by defensive attempts to withstand the assault on existing levels of federal support or salvage as much of it as possible. Not only was the federal mental health program cut, but so were all the supporting services, including Medicaid and cash assistance (both Aid to Families with Dependent Children [AFDC] and Supplementary Security Income [SSI] for the aged, blind, and disabled). The mental health program received the same treatment as many of the public health programs; it was put into a block grant with other programs[33] and the sum of the previous allotments to these programs was reduced, as described earlier (see Chap. 4). In his 1982 State of the Union Address, President Reagan included this block grant as one of the forty-three federal programs he wanted turned over to the states by 1984 with complete freedom for them to continue or discontinue them as they wished. The amounts authorized for the entire block grant in the Reconciliation Act for fiscal 1982 were below the total requested in the Carter budget for the three component programs, but the 1983 actual appropriation was well above the Reagan authorizations for 1982, 1983, or 1984. After a decrease of 20.8 percent from the $540.5 million appropriated in 1981, Congress appropriated $777.5 million for 1983 (Child Welfare League of America, 1/10/83), 82 percent higher than the 1982 appropriation and 44 percent higher than the 1981 one (Palmer and Sawhill, 1982), the last pre-Reagan appropriation.

SUMMARY AND COMMENTS

As of 1980 the state role in direct health services continued to be primarily invested in the state mental hospitals, but it was also heavily intertwined with the care of patients discharged from mental hospitals. Their care was largely being provided by the private sector with federal and state governments paying for much of it, the state's share varying greatly from state to state. This arrangement has continued.

In keeping with the general post–World War II growth of a consensus that certain services, health care in particular, constitute a basic human right and should be equally available to all who need them, the idea of "two-track" medicine fell increasingly into disrepute. This view was reflected in a shift in the mode of providing general medical care to the poor and otherwise medically indigent from direct service in public institutions to buying it in the "mainstream" of private practice, including the use of private hospitals and private fee-for-service psychiatrists. The deinstitutionalization movement was not, therefore, based only, perhaps not even mainly, on technical professional perceptions of desirable psychotherapeutic techniques and management of mental health problems. It was also part of the general movement to improve the quality of health care for the poor and near poor, and the perception that the best way to do this was by increasing their access to private providers while diminishing the role of public providers, thereby reducing the extent of the inferior track in "two-track" care.

The preference of the mental health movement for using private providers, even when the financing was largely governmental, was perhaps even stronger than that of reformers in other aspects of health services because of the special historical experience with the asylum and the state mental hospital and the rapid growth of private office-based psychotherapy in the United States. Furthermore, because a strongly held preference for nongovernmental provision of services often carried with it a general view of the undesirability and inefficiency of government "intervention" and regulation whenever the question of costliness arose, the underlying a priori assumption was that private operation and service are inherently superior to those of government because they are assumed to rest on laws governing a hypothesized free, competitive market. If one accepts these assumptions, then clearly every service that can be provided the poor, the near poor, and the medically indigent by means of nongovernmental instrumentalities can be expected to be better provided by the that very fact alone. It follows naturally that persons truly interested in bettering the health services of the poor, the true re-

formers in this view, will therefore favor providing access to the mainstream of medical and mental health care used by well-to-do and well-insured persons. Thus, many mental health advocates,[34] mental health professionals, and public administrators and legislators, saw community-based services—preferably by private providers—as likely to achieve better quality of services and at the same or perhaps lower costs than public providers would. Thus, the desirable future for the state mental hospital could only be virtual if not complete obliteration both because it was based on direct public provision and because it had a history as a place of incarceration rather than treatment.

But experience with the deinstitutionalization program uncovered a number of pitfalls in applying this a priori reasoning to de facto policy formulation. First, the mainstream mode of providing health services, and especially mental health services, does not offer the same advantages to a poor person with inadequate social supports as to a well-to-do person. Merely offering to send a disadvantaged person to a therapist even a good, mainstream one, might not provide adequate care given such a person's other life problems.

Second and closely related to the first point, the cost of providing care in the private sector, if the scope of services is really to be comparable to that provided in the public sector and the quality of care comparable to that provided to private paying patients, has not been shown to be less. There is every reason to expect it to be more costly. Most programs for health care for the poor using private providers have not been able to pay market rates of reimbursement. Many private providers have refused to accept participants in these programs as patients or have accepted only token numbers. Those that "specialize" in serving these clients are often not representative of the best among private providers. Contracting with the private sector, especially the for-profit portion, to provide support services at bargain prices for a particularly vulnerable group of persons presents a temptation to take advantage of them—a temptation that has too often proved irresistible.

Third, the motivations and incentives in the private sector, including much of the nonprofit portion, have impelled well-trained therapists toward private office-based practice, reimbursed on an hourly fee basis. This has tended to leave in short supply the personnel needed to treat and care for the more seriously ill persons who need care in a residential environment. Preventive services for persons who are not seriously ill and who can find their way to appropriate help may indeed best be carried out in a community environment with ambulatory modalities of therapy, perhaps along with intermittent short-term acute hospitalization. But unless one believes that all serious mental illness can be prevented by timely and appropriate community-based therapy, some persons will continue to be seriously ill and will need good long-term inpatient treatment for chronic illness, perhaps with close supervision and follow-up in the community during periods of remission. The private sector has characteristically avoided treating most such persons, whether the illness be ''mental'' or somatic.

Fourth, although state mental hospitals were very unsatisfactory places for appropriate mental treatment in 1945, Gruenberg's idea that they be upgraded and their programs reconstituted to make them the centers of truly coordinated community mental health networks was never tried when increased public funds became available. While it is true that many publicly provided health services for the poor, such as mental health care, have not been of acceptable quality, if one accepts his hypothesis that the cause has been primarily insufficient funding, it seems highly questionable that paying the same or less for these services in the private sector will result in more nearly adequate services for seriously ill persons. If public direct-service facilities are indiscriminately curtailed and funding for private care is not adequate, it is only reasonable to suppose that persons will be unable to obtain care of any kind, whether in the public hospital or the community mental health system. They are likely to be the most helpless and the sickest people. It seems that this has happened in many places although the extent of the problem has been difficult to fully measure. The growth of homelessness, for example, is a serious national problem that is believed to be significantly associated with mentally ill persons who have not

been accommodated in treatment centers. A dilemma of mental health reformers has been that their very efforts to improve mental health services has contributed to the closing and reduction of many needed mental hospitals, and after decades of unreservedly assailing these institutions they were forced into having to oppose further reductions. One wonders if the reformers' campaign for privatization of public services for disadvantaged persons has brought improvement commensurate to the efforts expended or whether at least part of the resources used in campaigning for privatization would not have been better directed toward striving for improvement in the public services. Perhaps the arguments of critics like Gruenberg deserve more attention than they have received.

We shall find that similar developments occurred in other health services programs for poor and disadvantaged persons. The general course of these developments has often been that existing services provided by the government for disadvantages groups are attacked by well-meaning reformers as being of poor quality (which they usually are). A large part of the cause of this poor quality is represented to be the government operation of the programs. Therefore, making the target populations eligible for mainstream private sources of service is seen as the best solution. Attempts are made to implement this change by quickly and sharply reducing the government service facilities and *declaring* (but not adequately paying for) the former clients to be eligible for mainstream services. The mainstream sources of service are not reimbursed at market rates and most refuse service to program clients, the old direct-service institutions have been destroyed or crippled, and much of the former clientele of the government program finds itself entirely without needed service; others find themselves with worse services than before the ''reform'' efforts were started. In effect, well-meaning reformers turn out to have worked together with those who seek to reduce all public services to the poor on ideological grounds.

This dilemma, faced by many social reformers and advocates in the health field, is a central thread running through the politics of all the programs aimed at providing better care for the poor. It will be more thoroughly discussed in subsequent chapters dealing with local public hospitals and "welfare" programs of medical care for the poor. The developments in the mental health services area provide a particularly good illustration of the issues involved in the arguments over government direct services versus nongovernment providers for such programs.

NOTES

1. Of all United States hospitals there were only 158 nonregistered hospitals with about 19,000 beds in 1980 compared with 6,965 registered hospitals with about 1.4 million beds.

2. The American Hospital Association classifies a hospital as short-term if the average length of stay is under thirty days or if over 50 percent of all patients admitted stay less than thirty days.

3. Or equivalently, 18.5 percent of the average daily census. The average daily census is the average number of patients in hospitals on one day. For the year, it is equivalent to the number of patient days divided by 365.

4. These averages are based on number of beds expressed in thousands rounded to the nearest tenth of a thousand, as used in Table 6-1.

5. The data used in the annual AHA Statistics and those in the *Report of the Commission on Public-General Hospitals* differ in the way they classify hospital sponsorship. The AHA statistics use "control" (i.e., managerial authority) as the sponsorship criterion and the commission study uses ownership. In 1975, for example, there were 197 nonfederal short-term hospitals that were publicly owned but managed by private organizations and 37 privately owned hospitals that were publicly managed. While this creates difficulties in using the two sets of data together, these difficulties are not of a magnitude that could obscure the main features discussed here. I have used the AHA statistics for overall description and the commission data selectively, where appropriate, for certain details not given in the published AHA statistics. The data on the forty-four state university hospitals cited here provide an illustration of the latter usage.

6. In most of these statistics, data for county psychiatric hospitals are combined with those for state psychiatric hospitals. The magnitude of the service data applying to the county institutions is small and does not materially affect the conclusions drawn from the data. In 1986, for example, the 285 state mental hospitals [excluding U.S. territories] listed by the NIMH included twenty-one county mental hospitals, all of them in New Jersey and Wisconsin (Sunshine, et al., 1990). The term "state mental hospitals" will henceforth therefore nearly always include county mental hospitals.

7. The percentages were 33.7 percent "no charge," 16.8 percent "personal payment," 9.5 per-

cent Medicare and Medicaid, 28.6 percent "other government payment," and 11.2 percent Blue Cross and commercial insurance. The state share had increased by 1986, when the NIMH reported the distribution of sources of revenue for state mental hospitals to include 78.4 percent from state funds and 11.2 percent from Medicaid (Sunshine, et al., 1990).

8. Somewhat later, a similar campaign sought to separate the *physically* ill into public medical hospitals—see Chapter 7.

9. The original and still one of the dictionary definitions of an asylum is "a sanctuary or inviolable place of protection."

10. Robert Felix, then chief of the Division of Mental Hygiene of the Public Health Service and later the first director of NIMH.

11. The development of this community mental health center network over the next three decades and beyond is clearly not an example of state-"operated medical care services," consisting as it does of services provided locally, mostly by private-sector professionals, supported by federal-state funding and monitored by the states. As such it perhaps belongs more naturally under a chapter in Part III, which deals with government payment to private providers for medical care services. As noted in the preface, however, I have decided to place the discussion of this system here under state-provided direct services because it developed in reaction to the state mental hospital system with its history an extension of that system's history. Furthermore, the relationship of the two systems—the state mental hospitals and community mental health centers—remains a unified vital policy question. It therefore seems more sensible from the point of view of understanding the role of government in the provision of mental health services and the policy questions surrounding it to treat the local community ambulatory portion of these services here.

12. This citation and much of the description of these acts is taken from the 1977 Report to Congress by the GAO Comptroller General (U.S. Gen. Accounting Office, 1977). It will not be further cited in the next few paragraphs.

13. A few definitions are in order here. *Mental illness* is defined as "an affliction resulting in a disturbance in behavior, feeling, thinking or judgment to such an extent that a person requires care and treatment." *Mental retardation* is defined as "significant subaverage general intellectual functioning which originates during the developmental period (between conception and age 18) and is associated with impairment in adaptive behavior." *Mentally disabled* includes the mentally ill and the mentally retarded. *Developmentally disabled* includes disabilities "attributable to mental retardation, cerebral palsy, epilepsy, autism, conditions closely related to mental retardation, or dyslexia" (U.S. General Accounting Office, 1977). These are all held to originate during the developmental period as in mental retardation.

14. These five mandatory "essential elements" of service were: (1) inpatient services providing twenty-

four-hour care for treatment of acute disorders; (2) outpatient services; (3) partial hospitalization services such as day care, night care, and weekend care; (4) emergency services twenty-four hours per day, which had to be available within at least one of the first three services listed above; and (5) consultation and education services available to community agencies and professional personnel.

In addition, as a long-term goal, each center would also at some future time need to provide five additional services, namely: (6) diagnostic services; (7) rehabilitative services, including vocational and educational programs; (8) preinstitutional care and aftercare services in the community, including foster home placement, home visiting, and halfway houses; (9) job training; and (10) research and evaluation on program progress (Kramer, 1969).

15. Gruenberg and Archer, advocates of such a partnership (1979), assert that the 1955 joint commission report to the president was interpreted by "the NIMH leaders responsible for providing guidance and direction to implement the report" as placing its main emphasis on "upgrading the state mental hospital system to a therapeutic level." But these leaders opposed aid to the mental hospitals and instead "NIMH personnel drafted legislation to create a system of community-based mental health services apart from the State hospitals" over the objections of "state mental hospital directors and state commissioners of mental hygiene. . . . The NIMH advocates won out with President Kennedy . . . by persuading him that the Joint Commission had been wrong in focusing on improving mental hospitals" (1979).

16. The NIMH term "number of episodes of care" is the sum of the number of persons under care at the beginning of the year plus "additions" (new admissions and readmissions) during the year. This number of episodes is therefore larger than the number of different persons served because one person may be admitted several times to the same facility. Omitted from the table are episodes in psychiatric services of all federal agencies other than the VA (e.g., PHS, Indian Health Service, DOD, Bureau of Prisons etc.). All episodes in private office-based practices of mental health professionals, general medical practice and clinics, and other health centers, general hospital medical services, nursing homes, and other settings are also excluded (Redick et al., 1990).

17. See Table 6-2, notes e and g.

18. Data on source of referral to CMHCs have appeared intermittently. In 1974 for example, 4.1 percent of their referrals came from a "public psychiatric hospital." By contrast, 41 percent came from "self, family, or friend (NIMH, 1979).

19. In this case direct care constitutes both public and private direct provision. The other-than-direct care comprises research, training and fellowships, facilities development, management expenses such as insurance, and some other items.

20. This pattern has not changed over the years. As late as 1986 the percentage distribution of the sources of state mental hospital revenues included: state funds, 78.4 percent; Medicaid, 11.2 percent (including state and local share); and client fees, 4.3 percent (Sunshine, et al., 1990).

21. The real (i.e., inflation-adjusted) amount spent annually for state mental hospitals has been fluctuating over the years but it was higher than in 1967 for each year thereafter. The picture is clouded for real total expenditures, but in any case it is clear that there was no dramatic reduction in these real costs.

22. A 1977 GAO report defined the goals of deinstitutionalization "as the process of (1) preventing both unnecessary admission to and retention in institutions, (2) finding and developing appropriate alternatives in the community for housing, treatment, training, education, and rehabilitation of the mentally disabled who do not need to be in institutions, and (3) improving conditions, care and treatment for those who need institutional care. This approach is based on the principle that mentally disabled persons are entitled to live in the least restrictive environment necessary to lead their lives as normally and independently as they can." This complex of objectives is what I mean by the "deinstitutionalization program" in contrast to the word "deinstitutionalization," which by itself implies only getting patients *out of* mental hospitals. The program heavily stressed getting patients *into* appropriate settings.

23. The primary discussion of these programs is in Chapter 10 and the connection with deinstitutionalization is further treated there.

24. Aged, blind, permanently and totally disabled, and families with dependent children (AFDC).

25. The original Social Security Act required that the welfare recipients receive all their benefits in cash. Giving any part of the welfare grant "in kind" including in the form of services was prohibited. The services provided for under these titles departed from this principle in much the same way that Medicaid did for medical services.

26. *Wyatt* v. *Stickney,* 1972; *United States* v. *Solomon and Welsch* v. *Likens,* 1974; *New York State Association for Retarded Children* v. *Carey,* 1975; *O'Connor* v. *Donaldson, Dixon* v. *Weinberger,* and *Horacek* v. *Exon,* all in 1975.

27. Special Health Revenue Sharing Acts of 1975, Community Mental Health Centers Amendments of 1975, and Developmentally Disabled Assistance and Bill of Rights Act.

28. A 1969 study by NIMH found that only 7.1 percent of the patients discharged from state and county mental hospitals were referred to a community mental health center; 37.6 percent were discharged with no referrals at all (Redick, 1971).

29. Similar attempts were made to discontinue state institutions for mentally retarded persons, but parents of patients in these institutions along with interested other people were instrumental in getting the state legislature to pass a law prohibiting the closing of such institutions without specific legislative sanction. Governor Ronald Reagan's veto of the bill was

overridden by the legislature—the first such overriding of a veto in California in twenty-eight years.

30. Gruenberg and Archer attribute some of what they consider to be the inappropriately heavy shift away from caring for the seriously ill in mental hospitals to inadequate community psychiatric services to the growing dominance of psychiatrists trained with support of postwar training grants primarily at university centers and ambulatory clinics rather than state mental hospitals. One of the factors that contributed importantly to this switch in training sites, according to these authors, was the ''migration of hundreds of psychiatrists from Nazi Germany'' into the United States in the 1930s who heavily influenced United States psychiatry ''to develop . . . psychoanalytically oriented services'' and that ''their amalgam of university psychiatry and psychotherapeutic office practice laid the foundation for psychiatric careers unconnected with mental hospitals. . . . These hospitals, which provided the bulk of the psychiatric training before World War II, could not compete with the universities for the most highly qualified residents.'' The psychiatrists produced by these post–World War II training programs saw their role as redefined by a number of European psychiatrists, most particularly Sigmund Freud, a role that viewed the psychiatrist as one ''who helps the patient to struggle against his disordered functioning, rather than that of a doctor who diagnoses it and prescribes treatment. Freud also evolved the principle that, like a music teacher charging by the hour, the therapist sells his time, knowledge, skill and attention. This put the office practice of psychiatry on a commercial basis'' (1979).

31. This tendency for the deinstitutionalization movement to neglect the seriously disabled was also noted with respect to the mentally retarded in a GAO report. Particularly in the vocational rehabilitation program, the report noted,

more emphasis needs to be placed on the more severely mentally disabled if the deinstitutionalization goal is to be achieved.

For the mentally retarded, vocational rehabilitation has been primarily directed toward the less severely retarded (or those who may not be retarded) and apparently toward those in the community *instead of those in institutions* [emphasis added]. In previous years, rehabilitation for the mentally ill often focused on drug addicts, alcoholics, and those with behavioral disorders. These forms of mental illness were not categorically considered severe disabilities by the Rehabilitation Service Administration under the Rehabilitation Act of 1973 as amended (29 U.S.C. 701).

But the Rehabilitation Act of 1973 did require that states give first priority to persons with the most severe handicaps in their state vocational rehabilitation plans and ''RSA [Rehabilitation Services Administration] has told the States to focus on persons on public support, such as the institutionalized mentally disabled. . .'' (1977).

32. The core service agency could be ''a [general] hospital, community mental health center, a sheltered workshop, a rehabilitation center, a transitional living program, or some other service organization.''

33. More specifically, the activities of the community mental health centers and those of the new Mental Health Systems Act were combined with the Alcohol Abuse Act into the Alcohol Abuse, Drug Abuse and Mental Health block grant under the Omnibus Budget Reconciliation Act of 1981 (P.L. 97-35). (Some of these are my short titles. See Chap. 4 for the complete titles.)

34. One school of thought whose writings enjoyed considerable popularity in the 1960s and 1970s based its opposition to the mental hospital on the premise that it was used primarily to forcefully incarcerate persons who were only different from the majority but were stigmatized as being dangerous and criminal. One of the principal articulators of this view was the psychiatrist Thomas Szasz. He asserted that only a private psychiatrist retained by the patient can really be trusted to represent the patient's interest. Any mental therapist paid by the state can be expected to betray the patient's interest and serve the purposes of the state (1970).

Local, Government-Operated, Direct Health Care Programs

This chapter deals with the *direct* provision of health services to the poor by the public hospital and its predecessor institutions, primarily addressing inpatient services but unavoidably treating the ambulatory services provided in the public hospitals, and how the need for better ambulatory services affected the public hospital. The next chapter focuses on the public ambulatory care systems that *use public payment* to the private sector to provide medical care to the poor.[1]

The American Hospital Association reported that in 1980 there were 1,742 local, government-operated[2] hospitals, representing 25 percent of all hospitals and about 63 percent of all government hospitals. Of these, 1,701, or 98 percent, were short-term and the rest were long-term. They carried a total average daily census of 144,000 patients, or 13 percent of the total hospital patient census; 90 percent of this average census was short-term and 10 percent was long-term.[3] Table 7–1 gives further detail on the distribution of local government hospital services by type of service for 1980. It should be noted that less than 1 percent (3,600) of their entire average daily census is served in specialized psychiatric hospitals, which numbered only fourteen of the more than 1,700 local government hospitals.

The 1975 distribution of local government hospitals cross-classified by type of private or governmental unit sponsorship (''control'') and ownership is shown in Table 7–2. In earlier years, when the AHA annually published the number of beds, the average daily census, and the number of admissions and outpatient visits, all broken down by the four categories of local public hospital control—county, city, city-county and hospital district—the data indicated that city and city-county hospitals were larger than county hospitals.

The data in Table 7–2 show that county hospitals made up 46 percent of all hospitals operated by local governments in 1975, followed by city hospitals, which made up about 18 percent of the local government hospitals. When one adds the city-county hospital, almost 70 percent of all public local public hospitals have been included.

The county hospitals in predominantly rural counties constitute a heterogenous mix. In some places these hospitals serve a substantial portion of the paying patient population, for they are the only or at least one of the very few facilities available in their areas. Many of the hospitals run by specially constituted, state-chartered hospital districts are of this type. This chapter will not address the problems faced by these hospitals, but rather will focus on the urban public local hospitals in the largest 100 cities, whether under county or municipal ownership.[4] These hospitals have been the last-resort source for health care for the residents of large urban centers who could get care nowhere else. They have been facing problems that in large part reflect the growing ills of our core cities, and their pattern of financial support and style of operation bear the telltale marks of their origin (Burlage, 1967; Cooney, Roemer, and Ross, 1971; Hospital Research and Education Trust, 1978). Again referring to Table 7–2, we see that in 1975 there were ninety such hospitals.

The urban local public general hospital[5] was for many years the main source of inpatient hos-

Table 7–1. Operating and Capacity Statistics of Local Government Operated[2] Hospitals by Type of Stay and Service—1980.

	Hospitals		Beds		Average daily census		Admissions		Outpatient visits	
	No.	Percent[a]	No. (000)	Percent[a]	No. (000)	Percent[a]	No. (000)	Percent[a]	No. (000)	Percent[a]
Short-term	1701	97.6	183.8	92.0	129.5	90.3	6563.0	99.5	41001.0	99.5
General	1687	96.8	181.3	90.7	127.5	88.9	6547.0	99.3	40764.0	98.9
Psychiatric	8	0.5	1.7	0.9	1.4	1.0	8.0	0.1	158.0	0.4
Other	6	0.3	0.8	0.4	0.6	0.4	8.0	0.1	79.0	0.2
Long-term	41	2.3	16.0	8.1	14.0	9.7	23.0	0.3	210.0	0.5
General	2	0.1	0.4	0.2	0.3	0.2	1.0	0.0[b]	4.0	0.0[b]
Psychiatric	6	0.3	2.7	1.4	2.2	1.5	3.0	0.0[b]	39.0	0.1
TB and other respiratory diseases	1	0.1	0.1	0.1	0.0[b]	0.0[b]	1.0	0.0[b]	4.0	0.0[b]
Other	32	1.8	12.8	6.4	11.5	8.0	18.0	0.3	163.0	0.4
TOTAL	1742	99.9[c]	199.8	100.1[c]	143.5	100.0	6586.0	99.8[c]	41211.0	100.0

Source: AHA, 1980.

[a]Of total local government hospitals.

[b]Not zero but less than .05.

[c]Total does not add to 100 percent due to rounding.

pital care for the urban poor and near poor and its outpatient clinics also provided much of the ambulatory medical care used by these populations. The public hospital is an outgrowth of the poorhouse and has inherited part of the stigma attached to that institution.

When private health insurance and public medical care programs made private hospitals available to many people who had previously used public hospitals, the role of these public hospitals became less important. It did not, however, become negligible, because many persons were left without coverage for medical care by either private insurance or public reimbursement programs. The public hospitals that were obligated to serve those who cannot pay continued to be a necessary part of the spectrum of medical care providers, but their place in this spectrum became less well-defined in the public mind and was the subject of many political battles.

EARLY DEVELOPMENTS

For centuries publicly provided or guaranteed medical care has been part of the aid given the poor for survival—food, shelter, and clothing. The conditions under which "paupers" could obtain medical care were the same as those that made them eligible for "relief." It is therefore

necessary to consider these general conditions in any attempt to understand how the poor received medical care.

Early organization of care for the poor in the United States was heavily influenced by British institutions, which have left their mark to the present day. The means adopted by localities in early America to care for the poor differed from place to place, but the two main instrumentalities were the poorhouse or workhouse to which all paupers unable to sustain themselves had to move, and provision of "outdoor" (home) relief in cash or kind to paupers to enable them to continue living in the community. This system had important parallels to the English Elizabethan Poor Law public assistance system: it was local in administration, it used both institutional "poorhouse" facilities and "outdoor relief" resources that assisted qualified poor persons in their homes, and this outdoor assistance was usually restricted to persons who could not work, the "worthy poor," depending on the locality.

The social philosophy of the 1800s recognized only certain classes of society as "worthy poor." Generally these were persons unable to work through no "fault" of their own and therefore entitled to assistance from public and charity from private sources. If institutionalized, they received maintenance care, including some

Table 7-2. Distribution of Community Hospitals, by Control[a], Type of Hospital, and Ownership, 1975

Control	All community hospitals	Total		University		Urban		Other metropolitan		Rural	
		Public	Private	Public	Private	Public	Private	Public	Private	Public	Private
State	75	75	0	40	0	6	0	8	0	21	0
County	767	750	17	0	0	26	0	103	5	621	12
City	307	304	3	0	0	27	0	73	0	204	3
City-county	62	61	1	1	0	5	0	14	0	41	1
Hospital district or authority	534	518	16	0	0	19	0	130	3	369	13
Private, not-for-profit	3,220	196	3,024	4[b]	21	7	673	28	1,077	157	1,253
Private, for-profit	714	1	713	0	0	0	205	1	291	0	217
Total	5,679	1,905	3,774	45	21	90	878	357	1,376	1,413	1,499

Source: Hospital Research and Education Trust, 1978.

[a] As stated in note[2], the AHA has classified community hospitals as public only when controlled or managed by local, state, or regional government. This report defines public hospitals on the basis of ownership rather than control. This table shows that 197 community hospitals are publicly owned by not-for-profit or investor-owned organizations and that 37 privately owned hospitals are controlled by public organizations. These conditions occur because of delegation of management to other organizations, transfer of ownership in order to use public capital financing instruments, participation in multi-institutional arrangements, contractual arrangements for management by companies specializing in these services, and interpretations of the law concerning ownership (see following footnote).

[b] The four public university hospitals that reported control by private not-for-profit corporations are owned by private not-for-profit corporations that were chartered prior to their territories' achieving statehood. They have interpreted their organizations as private not-for-profit because they predate the state. Patterns of financing and policy decisions are the same as for other publicly owned university hospitals.

medical attention at the poorhouse or alsmhouse to which they were consigned. The able-bodied poor, on the other hand, if they were not working were regarded only as unemployed, not unemployable, and they were meant to be accommodated in workhouses. In these institutions they were theoretically, in analogy with the English model, expected to work to earn their keep and be trained to better compete for private sector jobs. The main concern was to prevent such persons from acquiring the habit of being slothful and not exerting maximum efforts to find work of any kind at all times.

Actually, the terms workhouse, almshouse, and poorhouse were often used interchangeably in the United States. Although the English poor law "reform" of 1834 stressed the workhouse in its literal meaning as the place for all able-bodied poor, the trend in the United States was to put all persons who could not support themselves in local poorhouses whose function was "more custodial than deliberately deterrent." Part of the difference in degree of punitiveness between the United States and British poor law administration was very likely due to the lower relative levels of chronic unemployment in the America of the 1800s because of the recurring opportunities offered by the westward expansion of the United States (Leiby, 1978). I shall refer to the American institution as a poorhouse or alsmhouse even though some continued to be called workhouses or may have continued some compulsory work programs for able-bodied inmates.

The infirmaries of these poorhouses gave some form of medical care to their residents and where permitted, local poor persons who were not inmates of the poorhouse also turned to these infirmaries for care and some of them gradually came to be equipped with special sections for ill poor persons. "Many a modern general hospital under public auspices had its origin in a workhouse" (Goldman, 1945). For example, Bellevue Hospital in New York City evolved from a pesthouse[6] built in 1794 and a workhouse built some sixty years earlier. The Philadelphia General Hospital began as an almshouse in 1732 and the county public hospital in Valhalla, New York (Grasslands Hospital) began as an almshouse in the early 1800s (Goldman, 1945). The economically non-viable poor of a locality would be herded together into the poorhouses: children, men, women and old people, sick and well together. Many of them were chronically ill, and for many of them it was their illness and disability that were responsible for their pauperism in the first place.

It was common to contract the medical care of the residents out to a physician who was the lowest bidder for this "business" and who came perhaps once a week to see patients. Often the low-paying contract required the physician to supply his own medicine. The drive to remove the sick from these poorhouses to hospitals run by medical personnel and dedicated to treatment rather than incarceration was reformist in origin and intent. In California, for example, the establishment of county hospitals was part of this movement, and in many large cities throughout the United States public hospitals were developed in response to the medical needs of the immigrants arriving after about 1890. In addition, the triumph of scientific medicine by 1920 (see Shryock, 1979) following the bacteriological discoveries around the turn of the century, established a need for large numbers of "house" patients to meet the needs of medical research and physician training, and the development of public hospitals in many large cities was enhanced by their links with medical schools and research institutes. The political power of these schools and institutes did much to augment local governments' appropriations for local public hospitals. In the period between World War I and World War II the large urban public hospital became a medically prestigious institution in many a large city, particularly along the Middle and North Atlantic seacoast and the Midwest. Perhaps the most impressive system of local public hospitals was developed in New York City, and a brief description of some of its characteristics may be illustrative here. Although much of the following is based specifically on the New York City system, which was larger and more comprehensive than any other, elements of the system applied to other large urban centers as well, always with particularized local variations that sometimes were very substantial. Much of this account is based on Burlage's excellent study of the New York City hospital system (1967).

Before World War II, a substantial portion of

the clientele of the New York City public hospitals was medically indigent[7] with respect to hospital stays and perhaps also with respect to the more costly ambulatory diagnostic procedures and consultations, but was otherwise self-supporting, including being able to meet the cost of occasional routine visits to neighborhood physicians and prescribed drugs. For their regular care many persons used their neighborhood private physicians, who charged on a sliding-fee scale and referred patients to the outpatient department of the municipal hospital for consultations and diagnostic procedures that they could not afford to have done privately. This same private practitioner also often referred patients to the municipal hospital for inpatient care if they could not afford private hospitalization. In many communities the neighborhood practicing physician was likely to be on the attending staff of the local municipal hospital, assuming teaching duties and giving free service in the clinics. It was not uncommon for this physician to "look in" on his own referred patient either to participate in the treatment or to reassure him or her that he was in close communication with members of the house medical staff.

In some neighborhoods a prospective practitioner training at a municipal hospital could look forward to establishing himself in practice in the economically mixed neighborhoods of the population served by that hospital and continuing his affiliation with the institution. This would lead to teaching assignments and ultimately to membership on the medical board and committees of the hospital. Many of the teachers at the large urban public hospitals enjoyed wide prestige as innovators and researchers. It was before the days of the large-scale federal research grants, and the public hospital was a leading center of teaching and research. Burlage (1967) describes the situation in New York City in these terms:

Before World War II, the municipal hospitals had been generally quite eminent, sought after by residents and interns from throughout the nation. Among the medical and scientific breakthroughs pioneered in New York City municipal hospitals are the following: first appendectomy, first ambulance service, first caesarian section, first insulin shock treatment for mental illness, first use of cocaine for surgical anaesthesia, first heart catheterization, first organ transplants, home dialysis, and the Bellevue-Wechsler intelligence tests.

Although New York City had the most developed public hospital system, well-known and medically prestigious public hospitals were also developed in Boston, Philadelphia, Baltimore, Chicago, Cleveland, and other urban centers.

THE URBAN PUBLIC HOSPITAL AFTER WORLD WAR II

During and after World War II the picture in many of the older cities changed sharply. The rapid spread of private medical insurance was largely tied to employment and more particularly to employment in the higher paid unionized industries.[8] The rise in employment rates and in take-home wages and salaries induced a spread of relative affluence among the middle classes and unionized working people, many of whom moved to the suburbs. Into their former dwellings in the central city moved newly arrived people, most of whom were members of minority groups from rural depressed areas. They were largely very poor and not able or equipped to partake of the employment benefits available in the post–World War II boom economy because of both racial and ethnic discrimination as well as lack of skills. They often used the urban public hospital for all their medical care, both ambulatory and inpatient. The municipal hospital in the post–World War II years often found itself situated in a changed neighborhood and with a changed clientele. There was no longer much incentive for physicians to establish their private practices in the ghetto areas served by the public hospital, and many physicians who had been practicing in these areas moved their offices to the suburbs.

Furthermore, the growth of the extramural funding program of the National Institutes of Health made research money increasingly available, with most of it going to prestigious and well-endowed private voluntary as well as state-owned teaching hospitals and medical schools. The leading medical research personnel and teachers gravitated toward these institutions, compounding the difficulties facing the urban public hospitals in obtaining quality house staff (i.e., medical residents and interns). It was the latter, working "in tandem with attending staffs and a few full-time staff physicians" (1967) who provided most of the patient care. Turning again to Burlage's description of the postwar New York City scene:

[N]ationally the number of available internships and residencies is about twice the number of actual American medical school graduates seeking positions. A rising demand for hospital-based care, a great lag in the input of attending and full-time postgraduate physicians into hospitals, and a shortening of the internship period from two years to one put all the more pressure on the scarce available supply of interns. With the rapidly changing scientific scene, greater emphasis on biomedical research, and intense specialization and sub-specialization, this increasingly meant that those municipal hospitals unable to count on the prestige or professional opportunities of a medical school or major voluntary teaching hospital had to turn to graduates of foreign medical schools. There is some dispute over the relative quality of such foreign medical school graduates. Special examinations to certify foreign medical graduates for American house staff duty were established in 1960. It was correctly anticipated then that failures in these exams would cut even deeper into the number of available house staff in the municipal hospitals (1967).

The quality of the medical staffing and facilities in urban public hospitals deteriorated so much during the 1950s that in many places these hospitals faced loss of accreditation.

The Increasing Need for Medical Care

During this post–World War II period, the rising expectations of the urban poor, encouraged by Truman's Fair Deal and Kennedy/Johnson's Great Society programs and policy pronouncements, included the demand for accessible and adequate medical care. This need was being expressed largely as an increasingly urgent demand for primary ambulatory care. The utilization of all hospital outpatient departments increased more rapidly nationally than did their inpatient use, but the increase in outpatient load fell much more heavily on the public than the private hospitals. These trends are amply substantiated by the data on hospital utilization dur-

ing those years. For example, in the fifteen-year period 1953–1968, the ratio of outpatient visits to inpatient admissions for all hospitals went from about two visits per admission in 1953 to four in 1968. In 1953, 60 percent of all community hospitals reported having outpatient facilities; in 1968, 90 percent did (Cooney, Roemer, and Ross, 1971; AHA, 1969). Although the number of visits to outpatient facilities per population doubled during this period for all hospitals, the large urban public hospital carried a far greater outpatient load relative to its inpatient load than did the private community hospital. The UCLA study of the ambulatory services of fifty-one large urban public hospitals (Cooney, Roemer, and Ross, 1971) found that among the hospitals included in the study, the ratio of visits to admissions in 1969 was 14, more than three times the 4.5 ratio of a comparison group of 600 private nonprofit hospitals.

The rising demand for more and better services, particularly ambulatory services, that faced the public urban hospital in large cities by the 1960s coincided with the decline in quality and quantity of medical staffing resulting from their inability to attract top teachers and house staff in sufficient numbers. There was also a decline in quantity of other personnel and a deterioration in physical facilities. Both developments—the increase in demand and the decline in personnel and facility resources—stemmed from the same underlying phenomenon: the large cities were suffering from fiscal erosion (Shonick, 1979) reflecting the departure of middle-class taxpayers and the influx of a large needy population. Of the principal federal programs for helping the poor and medically indigent achieve greater access to medical care,[9] only the National Health Service Corps Act substantially helped some of the local public hospitals by providing some medical staff. The other programs did not have helping the local public hospital as a priority.

Accompanying these difficulties, the managers of municipal hospitals found themselves increasingly impeded by local government procedural intricacies and alleged use of federal monies from Medicaid and Medicare to reimburse the general funds of city treasuries rather than to finance improved care (Brown, 1970).

Remedies Proposed for the Ills of Public Hospitals

Different Viewpoints

The sad condition into which so many large public urban hospitals had fallen brought forth different reactions from various sources, the reactions depending on the general philosophic outlook of those voicing them. Some attributed the condition of the public hospitals to the very fact of government operation, reflecting the notions that good-quality medical care must be privately delivered in the "mainstream" of private practice, and that government organizations are by their very nature intrinsically inefficient and less effective than private ones because "bureaucracy" and "red tape" are particularly endemic to public operations. In this view, if hospital care (both inpatient and outpatient) of adequate quality were to be efficiently provided for poor persons, it had to be done by paying private providers. Adherents of this view were mostly concerned with providing existing services at lesser cost, which would follow from the assumptions about the greater efficiency of private providers. For others, the central concern was that the poor get the *same* quality of services as the rest of the population—for them, medical care was a right, not a privilege—and given the realities of the society, they favored the mechanism of subsidizing the poor and medically indigent to use the existing medical care system in the same way that paying patients did. In any case, whether the genesis of their position lay primarily in cost saving or abolishing two-track medicine, many people were increasingly calling for the discontinuance of special public hospitals for poor and medically indigent persons and substituting the use of the private sector, through government subsidy for persons who could not pay.

On the other side were those who felt that the best solution to the problem of the deteriorating public hospital was to increase support for it. Among these were persons who worked closely with the poor, who felt that single-minded attempts to get the "mainstream" of private, office-based, largely fee-for-service medical practice and the insurance-financed hospital to serve the poor adequately were doomed to failure. They doubted that the incentives built into the existing private-sector system could produce the type of motivation required to serve the poor. Many of these persons favored universal, comprehensive health coverage—either national health insurance or a government-operated system—but pending such a development, they could see no satisfactory alternative to continuing the public hospital's existence. Their aim was to improve its financing to enable it to better provide the services of the "mainstream" private sector and in addition provide the special support services required by poor populations to enable them to benefit fully from good medical care—services such as nutrition and health education, outreach, transportation, and home visits. One facet of the arguments supporting the continuance of the local public hospital was that it was needed to provide the entire community with special services that other hospitals found it disadvantageous to provide. If there were no public hospitals, and the service were perceived as being badly needed, then either private hospitals would need to be required to provide these services, or a perhaps very expensive and inefficient incentive system would have to be organized to induce private hospitals to provide them. Closely allied to this idea was the thought that local public hospitals were particularly needed for teaching and research purposes. Although some health care administrators and public commentators were advocating closing these hospitals,[10] most were still asserting in the late 1960s that the time for discarding the urban public hospital, despite the advent of Medicare and Medicaid,[11] had not yet arrived. Writers such as Ray E. Brown (1970) were pointing out that this institution was still the ultimate resource for persons and types of care not covered by any funding program and the only one that had ultimate community responsibility for handling all cases: "a large city . . . must have one hospital that cannot pass the buck."

Different Proposals

The increasing national interest in the problems of the poor in the 1960s intensified public discussion of the evils of the "two-track" system of medical care, with the urban public hospital being one of the areas receiving particular attention. Investigators were finding and writers were declaring the urban public hospital to be overcrowded, underfinanced, inaccessible, and providing care of questionable medical as well as humane quality. Many different solutions, reflecting the various different viewpoints as to the roots of these problems, were being proposed and some were being tried. Reports of early experiences with these solutions were appearing in newspapers and periodicals, a high point being reached in 1970 with the publication by the American Hospital Association of a special issue of its journal, *Hospitals,* dedicated to "The Plight of the Public Hospitals" (July 1). It contained articles discussing the then-current problems of the public hospital as well as a number of solutions that were being tried in various locales around the nation. One of these articles grouped these attempted solutions under five main classifications (Elwood and Hoagberg, 1970):

1. Affiliation contracts between public hospitals and medical schools or large teaching hospitals (affiliation);
2. Transfer of public hospital ownership to an existing organization, or to a specially created community board (divestiture);
3. Creation of hospital districts (hospital district);
4. Creation of state-chartered public benefit corporations (semi-autonomous with control of budget and personnel) that are responsible for providing care for the medically indigent (public benefit corp.);
5. Merger with other local governmental health agencies, mainly health departments, with the aim of using the combined resources to establish a comprehensive system of medical care, especially for the urban poor, (agency merger).

A sixth proposed solution, tried later in the 1970s, called for contracting only the management of the public hospital out to private management companies with the local government retaining full ownership of the hospital. The nature of this proposal and some experience with it will be discussed later.

For the present we note that the five earlier proposed solutions are couched in terms of organizational changes, including changes in ownership. They imply an assumption that the nature of the public hospital's plight is basically organizational, managerial, and medical-technological. None of them specifically calls for increases in financing that would assure increased resources as a sine qua non, that is, clearly identifies it as a necessary, although perhaps not sufficient, condition for improved services. The tone and emphasis of these proposals and the discussion around them strongly implied that the etiology of the public hospitals' problems was internal and organizational.

Affiliating public hospitals with medical schools and teaching hospitals would bring the high medical standards of the elite, largely private teaching hospital into the public hospital; transfer of ownership to a medical school or community board would relieve the hospital management of the impossibly onerous regulations dealing with personnel, purchasing, and central maintenance that local governments promulgate; setting up a special-purpose local government to operate the hospitals (a hospital district) would make management more financially responsible because it would have to be solvent, including perhaps raising its own capital funds through issuing bonds, and it also would be free of the general purpose local government's "red tape." The creation of a public benefit corporation, by special state charter, would again make management more financially responsible, and by making its charter require that it care for defined classes of medically indigent persons, the social mission of the public hospital would be safeguarded; and the merger of local public hospitals with local public health departments would provide both better public health and medical services by integrating the resources of the two local government agencies.

The greater financial responsibility that was expected to be forced on management by creation of either a special hospital district or a public benefit corporation was expected to follow from two circumstances. First, there would be no open-ended appeal for deficit appropriations to a city council or a county board of commissioners if the hospital expenditures exceeded its income, although the transfer agreement might include a preset fixed contribution by the local government to its operations. Second, if a hospital management were specially diligent and skillful in collecting its receivables it could keep the additional money collected instead of turning it over to the local government treasury's general fund. This, it was reasoned, would provide the incentive to make the strongest possible effort to collect the receivables instead of letting them slide. Although the fifth proposal is the only one that does not imply these "privatizing" or "operating like a private business" ideas, still, in most places where it was put forth it was presented as one that could produce more and better services without any additional money. Thus, this proposal, too, put the principal blame for the plight of the public hospital on organizational factors.

It should also be noted that each of the first four proposals calls to a lesser or greater degree for decreasing the direct responsibility for operation of the services by the local government. Only the last proposed solution predicates keeping the public hospital fully in the orbit of direct governmental control *and* ownership. The others all go in the direction of turning these hospitals over to control that is either private or that could be constrained to operate increasingly on a self-financing basis by reducing and even eliminating public contributions to the deficits in the future. It seems clear that forcing an institution serving the poor to rely more on "self-financing" must result in reducing services unless there really is a large amount of inefficiently used existing revenue (i.e., "fat").

Another force driving the transfer of ownership of the local public hospital away from local government was found to be the need for new and enlarged old medical schools for more teaching facilities and patients to meet the requirements of expanded enrollments. A number of public hospitals that were taken over by private organizations were given to medical schools, and one study (Koleda and Craig, 1976) found that all the public hospitals that were taken over by a private organization were in the vicinity of a medical school that needed them, and that no public hospital, no matter how troubled, was taken over if there were no such "needy" medical schools in the area.

Two of these solutions underwent prolonged trial—the affiliation plan (number 1) in New York City, and two different versions of the merger plan (number 5), one in Denver and the other in Los Angeles County. The experiences are interesting to compare since the affiliation type of solution is an example of weakening local government control and going in a more "private" direction, while the merger type exemplifies attempts to strengthen the institution by enhancing government input and control. The Denver experience, in particular, provides an example of an extensive effort to overhaul the public hospital via the latter approach, an effort that largely succeeded in achieving an integrated merger. The case of Los Angeles County provides an example of a large system situated in an area that grew into a true urban megalopolis only after World War II. The effort to improve the public hospital's services by merger was much more cautious and tentative than the Denver action and did not succeed in achieving a highly integrated merger. The differences in outcome between Denver and Los Angeles County are interesting and instructive.

An Experience with Affiliation—The New York City Hospital System

As of 1967, the New York City hospital system consisted of twenty-one hospitals operated by the Department of Hospitals,[12] which had been organized in 1929 after having been split off from the Health Department. The twenty-one hospitals

included seven major hospital centers which incorporate some special institutions within them and seven individual general care hospitals, three separate special institutions (cancer, chronic care, nursing). In 1965, there were about 5.2 million patient days (A.D.C. = 14,246) in 18,373 hospital beds and about 750,000 patient days of home care. There were also more than 3.2 million clinic visits.

These figures reflect the high per capita public expenditure for personal health care in New York City compared with the rest of the country. In 1961, it was $227 for New York City, with 30 percent coming from local taxes, compared with $146 nationally, of which 18.5 percent came from local taxes. The New York City government was directly providing the most hospital beds per capita and also the greatest public financial contribution per capita for private hospital care of all the large cities in the United States. Furthermore, the definition of medical indigency was set at a comparatively liberal level, so that only 20 percent of those receiving free City medical care was on welfare; the rest were not indigent—only medically indigent. In addition, the City had for many years had an arrangement whereby City patients were cared for in "City beds" of voluntary hospitals and their hospitalization charged to the City. Still further, the City was rich in medical teaching and research resources: it had, in 1960, seven medical schools and a large number of major research and teaching institutions of world renown. The City had many groups of citizens concerned with and organizationally involved in social betterment activity, and this activity had not ignored the muncipal hospitals.

Citizen social welfare reform groups, such as the Citizens Committee for Children and the Community Council, civil rights organizations, and low-income neighborhood groups have been deeply concerned with municipal hospitals. Taxpayers' groups such as the Citizen Budget Commission have demanded more efficiency in these City operations. Philanthropic and religious groups and the insurance plans, especially the voluntary ones such as Blue Cross, are especially concerned about increasing the City payments to, and decreasing the costs of, voluntary hospitals. And, in a city where the municipal hospitals play such a prominent part in the total medical care picture, they become deeply ingrained as a concern of the general population.

And yet public dissatisfaction with the care provided in these municipal hospitals continued to mount despite the relative generosity of New York City, the abundance of health care personnel and facilities in the City, and the active concern of its citizens. By 1960, the situation had become acute. A confluence of the problems specific to the municipal hospitals with those facing the medical care delivery system nationally and the New York City private voluntary hospitals locally seemed to point to the affiliation scheme as a natural solution. Again, Burlage has described this confluence clearly and well:

As neighborhoods changed from mixed income to poor ghetto, the density of institutional demand in-

creased but the hospitals had more difficulty finding medical staffs in their service areas. As more young doctors' career patterns shifted to specialities and super-specialties, the less advanced teaching hospitals were less professionally appealing. Since physicians could not treat their own private patients in the municipal hospitals and City sessional fees were very low, there was no direct economic incentive. The areas with the hard-core problems of poverty were seen by many physicians as unfathomable jungles, professionally and socially. The ghettos of poverty were becoming ghettos of medicine, except for the juttings of super-specialized centers seeking only a sample of "interesting cases." . . .

Some [municipal] hospitals faced even the loss of accreditation by the Joint Commission on the Accreditation of Hospitals; one actually had lost it. Threatened or actually ended were training program certifications in a number of specialties and even internship training programs were lost in some.

Harsh questions were being asked by the press and by citizen and medical groups about the quality of care in jammed and chaotic clinics, wards, and emergency rooms with treatment procedural difficulties and highly fragmented organization.

Voluntary Hospital Difficulties: At the same time the voluntary hospitals of the city had also faced great difficulties. Some of the smaller ones had been forced to close and others were threatened. Voluntary hospitals' financial condition had deteriorated, especially for capital expansion (p. 34).

Also, beginning with 1950 increased unionization of hospital employees had begun to create strong pressure for increased salary costs.

In 1960, Dr. Ray E. Trussell, of the School of Hospital Administration at Columbia University, proposed and widely publicized a plan of affiliation between the municipal hospitals and voluntary medical centers that could be expected to benefit both groups. Under this plan, the City would pay a number of prestigious medical teaching institutions to each adopt a municipal hospital, with such an arrangement being made for all municipal hospitals needing it. The teaching medical center would share its full-time teaching chiefs with the affiliated municipal hospital, thereby increasing the latter's prestige and consequent ability to attract high-quality house staff. In addition, the voluntary institution would rotate its own interns and residents through the municipal hospital, thus further improving its services. This arrangement would help the participating private teaching institutions by injecting City money into their depleted coffers and providing them with access to large quantities of "teaching material." The New York City government was convinced of the worth of this plan, and in 1961 Dr. Trussell was appointed Commissioner of Hospitals and charged with effectuating it. During his four-year tenure, implementation of the affiliation process was energetically pursued, and by 1965 ten of the eleven previously unaffiliated municipal general hospitals had been affiliated with voluntary teaching hospitals, some of which were in turn affiliated with medical schools. Since six of the municipal hospitals (four general and two cancer) already had affiliations with medical schools and leading hospitals predating the initiation of the "new" affiliation policy in 1961, the ten additional hospitals affiliated during the 1961–65 period brought to sixteen the number of municipal hospitals affiliated by 1965. These included all general municipal hospitals but one (Sydenham).

The impact of these affiliations upon the quality and quantity of the service provided by the municipal hospitals became the subject of numerous surveys, evaluations, and other writings. Two of the more comprehensive studies, expressing distinctly different views of the outcomes, are sketched in the following paragraphs.

Evaluative Studies of the Affiliation Plan: The Piel Report (1969) A report by a commission on the delivery of personal health services found that, after six years of affiliation, patient care was generally still of poor quality, both inpatient and outpatient. This was attributed almost entirely to an insufficient financial effort on the part of the City. The basic thrust of the recommendations was that the Affiliation Plan approach was entirely correct in concept, requiring only more City money to make the City hospitals replicas of the prestigious private teaching hospitals. This view is revealing of some of the tenets held as axioms by most of the Commission membership, many of whom were representative of humanitarian, liberal, and philanthropic segments of powerful community leadership. Their view of good medical care for low-income groups was formed by their association with prestigious medical researchers and specialty luminaries. The general recommendation underlying all the specific recommendations was that the only way to provide good medical care for the low-income population of New York City was to provide access for all to high-level teaching hospitals. The City should pay for whatever the academic medical leadership considered necessary to operate the public medical services like they ran their units in the private teaching centers.

This formulation implied that access to sophisticated services operating on the frontiers of medical knowledge was the top priority of medical care for the poor. It failed to strongly address the needs for routine primary care, preventive services, and access to good community hospitals that were priorities for ghetto dwellers and low-income persons generally. And it did not address the fact that many poor persons needed social support services in order to be able to benefit from the medical care they required, a point by now familiar to us from the deinstitutionalization story. And, crucially important, the Commission apparently had no inkling of what their recommendations might lead to in the way of costs.

Evaluative Studies of the Affiliation Plan: The Burlage Study (1967) The conclusions of this study were rather different from those of the Piel Commission. Because the Piel report was the product of staff work and input from a commission of citizens with varied views and interests, one might therefore tend a priori to credit it with greater objectivity than the work of a single investigator. But the differences between the two evaluations have more to do with differences in viewpoint than with different degrees of objectivity. The facts that both reports cite seem objectively reported, but each chose to stress different facts and to interpret the same facts differently. For example, both the Piel report and the Burlage study recommended complete reorganization of the City's health services under a central health administration and a regionalized plan for medical care that would:

1. Establish a network of primary care centers clustered about community hospitals which, in turn, would be clustered about a teaching hospital.
2. Reintegrate community physicians into hospital staff.
3. Use public and private facilities in tandem but under strict accountability to government

auditing, both as to expenditures and services, with all arrangements to be made public.
4. All such arrangements were to be made to fit
an overall plan arrived at by City planning
bodies.

Despite the apparent similarities in the recommendations, however, the emphasis in the
two reports was different, with the priorities being increased support for high technology in the
Piel report, and outreach and neighborhood clinics in the Burlage recommendations.[13] The writing of Burlage contributes to our understanding
of aspects of the functioning of the Affiliation
Plan that are absent from the Piel Report. It is
useful to counterbalance the viewpoint of academic medicine, which informs the delibera-
tions of most blue-ribbon bodies like the Piel
Commission despite the inclusion of representatives from other societal sectors, with the
wider view of the social scientist and social
commentator who attempts to answer the basic
question: "Why did the apparently bright promise of the plan fall so far short of its goals?"

In Robert Burlage's analysis of the dynamics
of the implementation of the affiliation plan in
1961, the new health commissioner, Dr. Ray
Trussell, is seen as working with the major philanthropic leadership of the city (what he called
"the corporate voluntarists") and the leading
medical specialists in the teaching hospitals and
medical schools ("the patricians") to weaken or
even end the influence of the local privately
practicing physicians who were the part-time
teachers and the medical leaders of many New
York City hospitals ("the practitioners"). This
move was part of the actions flowing from the
overriding priority accorded to upgrading high
technology to the neglect of everyday care and
outreach. Burlage's main findings were that:

1. The large new City expenditures brought increases
in the quantity and certified quality of physician staffing available and relieved some major physician staffing crises. The needed depth, actual service time, appropriate integration, and community outreach of
these new skills were usually not achieved.

2. The new research environment had mixed effects,
at best, on patient care. New major equipment items
bolstered a number of programs but in an uneven and
often unplanned fashion. An uneven and uncorrected

distribution of new and expanded programs was developed at different affiliated hospitals, most of them
concentrated on the inpatient environment or on specialized, research-connected clinic programs.

3. Some loose general indices of hospital program
improvement and of quality of care—autopsy percentages, prenatal care neglect, death rate—have
shown quite generally mixed and in some cases
deeply disappointing results.

Burlage thus implied that the New York City
experience with the Affiliation Plan indicated
that supervising the delivery of day-to-day
health care to a disadvantaged and weakly empowered target population is not the strong point
of the teaching hospital and medical school and
their leading personnel.

Further light upon the difficulties encountered
in attempting to implement the affiliation program is cast by two administrative officials of
the New York Municipal Hospital System, who
stated that "The limitations of the affiliation
programs were evident almost immediately. The
City found it impossible to respond properly to
the demanding needs [by the teaching hospitals]
for space, facilities, technical personnel and, indeed, materials" (Terenzio and Manning, 1970).
Within five years, many of the municipal hospitals were committing as much as 40 percent of
their budget to expenditures by the affiliated
medical school or hospital.

The affiliation program started with one hospital and
a $3 million annual expenditure in 1961; by 1967, it
had grown to 15 hospitals and a $130 million hospital
system. . . . Attempts to circumvent the city's administrative machinery through the use of affiliation controls brought abour major conflicts involving the Department of Hospitals, labor unions, the affiliates, and
officials of city government (Terenzio and Manning,
1970).

At the end of the 1960s the City resorted to
another of the principal solutions then in vogue
in addition to the affiliation plan—the public
benefit corporation alternative (number 4). In
1969, the state legislature established the New
York City Health and Hospitals Corporation
(HHC) to replace New York City's Department
of Hospitals. This public benefit corporation assumed administration of all municipal hospital
facilities in the summer of 1970 and was to be
"free of operational participation by City over-

head agencies." Its aim, according to the enabling act, was to establish a system "permitting legal, financial and managerial flexibility for provision and delivery of high quality, dignified and comprehensive care and treatment for the ill and infirm, particularly those who can least afford such services" (Isaacs, Lichter, and Lipschultz, 1982)[14] The agency's board of sixteen directors was given governing authority over twelve municipal hospitals with some 8,000 beds and a service spectrum ranging from long-term hospitals to emergency medical services. In addition, the agency was given authority over twenty-nine satellite ambulatory care clinics and four neighborhood family-care centers of the public health department with the aim of combining the primary-care clinics of the public health department with the inpatient and specialist backup available through the inpatient beds and outpatient clinics of the public hospital. Billing, accounting, purchasing, and financial planning as well as all reimbursement activities were assigned to the corporation. Service affiliations with teaching institutions were also continued, so that the public hospitals of New York City were now using three of the five types of solutions listed on page 222: affiliation contracts, (number 1) the creation of a public benefit corporation (number 4), and elements of the "merger" solution (number 5).

The results of these reorganizations as of 1980 showed little evidence of having "solved" or very materially improved the public hospitals' serious problems. The system was still underfunded and under constant criticism. It had had "seven HHC board chairpersons, three HHC presidents, two task forces, and one special assistant for health. Every HHC president has either been dismissed or forced to resign" (Isaacs, Lichter, and Lipschultz, 1982). A comprehensive and objective evaluation of the effects of the HHC system in some depth has been hard to come by. The assertions in defense of the HHC voiced by the corporation itself argued that management improvements producing efficiencies had indeed been made. Even if they were not clearly visible, without these improvements the condition of the hospitals would have been much worse given the national deterioration of the large public urban hospitals during those years. They also cited a 25 percent reduction in

beds between 1970 and 1981 with only a .4 percent reduction in the number of patients served, due to a reduction in length of stay resulting from "better management," and improvement in nurse staffing due to better personnel practices. Critics of the corporation noted that the system was still overspending its budget, that the board was not independent of the City government but was "directly controlled by the mayor [resulting] in poor quality care, mounting deficits and costly decisions involving the location and design of new facilities and the closing of old ones. . . . " (Health Policy Advisory Center as cited in Isaacs, Lichter, and Lipschultz, 1982). In addition to the rate of turnover of top staff and governance, the reductions in staff and resources were constantly attacked by employee organizations, consumer advocate and left publications, and academic writers as evidence of continuing poor governance and lack of independence from City pressures to cut services. One thing is certain: New York City put more money and effort into trying to improve its public hospital system than any other place in the United States, yet there is no clear evidence that use of the affiliation plan, the public benefit Corporation, and a very weak version of the merger plan, introduced cumulatively and applied together, succeeded in substantially solving the "plight" of the City's public hospitals.

An Experience with a Fully Implemented Merger: The Denver Department of Health Services

The Denver experience with the merger (number 5) solution to the plight of the large urban public hospital is of particular interest because it is a case of the merger plan apparently successfully implemented and maintained over a period of years. In 1963, Denver's municipal hospital, Denver General Hospital, found itself in dire straits.[15] Its dilapidated buildings were beyond practical repair, its ties with the University of Colorado medical school had been severed, and it was being proposed that the City discontinue its relationship with the public hospital and have its functions transferred to the Colorado Medical Center, i.e., that a "divestiture" solution (number 2) be tried. The question of retaining full City control of the public hospital became an election issue in the mayoralty race, which the candidate favoring retention of the hospital won. In 1964 the new municipal administration, fortified by the passage of a bond issue to build a new hospital, started a restructuring of municipal medical care services.

The Denver Department of Health and Hospitals had already been formed by amalgamating the two previously separate Health and Charities Department and the Hospital Department in 1950, but this largely pro forma merger was what one writer on organizational matters has called a "loosely coupled" consolidation (Weick, 1962) denoting a union of public organizations that is only weakly integrated. The Denver merger described here is not the original loosely coupled union established by law in 1950, but rather the implementation of a policy to turn that nominal merger (enunciated policy) into a firmly coupled merger in the 1960s (actual or de facto policy). Beginning with 1964, the resources of the Health and Hospital Department were expanded and used to establish an integrated system comprising a network of comprehensive and satellite neighborhood health centers backed up by the resources of Denver General Hospital for specialty consultation and inpatient treatment.

The goal of the Denver health program since its inception has been to provide comprehensive, family-centered, continuous health care to low-income Denver residents in facilities that are conveniently located and that are staffed with indigenous personnel and with health professionals responsive to the patients' needs (Cowen, 1971).

The financing for expansion of resources was obtained by skillfully combining several federal grants, principally federal Neighborhood Health Center grants and National Institute of Mental Health grants for community mental health centers[16] (construction and initial staffing). Two large comprehensive neighborhood health centers and eight small satellite health stations had been established in the city by 1969, and with the completion of a new municipal hospital structure and the reestablishment of teaching affiliations with the University of Colorado Medical School, a basis for technical excellence was firmly established. The number of full-time staff physicians at Denver General rose from ten to

forty-seven during 1965–1970. The main difference between the arrangements made with the medical school in Denver and those made by New York City in its affiliation program was that managerial control of all operations was kept firmly in the City Department's hands. Cowen felt this to be a crucial point if such an arrangement is to result in better patient care.

[H]iring and firing of all staff (including professional personnel) must be retained by the health care delivery agency . . . professional standards must meet or exceed those of any medical school. . . . Such standards and hiring practices will permit a strong patient care orientation which is necessary to develop a program that is acceptable to the community; a program that is professional, cost-effective, and is still a fine teaching environment (1971).

The financing mechanism required to institute and operate an integrated total system by using funds from a number of different categorical grants was not a simple matter of merely using the different financing and reporting arrangements of all the separate categorical programs to pay bills. That would have resulted in an accounting system, and especially a disbursing system, consisting of a myriad of different closing dates, different accounting and statistical criteria, separate personnel systems, and many other differing operational modes that were not sufficiently compatible to permit the efficient running of an integrated system. The agency's heads battled and negotiated tirelessly with HEW to issue a waiver permitting a consolidated grant constituting the total of all the categorical health funds to which Denver was entitled that could be used as a single pot of money, and in 1973 the Department of Health and Hospitals "obtained a HEW agreement . . . to award a consolidated grant, the first of its kind in the United States" (Isaacs, Lichter, and Lipschultz, 1982). By the early 1970s, Denver was widely perceived as having instituted a public system of direct health services of low-income persons that was coordinated, comprehensive, and of good quality. However, the financial underpinning of much of the program was based on federal grant-in-aid programs whose support the Nixon administration was attempting to cut. At first the financial difficulties that the federal fund reductions would have caused were averted by increased funding from the city and the state. "In 1971, federal grants accounted for 43 percent of the total budget of $29 million. By 1974, federal aid had decreased to 22 percent of a $40 million budget. . . . With federal funds for health declining, the City of Denver assumed a greater share of the burden. . . . The city's contribution rose from $11.4 million in 1969 to a high of $18.6 million in 1972. . . . " (Price and Cohn, 1978). When the city's share begain to decline, the state of Colorado increased its support. The state's special medical indigency (MI) program, passed in 1975, allocated about 90 percent of its funds for acute care directly to the Denver Health and Hospitals (DHH) program rather than for payments to the private sector.

Another factor that helped maintain financial support for the DHH was the fact that Colorado's expenditures for acute indigent medical care were never as heavily channeled through Medicaid as in some other states and therefore were directed less to the private sector. Established in 1969, the Colorado Medicaid program limited eligibility to the minimum required classes of person (see Chapter 10), excluding virtually all but the mandatory recipients of federally subsidized cash assistance income support from its acute-care benefits. Other persons who needed help paying for medical care were assisted by the state's medical indigency program, but most of its money was also funneled through the Denver Department of Health and Hospitals. In contrast, in 1976 only about 5 percent of the money spent by Medicaid in Colorado went to DHH. Most Medicaid money went to private providers. Medicaid funds made up only 12 percent of the total revenues of DHH in 1981 (McGeary et al., 1982). In the same year "half of DHH's patients qualified for the MI program" (McGeary et al., 1982).

The ability of the City of Denver to maintain its relative generosity toward its public health care system was aided by its continual annexation of newly developed adjoining areas, which helped prevent the loss of the middle-class tax base from the city. The ability to annex contiguous towns in the expanding suburban fringe came to an end, however, with the passage of the Poundstone amendment to the state constitution in 1974. With further annexation of suburban territory prohibited, the problem of local financial support for health services became increasingly serious as the limitations of the Denver tax base began to more closely resemble those of other large cities. At first the state MI program, originally passed as part of the political compromise entailed in support for the Poundstone amendment, helped make up for the erosion of the local tax base. In 1977, however, an annual limit on increased state spending was imposed by state law and "the recession . . . cut tax receipts significantly while increasing welfare expenditures, and there have been no [State] surpluses for [local] tax relief in 1982 or 1983" (McGeary, et al., 1982). The City of Denver was also adversely affected by the recession, especially the reduction in revenues from its sales tax (its principal tax), so that other tax rates had to be raised. Despite the turn to more vigorous billing and collections from patients and third parties by DHH, its cost to the City rose sharply in 1981, and sharp cuts in services and personnel were imposed by the mayor in June of that year as well as in the 1982 budget. The main impact of these cuts was on general outpatient and community mental health services. Other reductions involved dental, nutrition, and social services, "thus drastically changing the shape as well as the level of services in the NHP [Neighborhood Health Program—the ambulatory care centers]. . . . Services of Denver General—emergency, ambulatory, and inpatient—were virtually untouched" (McGeary et al., 1982).

The Denver experience provides a good example, perhaps the best one, of a merger of the public hospital with other local governmental health agencies (particularly the health department) to provide a comprehensive system of medical care for the poor. A number of aspects of this experience are particularly instructive. One is that this solution entailed managerial and organizational changes to improve the operations of the public hospital within the framework of maintaining full government operation and ownership, but these changes required having an adequate central fund for effectuating them. Furthermore, the changes did not involve improving the public hospital as a free-standing institution but rather transforming it into the inpatient and high-technology consulting backup component of an integrated health care system that was predominantly focused on delivery of primary care away from the hospital. This seems paradoxical on its face, but it is not. The main objection to the public hospital as the main source of medical care for poor persons is its characterization as a provider of second-class care. The "mainstream" paying patient gets most of his or her care in a doctor's office, with the hospital used only for inpatient and high-technology consulting backup. Furthermore, the paying patient receives her prenatal and postpartum care in the obstetrician's office and not in a hospital (or public health) clinic. Similarly, her children receive their preventive immunizations in the pediatrician's office. not in a hospital (or public health) clinic. The physicians she sees are in full-time practice with their training completed, not "students" (interns and residents). These features and a number of other similar ones were incorporated in the Denver Neighborhood Health Program. They were implemented in the course of a long, bitter, and skillfully conducted struggle by the builders of the system to force all moneys from categorical grants into a common pool and to run the system like a good HMO with services attuned to patient needs on an integrated basis. However, the failure to duplicate this system elsewhere points to the uniqueness of the circumstances allowing it to happen and suggests that it could not become a general occurrence without basic changes in national governmental policies. The nature and causes of the ultimate decline of its local funding base strongly corroborate this supposition.

An Experience with a Partially Implemented Merger: The Los Angeles County Department of Health Services

The public hospitals of Los Angeles County constitute a third example of the attempts to solve the problems of the large public urban hospital—again by merger (number 5). Los Angeles County is much larger and more populous than Denver, with 7 1/2 million persons compared with Denver's 700,000. It is more akin to New York City in population size. But many of the specific conditions prevailing in this system were quite different from, and the problems less acute than, those in the New York City hospital system as it faced the 1970s. The Los Angeles

system had for many years maintained a de facto and later a de jure affiliation with a major medical school and had more recently affiliated with a second one. It was better funded than most public hospitals in urban areas, and had had little difficulty in obtaining quality house staff. Yet dissatisfaction with the care given patients had been expressed repeatedly by the house staff and by some community groups (Los Angeles Times, 1970; Times Picayune, 1969, 1970).

Background of the Two Merging Agencies The Los Angeles County public hospitals, located in a county that was largely rural until World War II, represent a prototype of the origins and development of such hospitals in areas that only developed into megalopolises after World War II. Over the period during and shortly after World War II its population more than doubled, and much of the county that had been rural became urbanized or suburbanized. The need for comprehensive public health services, including publicly provided health care in the rapidly urbanizing areas, began to take on the characteristics and magnitude of the needs in the older urbanized areas of the country, and pressure began to build for some revamping of existing services to make them more comprehensive and of greater depth countywide.

Like most other county hospitals, those in this system had evolved from the alsmhouse and poor farm whose inmates were mostly ill. The California Poor Law of 1855 encouraged some counties to establish county hospitals by offering state grants-in-aid, and in 1903 jurisdiction over the county hospitals in California was placed under a State Board of Charities and Correction after

a survey found that the sick poor of five counties were still cared for on a contract basis although this policy had been condemned as early as 1874 by the State Board of Health and had been prohibited by the County Government Act of 1897. The Board reported in 1908 that many County hospitals were still 'only poor poorhouses' and recommended standards for their operation.''. . . . By 1934 the wealthier counties in the state had segregated the able-bodied aged from the sick and placed them on a county farm or in a home, while in the less affluent counties the county hospital [still] served both as a home for the aged poor and as a hospital for the sick (Stern, 1946).

Thus, the establishment of county hospitals in California, as in some other parts of the country, was substantially motivated by humanitarian considerations to provide a special place for treating people who were physically ill, in much the same way the mental hospital had originally been intended to provide "moral treatment" for the mentally ill. In 1937, Section 17000 of the state's Welfare and Institutions Code mandated the counties to "relieve and support all incompetent, poor, indigent persons, and those incapacitated by age, disease, or accident." California law also authorized the board of supervisors (which served as the executive as well as legislative body) of each county to establish and maintain a county hospital, and most of California's fifty-eight counties chose to establish county hospitals as their way of meeting the obligations under Section 17000 (Roemer and Shonick, 1980). By 1960 there were sixty-six county hospitals in California located in forty-nine of the fifty-eight counties. The nine counties with no county hospital had very small populations.

Events Leading to the Merger The California law[17] under which the state elected to enter the Medicaid program (called "MediCal" in California) provided that counties could opt to be reimbursed by the state for all future increases over its 1964–1965 net costs for treating persons in county or contract hospitals. The state thus assumed the rise in net costs of county hospitals, and the Los Angeles County government saw it as an opportunity to expand its medical care services into a unified system. If the Public Health Department's local health centers were made an integral part of a single county system along with the county hospitals, the argument could be made that the cost of upgrading the personal health services of the fifty-odd local public health centers to full-scale ambulatory primary care centers was really part of upgrading the outpatient services of the county hospitals and therefore should be met by the state under the 1965 "county option" law.

Formulating county legislation to effect such a merger was facilitated by two previous reorganizations, which had established a larger countywide public health department and an in-

dependent county hospital department. A reorganization in 1964 had merged the comparatively small County Public Health Department[18] with the larger and previously independent Los Angeles City Public Health Department, and a 1966 an amendment to the Los Angeles County charter split up the Department of Charities, which had been administering the hospitals since about 1850, into separate Departments of Public Social Services, Hospitals, and Adoptions. The County now had a large unified public health department with a large independent department of hospitals to match, making it administratively straightforward to draft an ordinance merging the two into a single countywide health services department if the political circumstances were favorable.

By 1972, the County Department of Hospitals was operating eight hospitals and a number of special centers and bureaus that operated special programs. Of the eight hospitals, three were acute general hospitals, each affiliated with a major medical school, and five were special hospitals providing rehabilitation and other types of postacute care both on an inpatient and outpatient basis. Although Los Angeles County also had contracts with private hospitals for the care of indigent patients, the contracted services were limited to initial emergency care; after stabilization the patient was moved to a county facility and the public facilities were heavily overtaxed. There had been many instances of well-publicized complaints about the serious problems of inaccessibility of the main acute facilities and outpatient clinics that served enormous geographic areas. New York City, with a much smaller area, had twenty-one municipal hospitals, many of them with large primary-care centers. By comparison there were only three copmrehensive primary medical care centers in Los Angeles county, one of which had only opened in 1972. If one could convert most of the fifty public health neighborhood centers to provide general ambulatory medical care, and if these centers could be integrated with the hospitals in a referral network, it seemed reasonable that access to ambulatory care would be materially improved.

The technical facilitation of a merger act by the prior reorganizations, the mounting pressure on ambulatory facilities, and especially the promise of financial support implied by the county-option law all combined to point to a merger-type reorganization as a solution. This was not lost on the affected policymakers. A county-sponsored program review of the County Public Health Department by a consulting group of the American Public Health Association had taken place in 1969, and among its recommendations were that closer liaison between the public health department and the department of hospitals be developed. An ad hoc committee of local experts, known as the Bauer Commission after its chairman, also issued a report calling for closer organizational ties between the two departments to improve the provision of integrated health services. While not recommending a detailed plan for implementing such integration, the Bauer Commission recommended that the overall goal of the reorganization be to end "fragmentation" of personal health services by combining the departments of mental health, public health, and hospitals. The objective of the merger should be the creation of an integrated, community-based, personal health care delivery system, regionalized by geographic area, and including hospital-linked neighborhood health centers, specialty clinics, and hospitals. After much political maneuvering,[19] the Departments of Hospitals, Health, and Mental Health (as well as the 23 person staff Public Health Veterinary Department) of the County of Los Angeles were legally merged to form the Los Angeles Department of Health Service (DHS) in October 1972.

The Merger Experience The main aims of the new structure were twofold. First, the neighborhood facilities provided by the more than fifty health department centers would be used to strengthen the outreach of the county's medical services and improve their accessibility to its clients. Second, the expertise, personnel, and facilities of the hospitals would be used to provide these neighborhood health centers with the inpatient and specialist outpatient resources required to operate a full spectrum of medical care services. The plan proposed dividing the county into five semiautonomous regions with each regional directorship responsible for providing a wide range of health care to residents of the region.

However, the passage of the merger decree was almost simultaneous with the beginning of a trend in California state policy to reduce state support for county health services. The state "county option" law of 1966, which had been expected to finance much of the cost of the reorganization and expansion of services, had been repealed by the 1971 MediCal Reform Act, passed at the initiative of the then Governor Reagan. To compensate for the loss of state payments to counties for expanding their publicly provided direct health care systems under this law, a new class of eligibles for MediCal (called medically Indigent Adults–MIA–), for whom there was no federal cost participation, was established. However, the counties were required to pay about half the state's share of MediCal costs in California[20], and now not only did Los Angeles County find itself committed to supporting an expanded county health system at the same time that its expected resources were reduced by the ending of the state "county option" subsidy, it also faced additional demands on the county budget by the state to help for the MIA-fueled increase in MediCal utilization, much of it with private providers. Also in 1972, the state made retrenchments in payments to the counties for helping to pay for local health services that were in addition to the ending of the "county option."[21] As a result, while total gross expenditures of Los Angeles County for health care services rose 150 percent between 1969 and 1976, the county costs net of state reimbursement rose almost 270 percent. Local taxes in Los Angeles County, especially the property tax, were bearing an increasing share of the burden of financing local health expenditures. By 1976 health service costs in Los Angeles County were consuming 42 percent of county tax dollars compared with 24 percent in 1968.

The financial bind in which the county found itself was perhaps the major cause of the severe strains and stresses suffered by the newly merged organization during the crucial early implementation period. These worked to tear it apart. The Department of Health Services became a principal target of some of the county supervisors as they viewed with dismay the newly adopted responsibilities in face of sharply reduced state funding. There was constant harassment and public criticism from some supervisors of the department's operations as being inefficient and ineffective. The all-important element of strong political support from the local government that played so important a part in allowing the public system to develop its merger in Denver was clearly lacking. In its place was a constant stream of hostility. Public criticism from the press, community groups, and hospital house staff was also widespread.

While these external pressures were likely the more serious ones working against a successful transformation of the formal merger into an actual working system, there were also significant internal pressures operating to weaken the implementation of the merger. Chief among these was strong staff resistance to the merger, especially from public health and mental health personnel. The leading personnel of these formerly separate agencies had opposed the merger during the period when it was being negotiated and consequently the major staff participants in the preliminary planning for the merger had been personnel of the former department of hospitals. As was to be expected, when the merger was decreed hospital administrators dominated the leadership of the merged agency—in particular, the director of the consolidated agency was a hospital administrator. The public health professionals were disgruntled and pointed to the lack of knowledge of public health issues on the part of the top administrators of the Department of Health Services. Both public health and mental health personnel objected to what they felt was an unduly large share of the agency's total resources going to the hospitals. In 1972, 80 percent of the budget and some 85 percent of the personnel went to the hospitals. Public health and mental health administrators who had been in prestigious positions in the former separate health agencies now found themselves with greatly reduced influence and overshadowed by a new breed of administrators who were often schooled only in public administration or management theory.[22] The resistance was evident not only in a lack of enthusiasm for proposals and instructions emanating from central administration; it also occasionally surfaced as active

resistance that sought the aid of local government officials and members of the county commissions.[23]

Each of the previously independent county departments had had its own citizens' advisory commission. These were not abolished and replaced by a single DHS commission in the merger reorganization. Attempts to consolidate the commissions were impeded largely by the fact that they were an important source of political patronage in Los Angeles County. They were kept on as separate commissions and lobbied for larger shares of the total merged agency's resources for their own divisional constituencies. The public health commission (a weak analogue of a model board of public health), for example, echoed the viewpoint of top public health staff that the hospitals were using funds that belonged to public health. Over time, these views led to an increasingly overt stance by both the public health and mental health commissions favoring withdrawal from the merger. The mental health professionals, in addition to their complaints about not receiving their fair share of resources also objected to what they saw as an increasing imposition of the "medical model" on mental health services. They attributed much of this to the domination of the department's administration by hospital people.

In 1975, only three years after the merger had been enacted, the Board of Supervisors adopted a motion to reexamine the value of the merger but decided after much discussion and investigation by staff of the DHS and other county administrative offices to continue it. However, in April 1978 mental health was separated from the merged department and reconstituted as a separate department. Later the merger between public health and the hospitals was partially uncoupled by putting the free-standing ambulatory centers under the public health structure with the hospital outpatient services under hospitals, and the hospitals thereafter operating more as loosely affiliated parts of a separate hospital department. The Department of Health Services became more akin to a loosely coupled organization than an integrally merged public health/public hospital system.

Thus, Los Angeles county's experience with merger was not a fully successful one in setting up a publicly provided medical care system with widely accessible and comprehensive personal services, integrated horizontally across types of services (such as pediatrics, internal medicine, etc.) and with services coordinated vertically up and down the functional ladder from preventive personal services to tertiary care and long-term care. A systemwide comprehensive ambulatory service system had not been fully launched by 1978, and meaningful integration of free-standing primary care service with hospital backing had not been achieved. The strains on the system tore it apart before it could be substantially implemented. Why was the experience different from Denver?

The primary factor in the Los Angeles experience was the fact that the merger came too late. The funds to implement it would probably have been available during 1967–1971, but sufficiently strong sentiment and forces for decreeing a merger and building a unified system by pooling all available funds were lacking in Los Angeles County during these years. The County is geographically very much larger than Denver and at that time had about four times as many people. This by itself was a factor. More to the point, however, Denver entered the 1960s with a pro forma merger already in place, a new leadership of the merged department that had a strongly held vision of what a good medical care system should be like, local government prepared to support its decisions, and during a period when the system of state grants was in full flower. The public hospital was in disarray, with a weak leadership with its teaching affiliations being monitored for quality, and the public health department was even weaker, having been the subject of special APHA efforts to upgrade it. Thus the Denver Department of Health and Hospitals had little internal opposition from professional public health and public health leaders fighting to protect their turf, nor did they have to face opposition from medical school teaching chiefs who saw the public hospital primarily as a source of teaching material. The builders of the Neighborhood Health Program in Denver were able to pool their categorical grants, overriding whatever categorically minded leadership in public health opposed it; make the ambulatory system the center of the services with the hospital as backup, overriding

opposition, either actual or latent, from powerful hospital and medical school teaching chiefs; and get substantial city and state financial support. However, it should be noted that when Federal and especially state financing diminished, the system deteriorated.

In contrast, almost all these factors were reversed in Los Angeles. The organization of publicly delivered direct health services before 1964 had consisted of the typically separate county health department whose jurisdiction lay outside the large cities; the city health department in the big cities of the county that were independent of the county health department; and a county department of charities that had authority over the public hospitals. The long process, begun in 1964, of formally unifying the county's health services did not end until 1972. This process was carried out in the face of health department leadership strongly organized along categorical lines and public hospital leadership strongly tied to medical school teaching leadership. Neither of these groups had a strong positive vision of an integrated public service system along Denver lines. The process of merely achieving formal unification in the face of all that had to be done used up all the valuable time during which liberal state funding was available. And during all this time there was no single agency that could even attempt to pool categorical funds even if that had been desirable. With the enactment of the merger, the implementation process began with the expected increase in state funding being eliminated and the surfacing of internal disagreement among professionals that impeded any true pooling of available funds to build a unified system.

Thus, the experiences with affiliation indicated that technical excellence in the form of medical school hegemony over the program was not the answer to the plight of the public hospital. A merged public health/public hospital system was shown to be a good answer in one place, but the conditions needed to establish it suggest that a Denver solution would be impossible as a general solution under existing conditions. Comparing the Denver and Los Angeles county experience, the possibility of establishing a merged public system seemed to depend on the availability of increased local, state and federal funding; a local government that actively supported the idea; a relatively weak public health department, public hospital, and medical school influence; and skillful executive leadership. The leadership would have to be dedicated to the idea of an integrated service, with a vision not restricted to one or another specialized aspect of health service provision and knowledgeable in the issues of health provision policy. A reading of these prerequisites clearly indicates how unlikely it was and is that they will be found to exist in many other places, in fact, even in one other place. If such systems were to come into being in many places they would need strong state or federal support to provide at least some of the prerequisites, especially reliable funding. It should be noted that the oustanding elements of the Denver experiment did not survive the serious reduction in funding. The major difference between Los Angeles and Denver, then, may be that Denver had a grace period between setting the integrated merger into motion and the national funding decline whereas Los Angeles County did not.

Experiences with Outright Divestiture

All through the 1970s the problems that had been afflicting the large urban public hospital and some rural county hospitals continued and worsened. Underfunding remained endemic, service levels and quality continued to be deplorable, and duly deplored, and staffing problems continued (Los Angeles Times, 1970; Goldberg, 1972; Herald Traveler, 1970; Times-Picayune, 1972; Health Policy Advisory Center, 1973). While some local governments continued attempts to improve public health care services by merger, affiliating with prestigious teaching institutions, and tightened control, others were attempting to divest themselves of their public hospitals entirely, and many actually did so. The continuing cutbacks in Medicaid were a contributing cause of the financial distress of these hospitals. At the same time, private voluntary hospitals were experiencing a decline in occupancy rates for the first time since World War II. This may have contributed to the pressure to compete for Medicare and Medicaid patients and to a desire by the private hospitals to curtail the activities of the local public hospital. At any rate, there seemed to be pressure to close down public

hospitals of all sorts during the early 1970s, paralleling the closure of some state mental hospitals. The divestiture solution (number 2) came in several versions but all called for tranferring ownership of the hospital to other organizations such as medical schools, nonprofit community boards, and quasi-public organizations; or simply closing the hospital altogether. Divestiture was meant to answer the criticisms that the public hospital constituted the second and inferior track of a two-track system of care, on the one hand, and on the other, it was preferred by persons who opposed government operation of health care systems either on ideological grounds or simply to reduce the local government budget. Holders of both points of view felt that government "should not be in the hospital business." Some variants of divestiture called for a compensatory expansion by the local government of its other medical services activities, activities that did not involve owning or operating a public hospital. It might take the form of expanding the direct primary care services of the local government or paying for medical care for expanded classes of beneficiaries to nongovernment providers. Some other variants also required the organization taking over the public hospital to give some form of assurance that special attention would be given to accommodating poor patients, especially those for whom the county might be responsible. Many of these requirements were minimal and the provisions for enforcing them weak.

One of the best known trials of a compensatory variant of proposal number 2 was the so-called Project Health carried out in Multnomah County, Oregon.[24] In 1973, Multnomah County Hospital, located in Portland, Oregon, became a state-owned hospital attached to and operated by the University of Oregon medical school. The previous financial contribution by the county to the former local public hospital was combined with funds from other public sources and the total used to establish Project Health. The program helped to pay for health insurance for low-income persons not eligible for Medicaid.[25] Eligible persons who decided to enroll in Project Health could choose membership in a number of plans, ranging from prepaid plans of various types through an "episodic care program" under which enrolees could use private physicians and hospitals who were paid on a fee-for-service basis. The plan became fully operational in early 1976, and the financing, at its peak in 1980, came from the county (48 percent), a United States Public Health Service community health center grant (23 percent), federal and state Medicaid contributions under a special waiver arrangement (26 percent), client payments (2 percent), and provider refunds (1 percent). After 1980, funding sources atrophied as part of the general retrogression of government support.

By 1982, county funds accounted for fully 83 percent of the total budget, and these were 25 percent below 1981 levels. The program was left with three of its previous six provider choices as well as the episodic care program, which was rechristened "Multicare." Multicare differed from its predecessor episodic care program by confining the source of primary ambulatory care for its beneficiaries to county operated clinics and neighborhood health centers but continuing to pay for inpatient and speciality care from those private providers who agreed to sign contracts with the county.

It is interesting to note that both Project Health and the Denver Health and Hospitals Departments embarked on their expanded programs by pooling the funds from different granting sources into a single pot to run an integrated program. Denver used it to create a government-owned and -operated program and Multnomah to create what it called a "consumer choice" program. Actually, however, each program denied some choice to medically indigent persons: in Denver the eligible medically indigent population did not have Denver money available to use a private provider; in Multnomah County this population could not use a government-supported local public general hospital because there no longer was one. Both had to curtail program benefits when their funding sources atrophied, but Denver continued to have a public hospital and Multnomah County did not.

As has been noted, one of the developments motivating the adoption of the "noncompensatory" variant of divestiture—simply giving the public hospital away—was found to be the need of newly established as well as expanding old medical schools for more teaching facilities. I have referred to macro-type empirical evidence for this contention. Perhaps the most detailed ac-

count of one such closing is provided in the monograph by Edward Sparer (1974) that describes how the need for patients by the in-house medical practice of a prestigious medical school contributed to the decline in patient load and ultimate demise of Philadelphia's public hospital. In this case, the medical staffs of five medical schools were guiding and managing the medical services of Philadephia General Hospital under affiliation contracts with the city. Of these, the University of Pennsylvania was the most important. In the 1970s its teaching physicians, who were also serving at Philadelphia General, directed many public hospital patients to the medical school's Hospital of the University of Pennsylvania (HUP), because the medical practice groups at the medical school were suffering a drop in clientele. As the public hospital deteriorated more rapidly during the post–1970 period, partially as a result of such rerouting of patients, the diversion became increasingly more justified on the grounds of being in the patients' best interest, and subsequently the public hospital was closed because of insufficient utilization. The medical school practice of requiring that faculty members earn some or most of their salaries through their departmental practice was shown to have put pressure on them to maintain a high level of client patients in their medical school practices. The implication of Sparer's study is that a conflict of interest may be set up when these physicians have major administrative responsibilities over the medical program of a public hospital in the face of a declining patient load at their teaching institution.

In California, between 1970 and 1973, eight county hospitals closed or were being considering for closing, two had been transferred to university medical schools and one to a private corporation, and San Francisco General Hospital was being considered for transfer to a quasi-public corporation similar to the New York City operation (Health Policy Advisory Center, 1973). By 1980, there were only thirty-seven county hospitals left in California of the sixty-six that existed in 1960; only twenty-nine counties of the fifty-eight still had a county hospital, whereas in 1960 forty-nine counties had had at least one hospital.

Some other divestiture solutions were attempted in the 1960s: in 1968 Newark City Hospital was placed under the control of the New Jersey College of Medicine and Dentistry; in 1967 the King County Hospital of Seattle (Harborview) was placed under control of the University of Washington Medical School; and in 1962 the public hospital of Kansas City, Missouri, was put under the control of a public benefit corporation. Other instances can be cited (AHA, 1970).

Subsequent Developments

The Commission on Public-General Hospitals Report

By 1975, the organized hospital industry itself had become sufficiently concerned about the public hospital to establish a commission[26] to study the problem of the future of public hospitals. This Commission on Public-General Hospitals issued its report in 1978, *The Future of the Public-General Hospital: An Agenda for Transition,* with an accompanying volume of commissioned articles, *Readings on Public-General Hospitals.* The purview of the report was more extensive than that of this chapter and the definition of "public-general hospitals" was therefore correspondingly broader. Using AHA data, the Commission found that in 1975 there were 5,679 community hospitals[27] in the United States. Of these, 1,905, or 34 percent, were publicly owned[28], i.e., public-general hospitals. The Commission classified them into four types— university, urban, other metropolitan, and rural (see Table 7–2). Of these 1,905 public-general hospitals, 90 were defined as urban public-general hospitals. Their average bed size was 503, more than four times the average bed size of all public-general hospitals. This "urban public-general" type is the major focus of this chapter. In 1975, counties operated 26 of them, 27 were operated by cities, and 19 were operated by hospital authorities or districts. They were located in 63 of the 100 largest cities in the country and "by tradition . . . serve many patients who have no other source of financing for their health care. . . . Among all hospitals, the urban public-general hospitals, as a group, have the most serious and persistent problems" (1978).

Of the forty-five university-operated public-general hospitals, all but one were state-owned and in many ways the problems of their support pertained more to the question of financing medical education than to financing public medical care of the poor. "The future of these hospitals, like that of all university hospitals, lies in the ability to define their constituencies, to clarify their health profession education and community service missions, and to obtain support for them from planning agencies, third-party payers, the university, and the communities they serve. . . . In the long term, their future will be influenced as much by public priorities for health manpower development as by community health care needs" (1978).

The 357 medium-size "other metropolitan-area" public-general hospitals were located in cities other than the 100 largest and in suburbs within Standard Metropolitan Statistical Areas (SMSAs). They functioned very much like private community hospitals serving primarily paying patients. The Commission judged that "The future for these hospitals will be very much like that for other Community hospitals" (1978). A total of 130, or more than a third, of these hospitals were owned by special hospital districts or authorities.

Rural public-general hospitals are small; they averaged 70 beds in 1975 and 664 out of 1,413 hospitals had less than 50 beds. Although these 1,413 hospitals constituted almost three-fourths of the 1,905 public-general hospitals, they delivered only some 40 percent of the patient days. Most served as community hospitals for all residents in their areas, and in many places they were the only hospitals, with 369 of the 1,413 being operated by hospital districts or authorities and 157 by private, nonprofit entities. Most of the rest were operated by counties, some by cities, and a few by states. "For these hospitals, the future will be much like that for other rural hospitals—they will have to respond to pressures to provide more primary and long-term care, to establish linkages or share services with larger community hospitals that are not too remote. . . . " (1978). Thus, the problems of most of these hospitals stemmed more from their rural location than from their special orientation to the poor, although the two factors are closely related. Their problems are perhaps better addressed under the general rubric of rural health care.

As the preceding paragraphs indicate, the Commission's conclusions regarding the future of the three types of public-general hospitals other than the urban group indicated that it considered their problems to be not much different from private hospitals of similar type. The future of the urban public-general hospital, by contrast, was not seen to have a parallel in the private sector and had to be uniquely treated.

No set of hospitals in the private sector was charged primarily with serving the "unsponsored"[29] patient and delivering a heavy component of sociomedical services. The report found that although the ninety urban public-general hospitals delivered 13.2 percent of all inpatient services, they provided 28.9 percent of all hospital outpatient services in the cities in which they were located. They accounted for more than a fourth of the emergency visits, and in most places operated the intensive trauma care center for the area. They operated one-fifth to one-quarter of selected medical-social programs provided by urban community hospitals—21 percent of the psychiatric emergency services and about 26 percent each of inpatient and outpatient alcohol detoxification and treatment services. In some of these cities they delivered as much as one-third of all inpatient care and one-half of all outpatient care. And yet these hospitals represented only 9.3 percent of the community hospitals in these cities. The urban public-general hospitals were the training sites for almost one-fifth of the nation's medical and dental residents training in community hospitals.

The Commission also found that despite the existence of Medicaid and Medicare, "substantial numbers of Americans still cannot afford to pay for health care." Among such groups were: (a) the "so-called working poor"; (b) those with inadequate health insurance coverage; (c) the unemployed and underemployed who do not qualify for welfare; (d) the victims of Medicaid and other public assistance cutbacks; and (e) illegal aliens and nonresidents who are not eligible for public assistance. It is because of facts like these that the Commission judged the likely future of the urban public-general hospital to have no analogue in the problems of otherwise comparable private hospitals as the other classes of hospital in the public sector did. (Such considerations were also central to my decision to

focus on this class of public hospital in this chapter.)

One of the report's major recommendations for the urban public-general hospital states:

For the short term, the future of many of these hospitals is tied to the ability and willingness of federal and state governments to provide them with emergency financial relief and to share a greater part of the burden of caring for the unsponsored patient. For the longer term, they must become integral parts of the health care delivery system within their communities, providing needed services on a community wide basis rather than serving as separate providers for the poor. . . .

It is no longer appropriate for the public-general hospital to serve only the poor. . . . Once health care delivery programs are better integrated and are supported through an equitable general funding plan, there should be no reason to operate separate health facilities for the poor.

Thus, while the commission report unequivocally called for direct federal and state financial aid to existing urban public-general hospitals in the short run, its long-term solution envisioned a restructured future health care system that would be planned and regionalized, with the present urban public-general hospitals reconstituted differently in different places to meet the special needs of the regionally planned configuration. It is clear that these projections of the future were predicated on two important assumptions. At the time this report was written the Commission members apparently saw a future in which (1) local health planning would grow and become an integral feature of our health system; and (2) some form of "equitable general funding plan" that would give universal, comprehensive coverage for medical care would be legislated.

A later survey, done jointly by the American Hospital Association and the Urban Institute, of the experience of all community hospitals in 1980 with 100 or more beds and located in the 100 largest cities further documented the assertion about the central position of the urban public-general hospital in serving the "unsponsored" patient. It found that publicly owned hospitals constituted 13.3 percent of the 736 urban hospitals responding but delivered 38.2 percent of the "total care for the poor" (Hadley, Fedler, and Mullner, 1983). Even more trenchantly, "While private institutions provided the majority (about 70 percent) of Medicaid-financed care, charity care [that is, "unsponsored" care] was overwhelmingly the responsibility of public institutions, which provided 65 percent of the total." Very significantly, the report concluded:

Were fiscal stress clearly the results of mismanagement, inefficiency, or underuse, its occurrence would not cause great concern. Management could be improved; underused facilities could be closed or consolidated. In fact, however the best indicator of fiscal stress is not some measure of efficiency, management initiative, or occupancy, but instead, a hospital's volume of care to the poor.... If people without resources are to receive care, somebody else has to pay. [A]lthough inefficiency does not seem to be the cause of fiscal stress, greater efficiency could contribute to its solution . . . [but] whether costs can be sufficiently reduced without actually reducing service to the poor . . . remains questionable. Without some increased resources for hospitals serving the poor, reduced quantity or quality of service is probably inevitable" (Hadley, Fedler, and Mullner, 1983).

The earlier 1978 report of the Commission on Public Hospitals had already broken with the received wisdom of the day that called primarily for internal organizational changes in the public hospital to ameliorate its plight. As noted, the commission recommended that in the short run the solution lay in "immediate" financial aid as a sine qua non. But now in 1983 a major report, issued under the imprimatur of a leading "mainstream" research institute with hospital industry collaboration, specifically departed from deeply entrenched health services lore that the urban public-general hospital's problems are explicable mainly in terms of internal managerial factors, and attributed the root of its problems to insufficient funding.

The years after 1975 also saw the formation of save-the-public-hospital "self-help" constituencies consisting of hospital employee groups as well as organizations of the public hospitals themselves, who strove to disseminate the analysis of the "plight of the [urban] public hospital" as primarily due to external factors and not to management deficiencies, governmental red tape, or other efficiency factors. Some of the research, writing, and legislative testimony sponsored or disseminated by such groups gave these views greater visibility.

An example of the efforts of public hospital employee groups to rally public support for the continuance and enhancement of the urban public-general hospital in this fashion is the work of Professor Samuel Wolf and Hila Sherer at the Columbia University School of Public Health commissioned by the Coalition of American Public Employees.[30] Wolf and Sherer did a study of public hospitals in which they concluded that the following oft-repeated and widely disseminated arguments were invalid and even specious: the public hospital sector, including city-sponsored hospitals, is characteristically inefficient; there is no need for public general hospitals in what planners of the day were labeling "over-bedded" areas; if there were universal financing by the federal government with free choice of provider people would "vote with their feet" in favor of the private sector; the public hospital sector is ruining the cities' budgets; public hospitals, constituencies, and employees are uninterested in saving the public hospitals in their communities (1977).

An association of the leadership of public hospitals was formed in 1981 to defend the continuance of such hospitals. Calling itself the National Association of Public Hospitals (NAPH), it was created "to give a separate, distinct voice in national health care decision-making to large, urban public hospitals, their staff, and the patient population they serve" (Gage, 1983). The association's institutional membership was limited to large urban public hospitals. It issued materials on the urban public-general hospital, especially in the form of Congressional testimony.

The fundamental changes in financing and support of the large urban public hospitals recommended by the AHA 1978 commission report, the need for which was strongly corroborated later by the AHA-Urban Institute Study, were in the main unheeded by Congress and the President, and local governments continued to seek ways of relieving the financial burden caused by operating a public hospital. Beginning with 1975, they began trying the sixth "solution" (see page 222) more frequently—contracting the management of the hospital out to a private management company. The private management companies were for the most part subsidiaries or intregral parts of investor-owned ("for-profit") hospital chains. These firms were acquiring their own hospitals and also managing hospitals for other owners. In 1979, 36 companies owned or managed three or more hospitals each and operated a total of some 800 hospitals with 101,000 beds.[31] By 1980 they had grown to 38 companies with about 860 hospitals and 108,000 beds (Federation of American Hospitals, 1981). These chains of investor-owned hospitals (IOHs) contracted to manage both for-profit and not-for-profit hospitals. They had contracts with 191 not-for-profit hospitals (21,000 beds) in 1978 and with 264 hospitals (27,400 beds) in 1980. Although initially managing only private hospitals, during the 1970s they began to contract for management of public hospitals also. California was the starting point for this development, and by 1978 one company alone, National Medical Enterprises, had contracts to manage the public hospitals of six California counties. Counties in California turned to private management because there were supervisors who thought it would save money without undermining quality of care—another illustration of the ubiquitous nature of the presumption that the private sector is ipso factor more efficient than the public sector.[32] Other county supervisors, who favored continuing direct public services by maintaining their county hospitals, when faced with pressure to close the hospital or give it away, saw turning to private management as the best compromise available. Their reasoning was that management arrangements were temporary and therefore reversible; after all the climate might change at the end of the contract period. To supervisors wanting to divest the county of its hospital this also seemed like the best compromise available to them for the time being, for it was for them a step in the right direction.

A study of the experience of seven counties in California with this type of management contracting (Shonick and Roemer, 1983) found no evidence that true overall costs were reduced under contract management by private companies. In two cases, both semirural small hospitals, substantial reduction in net cost of the hospital *to the county* was accomplished. This was done, however, by shifting costs to patients who were insured by private insurance or sponsored by state and federal programs. This remedy was not available to the large urban public hospitals in

the study because they did not have sufficient paying patients to whom the cost of county patients could be shifted. Furthermore, with the institution of prospective payment and other reimbursement constraints by the public and later some private insurers, the prospect for this type of cost shifting was for it to dwindle or even vanish for all public hospitals. The study also found that administrative advantages did accrue to some hospitals from contract managements. These advantages, however, were largely confined to smaller hospitals in the more rural areas where local administrative expertise was hard to find, full-time executives difficult to pay for, and the administrative resources—both in personnel and technology—of a large management company were found useful. This supports the analysis of the Commission on Public Hospitals that the problems of the rural public hospital were centered more in their location than in the fact of their public ownership. In the two large urban public hospitals of the study, the contracts were discontinued after a brief period with both sides happy to be out of them. The multifaceted social and economic factors underlying the problems of these hospitals did not prove amenable to the contractors' managerial approach.

Summary and Reflections

The end of 1982 found the large urban public hospital in worse shape than ever. The economic recession sharply reduced state revenues, and the local tax revolt curtailed local government revenues in many places. The major sources of nonfederal revenue for support of the public hospital were thereby reduced. At the same time, the decline in federal categorical grants and Medicaid funds curtailed, or in some cases even eliminated, various health services to the poor provided at public expense by the private sector either through regular mainstream channels or through special facilities that were supported by federal categorical grants.[33] As a result many poor persons who had been receiving such services turned to the public hospital, wherever there still was one, and more were likely to do so in the future. The combination of increased need for and decreased supply of public hospital services not only left more low-income persons without access to medical care; it also increased the strain on the public hospitals' capacity and further diminished the quality of their services.

The experience of the postwar period supports a number of conclusions. The plight of the public hospital was not rooted in managerial or medical technological failings; these were the consequences of the "plight" rather than its causes. The root cause was a lack of a reliable source of ongoing and adequate financial support. Local efforts to solve the problem by bringing in high-level medical expertise or business-oriented management may sometimes have helped for a time. But they did not make a substantial permanent difference in any locality and certainly not in the general condition of the public hospital throughout the United States. At least one trial of reorganization that was well financed over a number of years did demonstrate what could be done with adequate financing and energetic, knowledgeable leadership.

Because the underlying problem was the failure to establish a reliable and uniformly available revenue source across the country that would be proportional to the local need, the attempted local solutions to the problem consisted of various ways, some of them innovative and ingenious, to juggle funds and resources appropriated for other purposes to patch together a revenue base for the local public hospital. These included using categorical public health grants; manipulating cost report forms to obtain optimal Medicare, Medicaid, and Blue Cross rates; obtaining grants as neighborhood health centers for the outpatient department; and many others. One could demur that optimizing Medicaid reimbursement was a bona fide hospital operation, not "juggling funds." So it was for the private hospital for whom fee-for-service payment through insurance made up most of its patient revenues. But for most urban local public hospitals this source was of relatively minor proportions. (After all, a principal aim of Medicaid was to enable hospitalization of its beneficiaries in mainstream facilities.) Establishing itemized charge systems for the sole purpose of producing bills for individual patients, and "cost" accounting systems that were largely artifacts required by insurer reimbursement mechanisms, has not been an operating priority for most public hospitals. Therefore, despite the many clever ways that were found to juggle, the result was

only to make a very few public hospitals more viable then they would otherwise have been and usually only for a short time. Since juggling made funding dependent on gaming the idiosyncrasies of the current funding and reimbursement systems, when these systems changed, the clever arrangements wilted or collapsed. And the reimbursement systems were changing rapidly and at an increasing pace. Further, closer regulation and increased case management and payment review programs by insurers and Medicaid made fund and report juggling even more difficult.

What then is to be the fate of the local public general hospital? In attempting to formulate a reasonable answer it is well to begin by recognizing that the underlying question remains: How is medical care to be provided to low-income people who cannot pay for it?

Since the special public hospital for the poor would not be needed in its present role under a national health system[34] with universal access to all needed services, this discussion related only to the immediate and short-term future during which special health care systems for the poor are likely to be continued. The question then becomes: "What are the implications of using a system like Medicaid that pays private providers for medical services to low-income persons as against providing the services directly with government health service agencies such as local general public hospitals?"

Many persons who favor equal access for the poor prefer a pay-the-private-provider system on social equity grounds. They see in this alternative the potential for achieving truly equal access because it could give the poor access to the "mainstream" care used by the paying public. However, in actuality, it hasn't. As will be more fully discussed in Chapters 8 and 9, this equal access has never been achieved, both because Medicaid never covered all persons who needed it and because Medicaid has never paid the full "market" rate the private sector gets from privately insured patients.[35] In fact, eligibility for Medicaid was steadily reduced after 1980 to levels even below the earlier already restrictive levels by most states, and the payment rates were further decreased. If a payment system does not pay the going "market" rates for its clients, they will not have equal access to private providers.

At this writing there is no expectation that government pay programs intend to extend their eligibility to include all persons not now eligible for Medicaid who have no other health care coverage or raise their reimbursement rates to market levels. In fact, many "cost containment" strategies in the health field have laid the major burden of cost containment on public programs, thus widening the disparity between what a provider can expect to get from a Medicaid patient and one covered by private insurance or Medicare. It is therefore not at all guaranteed that if we are to have special programs for providing health care for the poor, a pay-the-provider program will provide equal access to the private sector, even for the program's eligibles. Even a reasonably well-funded direct public provision program might in many cases provide care as good as or better than that obtainable by questionable access to the private sector.

If it comes to be recognized that a good public delivery system is at least as good as a pay-the-private-provider system that restricts eligibility and pays fees below the going market rate, then it may also come to be accepted that state and federal stipends for care to the poor should not all go to pay-the-private-provider systems but that substantial portions go to well-funded publicly operated systems.

NOTES

1. Chapter 8 also contains a fuller treatment of the background of medical care for the poor, including the general question of the provision of the necessities of life for the poor in which medical care is embedded.

2. There is a discrepancy between the number of hospitals that are classified as publicly owned and those that are publicly "controlled" or operated. Most hospitals that were involved in this dual sponsorship (234 in 1975)—that is, they were either publicly owned and privately "controlled" or vice versa—were rural hospitals. In 1975 197 hospitals were publicly owned but privately operated. The AHA data based on "control" therefore tend to slightly overstate the number of publicly owned hospitals. This may be of greater importance in more recent years than it was in 1975 because a number of large public hospitals have been operated under contract by private organizations. The American Hospital Association does not publish annual breakdowns of

hospitals cross-classified by control and ownership; unless otherwise noted, the data on such subdivisions in this chapter come from the special 1976 study of the Commission on Public Hospitals, which is discussed on pages 237–239.

3. See AHA, 1981.

4. Unless otherwise noted, whenever county and city public hospitals are discussed, it will hereafter be assumed that city-county hospitals are included.

5. Unless otherwise noted, the following discussion, through page 241, refers to this type of local public hospital.

6. The pesthouse was an institution for care of persons with contagious diseases. As late as 1927 there were still 98 "isolation hospitals" with almost 9,000 beds in the United States (Goldmann, 1945).

7. Medically indigent persons are economically self-supporting for their routine living needs but cannot afford some medical services they require. The term is relative depending on the patient's resources in relation to what medical services he or she requires. In today's high-technology and expensive medical care milieu, even quite well-to-do persons can soon find themselves medically indigent in the face of certain medical conditions.

8. Issues involving health insurance are discussed in greater detail in Chapter 9.

9. These programs were the amendments to the welfare provisions of the Social Security Act beginning with 1956, which allowed states to pay providers for medical services to their welfare clients with the expenditures being federally matched (see Chapter 8); the Medicaid Act of 1965, which provided for greatly augmented payments to providers for medical care of welfare recipients and some other classes of eligibles (see Chapter 10); the community health center and migrant health programs which provided federal funds for primary care centers in underserved areas (see Chapter 11); and the National Health Service Corps, which provided medical care personnel to medically underserved areas (see Chapter 11).

10. Cf. Martin Cherkasky quoted in AHA, 1969.

11. These programs are described and discussed in Chapter 10. I identify them very briefly here because they appear in various context in this chapter and in Chapters 8 and 9. Medicare is a federal program that became law in 1965. It pays for medical expenses of persons over sixty-five years of age (and some other groups). It is an insurance program with eligibility restricted to persons eligible for Social Security benefits. *Medicaid* is a federal program that became 1965 that pays for medical expenses of poor persons. The states share in these payments. In most states the only poor persons eligible for this program are those that fall in one of four categories: aged, blind, disabled, and families with dependent children.

12. Data and unattributed quotations relating to the structure, size, and utilization of the New York City hospital system that follow are from Burlage (1967).

13. These four recommendations, especially 1 and 4, were not implemented. There simply was not

enough City money available, given the huge increase in costs as more hospitals became affiliated.

14. Much of the immediately following factual description is from this source.

15. The account of these early years in the Denver merger is based largely on the writings of David L. Cowen (1970, 1971), who was manager of the Department of Health and Hospitals of the City and County of Denver during part of the period of the development of the merged system.

16. See Chapters 11 and 6 for a description of these federal grant programs.

17. Casey Bill, AB 5, 1966.

18. Most smaller communities in the County that had had their own health departments merged with the County's in 1964. However, two sizable communities, Pasadena and Long Beach, continued to maintain their own departments but contracted for selected services with the County department.

19. See Marshall, 1971, and Johnson, 1977 for accounts of this process.

20. The state mandated counties to levy local property taxes to cover the cost of the county's share in the state's MediCal costs.

21. These additional 1972 retrenchments included discontinuing state cost sharing for capital construction of health facilities, restricting eligibility for the regular (non-MIA) MediCal program, and reducing funding for mental health programs.

22. Much of the details in this description are from Cohn, 1977.

23. Public health officers from some of the health centers went directly to the Board of Supervisors and were successful in getting directives of the central administration countermanded.

24. The account of Project Health follows Danaceau in McGeary et al. (1982), and the quotations are from this source.

25. These were mostly persons under sixty-five years of age with no dependent children.

26. Actually the commission was established by the Hospital Research and Educational Trust (HRET),

an affiliate of the AHA, with foundation grant support.

27. Defined by the AHA as nonfederal, short-term, general and other special hospitals, excluding psychiatric, tuberculosis, and alcoholism and chemical dependency hospitals.

28. See note 2 for a discussion of the definition of "publicly owned."

29. The term "unsponsored" patient came to be used in the late 1970s in literature dealing with hospital problems in general and public hospital problems in particular. In the public hospital literature the term designates a patient for whom there is no formally recognized source of funding from which the local government can collect the major portion of the cost of the patient's care, such as the patient's own resources, private insurance, Medicare, or Medicaid. A substantial part or all of such a patient's care must be paid for by the local government.

30. Comprising American Federation of State, County and Municipal Employees (AFSCME), National Education Association (NEA), National Treasury Employees Union (NTEU), American Nurse Association (ANA), National Association of Social Workers (NASW), and Physicians National Housestaff Association (PNHA).

31. This section closely follows Shonick and Roemer, 1983, p. 21, and elsewhere.

32. There was one way in which a private management contractor could indeed save money. This was by replacing the government workers with good seniority and fringe benefits with his own new employees who generally had neither.

33. These were programs like the neighborhood health centers, the National Health Service Corps, and others that are discussed in later chapters.

34. The implications of legislating universal access will be discussed in Chapter 8.

35. It should be noted how similar this course of events was to the deinstitutionalization phenomenon, with its state mental hospitals on the one hand and community mental health services on the other.

III

Government as Payer for Medical Care Provided by Others

In this section the focus shifts from health services provided directly by government—whether "public health" or "medical care"—to payment by government to private providers on behalf of beneficiaries of government programs. For the most part, these purchased services have been medical care, which in currently fashionable economics terminology is said to be purchased by government in "the market." The main target populations of these programs have been the poor and the elderly, and the programs fall into the two broad categories of public assistance and social insurance.

The many policy ramifications of choosing to provide access by direct services versus provider payment mechanisms, and the further implications of choosing a public assistance versus an insurance system in the latter case are explored. They involve many questions of social equity as well as the quality and efficiency of the system. Chapters 8, 9, and 10 deal with the background of and more recent experience with government involvement in paying providers for health care for its targetted beneficiaries via "welfare medicine" as against social insurance. In Chapter 11 experience with a hybrid mechanism, the government-supported but privately administered neighborhood health center, is presented and analyzed.

8

Government-Reimbursed Medical Programs for the Indigent and Medically Indigent: The Period Before 1965

OVERVIEW AND BACKGROUND

The English Poor Law

As previously noted, medical services have been directly provided under government sponsorship in the United States only for specially identified classes of persons. Chapters 5, 6, and 7 deal with systems of care provided directly by government to such special populations as merchant seamen, American Indians, armed forces personnel and dependents, veterans, the tubercular, the mentally ill, and medically indigent persons. Of these groups, the last one is of special interest since much of the policy analysis in the field of health services studies has dealt with the question of providing needed medical services to those who cannot pay market prices for them. Since government in the United States has never agreed to provide for a minimally adequate package of medical services to all persons as a matter of right regardless of ability to pay, special programs have always been necessary for those who were unable to pay and were not entitled to existing direct services by virtue of being members of one of the other special groups.

Eligibility to enter programs for the medically indigent had to be established by proof of poverty, i.e., a "means test," a point appropriately emphasized and well examined by Burns (1965). Making medical services available to such persons was perceived as part of the general responsibility of government to provide the necessities of life for indigent citizens, a function variously called "public assistance," "relief," or "public welfare." Since public assis-

tance medical care has been part of the total package of public assistance for living maintenance, the requirements for eligibility have generally been the same for both, especially before 1965. The responsibility for providing public assistance was, again, constitutionally vested in the states, which usually delegated its administration and much of its financing to local government, with the result that much general medical care has been provided for the poor by localities. The California state constitution, for example, explicitly places this responsibility upon its counties. Until 1935, the federal government played no role in helping provide for indigent persons except for emergency measures adopted during the early depression years.

In Chapter 7 the direct provision of medical care to the poor through local public general hospitals was examined. Although this chapter is mainly about service purchased by the government, I also revisit the more general question of providing access to government programs for medical care to the poor, whether directly provided or purchased, and the importance of the criteria set by public assistance laws for when these two modalities should be used. The public policy implications of using each are examined.

Historically, local attitudes toward providing medical care for the poor were characterized by the prevalence of means-test medical care, reflecting the influence of the English Poor Law on early American life. The early English Poor Law, a series of acts, beginning with the Statute of Laborers in 1349, which forbade almsgiving to able-bodied men (Handel, 1982), and culminating in the well-known Elizabethan Poor Law codification of 1601, established local responsibility for the care of the destitute. Its main features remained part of the public assistance philosophy of the United States for many years, with many aspects continuing to the persent day.

The Elizabethan Poor Laws requiring the locality or parish to care for its "worthy" poor reflected religious (largely early Protestant) views of morality. The "worthy" poor comprised those persons whose poverty was ascribable to a misfortune that made it impossible for them to be gainfully employed, such as widowhood with small children, physical disability, or enfeeblement due to old age. For these "worthy" poor, the parish had to provide some form of sustenance, but it should be noted that the blameless unemployed, those who were able and willing to work except that no jobs could be found for them, were also entitled to some aid, but only on a temporary basis. Furthermore, work of some kind by the recipient was required if assistance were given.

The 1601 law, the "first completely secular and comprehensive poor law," accordingly identified three categories of dependents—vagrants (including able-bodied persons for whom jobs existed but who did not work), the true (involuntarily) unemployed, and the unemployables—those who were disabled or helpless.[1] The local parish was required to provide food and shelter for the unemployables in almshouses or "sustenance" for them in their own homes and see to it that able-bodied truly unemployed persons were put to useful work. Vagrants or other able-bodied persons with no means of support who refused to take available work were to be jailed. The law also decreed legal responsibility of closest relatives to support their pauperized kin. Since each parish was responsible only for its own "worthy" poor, it was deemed perfectly proper for a designated period of residence in the parish to be stipulated as a condition of eligibility for any aid.

The funds for meeting these requirements were to be raised locally through taxation or from philanthropic contributions with tax exemptions granted to persons giving to philanthropy for these purposes. The amounts raised from philanthropy contributed over 90 percent of the funds used to administer the Poor Law.

This English precedent established a clear pattern: work relief for the unemployed, almshouse or outdoor relief[2] for the helpless, and punishment for those who would not work, all financed largely by philanthropists who therefore had considerable say on how the funds were to be used.

According to Blanche D. Coll's account (1969), both the church-administered charity of the Middle Ages and the local secular government-administered Elizabethan Poor Laws acknowledged each stricken persons' right to assistance. The earlier church-administered feudal concept regarded need as a "result of misfortune for which society, in an act of justice, must assume responsibility," and the Elizabethan Poor Law "acknowledged the presence of involuntary unemployment. . . . It was [not until] late in the 17th Century, when the pursuit of wealth became a moral virtue, that dependency became a vice . . . implying that the able-bodied [were] brought to destitution by individual fault. . . a set of mind that, by ignoring the facts of the Industrial Revolution justified the insecurity it created." After 1660 the publicly expressed attitude toward supplicants for public assistance hardened. With increasing assertiveness and fervor, the theology of leading Protestant denominations linked the personal characteristics that promoted commercial success with religious rectitude and divine grace. "Calvinism and the sects springing from it . . . [were providing] a rationale for the capitalism growing about them. The economic virtues of industry, sobriety, and thrift were accorded a prominent place. Wealth, wisely used, became a mark of virtue . . . poverty—but, most particularly, dependency—came to be regarded as a failure of character" (Coll, 1969). Other branches of Protestantism, such as the Lutheran, preached that persons should live in a manner pleasing to God, and this could be done only by laboring dutifully at one's "calling." "The only way of living acceptably to God was not to surpass worldly morality in monastic asceticism, but solely through the fulfillment of the obligation imposed upon the individual by his position in the world" (Weber, 1958). The more austere Calvinist branch of Protestant thought preached that man could not earn salvation since God had predestined some—those who had divine grace—to go to heaven and some to hell. But a man's condition on earth was a sign of whether he had divine grace or not. If he was poor without visible good cause, it was a sign of a lack of divine grace. This view "was accompanied by an attitude toward the sin of one's neighbor, not of sympathetic understanding based on consciousness of one's own weakness, but of hatred and contempt for him as an enemy of God bearing the signs of eternal damnation" (Weber, 1958).

Another example of this hardening stance was the Law of Settlement and Removal. Passed in 1662, it sharpened the provisions directed against "vagrancy," which referred to migrating poor persons who were without means or employment. It empowered a local parish to eject such persons and families from its jurisdiction who seemed likely to become dependent in the future. The preamble to the 1662 law asserted that its aim was to stop the migrations of large numbers of indigent people who were said to be moving to locales with more generous relief provisions. Coll points out that this assertion was not in fact true, and asserts that the law was only desultorily enforced. Its importance lay in its being "a telling illustration of the change [toward increased harshness] in attitude toward the helpless poor against whom it was used" (1969). Also during the period after 1660, workhouses for the poor came to be more strongly advocated in public discourse, as well as used more often in practice, and by 1800 "there were more than 4,000 so-called workhouses in England housing about 100,000 persons out of a population of 9 million" (1969).

Thus, a widely held perception that a very large number of the English poor were still in workhouses as late as 1800 is apparently greatly exaggerated. Much of the increased harshness toward methods of aiding the poor was by this time more evident in legal wording and public speeches than in actual application. Citing the work of the noted British reformers and social welfare scholars Sidney and Beatrice Webb, Coll writes:

The adjective "so-called" [workhouses] is used advisedly, for, no matter what their original purpose, these institutions had by this time [about 1800] become what Sidney and Beatrice Webb term the "general mixed workhouse"—a shelter for social outcasts.

Proliferate as they did, neither workhouses nor almshouses were the usual means of caring for the destitute during the 18th and early 19th Centuries. The basic system remained the relief of the poor in their houses, sometimes in kind, but usually by a small money payment (1969).

A serious attempt to substantially alter this situation had been made in the 1830s. Between 1795 and 1830 the costs of poor relief in Britain escalated greatly. From 1803 to 1818 they almost doubled, reaching in 1832 more than three times the per capita expenditure of 1776 and occasioning "numerous adverse comments beginning in the 1820's" (1969). In response to this dissatisfaction with the rise in taxes, the Poor Law of 1834, known as the New Poor Law in contradistinction to the Elizabethan Poor Law, which is the Old Poor Law, was passed, decreeing a harsher administration of poor relief. The main thrust of the New Poor Law as to crack down on aid to able-bodied persons that purportedly encouraged them not to work. A government commission investigating the relief system from 1832 to 1834 had reported that it found the recipients to include large numbers of able-bodied persons and the administration of the system to have been lax (1969). The commission's recommendations focused on abolishing all outdoor relief for able-bodied persons, especially the *supplementation of wages* of poor *working* persons—the so-called Speenhamland system that had begun to spread among localities on 1795[3] (Coll, 1969; Handel, 1982). The 1834 amendment to the Poor Law did indeed ban all relief to the able-bodied except in a workhouse and established the National Board of Poor Law Commissioners, to administer the system across the country.

But again, despite the proclaimed intent of the Poor Law Amendment of 1834 to make relief in a harsh workhouse the only modality for public assistance to the able-bodied, in actuality outdoor relief continued to be the main means of granting them assistance, including in some places supplementing the wages of the working poor under the "Speenhamland system." Coll notes:

The workhouses—more accurately termed almshouses—of the 19th Century were cut from the same cloth as those of the 18th, and about the same number of persons were living in them as before. In a 3-month period in 1844, for example, 234,000 persons were in almshouses, as compared to 1.2 million in receipt of outdoor relief. In 1850 there were a million persons receiving relief, but only 110,000 were in almshouses (1969).

Another writer on social welfare largely agrees, observing that:

In 1854, twenty years after the enactment of the new law, 84 perent of paupers were still on outdoor relief. Nevertheless, the number of people in workhouses was substantial, particularly after the relief policy was toughened around 1870. An 1898 census showed that 216,000 people were in workhouses on the day of the census, and it was estimated that about three times that number spent some time in them in the course of a year. . . . The 1834 Poor Law remained in force until 1929; only then did the workhouses disappear. Also in 1929, the Poor Law Boards of Guardians were abolished and their functions turned over to the county government, and the term *poor law* disappeared, and was replaced by the term *public assistance* (Handel, 1982).

Perhaps the most important point about this "workhouse" versus "outdoor relief" question is that the 1834 law did bequeath to the then current as well as subsequent U.S. relief programs an ideology and rhetoric that were widely used to defend reductions in welfare outlays, including the medical care provided under them, especially with respect to tightening the eligibility criteria. Many of the public welfare (including public medical care) practices and ideas formulated in the 1800s in the United States were based on the excessive credulity eagerly accorded the reports of the English experience. A main feature of this rhetoric calling for harsher treatment of public welfare recipients was the practice of greatly exaggerating the numbers of able-bodied persons relying on charity. [T]he British public was led to believe that most recipients—perhaps as many as a million—were able-bodied persons and their families. About 300,000 able-bodied persons was undoubtedly closer to the mark. The bulk of 'paupers' were incapacitated—aged, disabled persons and dependent children. Moreover, it was subsequently discovered that as much as 50 percent of relief given to the so-called able-bodied had been granted because of illness" (Coll, 1969). The lament over the extent of "welfare

abuse" and "welfare cheats" was to echo and re-echo through American social welfare history right up to the present, while investigation after investigation would announce the same findings as those noted by Coll with respect to nineteenth-century England.

A second loudly proclaimed principle of the new 1834 English austerity that found its way prominently into United States welfare practice was that of "less eligibility," which asserted that the condition of persons receiving relief should always be kept at a level less desirable than that of the lowest-earning employed person. The proclaimed intent of this principle was to discourage low-income able-bodied workers from electing not to work. But again, most persons receiving relief in England were unable to work, and the accusation of choosing not to work "was perforce extended indiscriminately to all persons dependent on public assistance—the young and old, the sick and disabled, the unemployed, and the underpaid" (Coll, 1969). Although it was claimed that the "worthy poor" were not the intended objects of the "less eligibility" principle, they constituted most of the relief recipients, and the tax savings promised from increased austerity in the Poor Law could only be accomplished by reducing their allotments below the lowest levels paid to any employed persons.

In all of the English Poor Laws, the sick were considered part of the "worthy poor" if they were chronically ill or disabled, and families rendered temporarily destitute by illness were also often eligible for some outdoor relief. Those in almshouses who became ill were also accorded some medical assistance. All the arguments used to denounce and exaggerate cheaters on public welfare rolls were used against recipients of public welfare medicine in the Untied States with the same results. Funds were constantly cut to the bone (and beyond) and kept at an absolute minimum over time. Thus, the heritage of the English Poor Law tradition comprised the ideas of restricting eligibility to the worthy poor, requiring financial responsibility of relatives for care of "incompetent" persons, local administration and financing, residence requirements for eligibility, and the principle of less eligibility. Special stress was laid on not corrupting able-bodied paupers by undermining their instinct and desire for gainful work through granting them relief.

Poor Relief and Medical Care in the Early United States

With the early American residents in the English colonies bringing many of the British ideas and practices to the new settlements in colonial America, Elizabethan-type poor laws prevailed in a number of the colonies. Basic features common to these colonial laws attested to their English lineage. The distinction between the helpless and able-bodied poor of English law is clearly evident in the restriction of eligibility to the "lame, impotent, old, blind and such other among them being poor, and not able to work" (Coll, 1969). The strong emphasis on local residence requirements reflected the spirit of the English Law of Settlement and Removal. A great deal of time and money were spent litigating the question of which locality was responsible for the care of given dependent persons. It was not until 1969 that the Supreme Court declared residence requirements to be unconstitutional *(Shapiro* v. *Thompson).* A third English feature found in early United States poor laws was the financial responsibility of relatives for support of poor parents, children, and other defined kin.

As had been the case in England, providing for care of the sick among the "worthy" poor was looked on as part of the locality's responsibility under the poor law, and a number of colonial legislatures passed laws to this effect. For example, the Rhode Island assembly in 1662 included the indigent sick among those who were to be maintained by towns. A typical poor law of the colonial period is the one passed by Connecticut in 1673 making every town responsible for caring for the sick or destitute who had lived in the community for three months or more. Generally, the fact that persons were ill qualified them as "worthy," provided the illness was sufficiently severe and protracted to be effectively disabling for gainful employment.

The states of the new government established after the American Revolution largely continued the Elizabethan poor law pattern of legislation. However, there were challenges in the state courts contesting the extent of the state's obligation to provide for medical care as part of its responsibility to care for its "worthy" poor under the Constitution's police powers. The state courts generally held the state responsible for providing medical care to the poor for serious conditions.

But the sentiments for increased harshness toward aiding the poor in England expressed in the 1834 Poor Law amendments and the philosophy behind them were echoed in the United States. As the United States became increasingly industrial, concerns increased about able-bodied paupers not seeking out available jobs because they were living on relief and thereby distorting the labor market. Public writing and speechmaking on the question of public assistance increasingly stressed the evils of economic dependency, especially the danger of character deterioration of the dependents. An aspect of this attitude toward public assistance that assumed importance during the period 1860 to 1900 was a movement that came to be known as "scientific charity" (Leiby, 1978; Coll, 1969). Its underlying philosophical rationale was Social Darwinism. Mechanically adopting what Herbert Spencer, an "English engineer-turned-sociologist" (Coll, 1969) thought Darwin's theory implied[4] about society, the phrase "survival of the fittest," which Spencer coined, was used to underpin arguments for reducing aid to the poor to minimum levels. According to this argument, giving financial assistance to poor persons (especially the able-bodied) tends to increase their dependence on charity and undermines their drive to compete in the market to achieve economic self-sufficiency. It also tends, Spencer asserted, toward "the artificial preservation of those least able to care for themselves" (Coll, 1969). A professor of sociology at Yale, William Graham Sumner, argued that the poor were idle and extravagant and to favor them was to favor the survival of the least fit (Coll, 1969). Tied to this view was an advocacy of less government involvement in relief activities because government relief tended to be profligate and to undermine society by giving money to people who with proper encouragement could otherwise be expected to become independent. This conception was reinforced by numerous exposés of corruption in local government at the turn of the century. Government assistance should not include outdoor relief, it was argued, because only in institutions could the public dispensation of alms be monitored to see that it did not operate to make recipients dependent.

The organizational realization of scientific charity notions was centered in the Charity Organization Society (COS) movement. The first society was founded in Buffalo in 1877 with ideas imported from England. By 1892 there were ninety-two such societies in various cities and towns. A COS would organize the charities of a municipality that were under voluntary (i.e., private) auspices in line with Social Darwinian ideas that pauperism was a disease resulting from personal defects such as laziness, deceitfulness, intemperance, improvidence, inefficiency, extravagance, and sexual vices. Ill-considered almsgiving had created a "mire of pauperism." The founder of the New York City COS, Mrs. Josephine Shaw Lowell, argued that "relief should be surrounded by circumstances that shall . . . repel every one, not in extremity from accepting it. . . . " Public relief was pejoratively different from charity, which had to be privately administered according to COS principles. Public assistance should exclude outdoor relief, for it "did great moral harm because human nature is so constituted that no man can receive as a gift which he should earn by his own labor without a moral deterioration. . . . " (Lowell, 1884). The almshouse or workhouse was the appropriate agency for "moral regeneration and training and all outdoor public relief. . . . "

Reaction Against Social Darwinism

The COS movement was successful in getting most East Coast cities to abandon outdoor relief, with Boston a notable exception. "Seldom, if ever, have the poor and the indigent been so vilified as in the 1870's and 1880's" (Coll, 1969). However, these stern views were not unopposed. Other writers and reformers were beginning to bring to public attention facts indicating that most paupers were not able-bodied and of those that were, most were unemployed because of cyclical unemployment in their industries and not because they were shiftless. The heartlessness of the scientific charity approach was attacked in the "scathing verse" of John Boyle O'Reilly, a

"Catholic journalist-reformer" of Boston, who wrote in 1886:

The organized charity scrimped and iced
In the name of a cautious, statistical Christ (Coll, 1969).

It is important to note that the scientific charity movement, based on voluntary (i.e., private philanthropic) charity and Social Darwinist ideas, did not get to the "States west of the Mississippi, [where] public welfare rather than voluntary charity has been the main means of assisting the indigent" (Coll, 1969). The Midwestern cities, Chicago, Cleveland, Milwaukee, and Detroit, by and large continued to give outdoor relief as well as maintain almshouses.

A countervailing movement against Social Darwinist notions developed, starting in the 1870s when the COS movement was still dominating the East, becoming powerful in the Progressive Era[5] immediately after 1900 and lasting until 1918. Known as the settlement house movement, this new trend among opinion makers and activists "centered its efforts on the poor [emphasizing the need for] improvements in economic and social conditions in contrast to the COS which centered its attention on personal failure and only occasionally on conditions needing reform such as slum housing and inadequate provision for public health . . . the issue of poverty amid plenty moved onto the center stage" (Coll, 1969). It was during this Progressive Era that settlement house workers, liberal economists, and others established concepts such as the poverty line and a living wage (as opposed to a subsistence wage) and began to develop methodologies for calculating them. These activities enabled researchers and publicists to delineate more clearly the size and shape of poverty in the United States. They also laid the basis for drawing up personal budgets to be used in determining the levels of public assistance needed to bring a family's living standard to a minimum standard of decency. The budgets included not only the cost of decent food, clothing, and shelter, but also of medical care, education, and recreation. This work laid the foundations for the administrative methods and philosophy that were later to be incorporated in the Social Security Act of 1935 for federally matched public assistance and into the Medicaid Act of 1965 for federally matched publicly assisted medical care payments. Perhaps the most important ideological effect of the Progressives, as people with this philosophy often called themselves in that period, was to bring a "turnabout from the doctrine of personal fault to stress social and economic conditions as prime causes of hunger and squalor" (Coll, 1969).

An aspect of the campaigns for social services waged by the Progressives was their advocacy of *social insurance* against old age, unemployment, disablement, and death of the breadwinner. They derided permanent charity handouts as degrading and corrosive of human character just as much as the Social Darwinists did, but they rejected blaming charity recipients for their plight. The fault lay with society for not providing proper work to all who could work and *social insurance* as a matter of *right* to help those who could not work. The main objective was to avoid pauperism, not to punish it.

This clash of attitudes toward assistance for the poor would carry over, with different players, into later public controversies. Public medical care advocates and liberal or progressive commentators would recommend that the administration of public medical care be under a health agency rather than a public assistance agency, while medical societies and conservative commentators would prefer that public hospitals and other direct service organizations of local government be operated by welfare rather than health agencies, thereby making it clear that publicly delivered general medical care was a form of public assistance and properly subject to the standard of "less eligibility." The issue was also to be prominent in the later struggles over the form that universal national health insurance should take. One camp would advocate access to medical care as a right and objected to its use as a charity or public welfare handout to means-tested poor, while the other camp would advocate the use of means-tested medicine for the poor, with at best an increase in benefits. Universal national health insurance proponents would argue that access to medical care should be available to all under social *insurance* and not under private charity or a public welfare means-

tested dole, for any form of public assistance creates dependency, a syndrome that degrades human character; opponents would support proposals that would lead to continuation of two-tier medical care—the embodiment of "lesser eligibility" philosophy.

Over the years from 1800 through 1950 the state courts spelled out with increasing specificity the government responsibility for medical care for the poor. For example, in 1811 the New York state higher court reaffirmed the state government's responsibility to provide medical care for persons without resources, stating that if a "pauper" were sick, "medicine and attendance are as necessary as food."

The issue was last raised in California as late as 1917, and the California court held that "It has never been, nor will it ever be, questioned that among the first or primary duties devolving upon a state is that of providing suitable means and measures for the proper care and treatment, at the public expense, of the indigent sick, having no relative legally liable for their care." The responsibility of the state for providing medical care for the indigent was well established in all the state courts by 1920. For general medical care, the states in turn generally mandated this responsibility to the lcoal governments. As noted in Chapter 7, California, for example, made its counties responsible for the health care of poor persons in 1855, and in 1937 this obligation was broadened and codified in section 17000 of the state's Welfare and Institutions Code:

Every county and every city and county shall relieve all incompetent, poor, indigent persons, and those incapacitated by age, disease, or accident, lawfully resident therein when such persons are not supported and relieved by their relations or friends, by their own means or by state hospitals or either state or private institutions (Shonick and Roemer, 1983).

It is interesting to note that as late as 1937 the California state code still refers to residence and lack of kin support, in addition to disablement, as conditions of eligibility. By 1950 most states had laws that resembled California's in placing responsibility for the medical care of indigent people on local government, but outside California most counties in the United States had not elected to meet this mandate by having a public general hospital (Earle, 1952).

And finally in 1950 an expert in social welfare could write that:

Higher court decisions in different States appear to agree that the statutory public responsibility for the destitute includes not only medical services but hospital and nursing as well as food. The higher courts in many States have also held that the life of the destitute person must be saved and that if there has been no formal authorization for medical care, it may nevertheless be provided, and county authorities must accept the responsibility for paying the costs (Greenfield, 1958).

METHODS USED IN THE UNITED STATES TO PROVIDE FOR THE INDIGENT SICK

One method used to provide medical care for the indigent sick before 1965 was the local public general hospital. This institution was treated in Chapter 7 which dealt with the direct delivery of medical care by government—the subject of Part II of the book.

We have now turned to Part III, which considers medical care paid for by government, principally to private providers, for delivering medical care to a specified population—in this case the poor. Although some overlap with the previous discussion of the local public general hospital is unavoidable, the primary focus will be on other methods used by local government before 1965 to provide medical care to the poor, especially those who were on the public assistance rolls.

In the earlier years care of the indigent sick was part of public assistance in the case of the helpless or "worthy poor," along with food, housing, and clothing.[6] A noteworthy aspect of medical care provided for the poor is that although medical care for the welfare or "blameless" poor has been a part of their overall welfare entitlement, it was at times perceived to deserve greater attention than its other components. There has been little or no support for the proposition that "welfare" (i.e., public assistance) clients should be provided with food, clothing, shelter, transportation, and amenities that are comparable in quality to what middle-class persons have. Yet at various times it has been argued that medical care for the poor should be of "the best" (albeit without unnecessary "frills"). Sometimes this is formulated as a recommendation to abolish a two-track system of medical care. This was sometimes intended to mean offering universal access to private physicians and hospitals of the welfare recipient's choosing. Why this difference in perception? Is severely spartan health care any worse than severely spartan housing? Why have we not insisted that welfare recipients be supported at a level that would enable them to buy a middle-class house, drive a medium-priced car, and be able to eat good cuts of meat often? In actual fact, public assistance has rarely made single track medical care available to its beneficiaries but the limitations have been different in degree at different times. Much of the degree of restriction to special classes of provider can be deduced from the methods used to pay them. These and other issues will be explored in the next sections and in Chapters 9 and 10, but it is important to bear them in mind in what follows.

Earlier Methods Used by Communities

Almshouses

Reliable data are not available on the proportion of relief that was granted on an "outdoor" basis versus an "indoor" or institutional basis. Writers on this subject (e.g., Coll, 1969) generally agree that between 1850 and 1900 voices began to argue in favor of discontinuing almshouses (or poorhouses, workhouses) and using outdoor relief for general assistance along with special treatment-oriented institutions for mentally or physically ill persons. The development of ambulatory medical care systems for the poor receiving relief depended importantly on the development of outdoor relief. As long as relief was given primarily in the almshouse, medical care was also given there, but for those receiving outdoor relief, programs of ambulatory care became increasingly available after about 1850.

If no, or very little, outdoor relief was given by a locality, almshouses continued to house the indigent—the sick as well as the healthy. Because many indigent persons were poor primarily because they were not well enough to work, the sick usually made up a substantial share of the poorhouse population. For example, in 1873 a report on the condition of these institutions in Michigan estimated that for an average poorhouse population of 1,500 persons, the typical composition would include, in the terminology of the report, 250 insane, 125 idiots, etc.; 40 blind; 20 mute; and 300 epileptic and other deformities. It was also found that "34 Michigan counties delegated responsibility for the care of the sick to the superintendent of the poorhouse and his family and only fifteen counties reported physicians who were 'on call' or who made weekly visits." Similarly, "the early hospitals of California did not segregate chronic from acute cases." In general, sick, well, feebleminded adults, and children were all herded together in these almshouses. "The segregation of the sick from the well in the poorhouses has been coincident with the development of county general hospitals and special hospitals for the mentally disordered" (Stern, 1946).[7]

Use of the Salaried Public Physician

As early as 1736, we find a Dr. John Van Beuren receiving £100 per annum in colonial New York City to take care of the sick poor. For this sum, he also provided his own medicine. In 1820 Dr. John Cotton was paid $100 per annum in Rhode Island "to visit the sick at the asylum at least once a week . . . " and in 1835 we find Chicago employing a salaried physician. By 1866 this sole physician had been increased to three salaried physicians, each paid $500 per annum. By 1912 Missouri could report that 98 of 100 reporting counties employed county physicians. Courts have held that where regularly appointed physicians were not available in an emergency, any reputable physician could be called and poor law funds would recompense him (Stern, 1946)[8].

Contracting Out

The practice of leasing out the medical care of their indigent sick to the lowest bidder, a practice that brought increasingly bitter and frequent protest from reformers, was used at different times by different communities. The contract could be for treating the poor in almshouses, in physicians' offices, or in patients' homes.

Later Methods Used

The 1900s saw the organizational development of the county and municipal welfare department. It operated various domiciliary as well as medical care institutions for indigent persons and programs for contracting and paying for ambulatory medical care for their clients. The almshouse had become less important as a repository for all poor. The Spencerian position of the COS agencies and their "scientific philanthropy" philosophy was giving way to that of the settlement house social workers and leaders and the Progressive view that most poverty was not caused by the victim. The occupancy of the poorhouses was reduced by two developments: more of the able-bodied poor, especially widowed and deserted mothers, were being helped through outdoor relief, and many of the poor that were judged to need institutional care were being referred to specialized institutions dedicated to the care of their special needs. These were primarily the mental hospital, the tuberculosis hospital, the local public-general hospital, and the orphan asylum. The poorhouse became primarily a repository for the poor aged and "remained the last refuge for most aged persons until well into the 20th century" (Coll, 1969). Various arrangements for paying providers were used to provide medical care for the growing number of persons receiving outdoor relief and for those receiving the newer forms of mothers' aid "pensions." Some of the methods employed to reimburse physicians and hospitals are discussed in the following sections.

Payments to Physicians

Three main ways were used to pay physicians to care for relief clients.

Employment of Salaried Physicians The advantages of this method lay in its economy and ease of administration. Its disadvantages lay in the lack of choice of physician by the recipient and the inflexibility of the supply of physicians to meet a fluctuating load in demand. Also, this method often failed to attract the more competent physicians and the participating physicians were subject to political dictation and pressures to inappropriately curtail services.

The Panel System Under this method the welfare department contracted with a panel of physicians who agreed to serve its clients on a free-for-service basis according to a fixed fee schedule. In some instances, the local medical society was the contractee and the panel consisted of a rotating group of the society's members. This method provided the welfare recipient with some choice of physician since he or she could use any member of the panel. However, the better-qualified physicians often refused to participate, and the bulk of the care tended to fall into the hands of a relatively small number of less qualified, or at least less successful, practitioners. The administration of this system was usually heavily burdened by the red tape involved in determining eligibility for payment for each service billed. A limit was commonly placed on the type and amount of services that would be reimbursed without prior authorization, and physicians were burdened with an intricate task of record-keeping. It was common, particularly before 1935, for some physicians to serve as panel members for varying periods on a charitable basis, either with no reimbursement or for nominal pay. Much unpaid time was also given by physicians in free clinics for the poor.

Free Choice Under this system the welfare department of the locality issued a list of reimbursable services and their rates of reimbursement. Clients could use any physician willing to provide service at the stipulated fees. To facilitate locating such physicians welfare clients would sometimes be given a list of physicians who had agreed to provide care at the going rates. The method of payment to the physician under this system was usually fee-for-service but capitation was also sometimes used. In a few instances, welfare departments were able to purchase health insurance for clients, and the insured were required to use physicians who accepted the reimbursement rates as payment in full, but this arrangement was rarely used before 1956. "Few welfare agencies [had] developed

prepayment plans for medical care'' (Greenfield, 1958) before the passage of the Social Security Act and the amendments of 1956 providing for separately identified federal matching grants to the states specifically for medical care for welfare recipients.[9] After 1956 some such plans came into existence. Notable examples during the years 1956–57 were the seventeen Kansas counties that negotiated prepayment plans with the county medical society or a "substantial group" of participating physicians; the contract with Blue Cross and Blue Shield negotiated by the state of Colorado; and the contract for statewide physicians' services negotiated by Washington state.

Payments to Hospitals

As was noted in the discussion of the local public general hospital in Chapter 7, these institutions did not usually receive any fee-for-service payment for their care of nonpaying patients either inpatient or outpatient. Indeed, before 1965 the large public urban hospital was itself often operated by the local welfare or charities department and was directly financed via local government appropriations to these departments. But in some places, such as New York City, the city also paid private hospitals for their care of poor patients. Whenever a hospital was paid by the local government for indigent care, the payments were made by several methods:

Direct Payment to Hospital The basis for reimbursement commonly used one of four methods: (1) a negotiated rate, usually an all-inclusive per diem rate; (2) payment of the hospital's usual charges to the public; (3) reimbursement based on cost of providing service; and (4) a lump-sum annual contribution to the local hospital.

Direct Payment to Hospital from Patient's Welfare Allowance This method involves a patient who is a recipient of cash assistance from a welfare agency reimbursing the hospital from his or her cash assistance allotment which includes a (theoretical) amount for hospital care in its budget. In practice, this was rarely used, for "Reimbursement by the recipient is not widely favored by hospitals because collection is frequently difficult'' (Coll, 1969).

Insurance As noted under the physician payment section, in the later years of the period under discussion (1956–1965), some policies were negotiated by welfare departments with commercial, Blue Cross and Blue Shield, and independent insurers. Self-insurance, using pooled funds of welfare agencies, was also used.

It should also be noted that before World War II, ambulatory and hospital care provided by voluntary philanthropic agencies figured prominently in the medical care provided for the poor, but it was less important after the 1929 Depression than before. Before the Depression, the system of medical care for the needy "relied primarily on local government resources and the charitable services of physicians, voluntary hospitals, and voluntary health and welfare agencies. Like other systems of local relief for the needy, it foundered under the impact of the economic depression of the Thirties" (Coll, 1969).

Federal Grants-in-Aid to the States for Medical Care to the Indigent

The FERA Program

The Great Depression, signaled by the stock market crash of 1929, altered the dimensions of poverty. With the quantum leap in the number of the unemployed came a change in the perception of the roots of joblessness. The percentage of the labor force that was unemployed rose from 3.2 percent in 1929 to 15.9 percent in 1931 and reached a peak of 24.9 percent in 1933 (U.S. Bureau of the Census, 1960). With one-fourth of the United States labor force unable to find work, the question of the "unworthiness" of the able-bodied unemployed was seen in a new light. Persons who throughout their entire adult life had been successful earners as business persons or wage workers were not easily convinced that their sudden inability to find gainful work was due to a deep-seated flaw in their character. Existing public medical care programs for welfare clients and private voluntary programs for the able-bodied poor could not begin to serve the number of applicants now appearing.

The Federal Emergency Relief Administration (FERA), a temporary program initiated in May 1933 and operating until 1935 to provide economic help to the unemployed, included a medical reimbursement program for ambulatory care. The medical care program of FERA included the following provisions:

1. Patients were accorded free choice of practitioner.
2. Federal funds were used to pay for medical care according to a fee schedule set up in each state in consultation with organized medical, dental, and nursing professions. The program was federally financed but state administered.
3. Eligibility was based on satisfying the condition of being "unemployed"—i/e., having been previously employed. It was not meant to include the type of caseload carried by welfare departments, the non-working worthy poor.

This program was the beginning of an important change in viewpoint toward the medical profession's role in providing medical care for the poor. Whereas previously the idea had been commonly held that physicians should serve the poor largely without pay, or at least with greatly reduced fees (the so-called "sliding scale" for charges), this program signaled a change in this attitude, calling for full compensation for providers of medical care for the poor and leaving the financing to governmental initiative.

The FERA medical program was aimed at supplementing such medical services as were provided by existing community agencies. In general, acute care and life-endangering conditions were covered and eligibility was restricted to persons receiving unemployment relief under the FERA program. As noted above, this medical care program, like the rest of the FERA programs, was clearly meant to exclude the pre-Depression "regular" welfare case load, the helpless who needed public assistance permanently, or the paupers. Parallel systems of home and office medical care continued to be operated by previously existing local agencies, both governmental and voluntary, to serve persons who were not eligible under the FERA plans.

The FERA medical program had many gaps in coverage: it excluded hospitalization costs, with fifteen states restricting medical services to home and office calls for acute illness; there was almost no federal control of quality of service; and it excluded payments to clinics or their physicians. The public hospital, it should be particularly noted, received no help from this program, a precedent that was to be followed by all the subsequent pre-1965 federally financed social programs and that was to contribute so heavily to the later "plight of the public hospital" discussed in Chapter 7.

The Social Security Act of 1935

With respect to helping finance medical care for the poor, the passage of the Social Security Act again marks a watershed in the change of the federal role as it did in the area of public health. As noted in the chapters on public health, this act established for the first time in the United States substantial federal subsidization and regulation of important social welfare programs in four major areas: (a) old age insurance; (b) public health department support; (c) maternal and child welfare; and (d) cash public assistance to three categories of indigent persons—old, blind, and dependent children (deprived of one parent).[10] The provisions in (a) will be discussed in Chapters 9 and 10 on social insurance, and the provisions under (b) and (c) have been discussed in Part I, which dealt with public health. This section is concerned with the fourth program in the preceding list, (d), cash public assistance to three categories of person defining the "worthy" poor concept used by welfare or relief programs since the earliest days of the republic (and by the English poor law before them).

The 1935 act provided for matching federal grants to the states for money payments to qualifying welfare recipients. Aid "in kind" of any form was forbidden. The basic intention of this prohibition was to prevent assistance in the form of items like used clothing or furniture and surplus food commodities instead of money to buy the items in the market. However, it was interpreted also to prohibit the use of any part of the federal matching funds by the states to pay health plans, insurance companies, physicians, or hospitals directly under special arrangements for the medical care of welfare beneficiaries, since such an arrangement involved not directly giving the recipient the cash to dispose of as he or she saw fit. The purchase of medical care for public welfare beneficiaries with a portion of their assistance grants was thus seen to be a type of payment in kind. The only way in which federal government grants for cash assistance to public welfare recipients entered the medical care provision picture was oblique and ineffective. It could be allowed as an item to be added to the recipient's theoretical cost-of-living budget, drawn up by the welfare agency to be used as a basis for computing the cash allotment to be dispensed to welfare clients. This prohibition precluded arrangements by welfare agencies to prepay the medical care of their clients.

States and localities continued to bear the sole burden of welfare payments to indigent citizens who were not in one of the federal "worthy" categories. This residual welfare category was known as "general assistance." Localities continued medical programs for these welfare clients, sometimes with some state assistance, but there was no federal contribution to these programs. It should be noted that until a fourth category of persons, "permanently and totally disabled," was made eligible for federal matching in 1950, there was no way in which a poor person with continued or disabling illness could be eligible for federal matching, and he or she had to remain permanently on the relatively meager general assistance grant unless eligible for workmen's compensation, veteran's pensions, or a private pension.

In 1939 amendments to the Social Security Act made many widowed mothers with minor children eligible for assistance under survivor's *insurance*.[11] This left most of the remaining needy women dependent on federally matched *public welfare* under the Aid to Families with Dependent Children (AFDC) public assistance category with their eligibility based on the continued absence of a man. If a man could be found "about the house" such eligibility was endangered. Thus, the AFDC category was the only category of federally matched welfare assistance whose recipients were able-bodied. The failure to include the deserted mother, whether wed or unwed, under a mother's *pension*-type program along with other Social Security OASI recipients was to make the AFDC recipients the constant butt of the assault on the welfare system. These attacks usually sounded a call for the greater use of punitively deterrent measures, harking back to the COS days of "scientific philanthropy" with its emphasis on punitively discouraging immorality, maintaining less eligibility and stressing training the beneficiary for economic self-sufficiency.

A number of subsequent amendments to the Social Security Act widened the scope of persons defined as eligible for federal matching and increased the options available to the state and locality with respect to paying for medical care for their public welfare clients. Groups that had been opposed to all payments in kind, such as the National Association of Social Wokers and its predecessor organizations, became convinced that welfare clients would benefit from permitting welfare departments to negotiate directly with medical vendors, and provisions allowing these arrangements were added in subsequent amendments. An outline of the main amendments to the Social Security Act expanding eligibility and support for medical payments for public assistance beneficiaries in the years before 1965 follows:

1. *1950.* Two important changes were made in the Social Security Act pertaining to federally matched public welfare: (a) Welfare departments were permitted to use federal matching funds for cash assistance to negotiate for care with prepayment and insurance plans; and (b) a fourth category, "permanently and totally disabled," was added to the three originally eligible for federal matching funds for cash assistance.

The first of these two amendments did not immediately increase the medical care benefits of public welfare recipients as intended. Although states were now permitted to use federal matching funds to contract with organized health insurance systems for their public assistance beneficiaries, no additional money was provided for such expansion. The funds would have to come out of reallocating some of the existing cash assistance grant money or from additional (unmatched) state funds.

It was the second of these amendments, the one creating the newly eligible public assistance class of "disabled," that many mental health advocates and administrators hoped would provide an important missing link in the chain of services needed to make deinstitutionalization work (see Chapter 6). Because the disability of many of the persons in this category was mental, they would now be eligible for federally matched cash assistance grants that could be used to help support them to live in the community. However, many of these persons, as was noted in Chapter 6, really needed protected halfway houses of various types and not just cash, and under this amendment federal funds still could not be used to pay for supporting persons in institutions, a proviso that had been meant to discourage the support of care in the poorhouse.

Both the original prohibition of in kind support and of payments for institutionalized persons for many years prevented the federal welfare system from either buying into comprehensive health plans for their clients or supporting with individual grants or direct institutional assistance local public general hospitals or halfway houses. This situation is only one of many examples of the difficulty of preventing regulatory devices from producing collateral results not desired by the framers of thc legislation, and in fact sometimes producing perversely opposite results. Contexts change, and if regulatory measures are not kept current, unwanted results are likely to occur.

2. *1956.* Separate federal matching was provided for medical vendor payments with funds additional to those previously appropriated for cash assistance up to a specific per capita limit.[12] The requirement that all assistance payments to recipients be strictly cash grants with no money withheld for vendor payments was reinstated. These maximum additional amounts, which were matched 50 percent by the federal government, did not begin to pay for the cost of such medical payments to states with more generous programs.[13]

3. *1958.* Separately identified federal grants for medical vendor programs were eliminated and the additional amounts that had been separately granted to states for such payments since 1956, were incorporated into a single grant, raising the ceiling for total per capita matching by the federal government to $65 for adults and $30 for each child.[14] Each state was now free to give this money entirely as a cash grant or to subdivide it into cash grants and payments to medical vendors, and the base grant now had incorporated into it the additional amounts for making vendor payments. Although this folding in of funds weakened the financial incentive for the states to arrange for direct medical care pay-

ments to health plans or providers, by 1960 four-fifths of the states did have separately identified medical vendor payment provisions in their federally aided public assistance programs.

4. *1960.* After 1956 the states had wide latitude in setting up the medical vendor payment programs; they were free, for example, to set up programs with differing ranges of coverage for the four different welfare categories. In many states, the program for the aged category had been the most comprehensive of the four categories, even before 1960. Despite this fact, the Kerr-Mills Act of 1960 provided additional federal matching incentives for even greater expansion of medical programs for the aged category (old age assistance—"OAA") only.

Under the terms of this act (which were part of the Social Security amendments of 1960) a new welfare category was established: Medical Assistance for the Aged (MAA). Separate and additional federal matching funds were made available for medical vendor payments only on behalf of OAA welfare recipients. Federal matching percentages were made variable from state to state, ranging from 50 to 80 percent of total expenditures, the percentage depending inversely on the per capita income of the state. The initial maximum matchable expenditure was set at $15 per aged recipient per month, with no limitation on total state expenditure.

This act was an attempt to satisfy and thereby blunt public pressure for federally financed health insurance for the aged, such as was provided by the Forand Bill then pending in the House (see page 273f). It managed to stave off the passage of such insurance until 1965.

5. 1963. Increased Medical Care for High Risk and Low Income Mothers was passed in connection with the passage of the Mental Health and Mental Retardation Facilities Act of 1963 (see Chap. 6). Additional federal contributions for special medical care for mothers at risk for giving birth to mentally retarded children was provided. These were project grants that included prenatal care, delivery, and postpartum care. Also, Title V of the Social Security Act was amended to provide for special and additional financing of maternal and infant care for low-income mothers.

The movement toward providing access to medical care for all had been moving along several lines until 1965. There were privately paid physicians for those who could afford to pay or had private insurance; government direct service programs for specially singled-out groups; and private philanthropy and public welfare programs for the poor. I noted that beginning with the Progressive movement around the turn of the century, advocacy for social insurance as against either private philanthropy or public welfare was making its appearance. And after 1945, private medical care insurance (misnamed "health insurance") did indeed begin to take hold for employed workers. In 1965 two major pieces of legislation attempted to fill in the remaining access gaps for the entire population. Medicare provided health insurance for the aged and Medicaid provided a greatly expanded public welfare medical payment system for the "worthy" classes of poor and some near-poor persons.

NOTES

1. The material on the Elizabethan Poor Law in this section follows the formulation in Coll, 1969; unless otherwise designated the quotations are from that source.

2. Payments in money or goods and services (known as "payment in kind") to relief recipients living in their own or other private residences rather than in institutions.

3. In 1796 Parliament had passed a law allowing some public assistance to the *employed* working poor. A parish could elect to provide supplementary assistance to employed workers when wages fell below a specified subsistence level. The Speenkamland system is one part of English social welfare practice that was never generally adopted in the United States.

4. Darwin himself was not involved with this line of thought.

5. There was a Progressive Party on whose ticket Theodore Roosevelt ran for president in 1912.

6. However, over time health services for working poor and unemployed able-bodied poor began to be offered increasingly through various governmental agencies, the main one coming to be the local public hospital.

7. As noted in Chapter 7, many almshouses ultimately became local general public hospitals. This transition was closely linked to outdoor relief becoming the general modality for assisting the poor.

8. Stern cites additional references as sources for the information in this paragraph.

9. This is further explained under the discussion of the Social Security Act below.

10. It also, in effect, mandated the states to provide unemployment insurance.

11. The original 1935 act covered only retirement pensions under OAI, or old age insurance. In 1939 this became OASI, old age and survivor's insurance. Thus, in the first four years of Social Security there were no "widow's pensions." Only welfare was available if there was a minor child in the house and the widow was sufficiently poor to qualify for welfare in her state. Pensions based on disability were not added to Social Security until 1956, after which the *insurance* program was known as OASDI.

12. Initially $6 expenditure monthly per adult and $3 for each child.

13. New York state, for example, reported that average medical payments for welfare clients were $20 per month.

14. In 1950 the ceilings had been $55 per month per adult, $30 additional for the first child and $21 for each additional child.

9

Government-Sponsored Health Insurance: The Period Before 1965

WORKERS' COMPENSATION AND GENERAL DISABILITY INSURANCE

Background

The earliest entry of government into the health insurance field in the United States was through state-sponsored or -mandated insurance against injury associated with working conditions. Until the turn of the century, the courts rarely held a worker's injuries incurred on the job to be compensable by the employer (Somers and Somers, 1954; Elliot and Vaughan, 1978, 123; Williams, Barth, and Rosenbloom, 1973, Chap 21). Using English common law precedents, the state courts established two sets of doctrines defining employer liability for employee injury. The first set established the legal obligations of an employer to his employees with respect to providing for safety in the workplace: maintaining the work premises in safe condition, seeing that a workers' fellow employees were competent and of sufficient number to maintain safety, warning employees of unusual hazards inherent in the trade, and maintaining proper safety rules. The second set defined the obligations of workers to assure their own safety and established conditions that circumscribed the recovery of legal damages by an injured employee from his employer. This second set, the so-called employer defenses against liability, consisted of the doctrines of contributory negligence, the fellow servant rule, and the assumption of risk.

The doctrine of contributory negligence held that even when the injury was caused partly by some failure of the employer to meet his safety obligations, if the accident was in any part due to the employee's negligence[1], the employee was not entitled to damages. The fellow servant doctrine[2] asserted that an employer could not be held liable for an injury to an employee that was caused by the negligence of a fellow employee. The assumption of risk doctrine held that if the employment accepted by a worker entailed special or unusual risks that the employee could reasonably be expected to have known before assuming employment, he could not receive damages for injuries resulting from such unusual hazards.

The application of these doctrines resulted in a very small proportion of workers' injuries being recompensed through damages. "It has been estimated that not more than 15 percent of injured employees ever recovered damages under the common law, even though 70 percent of the injuries were estimated to have been related to working conditions or employer's negligence (Williams, Barth, and Rosenbloom, 1973:11). By the turn of the century, the sharply accelerating rate of injury and death associated with the work milieu was receiving widespread public attention. In an attempt to provide a better chance for such injured workmen to be compensated for their loss, a number of states began to pass "employers' liability statues" that limited the scope of the common-law employer defenses in specified instances. These laws did not reverse the fundamental common-law assumption that an injured employee could collect damages from an employer only if the latter could be proved to have been negligent, but they explicitly added more circumstances under which the employer assumed liability and thereby made negligence somewhat easier to establish. For example, some of these laws abolished the fellow servant doctrine, but often only for one industry. "By 1907, 26 States had enacted employer liability acts, with most of these abolishing the fellow servant rule while a few limited the assumption of risk and contributory negligence doctrines as well (Williams, Barth, and Rosenbloom, 1973:13). All railroads engaging in interstate commerce were placed under such employers' liability law by the federal Employers' Liability Act of 1908.

The employers' liability statutes did not effectively meet the dissatisfaction of labor, some of industry, and much of the public with the status of employee compensation for injuries. At best, damages could be collected only through costly and lengthy litigation, but in most cases the injury could not be shown in court to be traceable to a specific act of negligence on the part of the employer. The very nature of industrial work under existing technologies carried with it an inherent chance of injury, and the notion came to be increasingly held that the cost of compensating such injury should properly be considered a normal cost of production. This perception led to increasing support for basing compensation for injury solely on the degree of incapacity caused, the so-called doctrine of compensation *without fault,* which was the fundamental concept underlying the workmen's compensation laws. This philosophy had been written into law in Germany for certain industries as early as 1838, and by 1890 it was a firmly established principle there. Great Britain, the home of the employer common-law defenses, had gone through the employers' liability statutes phase in the 1880s and 1890s and passed its first workmen's compensation act in 1897. In 1906 these laws were extended to virtually all workers.

Reacting to industrial conditions in the United States, as well as to the developments in Germany and Great Britain, a number of states began to pass workmen's compensation laws shortly after 1900. New York was the first state to adopt such a law, in 1910, but it was declared unconstitutional by the New York State Supreme Court in 1911,[3] mainly on the grounds of its compulsory feature. And, although the United States Supreme Court ruled that such laws were constitutional, in 1917,[4] the "pattern of elective statutes had been set" (Williams,

Barth, and Rosenbloom, 1973, 18) by the laws passed in a number of states between the time of the New York state law decision of 1911 and the U.S. Supreme Court decision of 1917. By 1925, twenty-four jurisdictions had passed workmen's compensation laws, and with the passage of such a law by Mississippi in 1948 every state had one.

The Program in 1980

The Administrative Structure

In 1980 all fifty-six geographic jurisdictions[5] had Workers' Compensation[6] laws in effect. In addition, the Federal Employees' Compensation Act covered the employees of the U.S. government; the Longshoremen and Harbor Workers' Act covered maritime workers other than seamen and some other groups; and the Black Lung Program covered miners. The laws varied from state to state, but they all shared certain features. In all states the employer paid the entire premium. This follows the British system but is different from the German system. In the latter, the employee contributed to the premium, a feature that still held in East Germany in 1980. There were other features that most of the plans had.

In the United States, workers' compensation benefits include two broad classifications: cash payments to affect loss of wages due to inability to work and free medical care for conditions caused by work-related traumas. Since these benefits are associated with health conditions, both are features of the United States health care landscape and its interface with governmental authority. In calendar year 1980, some $3.9 billion of national health care expenses were for medical care via workers' compensation. This is less than 2 percent of the $219.4 billion spent in that year for personal health care and something just under 6 percent of the $68 billion of the personal health expenditures met by insurance payments. In the same year, $9.5 billion was also paid out in cash benefits for income maintenance (Price, 1983) and $8.7 billion was spent on administration and supervision, the overwhelming portion for administering the cash benefits; only $700 million went for administration of the medical program. In 1980 slightly over 79 million workers were covered by state laws.

Workers' Compensation insurance was carried by three types of insurers in 1980: private insurance companies, special funds run by the states themselves, and self-insurance by employers. In six states the law mandated the use of the state fund, while among the remaining forty-four states, eighteen had state funds but their use was optional with the employer; and in twenty-six states only private insurance carriers were available. In all but three states, large employers were permitted to self-insure. In twenty of the fifty-six jurisdictions, the state agency that administered the workers' compensation program was the state labor department; in twenty-seven it was a separate workers' compensation board or commission, and in five it was administered by the courts. The premiums were based on experience rating systems under which high injury rates led to a higher premium rate for an employer and vice versa. This practice was presumed to encourage employers to pay greater attention to employee safety.

Benefits

Cash indemnities were paid to workers who were disabled or to survivors of those who died on the job. Disability payments were made for temporary total disablement, permanent partial disablement, and permanent total disablement. The amount of the payment varied from state to state and depended on the nature of the disability and the number of dependents. It was scaled to the worker's wage level but was often additionally limited by maximum total dollar amounts and total time limits. Most commonly, the basic rate was two-thirds of the wages earned, subject to the further limitations indicated above.

Workers who were permanently and totally disabled were also eligible for Social Security payments and many of the larger firms offered privately insured group long-term disability insurance as an employee benefit. Many firms carried pension plans that included disability retirement provisions. Social Security disability payments were reduced if disabled workers were also receiving workers' compensation sufficiently large to bring the total of both payments to over 80 percent of their former wage. A sim-

ilar situation existed with respect to temporary disability. Private insurance programs financed by employers often paid the worker to maintain his or her income level during sickness. These included sick leave plans. Finally, for disabled low-income workers covered by workers' compensation there were also available welfare payments under Aid to the Blind and Aid to the Permanently and Totally Disabled categories, but the welfare payments, if any, could only be supplemental to bring the total income up to the welfare assistance maximum permissible income level.

Medical benefits were quite comprehensive, covering first aid, physicians, hospitals, nursing, drugs, supplies, and prosthetic devices. In 1970 "only 9 States limited the total medical care available for work-related injuries by specific dollar amounts or maximum periods (Williams, Barth, and Rosenbloom, 1983). An important area of ambiguity in defining eligibility for workmen's compensation has been the type of illness that may be covered. The general definition has been "personal injury caused by accident or arising out of and in the course of employment." While actual injury sustained on the job has nearly always been covered, the area of occupational disease has been treated very variably from state to state and has been a main source of dissatisfaction with the system. In 1972, forty-one states covered a wide spectrum of occupational diseases.

Continuing Problems and Review of Program Status After 1970

With the development of private health insurance, government-sponsored insurance, welfare medical programs, and the growth of special health-care systems like the Veterans Administration medical program, the functions and structure of the workers' compensation program came under scrutiny by both government and private bodies. The performance of the program was examined to see to what extent it had met its objectives and to what degree changed circumstances required changes in the program.

In a publication issued in 1983 the U.S. Chamber of Commerce held the objectives of the program to be to:

1—Provide sure, prompt, and reasonable income and medical benefits to work-accident victims, or income benefits to their dependents, regardless of fault;
2—Provide a single remedy and reduce court delays, costs, and work loads arising out of personal-injury litigation;
3—Relieve public and private charities of financial drains–incident to uncompensated industrial accidents;
4—Eliminate payment of fees to lawyers and witnesses as well as time-consuming trials and appeals;
5—Encourage maximum employer interest in safety and rehabilitation through an appropriate experience-rating mechanisms; and
6—Promote frank study of causes of accidents (rather than concealment of fault)–reducing preventable accidents and human suffering (U.S. Chamber of Commerce, 1983, VII).

Opinions have varied as to the degree of achievement of these aims and the value of continuing the workers' compensation program. As early as 1954, Herman M. Somers and Anne R. Somers in their study of the system expressed many misgivings and doubts about its values. And although by 1970 83 percent of employed workers in the fifty states and District of Columbia were covered by workers' compensation, fifteen states covered less than 70 percent. The noncoverage was due to exclusion of certain occupations, the noncompulsory nature of some state laws, and the failure of some employers to meet their legal obligations. "The occupations typically excluded from coverage, such as household workers and farm help, are disproportionately low income, less educated, nonwhite, and female—those least able financially of carrying the burden of disability by themselves" (Commission on Workmen's Compensation, 1972, 44). Only twenty-seven states in 1972 provided compensation coverage without exempting firms of small size, only seventeen states covered agricultural workers on the same basis as other workers, and the longevity of the "pattern of elective statutes" set between 1911 and 1917 was attested to by the fact that only thirty-one of the fifty states had compulsory coverage in 1972 (Commission on Workmen's Compensation, 1972, 45–46). It was largely because of these facts that eighteen years after the Somers and Somers study, when the National Commission on State Workmen's Compensa-

tion Laws issued its report in compliance with the requirements of the Occupational Safety and Health Act of 1970, its judgment was:

The inescapable conclusion is that State workmen's compensation laws in general are inadequate and unequitable. While several states have good programs, and while medical care and some other aspects of workmen's compensation are commendable in most States, the strong points are too often matched by the weak (p. 119).

The report went on to cite the findings of the Department of Labor on the degree to which the states met sixteen "conservative" recommendations for a good program. The results are shown in Table 9–1. The (majority) report recommended that support for workmen's compensation programs be continued but with strong efforts to improve them. The recommendations designated as "essential and particularly suitable for federal support to guarantee their adoption" by each state were:

1. Compulsory coverage.
2. Benefits should not be limited by occupation nor should employers of a small number of employees be exempt. Specifically, farm workers, household workers, and state and local employees should be included.
3. All work-related diseases should be covered.
4. Full medical care without time or money limitation should be covered.
5. Employees should be able to file in the state where injured, where hired, or where employment is principally localized.

Table 9–1. Number of Jurisdictions Meeting Sixteen Workers' Compensation Recommended Standards, January 1, 1972

Number of Standards Met	States (50)	Other States (6)	Federal (2)
13–16	9	1	1
9–12	13	4	1
5–8	18	0	0
0–4	10	1	0

Source: Commission on Workmen's Compensation, 1972, table 7.1

6. Temporary disability benefits should be at least two-thirds of the employee's average wage, but not necessarily above the state's average wage. No time or dollar limit should be applied.
7. and 8. Recommendations similar to those for "6" for death benefits and permanent disability benefits.

The report called for evaluation of the attainment of these recommendations by July 1, 1975, and "if necessary, Congress with no further delay should guarantee compliance."

By contrast, an industry view (U.S. Chamber of Commerce, 1973) held in 1973 that "a general consensus shows: Today—after more than 50 years of legal development—workmen's compensation is a valued institution in our industrial economy ... the worth of workmen's compensation is measurable in many ways other than valued assistance to disabled workers."

In light of these differing evaluations of the success of the program in achieving its goals it seems clear that a consensus on this matter was not achieved. Rather, the evidence indicates that the efficacy of the workmen's compensation program in achieving its objectives was being seriously questioned. When the laws were first advocated during the years 1900–1910, and passed mostly during 1910–1920, the provisions filled a clearly visible gap. With the passage of the Social Security Act in 1935 and the subsequent amendments, and the rapid growth of private health and other "fringe benefit" insurance after World War II, the void had narrowed noticeably. As I have noted, the creation of permanent disability pensions under Social Security insurance in 1956 and permanent disability as an eligible category (of the worthy poor) under federally subsidized public assistance had also filled part of the void, as did the existence of private insurance with sick leave provisions, medical care coverage, permanent and total disability insurance, and disability retirement provisions in pension plans. And there was a widespread feeling in labor circles that for serious injuries the large awards possible through litigation were to be preferred to the circumscribed benefits provided by workers' compensation

schedules. And finally, the promised decline in litigation mostly did not occur; for large unions it was no longer as important as it had been. They had access to their own legal staffs and consulting legal firms.

The usefulness of the medical service portion of the workers' compensation program has clearly depended on the extent to which it filled the gaps left by other programs. For example, the quite comprehensive medical care coverage, which in 1972 was provided without time limit in forty-one states (for injuries; only in thirty-six states for occupational diseases), is of this nature. However, the continuing widespread exclusions of certain categories of persons in these programs, such as farm workers, domestic workers, and casual workers, and the reduction of Social Security disability benefits for persons receiving workers' compensation, deny or reduce payments precisely to persons for whom other programs are nonexistent or inadequate.

It should also be noted that health care coverage for nonemployed persons and low-earning employed workers had been one of the major weak spots in the United States health care system and was likely to become more so. Since the workers' compensation program is entirely tied to employed status, it provides nothing for nonemployed workers. Its medical benefits thus became and were likely to become increasingly less relevant to the lack-of-access-to-care problem in the United States unless it especially focused on unmet needs among employed persons with poor health insurance coverage. In states where workers' compensation covered employed uninsured persons in large numbers, it remained an important source of care, but only of employees injured on the job. However, these workers with no or poor health insurance were (and are) concentrated in precisely those industries that are likely to be poorly covered by workers' compensation laws.

Finally, achievement of the anticipated effects of the experience-rating features of workers' compensation on work-related deaths and injuries is supported by the applicable statistics only for the earlier years (see Table 9–2). After 1960, however, the rates showed no marked decline. It should be noted that the overall rates shown average out trends that are quite different for specific sub-classes of industrial endeavor. The

Table 9–2. Trends in Work-Related Deaths and Injuries, 1930–1971, Selected Years

| | Deaths All Workers | | Manufacturing Injuries | | |
Year	Number	Rate per 100,000 Workers	Number	Rate per 100,000 Workers	Frequency Rate*
1930	19,000	—	—	—	23.1
1935	16,500	39	1,900	22	17.9
1940	17,000	38	2,000	19	15.3
1945	16,500	33	2,700	18	18.6
1950	15,500	27	2,600	17	14.7
1955	14,200	24	2,000	12	12.1
1960	13,800	21	1,700	10	12.0
1965	14,100	20	1,800	10	12.8
1970	14,300	18	1,800	9	15.2
1971	14,200	18	1,800	10	NA

Source: Commission on Workmen's Compensation, 1972, table 5.1.
*Frequency rate is the number of disabling injuries per 1,000,000 man-hours of exposure.

National Commission Report (1972) provides further detail and concludes that a definite connection between merit (experience) rating and safety record is difficult to demonstrate,'' probably because there are so many [other] variable factors that influence accident rates'' (1972). Some liberal and left-of-center reformers advocate the use of worker safety monitoring in the workplace with power to halt dangerous operations, a procedure used in Sweden. Failing the introduction of an alternative and better way of preventing injuries, however, one must at least consider the likelihood of the injury and death rates rising to former heights if the workers' compensation laws with their experience rating feature are abandoned.

During the 1980s, business voices were increasingly strident, calling for workers' compensation reform. They asserted that it had become very expensive and inefficient owing to high administrative costs and fraud brought about by collusion between attorneys and physicians. In California it has even been claimed that the workers' compensation program is responsible for business wanting to leave the state and for discouraging others from coming into the state. It is not clear to what degree these charges are unique to this facet of health insurance. There is the question of how much they reflect the perception of the national medical care system as costly and inefficient, a perception fueled by the sharpening business competition in the face of a prolonged sluggish economy.

General Disability Insurance

In an attempt to fill the gap in coverage of employed persons who become ill and whose illness does not meet the "appropriate work-related disease" requirements of the state's workers' compensation law, six jurisdictions by 1973 had passed compulsory laws covering temporary disability with no requirements for showing work relatedness. These jurisdictions and the dates of passage of these laws are: California (1946), Hawaii (1969), New Jersey (1948), New York (1949), Rhode Island (1942), and Puerto Rico (1968).

The laws provide cash benefits only. California had also provided hospital benefits, but these were discontinued as of December 31, 1978.

CONTROVERSY OVER SCHEMES OF GOVERNMENT-SPONSORED HEALTH INSURANCE FOR GENERAL MEDICAL CARE

I have noted that insurance against the costs of sickness has two aspects: protection against income loss due to a breadwinner's illness, and protection against the costs of medical care required by the illness. In the first twenty years of the 1900s the main cost of illness to the employed sick person and his or her family was the loss of income because of not being able to work. The medical expenses of the illness were often secondary. After 1920, the medical expenses of the illness rose more rapidly than the income lost, and meeting the cost of medical care became increasingly important (Falk, 1936; Davis, 1937). The discussion of workers' compensation legislation in the previous section described the coverage of these two facets of illness insurance when the illness is job-related. This section focuses on government-sponsored insurance for the costs of *general* medical care, that is, treatment for illness or injury that is presumably not job-related. Clearly, maintaining the income of working people when they are ill is related to the total general health insurance picture, but this aspect of the question will not be considered here.

The Early Period: 1900–1932

Schemes of government-sponsored general health insurance were discussed and debated almost continuously in public life with varying rates of intensity during the entire period of 1900–1965. The question of government-sponsored insurance for personal health services came to the fore as a major issue during the years 1912–1920. This period witnessed a surge of reform and populist thought and activities resulting in the passage of a spate of national legislation including the first permanent national income tax, a flurry of environmental and food and drug control legislation, the enfranchisement of women, the introduction of the eight hour work day and the previously described laws compensating workers for the results of industrial accidents. In literature, Upton Sinclair, Lincoln Steffens, Ida Tarbell, and the other muckrakers were popularizing the need for conserving the environment, protecting the consuming and working public against excesses of the industrial system, defending the body politic against the abuses of political corruption, and regulating the activities of giant corporations.

One of the most important national political bodies pressing for legislation to accomplish these reforms during this "Progressive" period was the American Association for Labor Legislation (AALL), a loose conglomeration consisting mostly of liberal economists but also including civic leaders, labor leaders, and other professionals and intellectuals. This group had been notably successful in getting workers' (or workmen's, as it was then called) compensation laws passed in most of the states in which this type of legislation was an important issue, and embarked next on a campaign to get the states to pass government-sponsored general health insurance laws. By 1915, AALL had drafted a model state bill calling for protection of all low-income workers during periods of sickness by giving cash compensation, as well as offering inpatient and out-of-hospital medical care benefits to the workers and their dependents. At first this bill was favorably regarded by the American Medical Association, the American Hospital Association, many local unions, the National Association of Manufacturers,[7] and the first three state legislative commissions (California, Massachusetts, and New Jersey) that were appointed to study it. However, between 1918 and 1920, support was lost for the model bill, with several state-appointed study commissions reporting unfavorably. The state medical societies had opposed it all along and the national American Medical Association reversed itself in 1920, taking a position of implacable opposition. The legislation did not pass in a single state, and after 1920 the AALL turned its attention to unemployment and old age insurance, the issue of health insurance lying dormant until the 1930s.

It is interesting that while the national body of organized medicine was for a time in favor and its grass-roots elements in opposition, the converse held true in labor ranks. The local membership bodies of organized labor favored the proposal but the national leadership opposed it. By the end of 1918, for example, twenty-one international unions and eighteen state federations of labor had endorsed the proposal (Corning, 1969). Although the issue of national health insurance remained in limbo on the national political scene during the years 1921 through 1933, studies were proceeding, for the most part modest in scope and without public fanfare, to marshall facts supporting the need for some form of health insurance. Furthermore, a host of private social welfare institutions helped keep the reform impulse alive, among these the National Consumers' League, the National Conference of Social Work, the National Federation of Settlements, and the AALL. These organizations engaged in activities that included operating limited social welfare programs with philanthropic funds, lobbying modestly, conducting research, and engaging in public educational activities.

The most important piece of research to come out of this post–Progressive period was the report of the Committee on the Costs of Medical Care (CCMC), issued in 1932. The result of a five-year study, this report "amassed a veritable library of research data" (Corning, 1969), and its majority recommendations suggested fundamental changes in the organization and financing of medicine. Established in 1927 under the leadership of Dr. Ray Lyman Wilbur, a physician, president of Stanford University, and secretary of the interior under President Hoover, the CCML was financially supported by six private philanthropic foundations: the Josiah Macy Jr.,

Foundation, the Milbank Memorial Fund, the Russell Sage Foundation, the Twentieth Century Fund, the Carnegie Corporation, and the Julius Rosenwald Fund. This project illustrates the importance of the private philanthropies and foundations in funding health research during this era and the predominance of special research bodies outside the universities. The foundations together contributed about $1 million, "a very large sum in those days." The committee employed a full-time research staff of seventy-five technical experts in research and statistics as well as many temporary employees and chose five broad areas for intensive study:

1. Incidence of disease and disability in the population;
2. Existing facilities;
3. Family expenditures for services;
4. Incomes of providers of services;
5. Organized facilities for medical care servicing of particular groups of the population.

The final product consisted of twenty-eight reports, twenty-seven field studies, and a summary volume with recommendations. "Other agencies conducted studies along the same line, but in cooperation with the Committee" (Anderson, 1967, 19).

From the point of view of the topic at hand, the most important parts of the committee's findings were that illness and expenditures for medical services fell "unevenly onto families over a year so that a small minority experience severe illness and large medical expenditures" (Anderson, 1967, 19). Case studies of closed group practice plans using salaried physicians were cited by the majority of the committee as leading them to favor prepaid group practice as a form of organization, a view that was by no means unanimously endorsed by the committee. In fact, the opinions of the committee members varied widely, were strongly held and even more strongly enunciated on the subject of recommendations for the proper organization of the American medical care system. This is not very surprising when one considers the committee's composition. In addition to its chairman, Dr. Wilbur, the committee comprised fifteen private practitioners of medicine; 2 dentists from private practice; six representatives from public health; ten from medical and other health profession

schools, insurance, and professional groups; 6 social scientists, mostly economists; and nine "public" representatives (Committee on Cost of Medical Care, 1932). The final report and recommendations contained a majority and minority statement as well as individual statements by two members, Edgar Sydenstricker and Walton Hamilton, for whom neither the majority nor minority reports provided an acceptable umbrella. The two main reports formulated the fundamental "platforms" of the two adversary positions that were to contend in the political arena in the following years over the question of national health insurance.

The majority report recommended that the prevailing form of organizing medical practice in the American system of medical care be transformed to group practice[8] financed by insurance, the latter to be carried either by private or government agencies. Most of the signers holding this position personally preferred voluntary private insurance, while a smaller number favored compulsory government insurance on the grounds that European experience had shown that private voluntary insurance did not cover the most needy groups. The "private" proponents in this group of signers felt that the higher economic standing of the United States might make the voluntary principle workable. As noted, a compromise position that did not endorse either government or private sponsorship was adopted by the majority report.

The minority report categorically rejected group practice as a desirable mode of organization and stated that only solo, fee-for-service practice could provide the type of patient-doctor relationship ideally conducive to good patient care. Insurance was stated to be acceptable only if the plan were under medical society control, provided for free choice of physician, and used the fee-for-service method of payment. The focus of the minority report was on insurance for physician payment rather than on insurance for hospital care.

The American Hospital Association adopted an official position in 1933 against government-sponsored health insurance but strongly in favor of voluntary hospital insurance, thus joining the AMA in its opposition to government insurance. But in terms of actual activity, it devoted itself to aggressively sponsoring voluntary in-hospital insurance to protect the solvency of its members. In all subsequent legislative battles on the question of national health insurance through 1965, the association was to maintain its stance of supporting the AMA position but remaining in the background of the discussion.

The Depression Years and the Following Period Through U.S. Entry into World War II; 1929–1941

With the advent of the Great Depression in 1929, reform thinking and sentiment again came to the fore throughout the century. Under Herbert Hoover's presidency, the federal response to the suffering caused by the economic decline was to avoid introducing social programs that would give direct government aid to needy persons. The position of the Republican administration was that federal measures to alleviate the effects of the depression should be confined to providing incentives for industry to invest in production expansion. This, it was held, would lead to a sound recovery based on rising employment and industrial activity. For the remainder of President Hoover's term such measures were tried but proved of no avail and the depression grew worse.

The 1932 Democratic victory at the polls brought Franklin D. Roosevelt into office as president, elected on a platform that promised a "New Deal" to the people of the United States. He took office in March 1933 and in 1934 he established a cabinet "committee on economic security," charging it with the responsibility for framing legislation that was later to be passed as the Social Security Act. This committee considered all sorts of government insurance programs, but its main focus was on unemployment insurance and old age insurance (retirement pensions). However, health insurance was also being considered for inclusion in the forthcoming Social Security bill. The news that health insurance legislation was under consideration was met by a barrage of protest from the organized medical profession. Members of the committee on economic security, as well as other advisers to the president, were divided in their approach to this issue. Some felt that it was urgent to assure passage of the more basic forms of social insurance immediately and feared that the inclu-

sion of health insurance would endanger the proposed legislation for unemployment and old age insurance as well as public welfare assistance because of the opposition it would engender. Others felt that health insurance held so high a priority in the total needs of the country that it should be included in the "basic" package and that in the climate of strong support for the New Deal health insurance stood a good chance of passage, perhaps the best chance it would ever have. President Roosevelt personally decided on the course of getting the other social security measures passed first without risking the inclusion of a health insurance component. There were many subsequent government-sponsored studies and meetings on the subject, but during Roosevelt's years in office, no national health insurance bill was ever sponsored by the executive branch of the federal government.

After passage of the Social Security Act without a health insurance component, the president sent the final report of the committee on economic security dealing with health insurance, *Risks to Economic Security Arising Out of Illness,* to the Social Security Board with instructions to do further research on the subject. This was followed by I. S. Falk, associate director of the CCMC study and head of its research staff, being asked to join the Social Security Board's Bureau of Research and Statistics to work on health insurance. Simultaneously, the president formed the Interdepartmental Committee to Coordinate Health and Welfare Activities, which became "the focal point of leadership on Government health insurance and other health issues during the next few years (Corning, 1969, 44). In this manner, Roosevelt managed to placate both sides (not in equal degree, of course). Health insurance was not legislated, but government support for research and public relations activities on health insurance was provided.

Following their defeat in 1935, proponents of federal health insurance and some government agencies continued to conduct studies, publish findings, and hold conferences on the health status of the nation and the structure of the health care system. Some of the more important of these efforts were:

1. The National Health Survey[9], carried out in 1935–36 by the U.S. Public Health Service.

It gathered data on incidence of illness and attendant social and economic factors. Some 700,000 households in urban communities in eighteen states and 37,000 households in rural areas were surveyed. "The combined results of the Committee [on Costs of Medical Care] studies and the National Health Survey provided the basic data on health and medical care in the United States until the early 1950s. . . . The research was conducted outside of university auspices and was wholly public policy oriented" (Anderson, 1967, 21).

The main findings of the survey were that "The poor get sick much more often than the rich (47 percent more for acute illness and 87 percent more for chronic illness), and stay sick longer (63 percent longer for those on relief); the poor also get less adequate medical attention (for relief families, 30 percent were not receiving care for disabling illnesses of a week or longer, compared with 17 percent among families with over $3,000 in income); and upper-income families received 46 percent more doctors' visits per case. "The survey also revealed that annual mortality from accidents exceeded that of any other civilized country, as did the rate of infant mortality, and the researchers concluded that a large proportion of the population had no financial cushion to pay for the cost of medical care." (Corning, 1969, 45)

2. Studies and publications on the organization of medical care systems proliferated. By 1938 some fifteen books on health insurance and medical care organization had been published in addition to a larger number of public speeches and articles in magazines and journals (Corning, 1969, 45). In 1947 a series of books on medical care and related questions was sponsored by the Committee on Medicine and the Changing Order of the New York Academy of Medicine, and during the years 1945–48 Franz Goldmann published his book on public medical care, as well as one on voluntary medical insurance. Also in the 1940s, Nathan Sinai, Frederick D. Mott, and Milton I. Roemer were publishing studies in rural sociology and health.

3. A national health conference was convened in 1938. The three-day conference sponsored by the Interdepartmental Committee discussed the National Health Program, a five-point national health agenda drafted by the Technical Committee on Medical Care, a subcommittee of the Interdepartmental Committee.

The National Health Program called for expenditures of $850 million annually for:

a. Expansion of maternal and child health programs.
b. Federal grants-in-aid for hospital construction.
c. Grants-in-aid to states for direct medical care programs for:
   (1) recipients of welfare aid;
   (2) medically indigent (estimated at one-third of the population).
d. Grants to states to encourage but not compel statewide health insurance programs financed either by general revenues or social insurance taxes.
e. Federal initiatives to provide cash payments for illness-caused disability.

The general public reaction to the conference, even that of the AMA, seemed to range from conciliatory to favorable. However, in subsequent discussions with members of the Interdepartmental Committee, the AMA leaders announced their opposition to the health insurance provisions of the National Health Program (point d, above)—the nub of the controversial element in the program.

In 1939 the National Health Program was submitted to Congress for study, and Senator Wagner introduced a bill (S.1620) incorporating the program. The bill died in committee after very strong opposition by an arm of the AMA called the "National Physicians' Committee for the Extension of Medical Service." The AHA and ADA also directly opposed the bill. This brought to a close pre–World War II efforts to introduce national health insurance, promote state-sponsored health insurance, and to extend federal general revenue aid for medical care to welfare recipients and to the medically indigent.

World War II and the Early Postwar Period

During the entire period from 1935 to 1952 the debate on government versus private insurance raged. Opponents of compulsory government health insurance were propounding the notion that voluntary private insurance would adequately protect the United States population against the financial ravages of unexpected illness and proponents were pointing to its shortcomings. As Odin Anderson put it:

The establishment and growth of health insurance from 1933 to 1952, and the debates regarding the primary vehicle, voluntary or government health insurance, conditioned all the thinking on public policy problems. All other considerations such as level of costs, volume, quality and method of organization were subsidiary until the early 1950s. This was a free-wheeling period for voluntary health insurance, no doubt stimulated by the constant possibility of Congress seriously entertaining some form of government-sponsored health insurance in every Congress from 1938 to the end of the Truman Administration. . . . Previously collected data, and those from official sources relating to facilities, personnel, income levels, and so on, were worked and re-worked to justify government-sponsored health insurance in two major conferences sponsored by the Federal government in 1938 and again in 1948 (Anderson, 1967, 21).

In 1942 the Social Security board had "expressed support for a unified and comprehensive social insurance system, including health benefits" (Corning, 1969, 54). In the same year the Beveridge report in Great Britain, and a year later the report of the National Resources Planning Board in the United States, presented a vista of postwar security that would extend "from the cradle to the grave."

Private health insurance burgeoned during and after the war, initially as a consequence of the introduction of such insurance as a fringe benefit during the period of wartime government ceilings on cash wage increases. In light of subsequent developments, it is important to note a number of features of this rapid post–World War II expansion of private health insurance enrollment that left large portions of the population with little or no coverage for medical care.

First, the growth of such insurance left many types of health care services not covered for most persons, even for those who had some health insurance, and a substantial number of persons were not covered at all. In 1950, for example, only 12 percent of consumer expenditures for health care was covered by insurance (HEW, Social Security Bulletin, Feb. 1973).

Second, the health insurance policies were generally group contracts and concentrated on employed workers, mostly in the strongly unionized industries. They did not cover the population that was self-employed or worked for small businesses, and they did not touch most of the lowest-wage earners such as farm workers and domestic workers. And of course they provided no help to nonemployed persons.

Third, the aged were among the most inadequately covered. Their higher incidence of illness made them poor risks, while their low incomes rendered them unable to pay the high premiums for the special coverage they needed. By 1962, despite the special effort to cover the aged that had been made by the health insurance industry, only slightly more than half the population aged sixty-five and over had some type of medical care insurance and it was chiefly for hospitalization only.

The first of a serious of Congressional bills calling for compulsory national health insurance financed by payroll taxes was introduced in Congress as early as 1943. These were sponsored by Senators Wagner and Murray and Representative Dingell and have become known as the Wagner-Murray-Dingell bills. The first bill died in committee under the vigorous opposition of the AMA, the Pharmaceutical Manufacturers' Association, and other groups. The Truman-backed Wagner-Murray Dingell bill of 1945 was the first national health insurance bill to be officially supported by a president.[10] There now began a period of eight years of vigorous debate and maneuvering by opponents and advocates of national health insurance. The opposition was led by the AMA and the support by labor, liberal Congressmen, and various public figures in and out of the government, including a new coalition of government health insurance proponents organized in 1946—the Committee for the Nation's Health. This committee and other advocates of health insurance stimulated legislative support for the Wagner-Murray-Dingell bills by encouraging the writing of popular books (e.g., Malmberg, 1947), working with sympathetic legislators, and sponsoring public meetings and reports. Opponents of this legislation used similar approaches. The legislative tactics of the opposition were of three main types, several sometimes being used simultaneously. The most direct method was to achieve flat defeat of the bill, preferably by having it buried in a committee that never even considered it. A second line of defense consisted of backing a substitute bill that was less objectionable. A final line of defense was to get the objectionable legislation amended as it passed through Congressional labyrinths on the way to passage. Each of these approaches was used during the 1946–65 period on different health insurance bills.

In 1946 the Senate held hearings on the 1945 Wagner-Murray-Dingell bill but the House never did, the legislation being bottled up in the House Ways and Means Committee. An example of the back-up substitute bill tactic was the introduction by Republican members of the Taft-Smith-Ball bill calling for federal matching grants to help the "States subsidize private health insurance coverage for the medically indigent." This was a means-test bill and was unofficially supported by the AMA and opposed by the Administration. Since the Wagner-Murray-Dingell bill never came to a vote because of the success of the bottle-up-in-committee tactic, it was not necessary to advance the Taft-Smith-Ball bill legislatively, and it too never came to a vote.

In 1948 the Federal Security Administrator, Oscar Ewing, convened a National Health Assembly, "reminiscent of the 1938 National Health Conference" (Corning, 1969) to help mobilize support for the then-current version of the Wagner-Murray-Dingell bill that had been reintroduced into Congress. The bill failed to come to a vote in 1949 again. Paralleling the convening of the 1948 National Health Assembly, the AMA sharply stepped up its opposition campaign, assessing very member $25 in 1948 to set up a $4.5 million fund to wage a "national education" campaign. The AMA arguments according to Corning (1969) against these bills were:

1. The United States already had the highest standards of medical care the world had ever known; great strides had been made in the preceding decades and, while there were still deficiencies, these were being grossly exaggerated.
2. National Health Insurance would lead to Federal control of medical care which would undermine the existing system and help destroy free enterprise.
3. A universal health insurance system would be exorbitantly costly to operate.

4. It was unnecessary; private insurance was growing rapidly and was believed capable of doing the job.

The opposition was apparently more effective than the support. By 1952 President Truman virtually acknowledged defeat of the Murray-Wagner-Dingell bills by omitting a health insurance proposal from his State of the Union message, establishing instead a commission on the health needs of the nation to study the problem further and educate the public. Thus the pattern continued of legislative defeat followed by a return to research, education, and public advocacy on the part of health insurance supporters to help accumulate ammunition for a more propitious "next time."

Emphasis on Insurance for the Aged After 1952

With the election of President Eisenhower in November 1952, the advocates of national, universal, comprehensive health insurance accepted political defeat, and in 1953 they reduced their aims to that of health insurance for the aged under the Social Security system. This more limited goal, it was felt, was more attainable because of the growing political power of the aged and the demonstrated intractability of the problem of privately insuring this age group. Opponents of this measure strove to defeat it by providing increased private coverage for the aged on the one hand and supporting alternative legislation extending welfare medical care benefits (instead of insurance) for the aged on the other. During the years 1954–1957, the Eisenhower Administration supported several bills that would have helped private insurance companies offer improved medical care coverage to the aged, but none of these was passed. In 1957 the Forand bill, providing for federally sponsored medical insurance for limited hospital care and surgical and nursing home benefits for all Social Security beneficiaries, failed to become law. The bill was not successful, losing again in the face of the heavy opposition of the AMA after its reintroduction in 1959, and it was voted down in the House Ways and Means Committee in 1960.

Instead, Congress passed the Kerr-Mills Act

(p. 260), which established a fifth category in federal welfare assistance to the states—medical assistance to the aged (MAA). The federal government would match state expenditures for medical care up to a $15 average for each "medically needy" aged person per month, the matching proportion ranging from 50 to 80 percent, depending on the state's per capita income. No limit was set on the benefits or the total amount to be spent, and state participation in the program was optional.

A special subcommittee of the Senate Special Committee on Aging[11] issued a report on the Kerr-Mills Program in late 1963 which stated that "It was the intent of Congress that the MAA would provide broad health services to the many aged needing them but unable to afford them even though the individuals were not on welfare," and concluded that the operations of the Kerr-Mills Program "demonstrated conclusively that the congressional intent has not and will not be realized" (Subcommittee on Health of the Aging, 1973, 3). Some specifics cited to support its conclusion were:

1. By mid-1963 more than two-fifths of the aged resided in states that had no Kerr-Mills program.
2. After three years, the program was in operation in only twenty-eight states and four other jurisdictions, and "there is no reason to expect" that it would become a national program in the foreseeable future.
3. The degree of benefits varied widely from state to state, and they were typically "nominal, non-existent or inadequate."
4. Administrative costs were "too high," with a range that reached 59 percent of benefits in Tennessee.
5. The distribution of federal matching funds among the states was grossly disproportionate. Five states received 88 percent of all funds, although they contained only 32 percent of the nation's aged.
6. Several states shifted old age assistance (OAA) welfare clients to MAA to achieve the benefits of greater federal matching rather than increasing the number of elderly covered.
7. Stringent eligibility tests, "lien type" recovery provisions, and responsible relative provisions resulted in a total of only 148,000,

less than 1 percent, of the aged having received MAA assistance in July of 1963. "The welfare aspect of the Kerr-Mills program, including cumbersome investigations of eligibility, plus the requirement in most states that resources of an older person must be depleted to a point of near dependency, have further reduced participation" (1973, p. 1).

The emphasis on welfare means test features, including provisions holding relatives financially responsible, was probably the most objectionable feature of the program.

In 1964, President Johnson called for passage of a National Health Insurance Act for the Aged to be financed by payroll taxes, and in 1965 Congressman Cecil R. King and Senator Clinton P. Anderson introduced the King-Anderson bill covering hospital insurance in each house. Previous bills of this type had failed in 1962 and 1964, being heavily opposed by AMPAC (American Medical Political Action Committee), an arm of the AMA; the commercial insurance carriers; and the national Blue Cross Association. During 1961–64, in a last-ditch effort to forestall government insurance for the elderly, both the commercial insurance carriers and Blue Cross-Blue Shield ("the Blues") had begun new low-cost programs for the elderly. The "State 65" plans were sponsored by the commercials and the "over-65" plans by the Blues. Annual premiums of the State 65 plan were $210 in Massachusetts, $228 in New York, and $252 in Connecticut with a $100 annual deductible and 20 percent coinsurance. The Blues' over-65 plan at first offered a uniform national contract with a premium of $10–$12 per month, but they soon had to abandon the national uniform policy and let their member plans develop separate contracts that typically provided incomplete protection with deductibles and/or coinsurance. Even the special low-cost premiums were apparently too expensive for the elderly, for both types of plans made little progress in adequately insuring the aged. Federal subsidies for the Blues to cover the aged were discussed but never acted upon.

In addition to the King-Anderson bill of 1965 calling for hospital insurance for the aged to be financed under Social Security, two other bills were introduced as potential substitutes. These were:

1. The AMA-proposed "Eldercare" bill calling for a program operated by the states through private insurance carriers with premiums for the low-income elderly subsidized by state and federal tax revenues. The bill covered out-of-hospital physician payments, the AMA having severely criticized the King-Anderson bill for its one-sided emphasis on inpatient services.
2. The "Mills Bill," which revised the King-Anderson bill and was voted favorably out of the Ways and Means Committee.

The final "Mills Bill," which was actually passed after much "House-Senate conferencing and floor amending, became Title XVIII (Medicare) of the Social Security Act, combined aspects of both the King-Anderson and the Eldercare bills. Medicare Part A was essentially the revised King-Anderson bill for hospital insurance financed by payroll taxes. Medicare Part B provided a voluntary plan for ambulatory medical care insurance with part of the premiums paid for by the federal government from general revenues and part by the insured aged themselves. This portion took cognizance of the AMA's contention that "Eldercare" corrected the failure of the King-Anderson bill to cover ambulatory services.

Also passed was Title XIX (Medicaid), which amended the welfare provisions of the Social Security Act providing federal matching for medical programs for welfare clients to establish a greatly expanded program of paying for medical care for the poor.

The Medicare-Medicaid legislation of 1965 thus marks a watershed, both in the development of the national health insurance movement and in the financing of medical care for the poor, but universal national access to medical care would have to await another day. Still, the changes were sufficiently significant to make considering portions of this legislation in some detail worthwhile. This is done in Chapter 10.

THE RISE AND ROLE OF PRIVATE HEALTH INSURANCE

While this national struggle over government-sponsored health insurance was going on, the private health insurance industry was growing rapidly, especially during and after World War II, as I have noted. As more and more people were covered by private health insurance, it was to be expected that the pressure for government-sponsored insurance would lessen. The fact that private health insurance with its uniquely American form of sponsorship became so widespread before a government program was passed has had important repercussions on the structure of the United States health care system. The particular nature of the U.S. private insurance structure led to conditions that were later to be recognized as problems with respect to access, cost, utilization, and the ordering of priorities accorded to different types of services. Over time, government, especially the federal level, has become intimately involved with these problems. To understand the ways in which the heavy reliance on private insurance complicated national efforts to form a health care system accessible to all with good quality and acceptable cost, it is important to consider the workings of private insurance generally, as well as how these workings are adapted to health insurance.

Principles and Background of Commercial Insurance

The underlying concept of commercial insurance has been that the premium paid by the subscriber controls the financial risk of incurring unacceptably large losses. It was not meant to cover normally recurring expenditures of modest size, like small electrical or plumbing repairs, which were expected to be budgeted for out of current operating income. It therefore was not a vehicle for *prepaying* regularly anticipated expenditures during a specified period.

It is instructive to look at the principles and definitions asserted by professional practitioners and writers on the modern insurance industry as governing its operations (Vaughan and Elliott, 1978). A peril is defined as a mishap against which one is insuring; a loss is the cost to the insured if the peril occurs; and a hazard is a circumstance that increases the probability of the peril occurring. For example: a fire is a peril; the cost of replacing the burnt property is a loss; and an improperly exposed electric wire that increases the chances of a fire occurring is a hazard. The risk of a peril is the expected value of the loss, an actuarial concept that for an individual policyholder is calculated by multiplying the amount the individual is insured for by the probability that the peril will occur. Thus, if a house is insured against fire for $100,000 and the probabiliy of a fire of this magntiude occurring within the period covered by the insurance is one in 1,000, or .001 then $100,000 × .001, or $100, is the expected loss or risk. This amount is defined as the ''pure'' premium to be paid by the insured. If everyone in the insurance pool pays the amount of his or her own risk, the group as a whole will, in the long run, lose no more than the total premiums collected. A small chance of incurring a ruinous possible maximum loss has now been converted to a certainty of paying a business expense of $100.

The underlying assumptions of this arrangement are many. To be insurable under these concepts, a risk must be associated with perils that are clearly (consensually) defined outcomes (fires, automobile accidents, liability suits) and with losses that are clearly defined amounts. Furthermore, the peril should not be certain to occur in the period covered by the insurance contract nor should it be impossible of occurring. Since the estimated risk, which determines the pure premium, entails an estimate of the probability of the peril occurring, the insurer must take account of all observable hazards, circumstances that increase the chance (probability) of incurring a loss. In fire insurance a wood-frame house has a higher probability of burning than a stone house, and in car theft insurance a car kept on the street has a higher chance of being stolen than one that is garaged. The premiums for the situations with the existing hazards—wooden house, car kept on street—would consequently be higher than those in situations without them. It is not the preexisting hazard, the hazard that is present and visible before the insurance contract is signed, that worries the insurer. The added chance of a loss occurring due to this hazard can be duly estimated and the premium adjusted upward to cover the additional risk. What concerns the insurer more seriously are the increased hazards that have been observed to occur *after* the insurance contract is signed. The insured may now become careless about locking his or her car or repairing frayed, exposed electric wires because he or she knows

the loss will be reimbursed by the insurance company. In fact, an insured person in need of cash may even purposely cause a loss (e.g., set a fire) for the express purpose of collecting the insurance money. He or she may also act in collusion with service companies like automobile repairers to have the entire automobile repaired when only a small loss actually incurred as the result of an accident or vandalism.

These increased chances of a loss occurring that are deemed to result solely from the fact that the claimant has insurance are classified as moral hazards. They are added risks that would not exist in the absence of the insurance and consequently cannot be well estimated when the insurer evaluates the required premium. The insurance industry uses several methods to control moral hazard. To reduce fraud, companies often investigate claims, and to reduce carelessness[12] they often mount public prevention campaigns and offer reduced premiums to applicants with low loss records. But perhaps the main device used in the hope of deterring moral hazard is cost sharing. With this type of deterrent the insured is required to pay part of a loss. The main mechanisms are requiring the claimant to pay a specified initial amount of the loss, the ''deductible''; requiring him or her to pay a specified percentage of the loss, ''coinsurance''; limiting the reimbursement to a fixed maximum, the ''upper limit''; and excluding certain categories of loss (e.g., ''acts of God''), ''exclusions.'' Insurance theory claims that use of these cost-sharing devices is motivated mostly, perhaps solely, by the wish to control moral hazard. If replacing a loss is not entirely cost-free to the insured, he or she will be less likely to be careless and perhaps also to present fraudulent claims. Consumer advocates and other critics, however, have often asserted that a main objective of cost sharing is to allow a delusively low premium to be offered and thus reduce the apparent cost and inflate the stated maximum coverage of the insurance. This, they claim, is misrepresentation and impedes fair comparison of the true relative costs of competing insurance policies. Another assertion made by insurance companies is that the deductible form of cost sharing in particular contributes to economic efficiency because it eliminates processing of myriad small claims. Small losses cost more to process than they are worth, and such losses are more efficiently handled by the consumer out of his or her normal living budget. This argument does not of course explain the practice of applying the deductible even when reimbursing for large losses.

Neoclassical economists, with their preference for market mechanism that allow wide consumer choice on how to spend personal income, are generally strong advocates of cost sharing. On the assumption that many different types of insurance policies are available, consumers may choose to pay high premiums with low cost sharing and greatly lower their risk or low premiums with high cost sharing and thereby run higher risks. Generally the latter holds for consumers whose perception is that the probability of incurring a loss is or can be kept low because they are very careful persons. Economics literature abounds in talk of "risk takers" and "risk avoiders." Many economists also favor cost sharing because it is believed to curb moral hazard, thereby reducing uneconomic expenditures for avoidable losses.

The standard conditions prevailing in most commercial insurance transactions are reasonably well adapted to the application of these principles and practices. When an automobile is insured against theft one can clearly determine whether or not the car has been stolen. The price of its replacement can be determined in a clearcut manner based on the terms of the policy, and the use of cost-sharing devices may reduce the chances that the insured will leave the car unlocked or dispose of it merely to collect the insurance and buy a better new one. Similar considerations apply to fire and liability insurance.

But now, compare these circumstances and assumptions with those prevailing in insuring the cost of medical services on a fee-per-service basis. Hospital and physicians' charges, especially those of surgeons for inpatient services, are most unambiguously handled within the rubric of ordinary commercial insurance although there are very large differences in treatment prescribed by different physicians for the same patient conditions, even for many inpatient services (Wennberg and Gittelson, 1982). But as we move away from the better-defined acute illnesses requiring inpatient care and move toward ambulatory care of all kinds, especially that designated as preventive, the "peril" of standard

insurance usage becomes fuzzy. Since so many symptoms are self-limiting and self-correcting, that is, they "go away" if left to themselves, the choice is up to the person whether to save money by not seeing the physician or optimizing prevention by seeing him or her early. If the person has insurance covering such a visit, does it constitute "moral hazard" if the decision is to go earlier and thereby make more visits than would be made in the absence of insurance? From an insurance theory standpoint the answer is yes; any loss incurred merely because the insured had insurance is moral hazard. But from a public health prevention standpoint, what is the answer?

Some have argued that on business grounds alone, commercial health insurers, once they can be brought to recognize their own true interests, will encourage early visits to physicians because conditions caught in early stages will be relatively inexpensive to treat and may avoid later more expensive treatment of advanced conditions. This argument is true only for certain types of conditions and more generally for poor persons' care. Prenatal care may be expected to reduce expensive corrective care for all mothers and children, and good, prompt ambulatory care may be expected to reduce hospitalization for complications that can be avoided, like those associated with diabetes. However, for a large class of frequently diagnosed diseases, especially among middle-class persons, early diagnosis may lead to greater medical expense than finding the illness at an advanced stage. Many cancers are curable or controllable if found early, but the treatment can be more expensive than dealing with an advanced case resulting in early death. Other cases could be cited where early detection may increase medical cost, not decrease it. The main reason for advocating prevention and early detection is because it will save lives and lessen suffering, not that it is always or usually demonstrably cheaper. In any case, possible cost savings from an early trip to the doctor has not proved a persuasive argument against the widespread use of cost sharing by commercial health insurers to prevent moral hazard.

Or consider that most visits to the doctor by worried persons with symptoms result merely in a reassuring assessment that there is nothing seriously wrong, and that persons with health insurance may be more likely to make such visits. Should such visits be discouraged as moral hazard by the imposition of cost sharing? Again, from a social policy (i.e., public health) point of view, one must ask whether allaying anxiety is a "wasted" visit induced by the presence of insurance.

The *social* purpose of advocating health insurance for populations that have poor access to medical care is to *increase* their utilization. It is hoped that a certain number of doctor visits and elective hospitalizations would be induced by the presence of insurance. This has no counterpart in normal commercial insurance transactions. There are no desirable fires, thefts, or automobile accidents. What is the meaning, then, of labeling all medical care use induced by more insurance as "moral hazard"? What purpose is served by using cost sharing to reduce visits to the doctor that society wants to encourage by providing insurance? This is perhaps the most serious problem in adapting commercial-type health insurance to the social needs of financing health care. The structure of health insurance policies has not been able to divorce itself from the casualty insurance concept that utilization corresponds to losses and that a smaller number of "losses" is always better than a larger number.

Such considerations added to other criticisms raised during the 1945–1965 period of the increasing reliance on regular insurance mechanisms to finance medical care. They were an important part of the arguments for a national health insurance system under federal auspices. What was needed, it was argued, was *social* and not commercial insurance for health care, as all European countries had. It seemed strange to the ears of social insurance advocates to hear a visit to a physician labeled a "peril" like a fire, and one that results in a finding of no disease suspected of being a case of "moral hazard" or abuse of insurance. Equally unacceptable to the social insurance or public health view was the fact that while unneeded services are often prescribed by physicians to increase their income or that of a hospital (or simply because some physicians are not well informed about the efficacy of such services), the insurance type of thinking nearly always led to attempts to control

such overuse by penalizing the patient via cost sharing rather than attempting to control the behavior of physicians and hospitals.

The incompatibility of social insurance and commercial insurance concepts, especially the fear of utilization "abuse," had kept commercial insurance companies largely out of the medical care insurance business during the years 1890–1930 when other types of insurance business were flourishing. The major increase in personal insurance was in life insurance, which was being sold in small individual amounts to workers and which often paid little more than the cost of burial. This is not to say that there was no insurance for medical care, but the bulk of this insurance was offered by various fraternal organizations of workers and small businessmen who banded together to provide death and sickness benefits to their members. These organizations contracted with physicians to serve their members at a fixed reduced fee and sometimes also paid part of their members' hospital bills.

This type of health insurance sponsorship is what developed in Europe with the friendly societies in Great Britain and the Krankenkassen ("sickness chests") in Germany. They were outgrowths of arrangements made by the trade and craft guilds that emerged from the Middle Ages. In European capitalist countries this type of health insurance organization predominated right through their transformations into national systems with the assumption of control and regulation by the national government. The European systems began and evolved from cooperative arrangements among groups of persons. These fraternal associations were primarily concerned with finding physicians (or physicians' associations) who would agree to provide a package of services at prospectively negotiated payment rates. The U.S. commercial insurance structure, when it entered health insurance, was from the start concerned only with payment for specified services—"losses." Finding the provider and judging his adequacy or performance was not done by the insurer but left to the insured. The insurance company, as far as it could do so, strove to stay entirely clear of any considerations of access or quality assurance. The European systems sought to arrange for services; the American insurance companies were only provider paying mechanisms. Commercial insurance-company sponsorship of health insurance of the American type was unusual in Europe although it spilled over into Canada and has been used in Australia. The use of commercial insurance companies for health insurance in the United States was contrary to all earlier European experience and proved to be an impediment to introducing universal, comprehensive medical insurance.

The "Blues" and "Independents"

The advent of privately sponsored health insurance as a major financing mechanism in the United States is generally traced not to commercial insurance companies but to provider sources who established not-for-profit hospital service insurance companies. Early stirrings, first by individual hospitals and then by hospital associations, were visible as far back as 1929. These insurance companies were sponsored by hospitals and hospital associations to help keep the hospitals[13] solvent by encouraging working people to pay premiums in anticipation of possible future hospitalization. They were nonprofit, carried no insurance other than health insurance, and became known as Blue Cross associations. Similar organizations were later organized by medical societies to cover physician care, and these became known as Blue Shield societies. There were also other arrangements, but they played a relatively minor role. These were the "independents," so called because they were neither commercial insurance companies nor part of the "Blues." Some businesses had their own health plans with clinics, physicians, and hospitals for their employees. There were also a few groups of physicians that organized prepaid plans to provide physician services. For a fixed periodic advance payment, these groups of physicians undertook to handle all the medical needs (within a predefined list of services) of their subscribers. These were known as prepaid group practices (PGPs). The opposition of organized medicine to these independent forms of insurance structure was very strong and often became aggressively hostile. Company-sponsored medicine was condemned for being "contract medicine" and opposed because laymen hired physicians to work on salary. Prepaid group practice was also, and perhaps mainly, op-

posed because its clientele was restricted to using only physicians in the group, the "closed panel," which was anathema to medical society leaderships before 1960. All forms of private health insurance had modest enrollments before World War II.

The Post–World War II Growth of Private Health Insurance

The main impetus behind the rapid growth of private health insurance came with World War II. Prices and wages were controlled by the Office of Price Administration (OPA) and the War Labor Board (WLB), but corporate profits were not similarly controlled. Many unions were growing restive at the fact that the WLB controlled wage increases but not profits, and partly in response to the perception that the arrangement was unfair, the WLB permitted increases in fringe benefits—retirement, disability, life and health insurance—over and above allowable direct wage increases. It was argued that the purchase of insurance for workers would not put significant additional inflationary pressure on the economy. This enabled the unions, especially the large powerful ones, to negotiate employer-paid premiums for health insurance.[14] It was the beginning of the institutionalization of a system of special insurance benefits for a preferred segment of the population, those working in the strongly unionized industries and mostly for large corporations. As it matured, this system was found to produce many side effects considered undesirable by different groups of people. These will be discussed at greater length in Chapter 10; for now I only mention some of them. Three main groups were left out of this newly growing benefit system: the unemployable poor or the "welfare" population (the "deserving" poor); working people not employed by industries with good fringe benefits, notably including the working poor[15] and the unemployed; and the aged. Passage of the 1965 Medical/Medicaid legislation was later to attempt to remedy some of these omissions with Medicaid for the ("deserving") poor and near poor, and Medicare for the aged.

During and immediately after World War II, it was nonprofit Blue Cross that first grew by leaps and bounds in selling hospital insurance policies. Commercial insurance companies entered the field reluctantly at first, and until about 1955 had a lesser share of the private hospital insurance market than did Blue Cross. The Blue Cross coverage was typically for the cost of a hospital stay and sometimes included some physician services rendered in connection with it. Organized into local branches, usually one or two per state, Blue Cross was allied nationally with the American Hospital Association. Most hospitals became participating Blue Cross hospitals affiliated with their local Blue Cross society. The local Blue Cross negotiated rates individually with each participating hospital to be paid for service to Blue Cross subscribers. Typically the subscriber would pay the hospital little or nothing in cash, the bill being paid directly to the hospital by Blue Cross. The Blue Cross policy, therefore, offered the subscriber "service" benefits that were stated in terms of service units such as "120 days in the hospital." Commercial insurance company policies generally offered "indemnity" benefits stated in cash amounts such as "$200 per day for a total of 120 days in the hospital plus not more than $2,000 in ancillary services (X-ray, laboratory examination, etc.)." The commercials generally included elaborate cost-sharing schemes—deductibles, coinsurance, upper limits, and exclusions. Blue Cross used few cost-sharing devices, the main ones being upper limits to the number of service units covered and some exclusions. The most frequently used exclusions[16] were anesthetist, pathologist and radiologist fees, blood, and special-duty nursing. However, except for these exclusions, the payment to the hospital for its services usually had no deductible, no coinsurance, and no upper limit because the hospital fees were paid in full by Blue Cross per negotiated agreement with the hospital.

Blue Shield was organized by medical societies for payment of physicians' bills. It differed from Blue Cross in that the reimbursement was generally to the patient for fees that had been billed by the physician. Although in some cases the reimbursement was directly to the physician, there was no agreement in general with physicians for direct payment by Blue Shield without submitting a bill to the patient as there was in the case of Blue Cross and the hospitals. The payment schedules were often similar to those of commercial insurance companies with cost sharing common. The main services covered were surgeon's fees and other payments to physicians for in-hospital services. Thus, Blue Shield paid indemnity benefits as opposed to the service benefits of Blue Cross.

At first it was thought by some that Blue Cross in alliance with Blue Shield might develop into a system operating very much like a national health insurance system, a point developed by Somers and Somers (1961). Some Blue Cross leaders openly favored such a course and urged that Blue Cross strive to achieve this goal. Extending its eligibility to smaller groups and even individuals, Blue Cross attempted to apply the same premium rates across very wide groups of persons. This made it possible to cover aged persons and poor health risks for manageable premiums, but it also meant that the best health risks paid a slightly higher premium than their risk warranted. This type of premium rate setting, called "community rating," was an extension of the philanthropic system of hospital financing. As previously noted, part of that system required more affluent private patients to pay hospital charges that were above cost as a contribution to the care of poor patients. However, the use of community rating of premiums by Blue Cross was as short-lived as the hegemony of Blue Cross in the hospital insurance field. The commercial insurers were entering the field of health insurance with increasing vigor and by 1955 had pulled abreast of Blue Cross/Blue Shield, with each having about 45 percent of the private health insurance business.

The entrance of the commercials seems to have been motivated as much by their interest in their other insurance business as in the health insurance business itself. The rapid growth of private security benefits had produced a network of employee benefit plans with administrative offices that collected money from employers (sometimes also a contribution from employees), negotiated insurance contracts with insurers, and often were instrumental in administering the benefits. The employee benefit plans were run at first entirely by employers and later more often by joint employer-union entities; they were also, but infrequently, operated by unions alone. The employee benefit plan had much money to spend and many kinds of insurance to buy: life, pension, disability, unemployment supplement, and health. For many commercial companies life insurance was the big plum, with retirement pensions not far behind. It was often advantageous for them to include health insurance as a ''loss leader'' in a total package that might include as much as the entire insurance business of the employee benefit plan, even if they incurred an operating loss on the health insurance itself.

The advantages commercial insurers could offer in their health insurance policies were flexibility in writing multistate or even international contracts and rapid inclusion of specially desired new-type services, as well as lower premiums because of giving special rates to companies with relatively young workers. This rating system is known as ''experience'' rating in contradistinction to the community rating described earlier.

The Blues offered the advantages of the service benefits of Blue Cross, which generally meant less cost sharing and more ''first dollar'' coverage. Nearly all surveys of worker likes and dislikes found a marked preference for total coverage without cost sharing. But in attempts to meet the advantages held by the commercials in marketing to many of the large corporations, the Blues were increasingly forced to resort to experience rating, thus virtually eliminating the possibility of their evolving into something like a social insurance system in that it would include high risks at lower than their actuarially determined rates. In some places they even began to offer indemnity hospital benefits. The Blues also set up mechanisms for offering multistate contracts to large companies, but they continued to be less flexible than a single large commercial insurance company that could tailor a policy to the desires of a client out of its national office without needing to arrange agreements among semiautonomous local Blue Cross and Blue Shield entities in different States. They also remained less flexible in offering coverage for services that had not previously been part of the typical benefit package, such as optometry or physiotherapy on an ambulatory basis. As 1965 approached it became increasingly clear that private insurance was not going to be able to cover the workers in economically less favored industries, the unemployed, the unemployables, or the aged.

In addition to the service benefits of Blue Cross, the indemnity benefits of Blue Shield and commercial insurance, and the social insurance (either in indemnity or service benefits) of government, there was also the independent direct service type, which garnered from 7 to 10 percent of the total insurance business. Some voices had always been raised against the way medical care is provided under private reimbursement-type insurance, especially of the commercial variety. Such insurance did not meet the needs of persons who wanted to be a part of a health *service* system rather than be insured against the cost of fee-for-service payments to sundry unconnected and uncoordinated providers. The administrative problems of utilization ''abuse,'' the unpredictability of insurance coverage in the face of differing charges by different providers, and the excessive overhead costs resulted mainly, they asserted, from the anomaly of using commercial mechanisms developed only to control financial risk to finance, regulate, and control the delivery of health services whose first priority should be to deliver good care. Prepaid group practices were preferred by such persons. Bitter opposition by organized physicians, later joined by hospital associations and insurance companies, severely impeded the potential for growth of this type of health insurance that assures the delivery of services rather than payment for them. In recent years it has grown much more rapidly than before, and I shall discuss it in some detail in Chapter 10.

The question that again came to the fore was whether the country needed an overarching national system of social insurance or could continue to rely mainly on private insurance with government programs designed to fill in the gaps represented by uninsured and underinsured persons. Social insurance differs from private or voluntary insurance in that it superimposes on the commercial function of private insurance to control financial risk additional social purposes not related to strictly actuarial considerations. The difference on this point between social and commercial insurance speaks to the very basis of how the concept of "fairness" is seen. The two main contending views in the period after 1930 have been those of the neoclassical economists and those of social welfare advocates. The neoclassical economist lays primary stress on individual freedom to spend one's money as one chooses. The ideal society would allow each person the maximum freedom of choice compatible with not decreasing anyone else's freedom of choice, a condition called "Pareto optimality" after the Italian economist Vilfredo Pareto.[17] The main instrument for achieving optimality of choice is the market, which is to be maintained free and unfettered by the government. Indeed, keeping the market free is the principal function of government. The social welfare advocate argues that individuals have certain built-in ("are endowed by their Creator with certain inalienable . . . ") rights that supersede the requirements of complete market freedom. Included in these rights are or should be a minimally adequate level of food, shelter, and clothing and perhaps also education, medical care, and reasonable amenities. People who fail to win a sufficiently large share of the national wealth in the marketplace cannot exercise their fundamental right to these basic necessities. Their freedom to choose is of little benefit to them if their choices are too sharply circumscribed by insufficient money, even though the choices are freely available on the market at competitive prices. Of course there are many world views that lie between these polar alternatives, but for the purposes of the present discussion I believe it helps clarify the issues to consider the two positions in their pure forms.

The notion of fairness underlying commercial insurance is the freedom of choice in the marketplace, especially freedom from artificial non-market manipulations. Once an insurance company decides to offer a policy with certain benefits, the premium for that policy must be directly proportional to the benefits. A policy paying $10,000 if a stated loss occurs must, for a person of specified risk, cost twice as much as a policy that pays $5,000—no more, no less. If $10 were to buy $5,000 of insurance for a well-to-do person and a poor person could buy the same insurance for $2 then the payer of the $10 premium would be judged to be subsidizing the payer of the $2 premium. By the lights of com-

mercial insurance theory, this is considered to be unfair, and the state insurance commissioners, which regulate commercial insurance companies, would not approve it on those grounds. For social insurance such cross subsidization is not unfair; it is an avowed aim. Besides spreading the actuarial risks of the cost of illness or retirement living, it also seeks to guarantee basic economic "rights" to its clients. Low-income persons pay lower premiums and receive proportionately more for their money in order to achieve acceptable minimum levels of living. Because the benefits are not strictly proportionate to the premiums, many better-off persons as well as those who perceive themselves as being below-average risks would not voluntarily join the plan; social insurance is therefore typically compulsory and government operated. Participation in privately operated insurance is theoretically voluntary, and it is therefore often called voluntary insurance.[18]

RECAPITULATION: THIRD-PARTY COVERAGE OF MEDICAL CARE COSTS ON THE EVE OF PASSAGE OF MEDICARE AND MEDICAID IN 1965

In Chapter 8 the role of government in paying for the care of indigent and medically indigent persons, largely to the private sector, was addressed. In Chapters 5, 6, and 7 the direct provision of health services to special population groups, including indigent and medically indigent persons, was discussed. This chapter has dealt with the movement for and toward government-sponsored health insurance. By 1965 a considerable part of the population was covered for medical care expense by some form of third-party payer, that is, by some organization that would pay for or provide some or all incurred medical care expense. This system had been developing into its 1965 form since the turn of the century.

During these years many sources of care became further institutionalized in society serving various categories of person, defined by social and economic status. For purposes of defining eligibility for medical care coverage these were the affluent, middle class,[19] better-paid working people, lower-paid working people (the "working poor''), the unemployed and other persons who were employable but not working, (the "able-bodied" poor), and the disabled, "paupers," and other unemployables. Many of the unemployables obtained ambulatory care from special medical programs set up for them by local relief agencies and used local public general hospitals for their inpatient care. Some also used the outpatient departments of these hospitals for their ambulatory care. Unemployed and other nonworking persons not eligible for relief used the public hospital, both the outpatient and inpatient facilities, and private philanthropically supported facilities like clinics and voluntary hospitals. The employed lower- and modest-income people often had available the local private practitioner charging on a sliding scale and the voluntary and local public hospital, the former also charging on a sliding scale with the difference made up by philanthropic and governmental subsidy. The middle and upper classes used private physicians and were at first treated mostly at home. They increasingly came to use the hospital for serious illnesses as that institution developed into a house of scientific medicine and, even more after 1945 as private health insurance became widespread.

Most paid the full cost of hospital care, and the more affluent paid more than cost to help take care of unreimbursed care. In addition to these main avenues of care, there were government and some philanthropically supported services for persons specially categorized by service status or disease—veterans' facilities, state mental and tuberculosis hospitals, and special employer-sponsored medical plans.

The health services system in existence by the beginning of 1965 was greatly expanded over that of 1920. New features included the Veterans Administration health system and the extensive coverage by private health insurance. However, a central feature of the system, perhaps the central one, remained unchanged. This was the absence of a national system of health care with equal access to all and offering a comprehensive spectrum of services. The U.S. system of medical care still consisted of many different subsystems, each targeted at different eligibility groups and financed from different sources.

The premiums for employer-purchased health insurance were being paid to a substantial degree by the public. The payments for such health insurance were partially deductible as tax exemptions from federal income tax and partially passed on as price increases to consumers in a period when such increases were easily imposed. But workers in nonunionized and poorly unionized industries had minimal or no health insurance and did the best they could between paying out-of-pocket and using public hospitals. This poorly insured class of workers had low public visibility in 1965 as constituting a public policy problem.

Two classes of persons were perhaps most visible as still inadequately served, the poor and the aged. AFDC public welfare beneficiaries were becoming increasingly isolated politically, and their programs ever more subject to attack and cutbacks. And the care available under the different health care programs for the poor was unequal in quality both with respect to providers and very simple amenities. The aged were also not well covered by third-party mechanisms, either insurance or welfare-assisted programs. In 1965 the federal government made a major attempt to plug these two holes in the dike of health protection by passing Medicare to cover the aged through social insurance and Medicaid to cover the poor and medically indigent through enhanced public assistance. These are the subject of the next chapter.

NOTES

1. Established in *Butterfield* v. *Forrester* in 1809.
2. First stated in *Priestly* v. *Fowlen* in 1837 and reinforced by *Murray* v. *South Carolina Railroad Co.* in 1841 and *Farwell* v. *Boston and Worcester Railroad Corporation* in 1843.
3. In *Ives* v. *South Buffalo Railway Company*.
4. In *New York Central Railroad* v. *White*.
5. Fifty states and the District of Columbia, Puerto Rico, Virgin Islands, American Samoa, Guam, and the Trust Territory of the Pacific Islands.
6. In recent years the term most generally used is workers' compensation. I shall henceforth use this designation when referring to periods after 1970.
7. Paul Starr (1981) goes to some length to dispute the assertion that the National Association of Manufacturers supported government health insurance. He notes that it was merely favorably reported by a committee, not formally adopted as a position. However, it seems fair to me to characterize a favorable report by a committee of what has traditionally

been among the most conservative of the large business associations as indicative of the initial favorable attitudes toward government health insurance existing in many quarters that later turned to opposition.

8. The issue of group practice is tied to the question of health insurance. Part of the structure of an insurance system is the method of paying providers. If group practice becomes widespread then the question naturally arises about the desirability of forming large, multispecialty groups of salaried physicians who will offer to supply complete medical care to groups of subscribers for a fixed periodic fee. This did indeed happen as the first *prepaid* group practices began to form.

9. This should not be confused with the *Health Interview Survey,* later established by the National Health Survey Act of 1956 (P.L. 84–652), under which health and related data have been collected on a regular, periodic basis.

10. In the same year, it is interesting to note, a state health insurance bill sponsored by Governor Warren of California lost in the California state legislature by only one vote.

11. In 1956, Congress had approved $30,000 for the creation of a new Senate subcommittee on problems of the aged. This subcommittee later became the full-fledged Special Committee on Aging, a leading participant in the health insurance debate, although it had no power to initiate legislation. Its Subcommittee on Health of the Elderly issued this report (1963).

12. This is sometimes classified as ''morale'' hazard to differentiate it from the purposive fraud entailed in ''moral'' hazard. I shall not make this distinction in my discussion.

13. It is interesting to note that while European health insurance developed first for paying physicians, in the United States it developed first for paying hospitals. The European hospital is a descendant of medieval church hospices and has always been seen as a community establishment run first by religious orders and later by local governments. The private United States hospitals were established largely by charitable associations, at first mostly religious in sponsorship. By the 1900s, many of them had semi-

private beds for paying patients as well as philanthropic beds for private charity patients. Well-to-do patients used special private rooms for which they paid above costs as a contribution to the hospitals. If a patient wanted his own physician he had to be a semiprivate or a private paying patient.

14. The employers, for their part, did not much care what they paid workers during the war. Most large corporations were working entirely on defense contracts and were paid cost plus 15 percent. Additional legitimate costs only meant additional profits.

15. Many of these worked for small employers, and as medical care became increasingly expensive, the self-employed also began to feel the pinch of not having access to good health insurance.

16. The anesthetists, pathologists, and radiologists were often organized in what was known as hospital-based speciality practices. Although their patients were essentially ''captive'' in the sense of being supplied by the hospital, they insisted and often succeeded in billing the patient directly, in addition to the hospital bill, as though the patients had directly chosen them to be their doctors.

17. The detailed particulars of this notion are seldom, if ever, spelled out; it is offered more as a generalized concept or goal.

18. In actual fact, the conditions under which many of the better private insurance plans operate result in de facto compulsory participation. if the employer is paying the premium for insurance, nonparticipation is not a realistic alternative; and many ''closed shop'' union agreements automatically confer health insurance benefits on the worker. On the other hand, there are government insurance programs with voluntary participation. But the generalization about government health insurance programs predominantly requiring compulsory participation is valid.

19. This was always, and continued to be, an ambiguous classification. While it is highly correlated with income status, it is not identical to it. As used here it refers to the class of professionals, administrators, and business owners who are also in the middle-income brackets.

10

Medicare and Medicaid: Passage in 1965 and Aftermath

Until 1965 the efforts by the United States government to fill the gaps in medical care access were largely focused on public "welfare" medical programs and on local public hospitals. Access to many of these services, particularly those associated with public relief programs, was based on a means test and was therefore a special privilege bestowed by a magnanimous society upon designated categories of poor people. Attempts to convert the entire system to a national health care system with universal access as a fundamental right for all residents were consistently defeated. Except for relatively restricted areas like workers' compensation and temporary disability insurance, no government-sponsored health insurance legislation was passed. Even in these two types of laws, eligibility was still contingent on employment and in workers' compensation, the main program, services were covered only for injuries or illness that were work-related.

The passage of federally sponsored health insurance for persons sixty-five years of age and over in 1965 heralded a major departure from this pattern. At the same time, the enactment of Medicaid represented a major expansion in federal and state support of medical care for the poor, including an enhanced opportunity for states to pay for services to certain classes of the near poor as well. Because these two programs had substantial interlocking elements, and because taken together they were initially perceived as finally closing the gaps in access to medical care, I shall treat them together in certain contexts despite their quite different conceptual underpinnings: public (i.e., social) health insurance for Medicare and public assistance medicine for Medicaid. However, these differences remain real and will not be ignored. Because Medicare and Medicaid were at the center of health policy debates in the years after 1965, an acquaintance with the provisions of the original legislation is necessary for understanding these arguments as well as the rationale behind the subsequent amendments.

THE ORIGINAL 1965 LEGISLATION (AS AMENDED IN 1967)

Medicare

"Medicare" was created by that part of the Social Security [Act] Amendments of 1965 (P.L. 89–97) that added a new Title XVIII, which had two parts: Part A, Hospital Insurance (HI), providing mainly hospital care benefits, and Part B, Supplementary Medical Insurance (SMI), providing mainly physician care benefits. The hospital orientation of the act is indicated by the fact that the physician care part was called "supplementary" insurance. A summary of the main provisions of the original act, as amended in 1967, follows.

Part A—Hospital and Related Benefits

The major program features in this part were:

1. *Eligibility* All persons sixty-five years of age or older who were entitled to benefits under the Social Security or Railroad Retirement[1] Acts were eligible and *automatically* covered upon attaining age sixty-five. Persons who were over sixty-five but not eligible at the time the act was passed were blanketed in. All persons reaching the age of sixty-five after 1965 were required to

have a specified number of Social Security work credits[2] in order to be eligible.

2. *Benefits* These were measured in benefit periods that ended 60 days after discharge from a hospital or an extended-care facility. Benefits during one benefit period for a particular spell of illness included up to 90 days in a hospital, 100 days in an extended care facility, and home-care benefits for up to one year after the most recent discharge from a hospital or an extended-care facility. In addition (added by 1967 amendments), each insured person was entitled to a lifetime reserve of 60 days of hospitalization. Care in a psychiatric hospital was limited to a lifetime limit of 190 days[3] but only if the patient was certified by a physician as being "reasonably expected to improve." The same proviso held for care in a tuberculosis hospital, with the addition that care was covered for a patient if he or she were hospitalized in order to render his or her condition noncommunicable. Outpatient hospital diagnostic services were not covered under Part A. A minimum of three days in a hospital had to precede admission to an extended-care facility or eligibility for home-care services. Post hospital home health services included nursing care; physical, occupational, or speech therapy; medical social services; services of a part-time health aide and medical supplies; and use of medical appliances. Home health services were limited to 100 visits within one year of discharge from an approved facility.

3. *Quality Controls on Providers* Hospitals had to meet certain standards and the state could require licensing. The Public Health Service could consult with and advise states and the Social Security Administration, and it could conduct program studies and evaluations. Hospitals and extended-care facilities were required to establish utilization review committees consisting of at least two staff physicians and to conform to federal civil rights statutes. The intention of the legislation was clearly that an extended-care facility be an active, intensive restorative service. It was defined as an "institution primarily engaged in providing *skilled nursing* [emphasis added] and related services and rehabilitation services," was required to be under professional direction with every patient's treatment under a physician's supervision, and to have an arrange-

ment for transfer of patients with at least one hospital. Home health services were required to be administered in conformity with a plan of treatment drawn up by the patient's physician within fourteen days of the patient's latest discharge form a hospital or extended-care facility and to be provided by a public or nonprofit private "home health agency" primarily engaged in providing skilled nursing services and other therapeutic services supervised by a doctor or registered nurse.

4. *Out-of-pocket Costs to Patients* Subscriber benefits were circumscribed by a number of cost-sharing features.[4] For hospital care, a "front end" deductible was imposed on each stay[5] and after sixty days in the hospital, a per diem copayment charge was levied.[6] These per diem cost-sharing rates applied only through the ninetieth day, however. Thereafter, the patient would have available sixty days of the "lifetime reserve" if none of it had been used in prior stays.[7] There were no front-end deductibles for extended-care facility use, but after twenty days a daily copayment charge was levied.[8]

5. *Financing* Earmarked payroll taxes levied on both employers and employees were to be paid into a special trust fund administered by the Social Security Board. Disbursements were to be made from this fund to "intermediaries," insurance companies who reimbursed providers upon submission of a claim by or on behalf of the beneficiary.

6. *Reimbursement of Providers* Intermediaries were nominated by regional groups or associations of providers. There were separate associations for hospitals, extended-care facilities, and home health services agencies. Each individual provider could elect to deal directly with the federal government or choose an intermediary different from the one the group had chosen if it was satisfactory to the Department of Health, Education and Welfare.

The rates of reimbursement were to be based on "reasonable *costs*" [emphasis added]. Regulations for determining such costs were to be set by the secretary of the Department of Health, Education and Welfare subject to given stipulations specified in the act.

The intermediaries were to be paid the operating cost of administering the claims plus a service fee. Blue Cross was chosen as the intermediary for almost all hospitals and home health associations and for most extended-care facilities; in 1969 it was the intermediary for 87 percent of the hospitals, 54 percent of the extended-care facilities, and 77 percent of the home health associations (U.S. Senate Committee on Finance, 1970, Appendix F).

7. *National Health Insurance Benefits Advisory Council* A nineteen-member advisory council was to be appointed by the secretary of the Department of Health, Education, and Welfare to advise on matters of general policy and administration. The membership was to be a mix of persons "outstanding in fields related to hospital, medical and other health activities" and persons "who are representative of organizations and associations of professional personnel in the field of medicine," with at least one member "representative of the general public." Members were to serve for four-year terms with a maximum of two terms, and the council was required to issue an annual report.

Part B—Supplementary Medical Insurance

The main program features were:

1. *Eligibility All* persons over sixty-five years of age were eligible for participation in this program. Participation was *voluntary* and no history of having paid into Social Security was required.

2. *Benefits* These included physicians' services at any site, home health services (see hospital benefits for description) with no requirement for prior hospitalization, up to 100 visits per year. Also included were diagnostic tests, radiotherapy, ambulance services, and various medical supplies and appliances. A number of preventive services particularly important to elderly people were not covered at all; neither were any pharmaceuticals.

3. *Quality Controls on Providers* All services had to be certified as necessary by the patient's physician.

4. *Out-of-pocket and Premium Costs to Patients* The subscriber was at first required to pay one-half the monthly premium with the federal government paying the other half out of general revenues.[9] After July 1973, premium increases were limited "to not more than the percentage

by which Social Security cash benefits has been generally increased since the last Part B premium adjustment. Costs above those met by such premium payments will be paid out of general revenue in addition to the regular general revenue matching" (U.S. Senate Committee on Finance, 1973).

The front-end deductible was an annual amount[10] consisting of the first physician charges incurred that year that had to be met in full by the subscriber. After it had been met the patient was responsible for a coinsurance of 20 percent of the remaining "reasonable" charges for the rest of the year. There were also upper limits and important exclusions. A limit was set on the amount of psychiatric care that would be reimbursed and routine physical examinations and certain procedures were not covered at all. Eye refraction were excluded, for example, as were other preventive services such as immunizations, hearing aids or examinations for the purpose of fitting them, routine dental services, routine foot care (podiatry), and other such items. Pharmaceuticals were not covered at all.

5. *Financing* As noted in point 4 above, part of the monthly premium was paid by the subscriber and the remainder by the federal government out of general revenues. These premiums were also placed into a trust fund by the Social Security Board. As for Part A, the trust fund for Part B made disbursements to private insurance companies called "carriers" who reimbursed providers and were paid a service fee plus their cost of adminstering this program.

6. *Reimbursement of Providers* Carriers were chosen by the secretary of Health, Education and Welfare. They reimbursed the providers on a "reasonable cost" basis for institutional providers and on a "reasonable charges" basis for noninstitutional providers, who were mostly physicians. Reasonable charges were determined by, among other considerations, the "customary" charges of the physician furnishing the service and the "prevailing" charges in the locality. Note that the physician did not have to accept the "reasonable charge" as his complete payment and could bill the patient for an additional amount. If the physician agreed to accept the "reasonable charge" as payment in full,

he or she was then said to be "accepting assignment."

Medicaid

The portion of the Social Security Amendments of 1965 that added Title XIX to the Social Security Act established "Medicaid," which extended the scope of federal aid to the states for payments to vendors of medical care for the poor. In contrast to the national administration and the countrywide uniform eligibility provisions and benefits of Medicare, Medicaid was a state-administered program with eligibility requirements and benefits that varied greatly from state to state. States had a wide range of options with respect to their degree of participation, ranging from not joining the program at all (two states had not yet joined by 1973) to including a great many covered services and a range of eligible classes of persons. And yet, even this varied assortment was more uniform under the Medicaid legislation than it had been under the medical programs of the state welfare programs preceding it.

There were three types of population groups for which the federal government provided some type of matching contributions. For two of these the total outlay of the state was matched, but for the third none of the actual medical expenses were matched; only the program's administrative expenditures were. Inclusion of one of these eligible groups was obligatory if a state wished to join the program but inclusion of the others was optional.

Each state was required to submit an acceptable plan to HEW in order to qualify for this program. A requirement about a single state agency was included, but the agency was not specified. Every state was required to establish a medical advisory committee whose membership included consumer representatives.

Categories of Persons Eligible for Federal Reimbursement

The three types were:

1. *Categorically Needy* This was the obligatory class and included all persons receiving federally matched public welfare assistance. We recall from Chapter 8 that these were Families

with Dependent Children (AFDC), Permanently and Totally Disabled (ATD), Blind (AB) and Aged (OAA) and whose resources fell below welfare-stipulated levels of adequacy. State expenditures were federally matched 50 to 80 percent, depending on the per capita income of the state, averaging 55 percent across all participating states.

2. *Categorically Linked* This class was optional for inclusion by the state. Expenditures were matched as in 1 above. The class included persons who physically fell into one of the four federally assisted categories but who were ineligible for cash assistance because their resources exceeded federally set ceilings. This optional class was also often called the "categorically related." These persons were still the Elizabethan "worthy poor" but only with respect to *medical* indigency. If this extension to the *medically needy only* were opted by a state, it had to be extended equally across all four categories.[11]

3. *Not Categorically linked but Medically Indigent* This class was also optional for inclusion by states, but state operating expenditures were *not matched*. The federal government would match only the cost of administering this program, provided clients received services comparable to those provided to other groups receiving such services. These beneficiaries often included: (a) all recipients and eligibles for statewide *general assistance*; (b) all aged 21 to 65 who were medically needy; and (c) all whose income was above the federal maximum standard for determining medically needy under 2 above. This class of eligibles was confusingly sometimes also called the medically needy only, or the medically indigent adults. It was somewhat akin to the "able-bodied poor" of the poor law, and we note how meager was the federal contributory support offered for them.

Limits on Personal Resources of Categorical Applicants Used in Determining Program Eligibility and Recovery Provisions

I have referred to the federal ceilings placed on applicant resources in determining eligibility for Medicaid. The regulations defining these ceilings got to be indescribably intricate as the program went to ever greater lengths to screen out insufficiently poor supplicants. Some of the general features of these personal resource screening procedures will be of interest in later discussions of the program and the problems that arose with its administration.

The basic procedure was for the federal government to establish national personal resource ceilings for determining eligibility for the obligatory "categorically needy" classification for Medicaid. Any state could adopt the federal or a lower (i.e., more restrictive) ceiling for eligibility within that state. These ceilings were the same as the upper-income[12] limits set for eligibility for public welfare cash assistance.

The federal government also established a second income limit above the ceiling for public welfare eligibility below which a (categorically linked) client would be considered to be only "medically needy," that is, sufficiently poor to be eligible for Medicaid but not poor enough to be entitled to cash public assistance. This ceiling was originally set at 150 percent of the "needy" level, but after 1969 it was lowered to 133 1/3 percent. These are generally referred to as 150 percent and 133 1/3 percent above welfare level, respectively. Individuals who were in one of the four *physical* categories eligible for welfare were *unconditionally* eligible for Medicaid only if their income was below the *state's* public welfare income level; if their income was above the welfare income ceiling but not by more than 50 percent, they were eligible for Medicaid only if their state opted to have a program for them. These persons were the "categorically linked" group.

No liens were permitted on the property of the recipient before his or her death for care received before age sixty-five. For care after age sixty-five, action against the estate could be taken to recover costs only after the death of the surviving spouse if there were no surviving minors or handicapped children.

Benefits

States could receive federal matching for fifteen specified services in their Medicaid plan, but they were *required* to provide the first five services listed in Table 10–1 for the obligatory "categorically needy" eligibles except that skilled nursing home services could be limited to those twenty-one and older. These services

Table 10–1. Services Eligible for Federal Matching if Offered by a State under its Medicaid Program as Originally Enacted in 1965 and Amended in 1967

1. Inpatient hospital services (other than services in an institution for tuberculosis or mental disease).
2. Outpatient hospital services.
3. Other laboratory and X-ray services.
4. Skilled nursing facility services for persons 21 and over, and after July 1, 1969, early and periodic screening, diagnosis, and treatment of physical and mental defects in eligible people under 21. (After July 1, 1970, any eligible individual who was entitled to skilled nursing home services was also entitled to home health services.)
5. Physicians' services (in the office, patient's home, hospital, skilled nursing home, or elsewhere).
6. Medical care, or any other type of remedial care recognized under state law, furnished by licensed practitioners within the scope of their practice as defined by state law (such as podiatrists, chiropractors, naturopaths).
7. Home health care services.
8. Private duty nursing services.
9. Clinic services.
10. Dental services.
11. Physical therapy and related services.
12. Prescribed drugs, dentures, and prosthetic devices and eyeglasses prescribed by a physician skilled in diseases of the eye or an optometrist, whichever the patient may select.
13. Other diagnostic, screening, preventive, and rehabilitative services.
14. Inpatient hospital services and skilled nursing home services for individuals aged 65 or over in an institution for tuberculosis or mental diseases.
15. Any other medical care and any other type of remedial care recognized under state law and specified by the secretary, such as transportation to receive services, family planning services, whole blood when not otherwise available, Christian Science practitioners' services and care in Christian Science sanitoria, and skilled nursing home services.

Note: Services 1 through 5 were required to be provided for beneficiaries who received federally supported cash assistance.

were designated as the "basic five." For the optional "categorically linked," the states had a choice of providing either the "basic five" or any seven of the first fourteen services listed. If either inpatient hospital care or skilled nursing home service was included among the seven, physicians' services had to be provided for individuals while they were in a hospital or nursing home.

Free Choice and Quality Controls[13]

1. After July 1, 1969, states were explicitly required to allow Medicaid recipients free choice among qualified practitioners, medi-

cal facilities, and community pharmacies. The free choice of medical vendor included the right to choose an organized group practice of physicians as well as a solo-practicing qualified physician. The group practice definition covered not only the standard one of a voluntary association of three or more physicians working as a team, but also a consumer-sponsored prepaid group practice. In this case, a recipient could have his or her prepayment fees or dues paid to the group by the state Medicaid agency. There would have to be, however, an agreement between the state agency and the group guaranteeing that the care and services covered by the fees and dues were at least as comprehensive as those that would be obtained from an independently practicing fee-for-service physician.

2. Hospitals reimbursed by Medicaid had to be licensed or formally approved by an officially designated state standard-setting authority and were required to be certified under the Medicare program.

3. Skilled nursing homes had to be state licensed after December 1968 and after July 1, 1969, were required to make periodic medical evaluations of the appropriateness of the care provided. After July 1, 1970, the administrator also had to be licensed.

Coordination with Medicare

All aged who were insured under Medicare and were also eligible for Medicaid because of their low incomes had their hospital deductibles and copayments under Part A of Medicare paid by Medicaid. This process was described as the state Medicaid program "buying in" to Medicare. States were originally encouraged also to "buy-in" to Medicare Part B for all their low-income aged. For those classified as categorically needy (i.e., recipients of OAA[14]), the federal government paid one-half the premium, but for the aged medically needy only, the full premium was borne by the state. After January 1, 1970, federal matching was discontinued for medical care of aged persons whose care would have been met by Medicare if the state had bought in, making buying-in by Medicaid in effect compulsory for all categorically needy aged. Persons who are eligible for both Medicare and

Medicaid came to be known as the "crossover population."

Institutionalized Services in Intermediate-Care Facilities

An amendment to the existing Title XI of the Social Security Act in 1967 (P.L. 90–248) authorized federal Medicaid matching for institutional care in "intermediate-care facilities," (ICF) described as health care facilities for patients who needed institutional care but did not need the level of medical technology provided by a "skilled nursing" facility (SNF). The intention was to provide states with a less expensive alternative to skilled nursing care where use of such an alternative was appropriate. The federal matching for this program was on the same basis as the rest of the Medicaid matching.

Mandated Extension to All in Medical Need and State Maintenance of Effort

Under the categorical cash assistance programs, annual federal matching per welfare assistance recipient had always been capped by a fixed national maximum average annual amount per beneficiary. Such an upper limit had also applied to the federal grants to the states for welfare medical programs in the 1950s and early 1960s. The federal matching under Medicaid, however, for the obligatory categorically needy class of client (public welfare cash assistance recipient) applied to the *entire amount spent by the state*, whatever that turned out to be. The dependence of federal matching for the obligatory class of beneficiaries entirely upon what states chose to spend became one of the most politically controversial fiscal aspects of Title XIX. Even more important, the wording of the legislation implied that the inclusion of certain categories of "medically needy" persons being optional with the state was only a transitional phase, for the law proclaimed the intent that the states be providing comprehensive care and services under their Medicaid programs to "substantially all" the needy *and* medically needy by July 1, 1975. This proviso seems to have been intended as the ultimate "access-gap filler." Had it been implemented it would have eliminated the uninsured class of persons in the United States, for together with private health insurance, Medicare, and existing direct service government programs, the country would have had a universal access medical care system. However, the Anderson-Gore Amendment of 1969 advanced the required date for achieving a "comprehensive" Medicaid program to 1977, and the 1972 Social Security Amendments repealed this section entirely.

The original Medicaid legislation also required that states not reduce their contribution to medical assistance for the mandated compulsory class below levels existing before the initiation of the Medicaid program in the state.[15]

General Observations and Comments on Medicaid

The original Medicaid legislation represented a departure from the pre-1965 federal aid to states for medical payments on behalf of welfare recipients in four major respects. (1) It substituted a single program of medical assistance for the separate programs previously provided under the four categorical assistance programs and MAA. It therefore improved uniformity in administration, eligibility standards, medical services offered, and federal-state matching for all eligibles within a state where formerly there had been diversity in these respects among the different categories. (2) It offered many states a proportionately higher federal matching percentage for medical expenditures than they had received as part of the four previous basic categorical programs. (3) In states electing to participate in the optional programs it extended federally matched medical assistance to medically needy (only) persons in all four categorical assistance programs, thereby applying across the four categories the principle of optional state coverage of the medically needy first introduced just for the aged category by the Kerr-Mills Act. States were encouraged to exercise the option of providing medical assistance to the medically needy by this offer of federal matching. (4) Finally, there was the mandating of the *ultimate* extension of medical assistance to all others determined to be needy or medically needy by the states' standards of eligibility. It was hoped that the money saved by states and localities due to the assumption by the federal government of 50 percent or more of the costs of medical care for

the categorical poor would be used to finance care for the categorical medically indigent only as well as the noncategorical medically needy. The maintenance of effort requirements were meant to encourage this action and deter shifting of state and county savings on indigent medical care to other uses. We turn now to a consideration of the experience of the Medicare and Medicaid programs during the early years, 1966–1972.

EFFECTS OF PROGRAM OPERATION ON HEALTH SYSTEM 1966–1972

Medicare

By 1972 Congress and the administration were expressing serious concern about the rising costs of Medicare. The two main causes of this concern were the deterioration of the United States economy and the record of the Medicare program in its first years of operation with respect to costs and effectiveness. The effects of the first seven years of Medicare on utilization, prices, and expenditures for medical care are properly considered during two distinct periods: the transition period consisting of the years 1966 and 1967, and the subsequent five years, 1968–1972.

The Medicare program had been enacted to improve access to medical care for the aged, and one might reasonably have expected an increase in utilization if the program were effective. With the increased demand for services from the aged one might also have expected some increase in unit prices in the short run, both in charges (billings) and in average price collected, given the short-term fixed supply of providers. An increase in utilization and prices would of course mean a rise in health care expenditures, but ideally most of the increase would be due to the increased (appropriate) utilization rather than prices. What actually happened? This question was examined in a number of studies. Information about the two "warm-up" years, as well as data referring to the immediately preceding pre-Medicare years (the "baseline" years) comes mostly from special studies, many of them commissioned by the Social Security Administration (Donabedian and Thorly, 1969; Greenfield, 1968; Feldstein and Waldman, 1969; Lowenstein, 1971; Davis, 1972). Information relating to the later years was obtained mainly from a series of articles in the *Social Security Bulletin-* that analyzed operating data of Medicare (Wert, 1971; Wolkstein, 1970; Horowitz, 1972; Pettengill, 1972; Cooper, 1972).

There was a large percentage increase both in hospital and physician costs to the program in 1968 and smaller increases in the following three years. The initial spurt was larger in physician than in hospital costs (Wert, 1971, Table 5), which brought the ratio of per capita costs for hospitals compared with payments to physicians down from the 3.0 of 1967 to 2.3 for 1968.

Utilization

Hospitals and physicians constitute the main components of medical care expenditures. Their responses were not the same in all respects, to a large degree because they are covered by different portions of the Medicare Act.

Hospitals The studies dealing with Medicare's early effects agree that short-term acute hospital utilization by the aged, measured in patient days, rose at an annual rate of between 9 and 16 percent in the first year after Medicare and moved irregularly upward in the subsequent four years (Pettengill, 1972). There was a sharp increase in patient days between 1967 and 1968 that was due more to an increased length of stay than to a rise in admission rate (Wert, 1971). After 1969, utilization stabilized at something near 3,900 days per 1,000 enrollees in Medicare Part A.

There is considerable evidence that the increased utilization by the aged during the years 1966–1968 was partially at the expense of decreased utilization by other groups in the population (Pettentgill, 1972). Between 1965 and 1970 total days of hospital care per capita increased by 11 percent while the per capita bed supply rose only 7 percent, thereby raising the average percent occupancy in community hospitals from 76.0 percent to 78.8 percent in 1969 (Pettengill, 1972). Thus, during its first five years of operation Medicare benefited the hospitals by increasing their occupancy rates and partially altered their patient mix away from younger to older patients. Comparisons of the immediate post-Medicare period with the im-

mediate pre-Medicare period made by Feldstein and Waldman in a study of the effect on non-federal short-term hospitals over the first two years of Medicare (1969) corroborate these assertions. They concluded: "The proportion of hospital beds occupied by the aged . . . increased significantly in the second year of Medicare" (1969); and there was a moderate increase in occupancy rate the first year, this rate being maintained for the second year.

The immediate effects of Medicare did not, however, involve an increase in overall use of long-term facilities, whether in terms of long-stay hospital beds or extended-care facilities and nursing homes (Lowenstein, 1970).

Physicians Neither the immediate nor longer term effects of Medicare resulted in markedly increased rates of ambulatory utilization by the aged in these early years. In the first year of Medicare, the proportion of enrolled persons using ambulatory services remained unchanged, while the number of visits per person actually declined somewhat (Lowenstein, 1971). There was very little change in total ambulatory usage in the subsequent years either, but a shift in site of ambulatory care away from office visits to outpatient and home visits was discernible (Wert, 1971). An important contributing cause of the disparity between the very small increase in physician use on an ambulatory basis compared with hospital utilization during these first few years was the low proportion of aged enrolled in the voluntary supplementary medical insurance program (Part B) compared with the automatic enrollment in the hospital insurance program during the early years of Medicare. It is also likely that the greater cost sharing in Part B compared with Part A contributed to the disparity.

Prices

Price is sometimes given in health service statistics as an "asking price" in the form of charges "asked" (or quoted) by hospitals or physicians, usually in the form of billing. More frequently, the price is given in studies as the average actual price received. From the point of view of calculating the real cost of a service to an insurance program like Medicare, the price of a service is the average price actually paid out in claims. It is a computed quantity calculated by dividing total revenue by the number of units utilized. For a hospital, the realized price of a service is always lower than the asked or quoted price because of discounts allowed to some insurers and incomplete collections on bills known as "uncompensated care."

Hospitals In the early post-Medicare period both the hospital daily routine service charges and total per patient day income (realized prices) rose much faster than the overall Consumer Price Index and also faster than the overall medical care component of that index.[16] A large part of the increase in Medicare's costs was clearly due to increases in prices both of ancillary services and routine per diem services. Prices of hospital services rose more rapidly than utilization. In 1969 and 1970, the percentage increases in prices of ancillary services exceeded those in utilization by Medicare clients.

Feldstein and Waldman concluded that the BLS data indicated that hospital prices rose more rapidly after the introduction of Medicare than in other recent periods, and that hospital expenses per patient day in particular increased at a more rapid rate just after the beginning of Medicare compared with years immediately preceding Medicare 1969).

Physicians During the first five years of Medicare ending in 1971, physicians' fees (charges) rose 39 percent compared with only a 15 percent rise in the pre-Medicare five years ending 1965. However this 39 percent increase was only 2.6 times greater than the 15 percent rise registered during the pre-Medicare five-year period for physicians' charges, while the overall Consumer Price Index rose 4.5 times as fast in the post-Medicare period as during the five-year pre-Medicare period. In other words, physicians' prices at first rose more slowly than did the overall Consumer Price Index. There is, therefore, no evidence from these data that the coming of Medicare as such increased the rate of increase of physicians' charges in the first five years if the charges were adjusted for overall general price inflation.

Nevertheless, the secretary of the Department of Health, Education and Welfare in 1967 publicly expressed concern over the annual rate of increase in physicians' fees, and the staff of the U.S. Senate Committee on Finance in its 1970 report on Medicare and Medicaid asserted that "anticipatory bias" had been used by many physicians to raise their fees during the initial baseline Medicare period. At first glance the concentration of public pronouncements on physician fee increases compared with hospital costs, which rose more rapidly than the general inflation rate, seems inexplicable from this evidence, but the extent of the physicians' increased total *income* due to Medicare cannot be inferred entirely from the rise in fees per unit of service as expressed in the CPI. The average annual charge *per person* (meaning here actually collected physician income per patient) was estimated in one study to have gone from $66 in 1965 to $95 in 1967 (Lowenstein, 1971). While some of this increase was due to the rise in asking price per unit of service and some due to the assumption by Medicare of fees previously paid by other agencies, it still seems reasonable to assume that some of the increase also represented payment of charges that formerly were not collected in full or had perhaps been made on a sliding scale. Since the $95 charge per person in 1967 was met 47 percent out-of-pocket by the patient, compared with the $66 charge per person for 1965 having been met 81 percent out-of-pocket, the saving to the Medicare patient in ambulatory costs attributable to Medicare Part B was some 16 percent for that period.

Expenditures

The proportion of the health care expenses of the aged paid from public sources rose much more sharply than expected in the years immediately following the passage of Medicare. In FY 1966, public programs provided 31 percent of the expenses of health care for the aged. In one year, this proportion rose to 59 percent (35 percent from Medicare and 24 percent from other public funds). The percentage of the total spent on health care for the aged by Medicare alone in 1967 was larger than the total percentage from all public programs in 1966. The per capita expenditures for hospital care of the aged met by the private sector fell from $93 to $18 in these two years. Since hospital care (Part A) was by far the more important cost element in Medicare, congressional interest centered on the changes in costs and financial position of hospitals brought about by the new law. The Feldstein and Waldman study of the effect on hospital services of the first two years of Medicare operations found that in the first year, July 1966—June 1967, "net revenues rose substantially," and in the second year, "net revenues fell [from the first year level] but continued to considerably exceed pre-Medicare levels." The authors concluded that the increase in the hospitals' net revenue in the first year resulted from some greater utilization (quantity), a substantial increase in charges (prices), reimbursement by Medicare for some services to aged patients previously provided free or at reduced charges, and reduction in uncollectibles from aged patients. Their analysis further claimed that in the second year the added revenue was used to effect wage increases, to expand scope of services to patients, and to purchase additional supplies and equipment, thus accounting for the fall in net revenue in the second year of Medicare. The hypothesis that in 1966–67 Medicare was picking up charges previously met by other public sources and philanthropy was also substantiated by a Columbia University School of Public Health and Administrative Medicine study (CUS) (Lowenstein, 1971).

In summary, the available evidence indicates that the aged increased their hospital use in the early years of Medicare and then stabilized at a higher utilization rate reached in 1971. The new "steady state" level of about 3,900 patient days per 1,000 reached in 1971 by persons aged over sixty-five was 26 percent higher than the 3,100 patient days per 1,000 prevailing in 1965, the last pre-Medicare year (Lowenstein, 1971). The initial increase was partially at the expense of decreased rates of utilization by other segments of the population. Ambulatory utilization did not increase to any great degree, but this is not to say that physician visits did not increase, for we must remember that many physician visits are on an inpatient basis. Medical care prices rose steeply during the first five years of Medicare, more so for hospital than for physician reimbursement. It should be noted that some items not covered by Medicare (Part B), such as eyeglasses and prescriptions, rose far more slowly in price (Horowitz, 1972).

Price-deflated expenditures, a measure of utilization, rose for the elderly during the five post-Medicare years by 42 percent from 1966 through 1971. Yet although access to care for the aged was very much improved by Medicare, the cost savings to them were substantially diminished by cost sharing, upper limits, excluded services, and physicians' charges in excess of Medicare reimbursement schedules. Long-term care was scarcely affected, and access to health-maintaining and preventive ambulatory services was poorly covered by Medicare.

Effects on Private Insurance

After the passage of Medicare, both commercial and nonprofit health insurance carriers offered policies for subscribers over sixty-five that were meant only to supplement Medicare. These came to be called "Medigap" insurance, a striking recognition of the inadequacy of Medicare coverage alone as a gap-filling program. As of January 1, 1967, over 10 million aged persons were covered by such policies, according to a Social Security Board survey. The *Source Book of Health Insurance Data* of the Health Insurance Institute, a trade organization of insurance companies, states that in 1967, 9 million (48 percent) of the 20 million persons over sixty-five years of age carried such policies; commercial insurance companies carried 45 percent, the Blues 56 percent, and the independents 5 percent. About 80 percent of the number of aged who had had policies with commercial companies before Medicare carried commercial Medigap insurance after the passage of Medicare. The corresponding percentage for the Blues was 87 percent. The numbers of persons over sixty-five having private health insurance as of the end of 1969 are shown in Table 10–2.

The Social Security Board survey noted that

Table 10–2. Persons over Sixty-five Covered by Private Health Insurance, 1969

Type of coverage	Number of persons over 65 holding private Medigap coverage in 1969* (000)
Hospital. . . .	10,162
Surgical. . . .	8,840
Regular medical. . . .	7,703
Major medical. . . .	1,882

* Persons may be counted in more than one category.

many aged persons with Blue Cross-Blue Shield complementary (i.e., Medigap) coverage were complaining that they were paying almost as much for health care as before Medicare. Most of these Medigap policies covered the upper limits, exclusions, and cost sharing of Medicare. Very few offered affordable insurance for long-term care, which soon became the leading unmet health care need of the aged and remains so to this day.

Rising Criticisms of Medicare

The observed effects of the operations of Medicare on the health care system elicited criticisms from reformers, health professionals, analysts, and public officials. The critiques took two main directions. One addressed the shortcomings in service to beneficiaries (i.e., access and quality) while the other focused mainly on unnecessarily high costs (efficiency). While these two sets of critiques overlap to some degree, they are sufficiently distinct to treat individually.

Criticisms of Medicare based on its failure to service its target population more fully and appropriately centered on four points; (1) the deductible and coinsurance structure was affecting utilization in undesirable ways; (2) routine examinations and useful and desirable preventive and health maintenance services were excluded from coverage; (3) prescription drugs and some essential appliances were not covered; and (4) effects of reimbursement via "reasonable costs" and payment on the basis of "reasonable charges" were channeling some Medicare monies into accelerating price inflation rather than increasing access to care. It was noted, for example, that the criteria for physician reimbursement were often used in such a way as to render the Medicare reimbursement merely an addendum to the physician's pre-Medicare fee level because the patient could be asked to pay a considerable amount above the sum reimbursed by Medicare.

Criticisms dealing with inefficiencies of operation and supervision were typified by the hearings and staff report of Senator Long's Committee on Finance (1970), which included points such as the following: (1) hospital insurance costs were exceeding all actuarial estimates; (2) cost-based reimbursement should be abandoned in favor of methods that encourage cost control; (3) Medicare payment rates for physician services were often higher than those that the administering insurance carrier was paying for its own policy holders; (4) remuneration for "gang visiting" by doctors[17] in hospitals and allowances for multiple injections and routine laboratory tests should be curtailed; (5) the practice of billing Medicare under Part B for the services of a supervisory staff teaching physician in a teaching hospital and also collecting under Part A for the cost of the salary of this physician should be eliminated; (6) the committee identified providers collecting more than $25,000 annually in 1968 from Medicare (and Medicaid) and suggested regular reporting of detailed profile data on providers; (7) the staff was critical of the laxness in standards used to certify extended-care facilities, the "widespread failure" to apply utilization review, and the method of nominating intermediaries by providers; (8) the carriers were criticized for using the early Medicare Part B claims to establish baselines for "reasonable charges" for physicians; it was argued that the fees being paid by the carrier under its own most prevalent policy in effect at the time of passage of Medicare should have been used for these baselines.

In addition to this committee's criticisms, the Nixon administration was making known its preference for capitation payments to prepaid group practices and other HMOs, and a number of the national health insurance bills introduced in Congress contained clauses aimed at encouraging the development of this form of payment. The administration also testified in favor of increased cost sharing by patients and prospective payment to institutional providers.

These criticisms signaled a changing attitude toward Medicare in Congress, the administration, and in public writings and speeches. While the program was supported in general, changes were being called for. As Irwin Wolkstein, Deputy Director of the Bureau of Health Insurance of the Social Security Administration, noted (1970), the prevailing attitude in 1965, when Medicare was originally enacted, was that an insurance financing mechanism was being passed that abjured all but the most minimal regulation. Like its model, the private health insurance structure, it was to concern itself only with paying claims and not mix into any questions of quality of cost. The very first paragraph of Title XVIII stated:

Nothing in this title shall be construed to authorize any Federal Officer or employee to exercise any supervision or control over the practice of medicine or the manner in which medical services are provided, or over the selection, tenure, or compensation of any officer or employee of any institution, agency, or person providing health services; or to exercise any supervision or control over the administration or operation of any such institution, agency, or person.

When, after more than a year of hearings, the proposed *Social Security Amendments of 1972* (H.R. 1) were passed as P.L. 92–603, the sections concerning Medicare dealt, without apology or looking backward, largely with changes providing for cost and quality *controls*. Clearly, the federal attitude had changed from stressing its intention to exercise minimal "supervision or control" to emphasizing the need for them. The Social Security Amendments of 1972 marked the dividing line between two post-Medicare periods; the first was characterized by an almost single-minded concern with getting providers to participate in Medicare by quieting their fears that any strings would be attached, while the second was marked by a substantial reversal in attitude that now took a sternly critical stance toward providers and emphasized cost controls in Medicare. These amendments drew so clear a boundary between the two periods that they may justifiably be regarded as a watershed in the history of Medicare.

Medicaid

State Participation

As of March 1971, forty-eight of the fifty states had joined the Medicaid program. Alaska and Arizona were the only exceptions, reflecting uncertainty and anxiety in those states over assuming responsibility for the medical care of their Indian and Eskimo populations who were beneficiaries of the federal Indian Health Service (See Chapter 5). After December 31, 1969, the deadline for entering the Medicaid program set by Title XIX in 1965, these two states were denied federal matching for their medical assis-

tance programs. By 1975, Alaska had joined the program but Arizona never did.

By 1971, twenty-five states were participating on a minimal basis, offering the mandatory five[18] services and a few other services *only* to the obligatory categorical public assistance recipients, while twenty-seven others were also offering a set of services under Medicaid to the optional categorically linked medically needy population. The great disparity in state programs is illustrated by Wyoming, which offered only one service above the mandated minimum and then only to its obligatory public assistance recipients, and New York, in which not only was the obligatory class of welfare recipients entitled to fourteen additional services above the mandated five, but all the Medicaid services available to the obligatory public assistance population were also available to the categorically linked medically needy as well. In addition to the wide scope of services it offered, New York had one of the highest income eligibility ceilings for receiving public assistance so that the obligatory Medicaid-eligible class and the optional medically needy classes were larger than in other states.

Fiscal Impact on Federal, State, and Local Government

From the very first, widespread dissatisfaction was expressed with the cost of Medicaid. Because this was a public assistance welfare program paid out of general tax funds and not, like Medicare, an insurance program paid out of premiums collected as specially earmarked taxes, it brought out all the opposition that has for so long existed against putatively excessive doles to the helpless, reflecting an underlying antipathy to "welfare" malingering. This was particularly true of the increase in federal expenditures but was also true in many of the states and even localities, which some states mandated to share in state Medicaid expenditures.

Federal The open-ended obligation of the federal government to match all services the states might wish to provide for the two matchable classes of beneficiaries, and the optional nature of including the categorically linked under a state's Medicaid program made it difficult to estimate the future federal costs of this program. In other programs involving federal-state matching like public cash assistance, the federal government determined both a maximum grant per eligible person as well as the highest personal income ceiling for eligibility that it would match. This set a maximum total liability that the federal government could expect to accrue for matching state outlays, because it controlled both the possible number of eligibles and the maximum size of the matching grant per eligible. Federal expenditures for Medicaid, however, were much more open-endedly dependent on state decisions, an uncomfortable position for the federal government to be in. Thus, two main questions were involved: how many states would invoke which options among the optional "matchable" services, and how many would choose to include the matchable categorically linked group in their programs?

The ultimate sizes of the matchable population and services were virtually impossible to gauge accurately, but short-run expenditures estimates were made. In 1965, the House Ways and Means Committee estimated that "if all states took full advantage of provisions of the proposed Title XIX, the additional Federal participation [in fiscal 1966] would amount to $238 million." In 1966, Medicaid's first year of operation, total medical vendor payments were $1.9 billion, of which about half, or $962 million, may be supposed to have been federal funds, an increase of about $332 million over 1965. In the first three years of Medicaid's operation, total annual medical vendor payments rose from the pre-Medicaid 1965 amount of $1.3 billion (of which about $630 million was federal money) to $4.0 billion in 1968, a rise of 2.8 billion in annual outlay. The federal share rose about 1.4 billion.

The unanticipated size of the increases in vendor payments as well as the upwardly revised estimates of the size of future increases led to the passage of the 1967 amendments curtailing federal financial commitment. It was these amendments that reduced the personal income ceilings defining eligibility for the categorically linked medically needy from the original 150 to 133 1/3 percent of the AFDC eligibility level in each state and legislated a strong impetus, tantamount to a directive, for states to "buy-in" to

Medicare. In addition, a Medicaid payment category for care in a new class of facility, the "intermediate-care facility" (ICF) was established. An ICF was defined as a facility that provides "services beyond room and board but below the level of skilled nursing homes."[19]

Early in 1968, President Johnson called for the appointment of a Task Force on Costs of Medicaid and Public Assistance, which was to be a joint federal-state body charged with studying ways to improve reporting and estimating the cost of Medicaid. Reporting in June 1970, this body, the McNerney[20] Commission, noted that: (a) only 13 million of the 26 million poor (those with incomes below $3,500 for a family of four) and only 15 million of the near-poor (incomes below $4,500 for a family of four) would be covered by Medicaid by 1971; (b) less than thirty states had programs for medically needy persons (categorically linked) for whom federal matching was available; (c) two out of three children in poor or near-poor families were not being served by federally assisted maternal and child health programs *or* included in Medicaid programs; and (d) among the poor and near-poor, only a little over one-third of the persons below sixty-five years of age had private prepaid medical care or medical third-party coverage of any sort. In total, 30 to 45 million[21] persons under sixty-five had no insurance "to speak of." The commission recommended a number of changes in financing, population coverage, and operation of Medicaid that would have defined eligible persons more uniformly throughout the country, covered more people for more services, transferred the medical care assistance program under the public welfare category—Aid to Totally Disabled (ATD)—from Medicaid to Medicare,[22] included migrant workers under Medicaid, and changed the method of purchasing services to favor contracting for comprehensive health care packages.

It is instructive to note the nature of the commission's recommendations in response to its mandate in the face of a rising tide of calls for cost containment. The commission addressed itself primarily to noting shortfalls in the existing coverage of target populations. Recommendations for improved managerial efficiently were prescribed *within the context of correcting the shortfalls*. That is, *efficiently* was to be defined within a clearly defined normative[23] level of *efficacy*.

More in keeping with the single-minded cost-containment focus that was to dominate in later years was the previously cited report of the staff of the Senate Committee on Finance (1970), which also noted many problems facing the federal government in the operation of the Medicaid program. Some of the points made were: (1) There was "Congressional concern over rapidly rising Medicaid costs" with specific reference to the consistent tendency for experience to exceed estimates. (2) Medicaid's reimbursement procedures were criticized. The report noted that although federal regulations had prescribed that in general Medicaid should follow the same procedures set forth under Title XVIII for Medicare, using the Medicare "reasonable cost" determination method was unnecessarily costly for Medicaid and should be changed. This recommendation was an early intimation of a practice that was to become quite general in later years— paying less under Medicaid that under Medicare for the same type of services. (3) Disapproval was expressed over an Internal Revenue Service ruling (69–545) that a nonprofit hospital did not have to accept nonpaying patients in order to qualify for tax-exempt status. The committee staff noted that this requirement had been used by the states to get hospitals to accept lower Medicaid reimbursement rates than they would otherwise have demanded. (4) Strong criticism was aimed at the national administration of Medicaid by the Medical Services Administration of the Social and Rehabilitation Services. The report not only pointed out specific practices that could be improved but also strongly criticized the program's leadership. Many of the complaints dealt with the inadequacy of cost-control procedures in detecting abuses such as duplicate payments; improper rates, fees, and charges; poor utilization review; and violations of eligibility regulations. The need to strengthen quality control was noted, but the shortcomings in administration were strongly stressed.

The contrast between the orientation of the McNerney Commission report and the Senate Finance Committee report encapsulates the difference in approach to improving Medicaid. Senator Long's committee staff seemed interested almost only in cutting the cost of the program or at least slowing its rate of increase. While the formulation recommending that only "waste" and "mismanagement" costs be reduced does not necessarily imply a desire to cut access or quality, still there was almost a total lack of emphasis on the many persons Medicaid was meant to serve but in many states did not, and there was a less clearly expressed concern for improving the quality of services provided. There was also a push for paying less reimbursement for Medicaid clients than was being paid for Medicare (and certainly private insurance) beneficiaries, which was to continue and would serve to decrease the number of physicians and hospitals that accepted Medicaid patients. It seems fair to say that the McNerney Commission report was one of the last of the "old style" major evaluations that stressed service and access inadequacies. The Long Committee staff report was representative of a "new" approach that after 1970 was to stress cost containment.

States and Local Governments Among the twenty-six states that implemented their Medicaid programs early (i.e., they were in effect for all of 1967), the change in total expenditures for federally assisted medical vendor payments in the two-year period from calendar year 1965 through 1967 varied markedly from state to state. The variations stemmed from a complex of causes affecting the basic decisions made by state legislatures and administrators in initiating and establishing Title XIX state plans, as noted previously.

After 1967 the history of the Medicaid program in the states featured frequent cutbacks in services as they attempted to reduce costs, which were proving unacceptable to the state governments. The previously cited Senate Finance Committee report noted in 1970:

Increasing Medicaid costs have had a particularly severe fiscal impact on the States. Welfare costs typically constitute one of the largest items in the State budget, and vendor payments for medical care have represented an increasing share of welfare costs. In fiscal year 1965, just before Medicaid's enactment, medical assistance represented 25% of the total Federal, State and local welfare costs (excluding administrative costs). Over a four-year period, this percentage has risen to 41%. Looking at State and local funds only, medical vendor payments have risen over the four-year period from less than one-third to almost one-half of welfare expenditures (excluding costs of administration). In absolute dollar terms, the rise has been precipitous: from $764 million in State and local funds for medical vendor payments in fiscal year 1965 to an estimated $1,896 million in fiscal year 1968—a 150% increase within four years.

The report further noted that in its view, the states in scurrying about for ways to reduce costs had distorted legislative intent with respect to the Intermediate-Care Facility classification established under Title XI of the Social Security Act in 1967. Many states were arbitrarily reclassifying Skilled Nursing Facilities (SNFs) as Intermediate-Care Facilities (ICFs), and the status of their patients along with them to take advantage of the lower Medicaid reimbursement rates that could be paid to ICFs. The suspicion was that many patients who really needed skilled nursing were reclassified as needing only intermediate care to save state money—when savings should have been achieved by making the program more efficient. It was asserted that reclassification was being done "wholesale," without careful review matching the level of the facility with that required by the patient's condition. The Committee report contained a number of specific recommendations for procedures to improve Medicaid administration by the states. The term "improve" is used often, but as this example indicates, it was frequently only a code word for merely "reducing the costs of." These recommendations mostly followed the report's criticisms of the federal administration of Medicaid and its alleged failure to curb administrative abuses by the states.[24]

In addition to these deficiencies in program operation by the states, the staff report also pointed to a number of "actual and potential" other abuses. Examples of these are: ownership of facilities by physicians who were receiving large Medicaid payments for medical service and the sale of facilities at inflated prices to "nonprofit" groups made up of essentially the former owners. The new "reasonable cost" determinations for Medicaid reimbursement thereafter would include mortgage amortization payments to the previous owners (1970).

Thus, both Medicare and Medicaid were being faulted by Congressional leaders and public commentators for unnecessarily high costs, but the Medicare program was also being widely criticized for its incomplete coverage of the elderly. The Medicaid program, on the other hand, was being criticized almost entirely for being too expensive and badly administered. Comparatively little attention was being paid to the comprehensiveness and quality of the care actually delivered to its clients. The underservicing of many persons eligible for Medicaid and their inability to find physicians who would accept Medicaid patients, was increasingly ignored. National health policy with respect to medical care was moving toward where it was to end up by 1980, almost single-mindedly concerned with cost containment for both Medicare and Medicaid, but more for Medicaid. The 1972 amendments to the Social Security Act may be taken as the dividing line between the period that concentrated on increasing access and the new cost-containment period during which curtailment of access was often part of the drive to reduce costs.

THE 1972 AMENDMENTS TO THE SOCIAL SECURITY ACT: A WATERSHED

Taking cognizance of the operating history of Medicare and Medicaid and the changing climate of public opinion vis-à-vis these programs as the national economy began to subside from its 1946–1965 ebullience, the House Committee on Ways and Means, chaired by Congressman Wilbur Mills, proposed many changes in Medicare and Medicaid to contain costs. These were included in "H.R. 1," a bill introduced into the House of Representatives in 1971 to amend the Social Security Act. The Committee had held extensive hearings on this bill and produced a six-volume record (House Committee on Ways and Means, 1971) of testimony from the usual range of organizations and individuals who testify on matters they see as affecting their interests. It is particularly noteworthy, however, that representatives of the Nixon Administration testified often and at length. Their main recommendations with respect to Medicare and Medicaid were cost-control measures with emphasis on providing for capitation payments to health maintenance organizations (HMOs), increasing cost sharing in Medicare, and introducing it into Medicaid. The use of HMOs for providing total health care to an identified population for a fixed, periodic, prospectively paid fee shifts some of the responsibility for cost control to the provider; cost sharing shifts its onus to the consumer. These and other points pertaining to cost-containment matters will be discussed in more detail later, but for now the relevant observation is that the Nixon Administration's recommendations for cost control in these federal programs included both types of measures, those that shifted the burden to the provider and those that shifted it to the consumer. After a long period of hearings and a lengthy legislative history, the bill became law on October 30, 1972, as P.L. 92–603, the Social Security Amendments of 1972. This law made the most extensive changes in the Social Security Act since its passage in 1965, including incorporating into Medicare and Medicaid many of the cost-control recommendations made by the 1970 staff report of the Senate Committee on Finance and by the administration in congressional testimony and public statements.

One of the main changes altered the mode of federal-state sharing in the public cash assistance system. Beginning on January 1, 1974, three of the four classes of cash assistance recipients—the aged, blind, and disabled—were transformed into a completely federalized program, the Supplementary Security Income (SSI) program. Thenceforth, the federal government would pay monthly assistance grants directly to recipients to bring their monthly income up to a specified uniform national minimum. The AFDC cash assistance program remained a federal-state joint program with shared costs. However, the Medicaid program for the three categories under the new federalized SSI program remained with the states, continuing the federal-state cost-sharing arrangements obtaining before 1974, along with the AFDC class.[25]

The changes in Medicare and Medicaid, particularly the former, altered many reimbursement methods and instituted new regulatory methods. These became important features of the provider reimbursement system as well as the quality assurance and cost-containment aspects of the Medicare and Medicaid administrative systems over the next ten years. Many of the subsequent attempts to further rationalize and control the administration of these programs

dealt with efforts to adjust or fine-tune some of these 1972 changes based on how successful they came to be viewed in controlling costs. A number of the 1972 changes concerning matters that persisted as important issues warrant further comment here.

Changes to Medicare

1. Recipients of cash assistance under the Aid to Permanently and *Totally Disabled (APTD) category were rendered eligible for Medicare benefits* after having received APTD assistance for twenty-four months without needing to be sixty-five or over. Workers, who were the main beneficiaries, were included at any age, while widows and disabled dependent widowers became eligible only after age fifty. There were also certain other classes of new beneficiaries, affecting a relatively small number of persons. It was estimated that 1.7 million additional beneficiaries would be eligible immediately. This was the first time that any persons under sixty-five were made eligible for Medicare. As noted above, virtually all aged and most handicapped persons who were sufficiently poor could now receive Medicare as well as Medicaid benefits. Only the AFDC category remained entirely dependent on Medicaid for medical care.

2. Aged persons (i.e., those sixty-five years old or over) who were enrolled in Part B but were not eligible for Part A could now *voluntarily enroll in Part A* by paying a monthly premium to cover actuarially determined costs.

3. A number of changes in schedules of *payments by beneficiaries* were made, including limiting future premium increases in Part B to the percentage by which Social Security retirement benefits had been increased since the previous Part B premium increase.[26] Coinsurance under Part B for home health services was eliminated. These were two of the few provisions that improved benefits.

4. A number of provisions dealt with changes in health service *provider reimbursement* procedures. One that was to have important long-term significance concerned provision for capitation payments to Health Maintenance Organizations (HMOs). Medicare had been reimbursing HMOs for Part A care on a cost basis much like those used to reimburse other provid-

ers, with some adjustments to allow for the special bookkeeping problems that arose because HMOs did not normally keep records of the cost of each service rendered an individual patient. This amendment was an attempt to formally provide new mechanisms that would permit capitation payment for both Part A and Part B as alternatives to the old fee-for-service cost-reimbursement method.

Being paid on a capitation basis by Medicare was voluntary with each HMO and required a special contract negotiated with HEW. Two methods were authorized. One was a new *cost*-reimbursement contract under which payments to the HMO would be paid based on retrospective calculations of their year's costs of providing care to its Medicare subscribers.[27] The other was a *risk*-sharing contract under which those HMOs defined as ''established'' or ''mature'' could elect to be paid a retroactively determined capitation rate. The capitation rate for Parts A and B combined could not exceed the average cost to Medicare for its non-HMO beneficiaries in the area, the so-called *Adjusted Average Per Capita Cost* (AAPCC, see note 61). If the HMO's actual costs for its Medicare subscribers turned out to be less than the capitation rate it received for them, it could keep only part of the savings, but if its actual costs turned out to be higher, the HMO would carry the entire loss (McNeil and Schlenker, 1975).

Neither of these new options were widely taken up by the HMOs. The risk-sharing option, which was the desired one of the federal government, was particularly difficult to implement because few HMOs could qualify as ''well developed'' or ''mature,'' and those that could did not view the risk-sharing provisos as favorable to them. As late as 1979 there was only one HMO with a risk-sharing contract, but several had signed the new cost-reimbursement type of contract (Falkson, 1980). More widespread use of the risk-sharing capitation contract did not come until after the terms of these contracts were liberalized under the Tax Equity and Financial Responsibility Act of 1982 (TEFRA), which is discussed later in this chapter.

Other significant changes in reimbursement for all providers placed constraints on the items that could be included in a facility's calculation of its cost and limits on what physicians could

claim as their ''reasonable charges'' for reimbursement purposes. Limits were also placed on annual increases in payment rates for some types of facilities—skilled nursing facilities (SNFs), for example.

5. Another group of changes dealt mainly with increased controls over costs, utilization, quality of care, and abuses of the program and with the development of procedures for monitoring these factors. A particularly important provision was the requirement for establishing professional standards review organizations (PSRO) to assume responsibility for comprehensive and ongoing review of covered services. (This set of provisions also applied to Medicaid and established the precedent for formal national quality assurance requirements by Medicaid.) It should be noted that while a PSRO was required to review institutional services in its area, review of noninstitutional care was optional. The reviews had to cover both utilization and professional quality standards; use of existing hospital utilization review committees and medical organization quality review committees was permitted provided they were found to be effective.

Other provisions dealt with establishing penalties for fraud or reporting false information by providers. One of the more important of these provisions authorized the Secretary of HEW to undertake studies, experiments, or demonstration projects[28] dealing with *prospective reimbursement* of facilities, ambulatory surgical centers, intermediate-care (Medicaid) and homemaker services (Medicare); elimination or reduction of the three-day hospital stay before admission to a skilled nursing home required by Medicare; appropriate methods for reimbursing physicians' assistants and nurse practitioners; provision of day-care services to the aged; and the use of clinical psychologists.

6. A number of changes affected allied health and dental personnel. For the most part, these changes permitted Medicare reimbursement for services rendered by allied health personnel under certain conditions. These services previously had to be delivered by physicians to be reimbursable.

7. The rate of payroll deduction for hospital insurance (HI) for future years was increased beginning with calendar year 1973, as was the

amount deducted for old age, survivors, and disability insurance (OASDI).[29] A person making $10,800 (the maximum then subject to the Social Security tax) in 1973 would have $108, or 1 percent, deducted for health insurance. A person earning $40,000 would similarly have $108, or only .27 percent, deducted. The regressiveness of this tax (see note 36) had been raised in public debate, but the urgency with which it was raised increased with time as the increased cost of the program continued to be financed largely out of payroll taxes on a wage base that exempted much of the earnings of highly paid employees.

Changes to Medicaid

1. Perhaps the most significant change was the repeal of the two long-standing requirements of the law making it mandatory for the states to expand their Medicaid program from year to year while maintaining state effort and for these annual expansions to move toward a comprehensive Medicaid program with a 1977 deadline for complete coverage of all the medically needy. Thus was a form of universal medical care coverage conceived in 1965 and scheduled for 1977, canceled in 1972.

A number of lesser changes were also directed at cost containment. The procedural conformity of Medicaid to Medicare was strengthened, with many of the changes in Medicare also applying to Medicaid.

2. Notwithstanding the requirement of the previous paragraph, states were now *permitted* to develop their own methods of computing reasonable cost" Medicaid reimbursement rates for hospitals and maternal and child health programs even if these differed from those used by Medicare, provided these rates did not exceed the rates used under Medicare. It was hoped that this would result in substantially lower costs than those of Medicare. States were *required* to use cost-finding techniques approved by the secretary of HEW to establish "reasonable cost" reimbursement rates for skilled nursing facilities and intermediate-care facilities. The federal matching could be reduced by one-third for inappropriately long stays in all covered facilities as a penalty for states that failed to institute programs that effectively controlled utilization or to

conduct independent professional audits of patients.

3. Cost sharing and premium payments by Medicaid beneficiaries were cautiously introduced.

Cost sharing for the categorically needy (cash assistance recipients—the obligatory class) could be imposed but only for the optional service—that is, there could be no cost sharing for the seven mandatory types of service and such cost sharing was to be set at "nominal" amounts.

Beneficiary contributions to premium payments scaled to income level were made compulsory for categorically linked medically indigent persons (i.e., the "medically needy"). The imposition of cost sharing on noncategorical medically indigent persons (the federally unmatched class) was made optional and did not have to vary by income level.

4. Several changes provided higher matching percentages of federal support for state Medicaid administrative costs in order to develop better claims control systems and facility certification procedures.

5. Some provisions in the amendments dealt with making specified allied health personnel eligible for billing Medicaid directly.[30] Among these were optometrists, who were made eligible for Medicaid reimbursement under certain conditions, and chiropractors, who had also been made reimbursable under Part B of Medicare with the important difference that X-ray validation of the indication for chiropractic care interpreted by a physician was not required under Medicaid as it was under Medicare.

Recapitulation and Summary of the 1972 Amendments to the Medicaid/Medicare Legislation

1. Federal requirements for cost control were increased and the initiation or development of claims review, facility certification, and information-handling techniques was encouraged through various payment incentives.

2. There was a move toward unifying Medicare and Medicaid definitions and operations, mostly those involving review procedures. For reimbursing providers Medicaid was encouraged or required to use methods that paid less.

3. There was increased assignment of direct control responsibilities over Medicaid to the federal government.

4. The level of client cost sharing was increased, most notably by introducing it for the first time into Medicaid, but also by continuing to increase the rate of cost sharing in Medicare. The assumption was that the increased cost sharing, particularly in Medicaid, would reduce ''unnecessary'' utilization. To the extent that it reduced ''necessary'' utilization, it represented merely a reduction in benefits. The one exception to this trend was the removal of the home health care deductible in Part B of Medicare.

5. Some 1.7 million persons were expected to be shifted from Medicaid to Medicare as a result of the extension of Medicare eligibility to the APTD category below age sixty-five. This brought closer a situation in which complete dependence on Medicaid would be almost entirely for AFDC. For most SSI welfare clients Medicaid would serve primarily as a backup program for services not provided by Medicare.

6. There was a movement toward encouraging the HMO type of organization for health care delivery by making explicit provision for capitation payments by Medicare to such organizations. Provisions for Medicaid reimbursements to such organizations were already in Title XIX.[31]

7. A tentative and loosely structured start was made toward utilization and quality of care review of Medicare and Medicaid programs via the PSRO provisions.

8. The eligibility of certain types of health service providers for ''vending'' was extended and clarified separately with respect to Medicare and Medicaid. Under Medicare the insistence on licensed medical doctors was reduced only slightly, while under Medicaid wider latitude was introduced in making other providers like chiropractors eligible for direct payment from the state Medicaid program.

9. The financing of the increases in Medicare costs was largely through increases in withholding rates from wages and increasing the maximum taxable earnings.

10. The requirements for the states to work toward full coverage of their populations by Medicaid by a specified date were dropped.

In general, the emphasis on guaranteeing non-interference in the practice of medicine by the federal government implying minimal regulation and control that characterized the spirit of the original legislation was now clearly changed to its opposite, a call for increased regulation and control. These were most strongly applied to administration and cost-control procedures and more stringently to Medicaid than to Medicare; the introduction of quality-of-care and utilization review mechanisms was much more cautious and hesitating. The nation's de jure health policy had definitely abandoned the 1965 grand design that Medicaid would in some not-too-far-off future be the filler that would plug all the remaining gaps in our medical care system by providing access for all who needed medical care and had no means for paying for it.

CONTINUING NATIONAL DEBATE OVER GOVERNMENT-SPONSORED HEALTH INSURANCE

The passage of Medicare had removed one of the largest groups of ''uninsurables,'' the aged, from the exhibits demonstrating the failure of private health insurance to cover the entire population, and Medicaid was expected to remove the rest of the uninsurables—a large number almost immediately and the remainder within ten or twelve years. This done, it might have been expected that the national debate over federally sponsored health insurance would essentially end. It did not even subside. Two major long-standing, and in many ways conflicting, complaints about the inadequacy of the Medicare-Medicaid solution went on being made with the critical voices growing increasingly insistent and even raucous. These were the familiar criticisms that these programs were neither effective nor efficient: on the one hand too many persons were still left without reasonably adequate coverage; on the other hand, it was asserted, Medicare and Medicaid cost too much.

Of course, these two complaints are not necessarily incompatible. One could have argued that the health system as a whole was too costly precisely because of the absence of universal coverage and the efficiencies it would permit, but this argument was not to be strongly put forth by advocates of national health insurance until some fifteen years later. Although some advocates did indeed evince an interest in the cost-control question and argued that it could be more readily achieved under universal coverage (Trapnell Associates Study and see the Kennedy-Carter dispute on page 327, for example), those concerned primarily with effectiveness— the quality of care in Medicare and Medicaid and the persisting lack of access—generally called for improving the quality of the existing programs and enacting universal coverage as a matter of social equity, with whatever additional spending might be needed to achieve it. Most did not stress the cost-savings aspect, especially in the early post-1965 years.

By contrast, those concerned primarily with the costs of Medicare and Medicaid called for reduced spending, often paying scant attention to the issues of quality or access for lower-income persons. Of course it was true that full coverage would cost more than partial coverage, but the asserted increase in cost was usually presented by the "cost-containers" as being necessarily proportional to or greater than the increase in services entailed in universal coverage. They often slurred over two points implied in their caveat. The first was the arguable assumption that the economic inefficiencies in the existing system must necessarily remain in the process of extending access to all. The second was somewhat misleading in that the estimated increase in cost of *public* outlays for full national coverage was at times presented without presenting the estimated offsetting decreases in private expenditures. In any case, as we have seen, cost-containment forces handily won the day with the passage of the Social Security Amendments of 1972. The "increase-in-access" forces in Congress went along with this bill for the most part, the pressures for cost containment proving inexorable. Yet they continued and, if anything, intensified their battle after passage of "H.R. 1" for increased access through their sponsorship and support for bills that would establish a system of national health insurance (NHI) with universal access and comprehensive coverage of medical services in the United States.

Continued Inadequacy of Existing Coverage Despite Medicare/Medicaid

Looking at the evolving health care system that had emerged by 1970, we find that under existing *payment* subsystems (which reimbursed private providers almost exclusively), most people had medical care coverage of some sort. Workers injured on their jobs had workers' compensation; the aged had Medicare; the dependents of armed services personnel had CHAMPUS; and the "paupers" or categorically poor had Medicaid, as did some of the "able-bodied poor"—the categorically linked low-income persons in some states and the medically indigent noncategorically persons in very few states. In addition a number of direct-service governmental systems caught many persons who fell through the holes of the protective net of existing payment subsystems. Low-income persons in some places had access to one or more of the following: a local public hospital; a state mental hospital; a community or migrant health center; a community mental health center; a Veterans Administration, Public Health Service, or Armed Services hospital; free or low-cost services in voluntary hospitals or other facilities, or a local public health department clinic. But a sizable proportion of the population continued to remain outside all third-party coverage, whether by private insurance, government insurance, public assistance programs, or direct-service programs. Reasonably dependable data on this population are scarce for years as early as 1970, but a 1977 survey by the National Center for Health Services Research (NCHSR) found that 12.6 percent of the civilian noninstitutionalized population, or 26.6 million persons, had no third-party coverage of any kind, public or private. This figure is difficult to establish and requires special studies to obtain, for it seeks to identify persons who have *no* coverage under private health insurance, Medicare, Medicaid, CHAMPUS, Veterans Administration and armed services, workers' compensation or other sources. This is all quite aside from the question of *insufficient* coverage by any of these programs.[32] For many people who were eligible for some payment program, the coverage was so limited that resort to one of the direct-service systems was necessary to supplement the meager services paid for by their insurance or other type of third-party coverage.

Even for the majority who held private health insurance, the proportion of total medical expenses covered by insurance was, on average, rather small. This was because, first, persons who were counted as having private health insurance often had policies covering only some types of medical services but not others; and second, even for the types of services the policies did cover, the insurance paid only a part of the provider's charges. In 1970, for example, 154 million persons (76 percent of the civilian population) were covered by private health insurance for hospital care, and almost the same proportion had some insurance for in-hospital physician and X-ray and laboratory services (HEW, Vol. 41, No. 9). However, far fewer people were covered for other types of medical services. The further removed the usual site of a service was from the acute hospital inpatient environment, the skimpier the insurance coverage. Also, services delivered by personnel other than physicians were less well reimbursed (proportionately) than were physician services. Long-term services and those requiring more *care*, as opposed to intensive medical *treatment*, were more infrequently insured than those calling for short-term intensive medical treatment. Thus, 102 million persons, or 50 percent of the civilian population, had some kind of private health insurance coverage for physician office (and home) visits, but only 12.2. million, representing 6 percent of the civilian population, had some coverage for dental care. For nursing facility care the figures were 32 million and 16 percent, respectively. About 50 percent of the population had some private health insurance for prescribed drugs, private duty nursing, and visiting nurse service.[33] And because many persons had private health insurance that totally excluded coverage for many types of medical services while most covered services entailed cost-sharing features, the private insurance that people *did* have failed to cover a substantial part of their total personal health care expenses. In 1970, of the 42 billion dollars spent privately for personal health care by individuals, either directly out-of-pocket or through private insurance, only 37.5 percent, on average, was reimbursed by insurance. This low overall percentage was primarily

due to the very low percentages paid by out-of-hospital coverage but also to the lower percentages reimbursed for services given in the hospital by physicians and special-duty nurses compared with hospital service charges. Only 43 percent of the overall cost of physicians' services were covered, while a mere 4.1 percent of the cost of prescribed drugs (out-of-hospital) was met by insurance. For dental care it was 5.4 percent, and for all "other" services taken together (e.g., private-duty nursing, visiting nurse service, nursing home care, vision care, appliances), 4.9 percent of costs were covered, on average. Although the percentage of private consumer expenditures covered by private health insurance rose each year, it had reached only 44.7 percent by as late as 1979. (Until the present day, it has never exceeded 52 percent.)

Escalating Costs of Medical Care

We turn now to the second of the two major categories of post-1965 complaints—that Medicare and Medicaid fueled the fires of inflation with their profligate inefficiency. The proposed remedies of the "cost-containers" called for all manner of regulation of Medicare and Medicaid to control cost and utilization, such as those in the Social Security Amendments of 1972, as well as in further cost-containment measures being pushed by the Nixon and Ford administrations and advocates in Congress.[34] But the "access-increasers" in Congress were continuing to introduce various proposals for government-sponsored universal health insurance that focused on improving access over the same period, 1970–1975, during which the "cost-containers" were advancing proposals centered on controlling costs of existing programs. Consequently,[35] the cost-containment advocates also introduced their own NHI bills, to be held in reserve as less undesirable alternatives should one of the bills of the NHI advocates seem likely to pass. While all these ("reserve") alternative proposals would also have established universal access, none of them called for a *uniform basis of entitlement for all persons to a single, comprehensive system of medical care*. Also, they were strongly oriented to containing only government expenditures for health care, not necessarily all such expenditures.

The main features of many of these alternative proposals were the use of substantial cost sharing, an emphasis on catastrophic insurance that covered only expenses in excess of an expected "normal" annual amount, and a separate program for low-income persons. All these bills were introduced into Congress, but they were debated not on the floors of Congress but in the professional medical care and public health literature and in the public media, for they all remained bottled up in committees. There, much testimony was amassed at committee hearings for some of the bills and voluminous reports were issued by their staffs.

During this same period the federal administration was also pushing the health maintenance organization (HMO) as a preferred form of medical practice organization, mainly because of its purported economy of operation. In 1973 Congress passed a law providing federal assistance for HMO development. The federal government was also continuing to support the development of neighborhood health centers to help plug the gaps in access to service. The HMO Act of 1973 will be discussed later in this chapter and the neighborhood health centers in Chapter 11. I turn first to a consideration of the prototypical national health insurance bills that were introduced and widely discussed and the views of government's role in medical care that they represented.

The Post-1965 National Health Insurance Bills

Many "national health insurance" bills were introduced in each of the three biennial Congresses beginning with 1970, but none came to a floor vote. Prototypes of the main legislative proposals each represented a particular set of interests and provided significant insights into the attitudes toward national health insurance of its sponsors. The most forthright expressions of the self-interests of the sponsors appeared in the type of schema put forth in the health-industry and provider-sponsored bills. The American Medical Association, the American Hospital Association, and the health insurance industry each had bills in the hopper. More difficult to analyze are the proposals that more subtly and broadly

represented various societal values and philosophical views toward social welfare and other government policies. There were, during these years, comparatively few voices being raised flatly against national health insurance on the grounds that none was needed. As the bills died with the end of each Congress, they were reintroduced in the subsequent one. Some of the reintroduced versions were modifications of their predecessors, but in general the major outlines of the different types of ideas were retained. The following survey and analysis uses the specific versions introduced into the Ninety-third Congress (1972–1973) as particular examples, but either of the other two Congresses (1970–71 and 1974–75) would serve equally well.

The five bills presented here for analysis have been chosen because each clearly represents a particular view about how a universal, comprehensive national medical care system providing access in this country should be structured. Although they are intrinsically interesting from a purely historical standpoint, the main reason for this presentation is that the United States has still not solved its medical care access problem, even from the gross consideration of standard medical care being available to all, which *all* the main bills introduced in the early 1970s did. As we continue to grope toward a politically viable solution, the thinking and arguments behind previously presented proposals are useful to consider, for many of them were the distilled results of years of argument and amendment. They help clarify the implications of structuring a national system in one way rather that another and may thus increase our ability to make informed choices.

Salient Characteristics of Differing National Health Insurance Proposals

The six most important points on which the main bills differed among themselves were: (1) the basis for entitlement to service and the closely associated question of how access to medical care is viewed; (2) the sources of financing and the closely related question of how the "objectives" of a national health insurance system are viewed; (3) the types of services covered; (4) the basis and mechanism used for reimbursing providers; and (5) the use of mechanisms to directly and purposefully effect changes in the health delivery system over and above those produced incidental to operation of the system under the payment and entitlement structure.

Basis of Entitlement to Service This factor was perhaps the most fundamental one with respect to affecting the future direction of the United States health care system. The basis for entitlement illuminates the underlying philosophy of a national health insurance proposal perhaps more than any other characteristic, for it reveals how governmental assurance of access to medical care is regarded. The two main bases suggested for entitlement to service reflect two fundamentally different views on this question.

The first view holds that, in general, medical care should be regarded as just another commodity to be bought and sold in the marketplace. For these market consumers of medical care, the role of government is merely to protect the public safety by assuring the quality of the product and seeing to it that the consumer gets appropriate information for making informed choices. The role of government in *assuring* access to medical care should be to bestow it as a *privilege* on certain classes of people who cannot pay for care in the commercial markets, either through carrying private health insurance or by direct out-of-pocket payment. Society, through its governmental structure, decides which unfortunates are worthy of such beneficence and makes provision for it. The administration of such programs calls for establishment of means tests for determining eligibility for the nonmarket system. Government should also assure access to medical care for those who specially deserve it as an *earned right* or for whom it is deemed necessary to assure it because of special circumstances affecting the public interest.

The second view regards access to medical care either as a necessary part of societal equity or even as a *natural right*. It is a necessary part of social equity because it is a building block of social cohesion and community consciousness for the ''natural right'' advocates, it is in fact, part of the fundamental natural rights of all persons to life, liberty, and the pursuit of happiness. Government as the administrative arm of a so-ciety holding this view should provide equal access to a *single system* offering a comprehensive spectrum of medical services to all persons. Their eligibility is a *right* stemming from the simple fact of their humanity without further qualification, very much as the right to schooling and the right to police and fire protection are regarded.

By the 1970s the nation had already expanded its system of government support for access to medical care as a *privilege*, mainly for persons eligible for Medicaid. It had government-supported systems for persons who had *earned* the right to eligibility through special service to the nation and for the aged who had *earned* the right through contributions to the Social Security system during their working years. It also had government-supported systems for the mentally ill, for whom it was deemed necessary in the public interest. Now the question was whether the eligibility for government-supported medical care should be expanded to new classes of persons and if so, to whom and on what basis? The main question was whether all persons should be eligible on the same basis, i.e., on the basis either of community solidarity or natural right or whether there should be two classes of beneficiaries. One class would be eligible on the basis of ''paid-in right'' or insurance (e.g., payroll deductions) while the second class would be eligible on the basis of ''bestowed privilege,'' that is, worthy of public assistance by passing a means test. If universal coverage is established under the second two-tier version, the members of the means-tested group are more apt to be viewed as ''welfare'' recipients than insured. It is extremely unlikely that their benefits will be as good as the ''truly'' insured class unless a single set of covered services and a single schedule of provider payments are meticulously observed.

Although it was clear that politically powerful forces were continuing to oppose any further extension of government responsibility to additional groups of persons, as witness the failure of any of the insurance bills even to come close to passing, the actual NHI proposals all represented some form of extension, even those sponsored by groups who had opposed extension, like the AMA, the AHA and the Health Insurance Association of America (HIAA). Their proposals were clearly "reserve" bills to be pushed only if one of the less desirable bills came close to a vote. Most of the bills provided for enlarging the population covered by an expanded form of Medicaid. Only a few provided for covering everybody on a "natural right" basis rather than on a "bestowed privilege" basis.

Sources of Financing These include: (1) direct appropriations from the general fund; (2) payroll deduction contributions by employers, workers, and self-employed persons to earmarked government trust funds; (3) premium and cost sharing by beneficiaries; (4) indirect contributions by federal and state governments through tax exemptions for health care expenditures; and (5) mandating employer coverage of employees through private health insurance with means test coverage for the non-employed.

The influence of the financing method chosen upon the health system, while not as great as that of the eligibility basis, is considerable. In any case, the two issues are related.

It should be noted that establishing eligibility as a universal right to service in a single system does not mean that it cannot be *financed* from multiple sources, so long as access to the single system is without regard to the beneficiary's role in paying for its operation. In fact, a mixed financing system that comes partly from payroll deductions, partly from the general fund (with varying degrees of cost sharing) is a common mode of financing national health insurance systems with universal entitlement in many parts of the world. It was the financing system proposed by those national health insurance bills in the United States that called for universal entitlement as a natural right.

If the main source of income for the health insurance system is the general fund, the financing is at least theoretically progressive[36] because the most important revenue source of the general fund is the progressive federal income tax. But it should be noted that while the income tax is theoretically a progressive tax, in practice so many special tax exemptions have been enacted (so-called loopholes) that the degree to which the income tax is actually progressive has been debated.[37] A potential disadvantage of general-fund financing is that the resources available for health insurance are then subject to periodic appropriations by Congress in competition with other budget items. This can be a particularly serious threat in times of increased pressures for tax reductions.

To the degree that the insurance is financed by payroll deduction the financing is likely to be regressive if it follows the pattern of the Social Security, OASDI, and Medicare (Part A) financing of the past (see point 7, p. 301). These payroll taxes have consisted of a flat percentage on all earnings up to a certain maximum amount, with no further tax on earnings over this maximum. Both the flat percentage (a proportional tax) and the absence of tax on earnings over the maximum fail to impose a proportionately heavier tax responsibility on persons with higher earnings (which makes the entire tax a regressive tax).

An advantage of payroll deductions is that they generally go into a sequestered ("earmarked") trust fund and must be used only for health insurance. But if this fund is available only for benefits for those who have paid in, then universal coverage cannot be achieved without additional provision for nonearners. This often leads to a nonuniform medical care system that is not available on an equal basis to all persons.

There are pros and cons, therefore, for each of these forms of financing, which undoubtedly explains the prevalence of using a mixture of the two by well-developed universal access systems. The mixture seeks to combine the greater inviolability of the funds under earmarked payroll deductions with the greater progressivity of the general fund financing and the greater ease with which nonworking persons can be covered by the latter. The essential point in financing a national health insurance system from mixed funding sources is, again, whether eligibility is the same for all persons (i.e., based on "natural right") and is not related to the sources of financing. If some persons are eligible on a "paid-in-right" basis and others are eligible on a "bestowed privilege" basis, then a central question is whether the two funds are comingled into one common account for paying medical care expenses or whether the earmarked fund pays for the "paid-in" eligibles while the general fund pays for the "bestowed privilege" group. Congress and federal administrations are much more likely to reduce appropriations for a health insurance program if it can appropriate separately for the expenditures of lower-income persons. All this further highlights the centrality of the "basis of entitlement" issue.

The third possible source of financing is direct beneficiary cost participation through premiums and cost sharing. Its use has been advocated on quite other grounds than those used to promote payroll deductions or general-fund participation. While opponents of this form of financing have decried it as a covert way of decreasing the real value of the insurance premium and passing a disproportionate cost of the insurance program on to those persons who happen to get sick, its proponents defend this practice with arguments ascribing to it powers to improve system efficiency.

Advocates of cost sharing generally recommend it as a good mechanism for discouraging "unnecessary" utilization. "Unnecessary", translated into commercial insurance language, means an insured "loss" that would not have occurred if the claimant had had no insurance. Applied to health insurance this implies that any medical care or advice received by the insured that would not have been contracted for if it were not covered by insurance is "unnecessary" and comes under the category of what the insurance industry calls "moral hazard." (See Chapter 9, p. 275f.) Cost sharing will reduce moral hazard. The strongest advocates of the view that health insurance is or should be just another form of commercial insurance support so-called catastrophic coverage only, arguing that normal annual expenditures for health care should be budgeted for by individuals as part of the ordinary cost of living. They assert that it is unnecessarily expensive to require claims processing for regular, expected visits to the pediatrician and family physician (and perhaps also to the obstetrician for management of a pregnancy). Furthermore, exotic elective care should not be paid for by the premiums of other policyholders but by the person desiring it, a view illustrated by the exclusion of elective cosmetic surgery by nearly all insurance.

The sticking point lies in defining what utilization is truly elective in the sense of being medically useless or even more vaguely, "unnecessary." Is seeing a physician about a suspicious symptom that turns out to be "nothing" as un-

necessary visit? The fact that part of the purpose of making medical care insurance available to populations was often meant to *encourage* early or more frequent use of medical consultation makes this type of coverage unique among insurance items. By contrast, fire insurance is never meant to encourage the occurrence of fires. Health insurance is the only commercially insured peril that is meant to *encourage* the occurrence of (appropriate) "losses," like doctor's office visits. To the extent that cost sharing discourages early or sufficiently frequent medical consultation, it vitiates one of the unique purposes of health insurance. It is particularly difficult to conceive of certain prevalent forms of cost sharing, such as out-of-pocket contributions by the patient to the hospital bill, as having the effect of discouraging "unnecessary" admissions, particularly in clearly defined serious cases. In this instance, the coinsurance is more clearly seen as a form of diluting the risk-sharing feature of "pure insurance" since the person who suffers an illness pays an amount that the one who is not ill does not. Where cost sharing has been shown to affect utilization it generally reduced patient-generated utilization such as hospitalizations and laboratory tests. If the aim of enacting a national health insurance system is to introduce universal access to a single system of comprehensive health services, then cost sharing could be a perverse factor acting to perpetuate a two-tiered access system. Persons for whom the cost sharing is an affordable or even an inconsequential outlay would have different access that those for whom it was important enough to constitute a barrier, unless cost-sharing rates were tied to income—but then the means test is being introduced. It is also worth noting briefly at this point that by 1970 it had been quite clearly demonstrated that reduction in hospital use by group practice HMOs was effective in substantially reducing total cost while savings from cost sharing were as yet not well documented.[38]

Premium sharing[39] (in lieu of, *not* in addition to cost sharing) distinctly and openly reveals the percentage of the program's costs that is borne by its beneficiaries. It differs from cost sharing in that the degree of beneficiary participation in program cost is no heavier for persons who suffer illness. If the proportion of premium sharing is related to the beneficiary's income, it can constitute either a progressive or a regressive tax. Under a universal insurance system, premium sharing would have the effect of lowering the amount needed from other sources such as payroll taxes and general fund. The decision to use premium sharing would then depend on the political landscape of the moment.

Health insurance premiums may be financed indirectly by federal and state governments allowing them as tax deductions for businesses, individuals, or both. The fact that health insurance premiums have been allowed as business expense deductions from taxable income has had a marked effect on the growth of private health insurance. Both employers and unions, especially unions, have been more enthusiastic about private health insurance benefits than they otherwise would have been because an extra dollar paid the employee in wages is taxable to the employee, whereas a dollar paid through insurance premiums is not. Thus, both the employer and the employee derive advantage from the fact that the total value of the worker's benefits are worth more to him or her than the same amount in cash would be. This hidden government subsidy for private health insurance has often gone unrecognized in public discussions on the organization of our medical care system.

Finally, financing can come from mandating that employers provide insurance for their employees. For universal coverage this would require some provisions, perhaps from the general fund, for insuring noninsured persons. Mandated insurance will be discussed later when specific health insurance proposals are described.

Types of Services Covered or Benefit Structure I have noted that while all the main proposals would have established universal eligibility for health care, not all of them would made eligibility for all persons depend, either implicitly or explicitly, on the basis of natural right. Not all beneficiaries, therefore, would have had access to a single standard of service; some proposals would have created two tiers, separate and unequal.

It is all well and good to have everybody pronounced legally eligible for services under a national system, but if these services are few or exclude important types of service, the term "el-

igibility" must be understood as a limited right even if universal. All the national health insurance proposals covered most of the expenses for the more commonly used hospital inpatient acute services and some types of physician services. For these services the differences among proposals lay largely in the degree of cost sharing required. Where the form of cost sharing included coinsurance after a specified deductible, the coinsurance rate was almost never higher than 20 percent (with an infrequent requirement of 25 percent) of the bill.[40] Perhaps a more serious area of noncoverage was that of excluded services, types of medical services that were not covered at all. Some were covered very scantily, so sparsely that the insurance would pay no more than half of their usual cost. All the NHI bills excluded certain very important services. The types of services that were most likely not to be covered or covered only sparsely by most proposals were mental health care, prescribed drugs, appliances such as prosthetic devices, corrective vision care, and dental care. These constituted an important share of the medical care dollar[41], and omitting them from coverage was yet another way of making the premium cost of a plan appear smaller than it really was when considered in the light of how much of a person's total health expenditures was paid by the insurance. Furthermore, covering certain services, such as inpatient care, very fully and other services, such as ambulatory care, less fully can and historically did result in tilting the utilization pattern toward the better-insured services even when they were not medically preferable. One of the main complaints about private health insurance, as well as Medicare and Medicaid, had consistently been that their pattern of benefits drove the medical care system toward undue use of high-level technology and hospital care and away from preventive, health maintenance, and ambulatory primary care in general. For example, as late as 1990, Medicare Part B still excluded from coverage many services that the aged needed to help them stay ambulatory and well such as podiatry ("routine foot care"), examinations for fitting eyeglasses or hearing aids, immunizations, and preventive ("routine" physical) examinations.[42] And coverage of one of the most important areas of care for which access had always been very poor—long-term care, both in nursing homes and in patients' homes—was especially skimpy or entirely lacking in all the proposals. This omission was a particularly serious one for the elderly.

Basis for Paying the Provider The economic incentives built into the methods of provider payment used by a national health insurance system will affect the cost of the program and also encourage certain types of medical practices over others. They it will also influence the distribution and availability of health care resources by social class and geographic location of beneficiaries as well as the mix of medical specialties of physicians and its geographic distribution.

Broadly considered, there are two general categories of payment basis: fee-for-service and the lump sum, although there are many specific arrangements under each of these two broad types and they differ among themselves in the details sometimes in important ways. The fee-for-service methods, as the name indicates, pay a fee to the provider for each unit of service rendered each beneficiary. The lump-sum methods pay a fixed amount to a provider to care for a beneficiary or a designated population during a fixed time period regardless of units of service required. Obviously, speaking only from the perspective of "economic man", that is, of optimizing the provider's income, the fee-for-service payment basis may be expected to motivate the provider to offer as many services as possible and to lean toward prescribing the better-reimbursed procedures. It would, then, be expected to drive the system toward overutilization in general, and overuse of more highly reimbursed care in particular. If, as is often the case, the better-reimbursed procedures coincide with the use of expensive, high-technology equipment and other resources, then the fee-for-service method should also be expected to increase the average unit price of medical care. The lump-sum basis, on the other hand, may be expected to motivate the provider to render as few services as possible because it will not lower his or her income, and to shy away from prescribing treatment and diagnostic procedures that use expensive high-technology equipment and other resources because the cost of providing them will lower his net income. The physician provider may use the extra time left free by underservicing his or her existing "lump-sum" paid-

for patients in leisure-time activities or to acquire more patients for whom additional lump sums may be paid, depending on the details of the payment arrangements and the preferences of the physician. In any case, we would expect that this form of payment basis to drive the system to provide too few services per subscriber, that is, to move toward underutilization.

Table 10–3 presents schematically some of the main bases for paying providers that were in current use during this period of profusion of NHI bills in Congress. Among the payment methods that offer economic incentives for overutilization (Glaser, 1968, 1970) are paying hospitals on a fixed per diem basis (1, 2, 3 in Table 10–3) with the daily rate calculated on retroactive costs or on average charges. The same may be said about paying hospitals separately for each service (4), and less so for paying per discharge (5). Studies had shown a strong tendency toward higher utilization of hospital services under these payment arrangements when compared with systems that pay hospitals on a prospective *budget* basis (9) and physicians on a salary or capitation basis (10, 11, 12, 13).

Paying hospitals on a prospectively determined per diem *rate* (3) basis is a compromise between retroactive cost-based reimbursement (4) and the prospective lump-sum or global budgeting system of reimbursement (9). Experience with the compromise mechanism had shown some encouraging results. Yet while a prospectively determined daily rate at least avoids motivating the hospital to increase its costs to raise the daily reimbursement rate as it would if based on a retroactive cost calculation, it still retains the incentive for increasing utilization by admitting persons unnecessarily or by keeping them longer than medically necessary. Payment of a prospectively determined global budget, on the other hand, removes the incentive to increase either the unit cost of operation or the utilization.[43]

Similarly, paying physicians on a fee-for-service basis may be expected to motivate overservicing with too many procedures and visits. And if the schedule of fees paid is based on a usual, customary, and reasonable (UCR) criterion,[44] then prices may be caused to increase by decisions that are, at least implicitly, made collusively by and among physicians. Charging

Table 10–3. Some Bases for Paying Providers Used by Third-party Payers

Fee-for-services Bases

Per diem:

Hospitals

1. Arbitrary rate — Third party pays patient a set rate specified in insurance contracts. Patient pays the total hospital bill.
2. Rate based on retroactive costs calculation — Third party pays hospital its per diem costs computed retroactively for the current year at end of year.
3. Prospectively set rate — Third party pays hospital a per diem rate set at the start of the year. Methods 1, 2, and 3 are sometimes called "all-inclusive" per diem rates.

Per specified service item:

4. Hospital's charges — Third party pays for each billed item up to an amount designated by the third party's price list. Patient pays the rest. (Note: Payment basis 4 is often combined with one of methods 1, 2, or 3. In that case a per diem rate is paid for "routine services," including room and board and "routine" nursing, and per-service charges are paid for "ancillary services," such as X-rays, laboratory tests, pharmaceuticals, and the like. This combination of per diem payment for routine care and per-service payment for ancillary services is in contrast to the "all-inclusive per diem rate," a method of payment that pays a total single daily fee which, on average, covers the total costs of a patient's care.)

   Some insurers like Blue Cross and Medicare were paying hospitals the *cost* of the items billed to each subscriber rather than the amounts charged, but the costs were retroactively calculated.

Per case:

5. Discharge (after 1982 payment per type of discharge was used by Medicare) — Third party pays a preset fee per discharge. (After 1982 Medicare paid a differential fee depending on the discharge diagnosis (DRG) of the patient.) Note: These methods of payment are still fee-for-service, but they approach a lump-sum type of basis because they do not itemize charges for services.

Per price schedule:

Physicians

6. Relative value scale — Third party pays for billed services up to an amount listed in the third party's fee schedule. These amounts are most often based on an explicit or implicit form of weighting each service by its relative value as an appropriate charge. The basic dollar amount to be assigned to the item with relative value "1" is up to the physician. Many third parties set limits on the maximum level they will pay.

7. Usual, customary, and reasonable (UCR) — Third party pays the physician's bill if it meets the UCR criteria. "Usual" means it is the fee the physician charges all his or her patients, "customary" means it is within the range of what other physicians of similar training and in similar locations charge, and reasonable means the fee is both usual and customary.

8. Accepting assignment — Whatever the basis for computing the fees paid by the third party to the physician (e.g., 6 or 7 or a combination of the two) some third parties require that the physician accept the scheduled fee as payment in full for the service rendered. This means that he or she does not demand any additional payment from the patient. Accepting the third-party fee as payment in full is called "accepting assignment" on the part of the provider. Many third-party payers, especially private insurers, do not require that physicians eligible to receive insurance payment ("participating physicians") accept assignment. It has been an important issue in government-sponsored insurance in Canada and in Medicare in the U.S.

Lump Sum Bases

Hospitals

9. Prospective budget — Hospital is paid an annual total amount in appropriate installments to meet the operating costs of providing care for a target population. The amount is based on an approved operating budget for the hospital.

Salary:

Physicians

10. Pure salary
11. Base salary (plus variable amount) — Physicians are paid a base salary and share in the surplus of the organization if there is one. Kaiser Permanente uses a variant of this method.

312

Table 10–3 (continued)

Capitation:	*Physicians*
12. Pure capitation	The physician is paid a fixed periodic sum for each subscriber he or she agrees to provide care for. The agreement specifies the types of services to be provided but does not depend on how often these are provided.
13. Modified capitation	The physician is paid a basic capitation rate for each subscriber on his or her "list" and is reimbursed additionally for patients who are targeted by the insurance sponsor for special attention (e.g., the elderly) and for services that are specially targeted, such as preventive or health promotion. The main system using capitation is the British National Health Service.

prices higher than the insurance allows will result in the overage being disallowed as an insurance reimbursement in the current year but will cause norms based on prevailing charges to go up for the following year. However, while paying physicians by salary and hospitals a prospectively budgeted amount to service a specified population can be expected to provide strong incentives to reduce costs, it may also be expected to provide incentives to reduce services below a desirable level.

Thus, whatever method of payment is chosen, the economic motivation of the payment system will be either to overserve or underserve. If a national health insurance system is to meet standards of effectiveness (quality) and efficiency (low costs), no methods of paying providers will motivate them to be suitably concerned with both these criteria based on economic motivation alone. Regulation to institute proper monitoring of results will be required to verify publicly that appropriate services are provided for the payments made. Once a choice of methods for paying providers has been made, the main focus of the monitoring system needs to be in the proper direction for controlling the type of abuse to be expected from the use of these methods. The emphasis should be on monitoring overuse if the main incentives of the payment system are to overservice and on monitoring underuse if the main incentives are to underservice.

As the first of three examples demonstrating empirically the reality of this caveat, we recall that the 1972 Amendments to the Social Security Act included a provision for the establishment of professional standards review organizations (PSROs) to monitor the utilization rates and quality of service being received by Medicare and Medicaid beneficiaries, in hospitals and nursing homes. The thrust of these monitoring

organizations made up of local physicians, was the avoidance of unnecessary utilization, since the provider payment system being used by Medicare and Medicaid consisted overwhelmingly of fee-for-service payments to physicians and retrospective cost reimbursement to hospitals. Because these methods are prone to generate overservicing, the PSROs rarely concerned themselves with additional services that should have been provided but were not. On the other hand, the California Medicaid program (MediCal) had been using special HMOs to provide care for some groups of MediCal beneficiaries. These so-called prepaid health plans (PHPs) were required to operate at lower cost to the state than would be entailed in using the open market. There were widespread publicly voiced complaints that these PHPs seriously underserved their enrollees. Stringent corrective action was taken by the state to remedy the situation. The regulatory correction was met by the Waxman-Duffy Act, which focused on monitoring underservicing. As a last example, the Medicare program after 1982 began to pay hospitals a fixed fee per stay for specified diagnoses (DRGs). This system of payment clearly motivated hospitals toward influencing improperly short stays. Yet the monitoring by the PROs (as the successors to PSROs were called) of the appropriateness of care continued to focus on detecting inappropriately long stays, an improperly designed monitoring direction for this payment method.

On a different note, it should be noted that paying physicians fee-for-service on the basis of usual, customary, and reasonable (UCR) charges could be expected to skew the mix of medical specialties and the geographic distribution of primary physicians in undesirable ways. Subspecialists practicing in high-income areas would be paid the highest rates (as they indeed were under Medicare), further inducing a shortage of primary physicians generally as well as an overall dearth of physicians in low-income areas. HMOs would be particularly handicapped in their efforts to recruit physicians, both because of the high prices demanded by subspecialists and the shortage of primary physicians that would be encouraged by this system of payment. Again, experience corroborating both expected results had been provided under existing Medicare and Medicaid payment methods.

A final feature of the provider reimbursement system for physicians that could be expected to offer yet another obstacle to achieving universal access to comprehensive services is the question of whether the physician should be permitted to overbill—to charge the patient for an amount in addition to what the national health insurance system pays. If this excess patient payment were permitted, the achievement of a single-track system would be to some degree impaired. Persons with more money could see more expensive physicians, and it is likely that the physicians who accepted the government fee as payment in full would become the poor persons' physicians. They might even be motivated to see too many patients per hour to equalize their incomes with those of the physicians charging the higher rates. Again, this phenomenon was observed in the Medicare program, in which only about one-third of all physicians "accepted assignment," that is, agreed to accept the insurance reimbursement as payment in full. Some government health insurance systems have attempted to meet this problem by legislating that for physicians to be eligible for any insurance reimbursement ("participating" physicians) they had to accept the established health insurance fee in full payment—i.e., they had to "accept assignment." It was also observed that in the Medicaid program, which paid below market rates, physicians were setting up "Medicaid mills" to see perfunctorily a great many patients per hour.

Use of the Insurance Mechanism to Directly Affect the Health Delivery System Some National Health Insurance proposals incorporated explicit features to directly and purposefully steer the system toward certain modes of practice organization. Perhaps the main example was the spe-

cial benefits offered to persons joining HMOs and the priority claim on the annual health care budget given to HMOs under the most comprehensive of these proposals. Other proposals favored the open market fee-for-service system and still others favored systems of health care with hospitals as the core of the system. This type of explicit favoring of specific organizational modes was written into proposals when their sponsors thought that these ways of organizing medical practice were conducive either to furthering their own views of what would promote universal access and lower costs or would protect their own business or professional stakes in the medical care system.

In summary, the main issue advanced by the leading and enduring advocates of national health insurance was establishing universal access to a single, good quality system of care, and the entitlement provisions of any proposal therefore constituted the primary criterion from this point of view. However, financing sources, benefit structure, basis for paying the provider, and favoring particular practice modes could all affect the access. It is conceivable that a system that declared universal access to a single standard of care as its enunciated policy could establish and maintain this goal in the face of financing and other arrangements that in our analysis here contained economic and political incentives for a two-track system. Some European countries like (the former) West Germany and Denmark have done this. But the national ethos and the regulatory mechanisms need to be strong enough to counterbalance a system's economic pull toward qualitative stratification of services and maintain a single system.

Illustrative Health Insurance Bills Introduced into Congress 1972–74

As an empirical demonstration of how the preceding five criteria can serve to structure an evaluation of government health insurance proposals, this section briefly[45] analyzes a selected number of the proposals introduced into Congress during the years 1972 through 1974. These spanned the two years of the ninety-third Congress and the first year of the ninety-fourth. These analyses illustrate how they reflected different health care policy positions, including but not confined to how they stood on the five salient characteristics discussed above. In addition, the main outside organizational sponsor or interest group favoring the bill is given. Although none of these bills passed, they were widely discussed and debated in health policy circles. Many of the views they represent are deeply imbedded as practice in various sections of the health system and in the writings of scholars, commentators, and advocates to the present day. They continued to reappear in subsequent national health insurance plans and the debates that swirled around them.

Medicredit: The AMA Proposal Introduced in the House by Representatives Richard Fulton and Joel T. Broyhill (H.R. 2222) and in the Senate by Senator Vance Hartke under the name "Health Care Insurance Act of 1973" (S. 444), it provided, on a *voluntary*[46] participation basis, for personal income tax credits to offset the premium costs of privately marketed "qualified" health insurance policies. A "qualified" policy had to provide specified minimum benefits, and employers could take the full cost of their share of the premium as a business expense deduction only if the policy was qualified. Private insurance carriers would issue the policies and state insurance departments would certify carriers and qualified policies according to standards set by a federal board. The individual personal income tax credits were to be graduated from 100 percent of the premium costs for low-income persons down to 10 percent for high-income persons for "basic" benefits, and it would be 100 percent for "catastrophic" benefits. Medicare was to continue, but most of Medicaid would be replaced by a system of federal vouchers for buying qualified health insurance issued to persons with insufficient taxable income to enable them to use the income tax credits provided by the bill. Medicaid was to continue only as a residual program to pay for cost sharing in the benefit structure of policies bought by persons using vouchers. All U.S. residents were to be eligible, and physicians would be paid "usual and customary charges." Insurance premiums were to be paid from general tax revenues, deductions from workers' payrolls and by employers, contributions, with the workers' and employers' shares allowed as deductions from

income tax as provided by law—employers in full and employees on an income-graduated basis.

A great many cost-sharing features were called for, which were similar to those later used in Medicare, but the annual total cost sharing per family was capped by a specified maximum in any one year. The services covered were quite comprehensive and included dental care for children and home health services but excluded corrective eye care and prescribed drugs and devices, resulting in a large part of an individual's medical care expenditures remaining uncovered.

All persons were to be guaranteed financial access to health care by the federal government without directly affecting the existing delivery system in any way. Physicians and hospitals would be paid as before, and the physician was to remain the unquestioned arbiter of what kind and how much service the federal government would be billed for, so long as it lay within the broad range of services covered by the bill. The physician's fees were to continue to be determined largely by the profession and the onus of utilization control would be placed on the consumer by the extensive cost sharing.

Although this bill seemed to offer equal entitlement to care to all persons, the high cost sharing and the dual nature of the financing— one mechanism for those whose income tax was at least as large as the premium and another for all others—had the potential of reducing access for the working poor as well as the nonworking population. Also, future conflict between those on the lowest rungs of the economic ladder and those immediately above was very likely. The working poor would feel the pinch of the cost sharing and their contributions toward the premiums, while the poorest persons would have all these paid by the residual Medicaid program. This was inviting feelings akin to the longstanding doctrine of "lesser eligibility" on the part of the working poor, who might then demand that their benefits be equal to or greater than those offered to nonworking people.

These factors were likely to have led to congressional pressure to differentiate benefit structures, for the cost to the general fund was publicly evident only in paying for the vouchers of the poor, and the appropriation for this purpose would be under constant attack. On the other hand, the reduction in federal general tax revenue through the deduction of insurance premiums from taxable income by employers and from taxes for individuals was a hidden opportunity-cost type of contribution from the general fund and would not appear as an expenditure line in any social welfare program appropriation.[47]

The total lack of quality or utilization controls and the method of payment to providers were a continued invitation to rising costs through price increases, excessive utilization increases, excessive introduction and use of costly technology, or all three. With nearly all payments to physicians being "usual and customary charges," many providers might have been tempted to push charges up as quickly as possible.

In the political climate prevailing in federal government circles vis-à-vis cost control in 1973, it is unlikely that the sponsors of this bill seriously believed that it could pass. The bill included a clause that explicitly prohibited federal supervision and control of the practice of medicine, the manner in which services were provided, the selection or compensation of providers of services, or the operations of providers of services (Waldman, 1973). Such language was appropriate for the 1965 political climate but not for that of the 1970s, when the health laws that Congress passed, such as the Social Security Amendments of 1972 and the Health Maintenance Organization Act of 1973, were calling for control and monitoring rather than promising "noninterference." One is justified in assuming that this was an example of the retreat-to-a-second-line-of-defense ("reserve bill") tactic in the strategy of defeating an undesirable proposal such as the Health Security Act, to be discussed next. If that undesirable bill had advanced toward passage in Congress, then demands for hearings, votes on amendments, and other maneuvers around the Medicredit bill would have been available as a delaying tactic. If all these did not work, a third line of defense would have been to urge "reasonable" compromises between the two (Medicredit and whatever undesirable one was threatening) bills.

In brief, the Medicredit proposal called for a blank check for physicians to charge whatever they pleased and have it paid for directly or indirectly by the U.S. treasury, and yet it required extensive cost sharing. Except for the uninsured

who would have been insured (largely at public expense), the principal beneficiaries would have been physicians.

The Health Security Act: The Griffiths-Kennedy Bill Supported by Organized Labor Almost diametrically opposed to the AMA's Medicredit proposal in its stand on each of the five salient characteristics was the Health Security Act. This bill and its sponsors were the direct ideological descendants of a series of comprehensive-coverage bills introduced into successive Congresses beginning with the Murray-Wagner-Dingell bill of 1942,[48] and of a long line of advocates and campaigners for a national medical care system with universal access to a comprehensive set of services. This historical lineage included the campaigners for health insurance during the Progressive era, the liberal faction of the Committee on Costs of Medical Care, and some of the framers of the Social Security Act and subsequent social legislation. Many of its leading advocates were organized in a national coalition led by the "Committee of 100" consisting of labor (especially the unions in the mass-production industries that formed the original CIO), academics, and a wide range of social reformers and left-of-center activist organizations.

Introduced into the Ninety-third Congress by Representative Martha Griffiths (H.R. 22) and Senator Edward Kennedy (S. 3), the features that perhaps contrasted most with the Medicredit proposal were its cost-control features, its virtually total lack of cost sharing, its avowed purpose of changing the configuration of the health care delivery system, and its provision for expanding the supply of medical care to match the expanding demand for service. The proposed systemic changes called for greater governmental fiscal controls, encouragement of the HMO form of practice, increased consumer voice in operations and policy, and greater local area control over operations within regional and federal guideline constraints. All U.S. residents were to be eligible, coverage was to be *compulsory*, and benefits were to be very broad, including dentistry for children, appliances, corrective eye care, and even prescription drugs under certain conditions. Medicare would be abolished and Medicaid would remain available for those who could not afford needed services not covered by the health insurance. Financing was to be 50 percent from the federal general fund and 50 percent from a combination of taxes on employers' payrolls, employee wages, and self-employed persons' earnings.

The program was to be administered by HEW via a special national control board and HEW regional and local health service area offices. The national control board, as well as the regional and local offices, would have advisory councils to oversee their administration and hold hearings on grievances. An annual *global national budget* would be established following a specified formula and funds were to be allocated to each region on a per capita basis. The regions would allocate amounts from their regional allotment to local health service areas, also on a per capita basis. The calculation of the per capita amount for each region would be modified in the time-honored tradition of adjusting for differences in relevant conditions.

Providers were to be paid in various ways. Independently practicing physicians, dentists, and other professionals could be paid by fee-for-service, capitation, or salary. The total amount of money available for payment to each of these provider types would be fixed in advance each year, and if the fee-for-service claims threatened to exceed the funds allocated for this category of payment, independent providers' fees would be proportionately reduced. Hospitals would in general be paid by *prospective budgeting*, as would skilled nursing homes and home health agencies. HMOs, whether prepaid group practices (PGPs), physician foundations (medical care foundations or MCFs), or independent practice associations of physicians (IPAs), would receive periodic per capita amounts for ambulatory services. If they used inpatient facilities not owned by them to hospitalize their patients, they would receive reimbursement on a patient-day basis for the inpatient physician services they supplied; if they owned the facility, they could opt to have hospitalization costs included in their per capita payment per enrollee or be paid like free-standing hospitals—by prospective budgeting for operating the facility. Financial aid to help establish new HMOs or expand existing ones was provided.[49]

Money was provided for national planning and increasing medical resource supply for two years before the insurance program began. A percentage of the total income of the program (to reach 5 percent ultimately) was to be allocated to a health resources development fund. Included in such activities would be funds for training of various types of health personnel.

Some special restrictions on providers are worth noting. To quality as a provider of services, an individual or organization would be forbidden to practice racial or ethnic discrimination or to levy any additional charges over the insurance reimbursement on patients for covered services (i.e., overbill), and would be required to supply needed information and records. Hospitals could not refuse staff privileges to any qualified physician; skilled nursing facilities had to be affiliated with a hospital that would be responsible for their medical activities; and major surgery could be performed only by qualified specialists.

The progenitors of the Griffiths-Kennedy bill were clearly the Wagner-Murray-Dingell bills. The nature of its provisions bespeak such attitudes as the following: medical care is a public service to which all are equally entitled regardless of financial contribution or any attributes of person (i.e., it is a natural right); it therefore follows that the federal government's responsibility is to intervene actively in providing access to such services for all persons; the health care system should be changed to eliminate undue costliness and improve guarantees of quality. The wording of the bill made clear its approval of, perhaps even preference for, national planning and regulation to achieve its ends; it viewed consumers and the government as the primary voices in deciding how health services shall be delivered; and it implied that fee-for-service payment of reasonable charges to private physicians and reasonable costs to hospitals are not the only nor even the best ways of paying providers. On sources of financing, the attitudes expressed are less clear, since half the financing was to be from general funds and half from earmarked wage deductions at a time when it was evident that the wage deductions for Social Security were more regressive in distributing the tax burden than the income-tax-based general fund. As noted, in this respect this bill followed the pattern adopted by many European capitalist countries by seeking a compromise between the greater protection of the earmarked funds collected from wage deductions and the greater tax progressivity of using general fund financing.

The Comprehensive Health Insurance Act of 1974: The Nixon Administration Proposal Introduced into Congress on February 6, 1974, by Representatives Wilbur Mills and Herman T. Schneebeli (H.R. 12684) and into the Senate by Senator Robert Packwood (S. 2970), the Comprehensive Health Insurance Act of 1974 consisted of three parts: (a) the Employee Health Insurance Plan (E-HIP) mandating employers to *offer* specified minimally adequate private health insurance to their employees;[50] (b) the Assisted Health Insurance Plan (A-HIP) for low-income groups and high medical risks; and (c) the Federal Health Insurance (FHI) program for the aged, an expanded version of Medicare. Parts a and b of the program were to be run by the states, which would supervise both the employee and the assisted plans by regulating carriers and providers under federal guidelines. All membership was *voluntary on the part of the insured.*

The Employee Health Insurance Plan called for financing private health insurance through employer (75 percent) and employees (25 percent) premium contributions with temporary federal subsidies for some firms. Benefits included the fairly common ones such as hospital, skilled nursing facilities, physicians' services, and home health care. In addition, certain specified diagnostic services, prescription drugs, preventive care, and special services for children were included. Cost sharing was heavy, comprising an annual deductible of $150 per person up to $450 per family, a $50 additional deductible per person for prescription drugs, and a separate deductible for blood. There was also 25 percent coinsurance on the amounts that were covered, but total annual cost sharing was capped at $1,050 per person and $1,500 per family per year.[51] Cost sharing was not specifically earmarked for inpatient care or ambulatory care.

The Assisted Health Insurance Plan provided for federal and state general revenues sharing the financing of the premium costs of private insurance policies for low-income or high-risk persons. The benefits would be the same as under E-HIP, but cost sharing and premium charges to the insured would vary according to income. Persons would have to enroll *voluntarily.* The federal-state contribution ratio would be set by formula.

The Federal Health Insurance Plan retained Medicare, with extended benefits and cost sharing reduced to the levels of the other two parts of the plan. Persons over sixty-five not eligible for FHI could enroll in the Assisted Plan, and the existing administrative methods of Medicare were to be continued.

Under this proposal the states would have had major responsibility for program administration including approval of company policies and the benefits of other types of health plans as acceptable, certification and regulation of providers, and regulating insurance carriers. There were to be two kinds of participating providers, full and associate, with full providers agreeing to accept the fees set by the state as full payment (i.e., accepting assignment). Optometrists and dentists were permissible providers while chiropractors were not, and physician extenders were accepted as limited providers. Extenders' services were reimbursable if provided under the supervision of physicians or suitable medical organizations, but they could not bill separately.[52] Every employer had to offer prepaid plans as an option, if any existed in the community. The Assisted Plan and the Federal Plan were also required to offer this option. (This requirement was part of the Health Maintenance Act of 1973 discussed below.)

Some aspects of the Nixon administration proposal resembled Medicredit, such as its reliance on approved private insurance company policies and state program administration and its high level of cost sharing. It parted company with Medicredit on the issue of prepaid plans. While not encouraging them as directly as did the Griffiths-Kennedy Bill, it treated prepaid plans as equals, President Nixon being an avowed supporter of HMO formation. The E-HIP financing was almost entirely via wage deductions and cost sharing and as such was regressive, but again such financing shielded it better from the effect of budget slashes than reliance on the general fund alone would have done. Control of insurance standards and medical quality assurance was left largely to the states, but if the federal guidelines it called for had turned out to be specific and strictly enforced the control might have been largely federal. It might have caused certain states to become repositories of high-risk and poor residents raising the costs of health insurance to unduly high levels within those states. Also, many low-income persons might have elected not to join, leaving a pool of uncovered persons for local communities to care for.

The coverage was quite broad as far as included services are concerned, but the high level of cost sharing might have inhibited the use of these services to an undesirable degree. In any one year, a family of four, under an employee plan, would have had to spend $450 for medical services (or $150 per person) before receiving any insurance benefits at all for medical services, and $200 for drugs (or $50 per person) before receiving any drug benefits. Only after an individual spent $1050 or a family spent $1,500 would cost sharing have ceased in that year. To get a better idea of how high this cost sharing was, we note that in 1975 the average annual expenditure for personal health care was $522 per person.

The main drawback of this proposal was its built-in likelihood of producing a two-tier system of care as federal and state standards of quality control weakened to permit a lower standard for policies purchased for the A-HIP beneficiaries than for the E-HIP beneficiaries.

The Comprehensive National Health Insurance Act of 1974: The Kennedy-Mills Bill—A Compromise Proposal During the 1970s Senator Edward Kennedy was the most consistent and strongest congressional supporter and initiator of the series of comprehensive national health insurance bills culminating in the Health Security Act. There were two occasions when he collaborated with members of the House to sponsor compromise bills, in addition to having his own bill in the legislative hopper at the same time. He apparently felt that these bills were the best that could be expected to stand any chance of being passed at that time and that they would improve access sufficiently to warrant support. He introduced one such bill in 1974 with Congressman Mills, then the powerful chairman of the House Committee on Ways and Means and

the other later in 1978 with Congressman Henry Waxman. I shall discuss here only the first compromise bill, which combined some of the features of the Griffiths-Kennedy and the Nixon Administration bills and was introduced into Congress on April 2, 1974, as H.R. 13870 in the House and S.3286 in the Senate. It provided for *compulsory* participation and *universal* eligibility of all legal residents (i.e., access was viewed as a natural right); a national program with standard benefits to be administered by a newly configured Social Security administration; and health service resource planning and development. These were among the "Kennedy" features. On the other hand, cost sharing was substantial and private financial intermediaries were to be used; these were part of the "Nixon administration" features. Premium rates were to be nationally determined, but states would have contributed to financing and been responsible for enforcing standards, again a Nixon administration bill feature.

Benefit coverages were broad, similar to both the Nixon administration and Kennedy bills, and included prescription drugs, vision and hearing services, and dental services for children; and the bill provided for unlimited physician and inpatient care in the hospital. Although the cost sharing levels were lower than in the Nixon administration bill, they were still high—the annual family limit for out-of-pocket cost was $1,000 rather than $1,500. The maximum deductible was limited to two $150 deductibles per family with 25 percent coinsurance going into effect on all expenditures after that. There was no cost sharing for families with less than $4,800 income (which then would have automatically included all the poor—both working and not working), and cost-sharing for families with $4,800 to $8,000 income was reduced. Financing was to be mainly via payroll deductions (75 percent by employers and 25 percent by employees) and everyone was to contribute, including those on public assistance who were to contribute a suitable amount out of their welfare income. Supplementary general-fund financing was also provided to pay the premiums of the poor. Medicare would have been kept on with the addition of coverage for voluntary long-term care insurance for aged and disabled persons and for prescription drugs. The aged could have used

Kennedy-Mills benefits whenever these exceeded Medicare's. Medicaid would have been repealed as being no longer needed.

Operational characteristics were largely "Kennedy" type features. A special national Health Resource Development Board was to work on legislation and policy to increase the availability and adequacy of facilities, encourage the development of HMOs and other alternative delivery forms, and promote continuous health planning. *Prospective budgeting* was to be the payment basis for institutional providers, and quality and cost controls were built into reimbursement procedures.

The funding of the Kennedy-Mills proposal was quite regressive, largely because cost sharing was unduly heavy on lower-income groups despite the graduated rates for families earning $8,000 per annum and under, especially for those with earnings closer to the $8,000. This proposal seemed to be aimed at keeping direct federal costs low while providing universal coverage with broad benefits. It shifted a substantial portion of the cost to the user, and its greatest benefits seemed to lie in its coverage of "catastrophic" illnesses that exhausted the $1,000 ceiling on cost sharing.

The Catastrophic Health Insurance and Medical Assistance Reform Act: The Long-Ribicoff Bill: A Conservative Economics Proposal The final example is a National Health Insurance bill that represents a class of bills concentrating on covering the costs of "catastrophic" illness. At first glance one is inclined to say that this kind of proposal represents the attitude of neoclassical ideology toward health insurance—it should cover only truly unforeseen large losses and have a large deductible to reduce moral hazard. But since the bill also contained provisions for promoting the purchase of private insurance for first-dollar coverage, it is difficult to say whether the main motivation for the bill was ideological or aimed at confining federal financial involvement to catastrophic medical expenses.

The bill was introduced into the Senate (S. 2513) by Senators Russell Long and Abraham Ribicoff on October 3, 1973, and consisted of three parts. The first provided coverage for catastrophic illness, and entitlement for this part (the catastrophic plan) extended only to persons

defined in a specified manner as participating in Social Security, whether still working or retired. Covered services were the same type as those under Medicare, but insurance reimbursement would have begun only after a large deductible, expressed as an initial period of care. For example, hospital care insurance reimbursement would have begun only after the first sixty days of hospitalization within a benefit year (with a small additional front-end deductible for each stay). After a stay of sixty or more days in a hospital, one hundred days in a skilled nursing home would also be covered. The services of physicians and other medical care personnel would be reimbursed without time or service limit after a deductible of the first $2,000 per family per year. The program would have been financed in the same way as existing Medicare Part A, by payroll and wage deductions.

The second part of the bill was the Medical Assistance Plan, aimed at providing the benefits of the program to all low-income persons not then covered by Medicare. It was to be financed jointly from federal and state general revenues. It extended Medicare-type services to *all* low-income persons and supplemented them with catastrophic benefits where needed. Medicaid was to be discontinued but Medicare kept on and the administration of the program would have continued through the existing Medicare mechanism.

The third part of this bill, "Private basic health Insurance Certification," sought to increase the availability of adequate and reasonably priced private health insurance policies that would cover medical expenses before the catastrophic insurance was activated. It would have facilitated the offering of such policies by pools of private carriers as well as improved dissemination of consumer information about health insurance policies available in the open market. The plan called for *voluntary* certification by HEW of appropriate plans (a modified Nixon Administration bill feature) covering the basic medical care costs that were deductible under the catastrophic plan. To articulate with the catastrophic plan, a "certified" policy had to provide for at least sixty days of hospital care with a maximum deductible of $100, and ambulatory care up to $2,000 per year (the deductible for the catastrophic plan), with cost sharing not to exceed 10 percent. An approved policy could contain certain exclusion features, such as excluding certain family members or preexisting conditions. All federal and state antitrust laws that might impede the establishment of insurance pools for offering certified health insurance to the public were to be preempted.

As this brief outline indicates, should the political climate have become favorable to the enactment of a universal national health insurance law, this bill was another alternative to the Griffiths-Kennedy bill and would cost the federal government very much less money. At the same time, it would be more acceptable to those who viewed health insurance from the viewpoint of neoclassical economics. Its stress lay on catastrophic insurance for the rare but very costly event. The poor were to be covered by an expanded version of Medicare for which eligibility would be means tested. Most medical care expenses for nonpoor persons under sixty-five would continue to be covered by private health insurance, with government intervention limited to disseminating information about health insurance policies that met minimally adequate standards, presumably to satisfy the neoclassical economist's assumption of an informed buyer. Cost containment and quality assurance in most private health services were addressed minimally. The private health insurance industry would continue to be relieved of any responsibility for the difficult-to-insure cases—the poor and the very sick. Health care was thus being viewed as just another commodity to be sold on the market with government assuming responsibility for persons who could not buy at market prices.

In summary, the bills introduced into Congress in the period 1967–1975 proposing some form of national health insurance were introduced on behalf of different stake-holders with varying interests. Some were introduced on behalf of sponsoring forces that had wanted national health insurance for a long time. Others, perhaps most of the bills, were introduced for sponsors who did not favor national health insurance per se but wished to have their own bills in the legislative hopper in case a bill they found more objectionable began to advance toward passage. These contingency bills were designed to produce a national health insurance system that would tilt toward the sponsor's professional or business interests or be in accordance with the sponsor's ideological views.

All the bills in the representative sample presented here called for universal entitlement. Passage of any of them would very likely have removed a major problem from the national political arena, the existence of many persons who are not covered by any third-party payer or who are very skimpily covered. Because none of these bills were passed, these persons continued to present a moral and ethical problem for those who believe that care of the sick is a moral obligation of a good society. The persistence of this problem has also furthered public dissatisfaction with the health services system. But beyond the question of universal entitlement the proposals varied widely: on whether entitlement would be to a single health service system; how providers would be paid; who would pay for the program (how it would be financed); what services would be covered; and what form of medical practice organization would be favored; if any.

THE ACCELERATING EMPHASIS ON COST CONTAINMENT AFTER 1972

In the years after 1935, which saw a great expansion of the social welfare state, many government programs were initiated to soften the blows to individuals and families inherent in the workings of the market system. Social forces and ideas associated with World War II accelerated this development. With the economies of its main economic competitors in ruins, the U.S. economy boomed as it became the major supplier for reconstructing the war-torn capitalist countries. There was virtually full employment and large corporations granted increasingly generous fringe benefits to unions, easily passing the increased cost on to consumers as price increases. Most social concerns expressed in the media and social literature dealt with filling in the gaps for access to social services, with heavy emphasis on health services. Much of the justification for these programs was couched in terms of the waste to the nation of human resources ("manpower" was then the more common term) that were not productively employed because of poor health and education. (This is discussed in more detail in Chapter 11.)

In the late 1960s this national ambiance began to change. The economies of the other capitalist countries, especially those of West Germany and Japan, had been largely reconstructed and, of course, with the latest plant and equipment. They were beginning to import less from the United States and soon would become net exporters of finished goods to the U.S. The U.S. economy was beginning to feel the effects of the competition, and by the 1970s these effects were preoccupying the attention of business leaders, commentators, and government officials. By 1980, a well-known economist, prominent for his public writings and television appearances, would write:

Seemingly unsolvable problems were emerging everywhere—inflation, unemployment, slow growth, environmental decay, irreconcilable group demands, and complex cumbersome regulations . . . Do we need to junk our social welfare, health safety, and environmental systems in order to compete? Why were others doing better?

Where the U.S. economy had once generated the world's highest standard of living, it was now well down the list and slipping farther each year. Leaving the rich Middle East sheikdoms aside, we stood fifth among the nations of the world in per capita GNP in 1978, having been surpassed by Switzerland, Denmark, West Germany and Sweden . . . And on the outside the world's fastest economic runner, Japan, was advancing rapidly with a per capita GNP only 7 percent below ours (Thurow, 1980, 3–4).

Public discussion was turning away from the deficiencies of public programs in meeting human needs and toward a concentration on the need to cut costs to make more capital available for investment and to restore U.S. competitiveness.

While many social welfare advocates continued to press for national health insurance because of the continuing inadequacies of access after the passage of Medicare and Medicaid, others complained mostly about continually rising health care costs despite the "H.R. 1" reforms of 1972. In fact, the entire system of health insurance, both private and Medicare, was being criticized for escalating costs. Each year medical care prices rose more than the federal Cost of Living Index for other consumer prices, and much commentary asserted that medical services were overused, largely because of the skewed incentives of the provider payment systems used by many insurance programs. A number of publicly proposed cost containment proposals contended for public support alongside the introduction of the previously mentioned spate of national health insurance proposals aimed at increasing access. Because cost increases are a product of increased utilization, rises in unit prices, and the choice of more intricate technology over simpler therapy, demands for control of each of these factors were made. Cost-benefit and cost-effectiveness analysis ("technology assessment") attempted to indicate what rational controls might be placed on federal support for the proliferation of technology of unproven benefit. Utilization review, removing provider incentives to increase utilization, limiting facility resources, and making the patient more cost conscious were being advocated for controlling utilization increases. Prospectively negotiated fees and capitation rates were being urged for controlling increases in unit prices, a proposal that could only be fully effective if technology proliferation and utilization increases were already or simultaneously controlled. The question of controlling technology proliferation is discussed in Chapter 14, dealing with government support for medical research. In this chapter only the efforts to control utilization and price increase are considered.

Efforts to contain utilization took three major forms. One was to attempt direct control of utilization by reviewing hospital stays (and sometimes ambulatory service bills also) and retroactively refusing payment for excessive utilization. The most prominent early attempt to do this was the establishment of Professional Services Review Organizations (PSRO) under the Social Security Amendments of 1972 to review Medicare and Medicaid hospital utilization. The second approach was to reduce available resources, especially hospital beds, and hope thereby to constrain increases in hospital use. This was attempted largely through the certificate of need and health planning programs, which is discussed in Chapter 15. The third main method was to remove provider incentives to increase utilization by encouraging the growth of Health Maintenance Organizations (HMO).

The Movement Toward Health Maintenance Organizations

The Health Maintenance Organization (HMO): Types and Background

The health services literature distinguishes between two fundamentally different types of HMO, the prepaid group practice (PGP) and the individual practice association (IPA). The PGP was for years the prototype of the major alternative form of organizing medical practice in contradistinction to fee-for-service solo or small single-specialty partnership practice. It was bitterly opposed by local medical societies and made little headway for many years. After 1935, challenges to the hegemony of a single mode of practice cropped up in a few places, but only a small number of these survived and they enrolled only a small proportion of the total United States population. Some of the main ones that arose then, survived, and were still viable in 1950 were the Health Insurance Plan (HIP) of New York, the Group Health Cooperatives of Washington, D.C., and Puget Sound, Washington State, and the Kaiser Health Plan and Ross-Loos Clinic in California. After the Larsen Commission, an investigating committee of the AMA, found in 1960 that the Kaiser PGP was practicing good medicine, the longtime opposition of the medical societies became muted.

A new form of organization based on prepaid fees arose when the local medical society of San Joaquin Valley, California organized itself into a "Medical Care Foundation" (MCF) to counter the threat of expansion by the Kaiser Health Plan. Under this arrangement, subscribers enrolled as members of the foundation and went for ambulatory care to any physician who was a member of the medical society. The physician was then reimbursed by the foundation and hospital care was contracted for through private hospital insurance. The San Joaquin Valley Medical Care Foundation was the progenitor of the IPA form of HMO that proliferated in later years.

When the Nixon Administration expressed an interest in prepayment as a method of cost containment, a Minnesota physician, Dr. Paul Elwood, coined the name Health Maintenance Organization, of HMO. Its advantage over the name PGP was twofold: it defused the negative "buzzword" signals sent out by the use of the term PGP to many physicians and their societies; and it included the medical care foundation, which was a prepaid plan but not a group practice. Subsequently, any arrangement whereby prepayment was associated with private practicing physicians not organized into a single group came to be classified as an individual practice association (IPA). Some of these were "closed panel," meaning that only a limited number of physicians from the community participated, and others were open panel; the latter included the medical care foundation form. The fundamental distinguishing characteristic of the PGP was its provision of physician care via an organization of physicians practicing as a group, paid by salary, and serving a clientele that paid a capitation premium to a single central organization (the "health plan") for designated types of services to be used as needed.

In the course of developing federal assistance to HMOs after 1973 (described below under "The Health Maintenance Act of 1973," federal definitions were promulgated for purposes of administering this assistance. The old PGP was further classified into two groups: the staff HMO, in which the HMO is a health plan that hires its own physicians as paid employees who practice as a group, and the group practice or closed panel, in which the HMO is a health plan that contracts with a single medical group, partnership, or corporation of physicians for the delivery of medical care to its enrollees. An HMO was defined under the act as an organized system providing a comprehensive range of health care services to a voluntarily enrolled consumer population. In return for a prepaid fixed fee the enrollee is guaranteed a defined set of benefits, with the services themselves guaranteed to be provided by the plan. Note that the last proviso, in which the services themselves are guaranteed, is what really differentiates the HMO from regular health insurance as it did for the PGP before the term HMO was introduced.

The Health Maintenance Organization Act of 1973

The lower cost per patient of providing medical care via the prepaid group practice, which had been well established by investigators, sparked the interest in the HMO shown by the Nixon administration and some members of Congress. This interest is attested by such facts as the Nixon administration's using HEW funds (Section 314e of Public Health Act: page 98) to support the organization of pilot HMOs during its first term (1968–1972); the Kennedy health insurance bills strongly supporting HMOs; the 1972 amendments to the Social Security Act facilitating Medicare payments to HMOs; and passage of the Health Maintenance Organization Act in 1973, which authorized federal financial support to further the organization of new HMOs and the enlargement of existing ones.

The HMO Act made available grants and contracts for feasibility surveys; grants, contracts, and loan guarantees for planning the establishment or expansion of HMOs and for establishment and initial development costs; and loans and loan guarantees for the initial operating deficits of new HMOs in their first three years of operation. While grants, contracts, and loans were available to public and private nonprofit organizations, only loan guarantees were authorized to for-profit HMOs, and then only if they were to serve an "underserved" population. Only federally approved HMOs were eligible for assistance. The authorized appropriations totaled $325 million, as shown in Table 10–4.

Special provisions of the original act reflected a number of federal health policy principles with respect to supporting the restructuring of medical care practice:

1. Obviously, the very act of legislating assistance for the organization of HMOs indicated confidence in the virtues of this form of organization, at least among members of Congress and the federal executive. But it should also be noted that not-for-profit organization was strongly favored in the grant priority ordering.

2. Indians and migrant workers were included in the benefits of the act. Furthermore, the funds for operating health services provided to these two populations under various other

Table 10–4. Appropriations Authorized for HMOs, 1974–1977

FY	For: ($000,000)	
	Feasibility surveys, planning and initial development	Initial operating deficit (first three years)
1974	25	
1975	55	75
1976	85	
1977	85	

federal programs could be paid to HMOs if these existed in the area and segments of these populations chose to enroll. The wording for the two groups was not exactly the same. For Indian populations, "prepayment" was permitted, while for migrants, HMOs were mandated.

3. The definition of a federally "certified" HMO contained clauses that spelled out what Congress and the administration meant by a "minimally adequate" set of services. It stated that besides physician and acute inpatient service ("basic services"), the HMO "shall" also provide for "supplemental" service—choosing from something in the way of extended care, dental care, and the like—but the exact degree to which provision of any such services was compulsory was ambiguous. "Basic services" had to be available and accessible around the clock and the membership enrolled by community rating. Very significantly, one-third of the "policymaking body" was to consist of the membership, and if the persons an HMO served included an underserved population, this population was to be "equitably" represented. The HMO was required to provide for peer review of process and for ongoing quality assurance programs based on health outcomes. It had to provide for health education and medical social service and for continuing education of professional staff. It was also required to keep and make available statistics on costs, utilization, and style of operation. It is important to note that these "minimal" requirements represented a standard of care that was substantially above what most users of "mainstream" medicine could ever hope

to find in even very good fee-for-service practices.

4. Strong measures were taken to forestall two possible barriers to carrying out the intent of the law: (1) Employee benefit plans were *required* to offer an HMO as an option if a federally certified one existed in the area, a requirement that was to assume unexpectedly large importance in the development of HMOs. (b) State laws restricting certain medical practice modes, such as group practice, or requiring medical society approval for groups, were contermanded (''preempted'' by the federal government).

Health Maintenance Organization Amendments of 1976

It proved virtually impossible for the existing large, established, better-known HMOs to qualify for certification under the HMO Act of 1973 if they were to remain competitive with other health insurance. The Act's demanding requirements regarding open enrollment, community rating, and required benefit package would have raised the actuarial risk and operating costs for HMOs beyond levels they felt able to meet and still charge a marketable premium. As a consequence, very few HMOs applied for certification in the first three years after passage of the act. The federal certification of HMOs was in effect being burdened with the impossible task of singlehandedly beginning to remake the entire health care system into a model of efficiency, effectiveness, and equity.[53]

It was the recognition of how hobbling this requirement for perfection was to the program that led to the enactment of the Amendments to the Health Maintenance Organization Act of 1973 on October 8, 1976, as Public Law 94—460. The 1976 amendments relaxed the stringency of some of the 1973 requirements for certification to provide HMOs with greater flexibility, improve the administration of the program, and modify the parts of the original law that were placing federally certified HMOs at a competitive disadvantage with traditional insurance programs and health delivery systems. The new legislation eased some of the original act's more burdensome requirements regarding the benefit package that must be offered, open enrollment, community rating, the dual-choice provisions under employee health benefit plans, the availability of federal loan guarantees, and the organization of medical practice. The 1976 law made the supplemental benefits optional with the HMO but at the same time expanded the list of required basic services to include immunizations, well-child care from birth, and periodic health evaluations for adults.

Easing of 1973 Requirements for Federal Certification Adverse selection posed a real danger because HMOs had been required to enroll persons broadly representative of the various age, social and income groups within the areas they served and do so on an open enrollment basis. The 1976 amendments limited the open-enrollment requirement to those HMOs that had not incurred a financial deficit in a recent year *and*, either had been in existence for at least five years or had a minimum of 50,000 members, whichever occurred first, and an HMO had to accept no more than approximately 3 percent of its new members annually through open enrollment.[54] The provision in the original act that required prepaid enrollment fees (premiums) to be fixed uniformly for all subscribers (i.e., use a community rating system) without regard to the experience of any subgroup was substantially relaxed, and the secretary of Health, Education and Welfare was even given authority to waive the community-rating requirement entirely. Nevertheless, applications for federal qualification still had to contain assurances that the community-rating requirement would be met when appropriate.

The 1973 requirement that employers with twenty-five or more workers who offered a choice of health benefit plans include the option of membership in a qualified HMO if the HMO so requested was eased by limiting it to HMOs serving an area in which at least twenty-five *employees resided.* But at the same time, the new law also required employers to offer the HMO option first to the employees' union where one existed. (But if the union accepted the option, each employee still had the option of continuing with traditional health insurance.)

Coordination with Medicare and Medicaid The federal government's policy promoting HMOs through the HMO Act and the reimbursement principles on which the original 1965 Medicare act were based were contradictory in important aspects. By 1976 the federal HMO policy was to promote global prepaid fees for a complete set of covered services, while the 1965 Medicare reimbursement procedure was mainly concerned with fee-for-service reimbursements.[55]

The 1976 changes also included amendments to the Social Security Act that brought some, but not all, of the definitions of an HMO contained in the Medicare and Medicaid laws into conformance with those of the HMO act.

The 1976 amendments left unchanged a number of the requirements for an HMO to be eligible for using the special payment methods under Medicare laid down in the 1972 Amendments to the Social Security Act. A plan still had to have at least half of its enrolled membership composed of persons under age sixty-five and have an open-enrollment period during which it accepted Medicare beneficiaries to the limits of its capacity in the order in which they applied (with provisions for waivers and exceptions) to be eligible for special reimbursement as an HMO by HEW.[56] The HMO premium rate or other charge *made directly to Medicare enrollees*[57] did not need to be community-rated but could be based on the actuarial value of the Medicare excluded services plus cost sharing. The new law also continued to require that the services an HMO must provide to Medicare beneficiaries were at least those covered under Medicare's hospital insurance (Part A) and supplementary medical insurance (Part B) rather than the "basic health services" defined in the HMO Act.

Medicaid provisions were also amended to include a definition of HMOs that corresponded to the definition in the HMO Act in all respects except that "basic health services" were defined as referring to the five mandatory Medicaid services for Medicaid beneficiaries. Unless the provisions were waived, to be eligible for Medicaid reimbursement no more than half the enrollees in an HMO could be covered under Medicare *or* be recipients of Medicaid. The new law tightened up the provisions for federal matching payments to states for Medicaid services provided by organizations on a prepaid or capitation basis by requiring that such organizations be federally certified as HMOs.[58] This requirement did not apply to organizations that had contracted for the provision of services before 1970.

The Health Planning and Resources Development Amendments of 1979: Special Treatment for HMOs The original National Health Planning and Resources Development Act of 1974, to which these amendments refer, is discussed in Chapter 15, but the 1979 amendments to the Health Planning Act are treated here because they represented a further Federal encouragement of HMO development, mainly by giving HMOs certain exemptions from Certificate of need (CON) legislation. This legislation was part of the federal cost-containment efforts and required health facilities wishing to add to or alter existing capacity to obtain official permission to do so from the state's health planning agency. An HMO or a combination of HMOs was exempted from obtaining approval for three items—installing major medical equipment, adding institutional health services, and making large capital expenditures—that required prior mandatory review and approval for health facilities. These provisions applied only to the established, large HMOs.

California State Action on HMOs In 1975 the California legislature passed the Knox-Keane Health Care Service Plan Act, which went into effect in 1976, replacing the previous Knox-Mills Health Plan Act. Under Knox-Keane, all HMOs had to be licensed by the State Department of Corporations in order to solicit members and operate. The act laid down rules for solicitation and enrollment for an organization to be eligible as a health care service plan. These applied both to general plans providing general medical and hospital services and specialized plans; such as dental service plans.

HMO Status as of 1984 The results of the promotion of HMOs by the federal government were plainly visible if not sensational. In 1971 there were 39 HMOs serving 3.5 million people; in June 1984, there were 306[59] HMOs serving 15.1 million people, still slightly less than 7 percent of the American people. Of these 306 HMOs 180 were group practice[60] models and 126 were IPAs. A total of 194 were federally qualified, with 12.3 million members (Interstudy, 1985).

The Carter Administration

As President Carter assumed office in 1977, the issue of cost containment was continuing to grow in importance. The HMO initiative had not put a noticeable dent in cost inflation, mainly because no great numbers of new persons had joined HMOs, but also because many of the new ones were independent practice associations (IPAs). All the research on the lesser use of hospital care under HMOs had been done on Prepaid Group Practices (PGPs); IPAs and their predecessor Medical Care Foundations had not been found to have noticeably lower hospital use and the way HMOs were actually found to save money was through lower hospital admissions. President Nixon had put a price ceiling on hospitals which constrained their price increases while it was in effect, but after the cap was removed prices rose at a rate that more than made up for the period during which they were moderated.

The new Carter administration marked time on the question of national health insurance, taking the position that health care costs had to be controlled before federally sponsored health insurance could be successfully instituted. Opposing this view, Senator Kennedy pressed for passage first, arguing that costs could only be contained after passage of NHI, when the federal government would be able to more effectively exert control over both utilization and provider reimbursement. Toward the end of his administration, President Carter sponsored the National Health Plan Act (S. 1812), a proposal that ranked with the most cautious and conservative versions of previously introduced bills. It called for a two-tier system, one for the poor and aged ("Health Care") and another for the under-sixty-five, better-off working population. The Health Care part would include some 52 million persons: 16 million then on Medicaid, 14 million "near poor," and 22 million Medicare beneficiaries. The other part was to be administered by private insurance companies with premiums paid 75 percent by employers and 25 percent by employees and with heavy cost sharing. However, low-income workers would get partial subsidies for their share of the premiums. Maternal and child care would have been totally covered, with pregnant women receiving free prenatal,

delivery, and mother and infant health care for one year after birth.

Kennedy responded with the Kennedy-Waxman proposal. "Health Care for All Americans," embodied in H.R. 5191 and S. 1720. As previously noted, this was the second of Kennedy's attempts to get a compromise measure passed in the face of an administration that was resistant to the idea of a universal and comprehensive health insurance bill like the Griffiths-Kennedy Health Security Act. The earlier compromise (the Kennedy-Mills bill, p. 319) had been the heavy cost sharing; this time it was continuing the use of private insurance companies as fiscal intermediaries. Many of the comprehensive and national-planning features long associated with Kennedy sponsorship were still recognizable, however. Population coverage was universal, a wide spectrum of services was covered and this time there was no cost sharing and no limits, there was to be a national as well as local area annual budgets, hospitals were to be paid by prospectively determined budgets, and physicians by negotiated fees with no additional charges to the patient permitted. Medicaid was to be continued only for long-term care.

With the administration adamantly opposing the Kennedy-Waxman proposal, nothing stirred in Congress, but other voices were being heard. On the left, decrying the failures of Medicare, Medicaid, and private insurance to provide universal coverage or access to services that were comprehensive and efficiently administered, the supporters of the National Health Service Act introduced by Representative Ron Dellums argued that only a government direct-service system could provide care efficiently, effectively, and equitably. The Dellums proposal called for a national health service that would put all health care facilities under federal ownership and all health services under federal operation.

On the right, neoclassical economists and their adherents were calling even more loudly for greater reliance on market competition to control costs. Prominent among the advocates of competition were Professors Alain Enthoven of Stanford and Clark Havighurst of Duke; and Congressmen Richard Gephardt and David Stockman. Their central idea was that government regulation was responsible for the uncontrolled cost inflation by interfering with market competition and that all barriers to competition among health plans should be removed. These advocates differed in the specifics of their proposals but the common thread through their approaches was the need to increase price competition among health plans. Consumers should be made aware of their expenditures through substantial cost sharing, all special tax treatment that encouraged firms and employees to spend needlessly for rising health insurance premiums should be repealed, and all government regulation of price, quality, and service capacity should be discontinued because they served to encourage monopoly and increase costs needlessly (Havighurst, 1973). If the federal government wished to assure access to medical care to all, this should be done using methods that encourage price competition, such as allowing all persons a fixed federal sum for health care and thereby motivating them to comparison shop for efficient plans (Enthoven, 1980). But even this type of market-oriented proposal for creating universal access to health care was already an anachronism by 1980, for in 1981 the nation turned away from serious consideration of issues like enacting universal access to health care and toward a single minded concern with improving national economic and military predominance.

The Reagan Administration

With Ronald Reagan's inauguration in January of 1981, many of the doctrines of the right gained ascendancy. In the new administration they were perhaps most clearly reflected in the activities and statements of the Bureau of Management and Budget, headed by former Congressman David Stockman. Many of the regulatory agencies were weakened or dismantled, and the planning and medical quality assurance programs (PSROs) were gutted. But the essence of the "pro-competition" proposals, national health insurance in the form of a grant to each person to buy insurance accompanied by removal of all tax exemptions for expenditures over this nationally (adjusted) uniform amount, was never even introduced as a bill. The major trends that had emerged by the end of 1982 were large cuts in Medicaid and smaller ones in Medicare, and a sharply accelerated move by the fed-

eral government to introduce more radical cost-saving reimbursement methods into Medicare and Medicaid. There was also an interest in top corporate circles in directly controlling their medical care costs, especially through the use of corporate self-insurance as well as by forming regional coalitions of corporations to promote cost control. Because the developments after 1980 are outside the main time frame of this book they will not be discussed in detail, but a brief outline follows.

Changes in Medicare and Medicaid

The fiscal years 1981–1983 saw reductions in the provisions made for these programs—by reducing appropriations in 1981 and by changing provider reimbursement methods in 1982 and 1983.

The Omnibus Budget Reconciliation Act of 1981 (OBRA) This act (P.L. 97-35) had its greatest impact on Medicaid (see Chapter 4, pp. 110–111, for effects on federal public health grants). The main changes in Medicare, aside from a pro forma increase in the annual deductible in Part B from $60 to $75, consisted of reductions in a number of reimbursement items. A "routine nursing differential" that had been paid to hospitals was discontinued, for example. There were other relatively minor reductions.

The reductions in Medicaid were along two lines: (1) federal payments to states would be reduced over a period of three years; and (2) the states were given greater freedom to reduce and limit services in various ways as well as to devise their own payment systems. Newly allowed restrictions on the patient's freedom of choice (of provider) permitted use of such devices as locking in high user beneficiaries to specified providers and locking out offending providers (those seen as "over serving") from participation in the program. For the most part, permission to waive a state's obligation to abide by a specified Medicaid regulation had to be obtained from the Health Care Financing Administration (HCFA) of HHS.

The Tax Equity and Fiscal Responsibility Act of 1982 (TEFRA) While 1981 OBRA was directed more at Medicaid than at Medicare, TEFRA (P.L. 97-248) focused on Medicare. HMOs were given greater incentives to seek risk-sharing contracts (see note 55) with HCFA under Medicare. Under the previous 1972 legislation the risk-sharing contract had required that the contracting HMO be paid 80 percent of the average adjusted per capita costs (AAPCC)[61] and return one half of any savings over its actual costs to HEW. If the HMO lost money it absorbed the entire loss or carried it over to be offset by future savings. By March 1981, only one HMO was under a "normal risk contract" (Muse and Sawyer, 1982). The TEFRA legislation provided that risk-sharing contracts pay the HMO 95 percent of the AAPCC and the HMO could keep any "profit" derived from its actual costs being lower than the reimbursement. The HMO was required to use the excess for enriching the services offered its Medicare subscribers or for reducing their premiums. Organizations other than federally qualified HMOs, called competitive medical plans (CMP), were made eligible for obtaining these contracts. While not meeting all the requirements of the fully qualified HMO, the CMP still had to provide physicians' services using "primarily" its own employees or through contracts with physicians or physician groups.

Regulations implementing the risk-sharing contract provisions were published in January 1985 (Ellwood, 1985). By March 1986 "there were 114 TEFRA risk contracts with a total of 530,658 enrollees—about 2 percent of the total Medicare population . . . most of the contracts were with plans located in California, Kansas, and Massachusetts, while the people enrolled were concentrated in Florida, Minnesota, and California" (Lohr, 1985).

Other TEFRA provisions aimed at containing cost increases included: (a) For persons aged sixty-five to sixty-nine who continue to work for an employer with an employee health insurance plan, the employer's plan would thenceforth continue to be the primary insurer, with Medicare now being the secondary insurer (i.e., Medicare would pay only for those services covered by Medicare but not by the company plan). (b) Introduction of a form of cost-per-case (per stay) flat payment for some hospital bills and placing a ceiling on annual percentage increases in hospital revenues. This was the progenitor of the "DRG" reimbursement system described below. (c) Permitting states to require copayments for all Medicaid categories except for some specifically exempted classes like children under eighteen. (d) Replacing the Professional Standards and Review Organization (PSRO, see p. 301) by the Professional Review Organization program (PRO).

The Social Security Amendments of 1983 In terms of the impact on the U.S. health services system, the most important provision of this act (P.L. 98-21) was the establishment of a prospective payment system (PPS) as the basis for Medicare reimbursement of hospitals; they would be paid a prospectively determined rate per stay. These rates would be based on a classification of discharge diagnoses according to a system known as Diagnostically Related Groups (DRGs). All of the thousands of hospital discharge diagnoses listed in the official International Classification of Diseases (ICD) were assigned to one of only several hundred (originally 468) DRGs, and a flat reimbursement fee for each DRG was set. Originally these fees were based on a calculation of 1983 costs and an annual inflation factor was allowed each subsequent year. The fees were adjusted for regional differences in wage levels and for urban/rural location differences. The system was phased in over a period of three years, achieving full operation by October 1, 1986 (that is, for the fiscal year ending September 30, 1987).

A Prospective Payment Assessment Commission was established to review the operations of the PPS system and report to Congress.

Changes in the Private Health Insurance System

While all these changes were being made in Medicare and Medicaid during the 1980s to contain costs, private industry also continued its attempt to reduce its outlays for employee medical care. A large literature emerged on this general subject that cannot be dealt with in depth here, but these events of the Reagan administration period will be briefly summarized with some additional comments.

We recall the point made in the discussion on page 275 that the historical development and the configuration of the private health insurance system in the United States has largely determined the shape of the medical care system. This is mainly because the prevailing attitude that a privately sponsored medical care system is inherently superior to a publicly sponsored one means that the government system is largely a residual one. It consists of those services that the private sector has not seen fit to provide or serves people that the private sector has not regarded as desirable patients or insurance customers. Much of this book is devoted to identifying the subsystems that make up the public system, in particular the populations they serve and the circumstances under which these populations became (and some still remain) special target groups for these government medical care subsystems and thereby part of the residual population that does not and generally cannot receive its medical care through private health insurance. The extent of the private health insurance system is therefore an important determinant of the size and types of medical care programs provided by government—by subtraction, as it were.

A good deal of government's regulatory activity in the medical care field involves helping the private system to work better. The main stated purpose of such activities—licensing, quality assurance, resource development, expanding access, biomedical research—is to protect the public interest, but they serve also to protect and enhance the interests of private providers and industries and striking a proper balance between the two is often a delicate matter. (Witness the structure of the Medicare reimbursement mechanism, which uses private health insurance companies and the pricing practices of private-practice physician to establish its payment levels.) For both these reasons, it is important to identify and attempt to understand the import of changing trends in the private health insurance system in a work addressed to the role of government in health services. The development of the private health insurance system through 1980 was traced earlier in the section "The Rise and Role of Private Health Insurance" with this perspective in mind. During the Reagan administration private health insurance underwent a number of important structural changes that were already becoming evident in the 1970s.

Major purchasers of health care such as large corporations and union trust funds have been disturbed about spiraling health costs for some time. Until the late '70s, however, purchaser attitudes were typically polite, though concerned. The influence of a sluggish economy on corporate profits, competitiveness, and survival, however, changed this situation significantly. As one executive put it bluntly in conversation, "The fact that rising health care costs were the single largest growing expenditure in the corporate budget took on a new meaning for these corporations in highly competitive industries. . . ." The economic difficulties of the early 1980s, characterized by high unemployment, large federal deficits, and the concomitant lack of investor faith in the industrial sector[61] demanded that corporations aggressively seek out any and all tools for reducing operating costs. Bulging corporate benefit expenditures were a natural starting point (Barger, Hillman, and Garland, 1985).

Rising health care costs were part of the corporate world's increasing focus on lowering the cost of production and the concern of some corporate leaders and commentators with increasing capital accumulation for investment in modernizing U.S. industrial processes or shifting capital from declining to growing industries.

The changes made by corporations in their health benefit structure were many, including outright reductions in benefits, often in the form of increased cost sharing (Barger, Hillman, and Garland, 1985), which became increasingly feasible as organized labor retreated before the threats of layoffs and plant closings accompanying the increased foreign competition, including the transfer of U.S. jobs to third-world countries. But aside from these outright reductions in benefits, a central feature of the changes was the move by the corporations toward self-insurance which had already become evident in modest form in the mid-1970s (Barger, Hillman, and Garland, 1985).

The core of the self-insurance system was for the corporation itself to pay the health care bills of its employees instead of buying insurance from private insurances companies, whether Blues or commercial. This arrangement was expected to lead directly to increased corporate awareness and concomitant concern with lowering expenditures for medical care and thence to reducing unit prices as well as volume of use. It is true, of course, that this interest should also exist in theory in traditional health insurance, for high medical prices and a large volume of utilization are reflected in higher premiums. But the history of private health insurance had been one of insurance companies regarding themselves only as payers of (medically) authenticated bills. They had not moved to reduce the size of those bills largely because for many years they encountered little corporate resistance to the premium increases, and competition among insurance companies to offer lower premiums was not much in evidence.

A self-insured corporation can, and typically does, organize a health benefits office to perform a number of functions. Among these might be monitoring submitted claims for validity and accuracy; requiring second medical opinions for certain procedures; arranging for special rebates[63] for employees who participate in health enhancement programs; and arranging with groups of providers to give discounts to the corporation's employees.

Using self-insurance means the assuming of an actuarial risk by the client corporation, and this means having large reserves to support large drains upon company resources during surges of claims. Ordinarily this would imply that self-insurance is only for the very largest corporations. Furthermore, the efficient administration of claims payment requires a high degree of skill and experience, again, suggesting that self-insurance is only for the largest companies; and for the most part, self-insurance has been used by large enterprises. But one of the developments of the 1970s and growing in the 1980s was the use of special contracts between large insurance companies and corporations that permit modest-sized enterprises to use self-insurance. These are the Administrative Services Only (ASO) contracts and the Minimum Premium Policies (MPP). Under the ASO contracts an insurance company undertakes to do the claims processing and analyses for a corporation that is self-insured. The MPP policy assures the corporation that unusually high claims will be paid by the insurance company. This procedure is called reinsurance and is a common practice in the insurance industry. Because the extremely high claim is a rare event, the premium for this insurance is relatively low. In addition to the insurance companies, a number of consulting firms developed into third-party administrators (TPA), performing a range of health benefits ad-

ministrative functions under contract with corporations. The services might include claims administration, advice on benefit structure, utilization review and analysis, negotiations with provider groups for discounted rates, quality assurance and others.

Another of the more important results of self-insurance was the formation of groups of providers offering discounted fees to corporations. Nearly all of these were groups of physicians or hospitals. In return for the lower prices, the corporations were expected to induce their employees to use these providers, hence the term Preferred Provider Organization (PPO), by which these groups were known (Barger, Hillman, and Garland, 1985; Fox, Goldbeck, and Spies, 1984). The typical arrangement was for the corporation to offer specified health benefits, such as hospital and physician services, to its employees. The employee had to pay various amounts of cost sharing unless he/she used a preferred provider. If a preferred provider was used the employee paid a smaller amount of cost sharing, often none at all.

The PPO differs from the HMO mainly in that it has no enrolled client population. An employee can readily use a PPO physician for one visit and a non-PPO physician for another. It is thus difficult to accurately gauge the savings from using a PPO, especially reductions in utilization. ''As of late 1983, official estimates reported more than 120 PPOs either in existence or in developmental stages in the United States'' (Barger, Hillman, and Garland, 1985). Physicians and hospitals were the most frequent source of sponsorship, accounting together for 48 percent of the total 120. In February 1982 there had been only 4 PPOs (Barger, Hillman, and Garland, 1985).

Large private employers spent the 1975–80 period awakening to the general cost containment problem. Many became, to a large degree, supportive of the regulatory system that the Federal government and the states were adopting. They also began to take the first, rather tentative, stabs at cost containment, through benefits design changes and increased demands for the data needed to compare the price and utilization patterns of providers. By 1980, major employers had learned that federal regulation alone was not the answer, nor could most insurers and providers be counted on to make significant changes to systems that were, from their perspective, successful. Further, they came to recognize that benefit design changes and other measures they could take as individual companies would not be of such magnitude as to have a significant impact on community-wide utilization, reimbursement, or system capacity, principally hospital beds and high-technology equipment.

Faced with these facts, and insurance premium increases that often exceeded 20 percent, employers came to realize that cost management depended on the evolution of a strategy. A comprehensive strategy would have to integrate those cost-management activities that a company could undertake unilaterally and internally, such as benefit design changes, with those that the company could directly influence but which were external, such as hospital trustee education or contracts for utilization review. Finally, it became apparent that there remained major components of a strategy which could only be accomplished through collective action. Examples include alternative delivery system development, community health planning multiple employer utilization review programs, community education programs, and the utilization/price data systems upon which to base other cost-management actions. Coalitions, or local business groups on health, are the institutional response to the growing awareness of the need for collective action. . . . (Goldbeck, 1984).

To promote corporate efforts to control the cost of health benefits, employers were banding together in employer health care coalitions during the 1980s. A group of experts on the activities of business groups in the health field defined these in this fashion:

Coalitions are associations with purchaser representation whose primary reason for being is to promote local rather than national health care cost-containment efforts. It is regional, state, county, city, or other nonnational geopolitical boundaries that defined each group. . . .

There are two basic coalition models. There are coalitions that have, as equal members, most if not all of the major interests represented, in particular, both purchaser and providers. There are also those whose membership is limited to a specific interest (e.g., private sector employers) or a single comprehensive category, such as purchasers, which may include government and labor. . . . (Barger, Hillman, and Garland, 1985).

While unions and provider associations were represented on some of these employer associations, they appear to have been primarily under large corporation leadership and guidance. The initiative for organizing them came variously

from local business, local trade or other business associations; Health System Agencies (HSAs, see Chapter 15); insurers; national business, labor, or provider organizations; foundations; and government. They provided help to employer purchasers of health care through their health benefit analysis structures. This help concentrated on cost containment measures. The work of the coalitions involved informing their members about data availability for utilization and claims control benefit design, study of alternative delivery system, health education (including self-education about the cost issues and health planning) (Ellwood, 1985). By the mid-1970s there were only a "handful" of these local coalitions; by 1981 they had grown to about fifty and by early 1983 there were about one hundred (Ellwood, 1985).

Thus by 1983 or 1984 it was clear that large corporations were intervening directly to lower their health care costs. Some of the main approaches entailed promoting the use of alternative delivery systems, such as HMOs and PPOs. The large increase in corporate self-insurance was a leading mechanism through which the other measures were instituted. Increases in cost sharing were also used.

Standing back a bit from the canvas, we see that in the mid-1980s, after almost eighty years of national citizen activism advocating government-sponsored health insurance, some legislation that actually enacted such insurance, and the rapid growth of private health insurance, a large gap still yawned in access to medical care. In her survey of the problem of the uninsured population, Gail Wilensky found in 1988 that

the number of uninsured has increased significantly since the late 1970s but . . . the characteristics of the uninsured have remained surprisingly similar. The number of uninsured in 1980 was approximately the same as it was in late 1970s—about 26 million. There is some dispute about how much the numbers increased during the recession of the early 1980s, although most estimates indicate that about 34 million people were uninsured as of 1983.

The characteristics of the uninsured appear to be surprisingly stable: (1) about half of the uninsured are employed; (2) when their dependents are included, the employed uninsured account for 75 percent to 80 percent of the uninsured population; (3) most of the employed uninsured are low wage earners—69 percent earn less than $10,000; (4) despite the low wages, only 35 percent of the uninsured were in families below the poverty line, and one-third were in families more than twice the poverty line.

Clearly, the main gap fillers put in place thus far—direct government provision of medical care, government payment for medical care, and private health insurance—have not provided access to medical care for between 30 and 40 million people. Additional numbers have inadequate insurance. Furthermore, most of the uninsured are employed or dependents of employed persons. Will new gap fillers do the job? Part of the answer to this question rests on the reasons put forth for the failure of the past fillers to close the gap.

Certainly a major determinant of this failure has been the fact that much of our society has willed it. The antipathy toward providing government assistance to able-bodied poor persons is deeply rooted in centuries of religious, political, and social-Darwinist attitudes. Some of this antipathy extends even to medical care, but it takes the special form of providing much less than mainstream care rather than none at all. The "lesser eligibility" doctrine makes its presence felt in a particularly pervasive way with respect to this component of "living" standards.

Another factor has been the influence of special interests safeguarding their protected economic positions: the physicians, the hospitals, and the insurance companies. And a third has been the attitude of the large corporations that, unlike their European counterparts, never ceased to oppose comprehensive universal health insurance. Comparisons with other developed countries indicate that the latter factor may be a function of the weak condition of the labor movement in the United States compared with those in the other developed countries.

NOTES

1. Enactment of the Railroad Retirement Act predated the passage of the Social Security Act. It provided federal retirement benefits for railroad employees.

2. Measured in calendar quarters of work for an employee working for an employer subject to Social Security tax—i.e., working in "[Social Security] covered" employment. The required number of quarters was increased by three each year after 1968 until the stationary total number of forty required quarters of covered employment was reached. Forty quarters was thereafter required for eligibility, the same as for a retirement pension under the Social Security Act.

3. This provision was of some help to the state mental hospital, as noted in Chapter 3.

4. These have been rather generally defined in Chapter 9.

5. Initially $40, this amount rose steadily thereafter. It was in 1981 and $592 in 1990.

6. Initially $10 per day, this amount also rose steadily, to $51 per day in 1981 and $148 in 1990.

7. The per diem copayment on days charged to this reserve was $20 in 1968, the first year this benefit was available. In 1980 it was $102 and in 1988 it was $270.

8. In 1981, this was $25.50 per day and in 1988 it was $67.50.

9. The premium was increased many times from the original $6.00 ($3.00 paid by the beneficiary) until it stood at a total of $13.40 monthly ($6.70 paid by the beneficiary) on July 1974. In 1990 the beneficiary's share was $28.60, which represented only about 25 percent of the average total costs of the program.

10. $50 per year originally, $60 in 1973 and $75 in 1990.

11. There were two other classes that the states were mandated to include in Medicaid and three additional classes of person whose optional inclusion in Medicaid by the state would be matched by the federal government. They were a relatively small number and the description of their qualifications is very complicated. I restrict the description to the main classes of Medicaid eligibles: the categorically needy, the categorically linked and the medically needy only.

12. I shall henceforth use "income ceilings" in place of "resource ceilings" because (a) for very poor persons their resources consist almost entirely of their income, and (b) the term "income ceiling" is more widely used and generally understood.

13. Although in general it is the provisions of the 1965 Medicaid Act with its 1967 amendments that are being described, a number of program features added within the first five years following original enactment are also included.

14. We recall that old age assistance (OAA) was the public welfare cash assistance program for the aged poor.

15. The "maintenance of effort" requirement was also repealed by the 1972 Amendments to the Social Security Act, discussed later in this chapter.

16. Total hospital expenses per patient day consists of a "routine" daily service charge and charges for ancillary services such as laboratory tests and X-rays actually used. As noted in the text, the hospital's average *expenses* per patient day may be regarded as an approximate per diem (realized) *price* to a program such as Medicare that paid the *cost* of service to providers.

17. This refers to the physician visiting a number

of patients hospitalized in one facility and charging the same for each as for a single visit to a patient.

18. These are the first five services listed on Table 10-1. In 1969, early and periodic screening, diagnosis, and treatment (EPSDT) of physical and mental defects in eligible persons under twenty-one, and in 1970 home health services were added to the original basic five, so that by 1971 there were actually seven required services for the obligatory class.

19. This provision was not added to the regular Medicaid Title XIX of the Social Security Act but was instead affixed to various other portions of the Social Security Act, mainly Title XII.

20. Walter McNerney was then head of Blue Cross.

21. This figure persists to the present day (1992). See page 304 and note 32.

22. This was later done. See page 300.

23. This means that the existing inadequate level of coverage (efficacy) of the programs was *not* taken as a given; universal access by the target population was. This is in marked contrast to other approaches, which became more usual in later years, that examined gap-filling programs with the single-minded aim of finding ways to cut them, with perfunctory or no attention paid to whether a program's services needed to be maintained or even expanded to perform its mission. But this was just before the "watershed" year of 1972, and fully ten years before the beginning of the Reagan administration retrenchments.

24. These included standard items of cost control recommended for years by health services writers as well as items specific to the Medicaid program design: requiring fee schedules, adoption of a national drug formula for prescriptions, establishment of prior approval for specified nonemergency services, mandating the designation of a primary physician, instituting procedures to notify recipients of all payments made on their behalf, introducing cost-sharing not tied to income level for the medically indigent but only "wherever practicable," prohibiting payments of medical bills to collection agencies, and requiring states to maintain Medicaid fraud and abuse control units.

25. The AFDC category, it should be noted, was by far the largest category of federally supported welfare recipients and the one that received the most political abuse for harboring welfare "cheats." In this class were the unmarried and the deserted mothers and it contained percentages of minority women and their children larger than their percentages of the total population. This isolation of the AFDC category from the other three provided fuel for future attacks on the costs of the Medicaid program. Many, perhaps most, of the members of the other three welfare categories were eligible for Medicare as well as Medicaid.

26. The original Medicare Act provided for a 50–50 split in premium payment between the federal government (out of the General Fund) and the beneficiary. This limitation on increases resulted in the be-

neficiary's share of the premium falling to about 25 percent in later years.

27. In effect, this was the same as paying the HMO fee-for-service payments based on retroactive cost to hospitals and reasonable charges to physicians for services rendered the HMO's Medicare enrollees. This amounted to being much the same as the "reasonable" costs and "reasonable" charges payment methods being used by Medicare to pay all hospitals and physicians.

28. A number of these studies led to subsequent major changes in Medicare administrative practices. Best known of these is the institution of the prospective payment system for hospitals in 1983. (See p. 329). Changes in ways of paying physicians were made in the 1990s after a major study financed by the government.

29. The increases in payroll deduction rates for retirement (OASDI) are also relevant because the deductions for OASDI as well as for Medicare played a part in increasing the perception of wage earners that they were being heavily and regressively taxed for the benefit of the aged. Even though most polls showed that unionized wage earners favored the Social Security (including Medicare) program, the fact remained that wage earners perceived themselves as being increasingly pressed in meeting current obligations by a combination of rising inflation and taxes, including payroll taxes for Social Security.

30. In the jargon of government health services administration this became known as "vending" a particular class of providers, that is, classifying them as recognized vendors of services to the government.

31. The passage of the health Maintenance Act of 1973 further accentuated this trend. See page 324f.

32. Further research continued on this question, and by about 1985, a reasonably wide consensus had settled on an estimate of some 37 million persons being without any coverage at any particular time during a year.

33. As I have noted, even many of the aged purchased private health insurance in considerable numbers to cover the many gaps in Medicare coverage. For the aged poor receiving OAA, Medicaid paid the cost sharing, but of the others, 15 million persons, or 63 percent of the sixty-five-and-over civilian population had private "Medigap" insurance for hospital care in 1976 (Carroll and Arnett, 1981).

34. These are discussed below under "The Accelerating Emphasis on Cost Containment after 1972."

35. We recall the point made on page 303 that increased access and cost containment need not be mutually exclusive, but in the context of the economy and its resulting politics after 1972, they largely were. The cost-containers were directed at containing utilization even more than prices, and the access-increasers were not paying sufficient attention to cost-containment issues, including advocating cost-containment through price controls rather than access controls.

36. A tax structure is said to be progressive if higher earnings are taxed at a higher *rate*; it is said to be regressive if higher earnings are taxed at lower rates. If the tax rate is a constant on all earnings the tax structure is said to be proportional (Buchanan, 1970).

37. Since 1986, when the number of federal income tax rate brackets were sharply reduced and the maximum tax rate substantially lowered, the income tax has been even less progressive despite the closing of some loopholes, but it still retains some degree of progressivity.

38. These were later carefully investigated by the RAND health insurance experiment, which found that cost sharing did reduce medical care expenditures. What remains weakly documented is whether the reduction in utilization due to cost sharing is due to decreases in medically desirable or unnecessary services. See also page 275f.

39. Examples are the current practice of Medicare Part B and some commercial insurance in which the premiums are paid partly by the employer contribution and partly by deductions from employees' pay.

40. Actually, the coinsurance required of the patient was a stated percentage of the total fee "allowed" by the insurance system for specified services. If the provider were permitted to charge more than this "allowed" fee, the beneficiary would pay all of this excess, or "overbilling," as some now call it.

41. In 1972–73, of a total $375 per capita expenditure for personal health care, $84, or 22 percent, went for dentist visits, other professional services, drugs and medicines, and eyeglasses and appliances (HEW, Feb. 1974).

42. Pap smears were first covered as of July 1, 1990.

43. A *prospectively* set rate per (diagnostically classified) hospital stay, regardless of its length, will also reduce the incentive to increase utilization, but only partially, for although it reduces the incentive for long stays it does not reduce unnecessary admissions. It also introduces the necessity to set norms for appropriate stays for different diagnoses. This was later introduced in Medicare in 1983 as the DRG (diagnostically related groups) system, discussed later in the chapter. As of the early 1970s this method had not been used and therefore did not feature in the discussion of alternative plans for national health insurance.

44. See Table 10-3, method 7 for a definition of this term.

45. Detailed description of these bills may be found in Eilers and Moyerman, 1971 and Waldman, 1973.

46. The definition of *social* insurance (as opposed to private insurance) given by the American Association of State Health Insurance Commissioners includes the requirement that it be compulsory. There are many reasons for this, but this bill is one of several

examples that could be cited that called for government sponsorship for voluntary health insurance. This said, it remains true that an important feature of universal coverage government health insurance is its compulsory nature.

47. It was not until some five or six years later that the real but hidden public cost of tax deductions for health care expenditures would begin to become more prominent subject in health services literature.

48. The 1939 Wagner bill had called for state-sponsored health insurance whereas these bills proposed a national system.

49. Although the bill, like all the other NHI bills, did not pass, this particular provision did. It was enacted into law by passage of the "Health Maintenance Organizations Act" of 1973 (see page 324), some of whose provisions closely parallel this portion of the Griffiths-Kennedy Bill.

50. In later years some states (e.g., Hawaii in 1974 and Massachusetts in 1988) were to pass statewide health insurance laws whose underlying idea was mandating employers to provide insurance for their employees. National bills using this idea were being formulated by Senator Kennedy and Congressman Waxman in the late 1980s. In the 1990s, talk of "Health Care Reform" during the early Clinton administration prominently featured the employer mandating option.

51. We recall that imposing both an annual deductible and a coinsurance levy on the remaining expenditures was a feature of Medicare Part B and remains in effect without caps on annual totals.

52. In the language of welfare medical programs of that day, they were "vended."

53. If a piece of proposed legislation addresses a major overhaul of the entire health services system, such as the introduction of universal, comprehensive national health insurance, it is appropriate also to call for significant corrections of numerous structural weak spots in the existing system (although even then too many structural changes attempted at once may not be feasible and defeat the entire enterprise). But when the legislation calls for a proposed change in only one facet of the system, and as in the case of the HMO Act, the adoption of the change is made voluntary to boot, attaching many other required corrections of the system to the main proposal may dim or even extinguish the prospects for effective implementation. One gets the impression that the drafting of legislation to effect a modest structural change often turns into an exercise for an idealistic staff to draft a plan for a new world order in health services. But the setting of impossibly ambitious goals for subsystems like HMOs, community health centers (see Chapter 11) or local health planning agencies (see Chapter 15), without altering other crucial elements of the system in which they operated, was partly responsible for the difficulties these programs were to encounter as their administrators wriggled and squirmed to bend the regulations into some measure of feasibility.

54. The method of calculating this percentage was precisely indicated in the Amendments.

55. Some Medicare beneficiaries were enrolled in Group Practice Prepaid plans (GPPPs, as PGPs were called) under the original 1965 Medicare Act but most of these were not comprehensive plans. Under that act, hospitals and other Part A providers were paid by Medicare through the ordinary fee-for-service cost-based reimbursement methods using intermediaries. Physician services were paid for by a monthly capitation payment to the PGPP based on average costs of ambulatory services for Medicare beneficiaries to the PGPP. Enrollees were also reimbursed by Medicare for use of out-of-plan providers despite their membership in PGPPs. As noted previously, the 1972 amendments to Medicare did set up a payment mechanism by which Medicare could make a single capitated monthly payment that covered all Medicare services provided by the plan for its beneficiaries (by signing a so-called "risk contract"), but the health plan had to be a certified HMO and not just a PGPP to be eligible for such a contract (Muse and Sawyer, 1982).

56. That is, via a cost-reimbursement contract or a risk-sharing contract.

57. HMOs could charge premiums to their subscribers who were Medicare beneficiaries for those services the HMO provided that Medicare did not cover. These premiums were analogous to buying supplementary Medigap insurance from the HMO.

58. Exempted from this requirement were organizations that had received community health center or migrant health service grants under the Appalachian Regional Development Act.

59. This number had grown to 337 by December 1984.

60. These include group models, staff models, and network models.

61. The average adjusted per capita cost (AAPCC) for an HMO is "the average per capita costs for all Medicare beneficiaries" adjusted for the specificity of its service area by a geographic index and for the characteristics of its membership by considering its age, sex, institutionalized status and welfare status composition (Muse and Sawyer, 1982).

62. The conditions returned in even greater force in the early 1990s. (This is my footnote.)

63. These mostly took the form of reducing or forgiving the cost sharing required of the employee.

11

The Government-Supported Community Health Center

INADEQUATE ACCESS TO PRIMARY AMBULATORY CARE: A PERSISTING PROBLEM

By the 1960s it had become commonplace for writers, activists, and political figures to note that decreeing entitlement to health services was not the same as providing access.[1] For entitlement to be synonymous with access a crucial link was required—provider availability. For many "entitled" population groups this link has often been weak and sometimes even missing entirely. Availability has financial, geographic, and social dimensions while entitlement alone speaks only to legal (i.e. de jure) eligibility for a program's benefits. Full entitlement in a provider reimbursement program, for example, includes, the government being prepared to pay the prevailing market price for service to its eligibles if need be, and services being made available in areas where there was a shortage of private providers even at reimbursement rates equal to those paid by good health insurance.

The local public hospital had developed into the ultimate source of general medical care for low-income persons who could not find a suitable private provider, but even such hospitals were not accessible to many persons who needed them, whether or not they had entitlement from a government reimbursement program (see Chapter 7). For many medically needy persons the local public hospital was too far away, and in many localities there simply was no general public hospital for poor persons. Furthermore, the primary ambulatory care available in many local general public hospitals was often deemed to be inadequate and inappropriate for large numbers of poor people. In large cities the medical services of the outpatient department were usually controlled by a medical school or by postgraduate programs of a teaching hospital. The organization of the ambulatory services in such outpatient departments stressed specialty and subspecialty clinics while continuity of care, waiting times to see physicians, and travel times to the outpatient clinics were all said to suffer from the dominating influence of specialty medicine, concentrating on "interesting" teaching cases and acute episodic care to the detriment of ongoing management of patients' health problems. The low-income populations that used the public hospital's outpatient department had special need for social supports to render medical care effective, a need that was becoming more urgent as the proportion of the population of the inner city that was minority, permanently nonworking, or sporadically employed poor grew. Many poor persons were seen to be poor because of correctable health problems that persisted or worsened because they were poor. They needed health care that included adjuvant support services like social work, health education, and home visiting (all often including communication in languages other than English), which were not sufficiently stressed in many outpatient departments. One response to this perceived need was the federal attempt to get local public health departments to increase their provision of *general* medical primary care. But this project met with limited success because of many factors discussed in previous chapters. (See Chapters 2 and 7) Chief among these were the short-term, limited nature of the federal commitment and the historically formed structure of the local public health department, reflecting the attitudes of public health officers who agreed with the commonly accepted limiting of their scope of function to "preventive" activities.

Hopes were raised by the passage of the Medicaid Act in 1965 that many of the remaining shortfalls in providing access to primary ambulatory medical care would be remedied. A low-income person who had not had access to a convenient and appropriate source of primary care could now be expected to be able to use private physicians, seeing them either in their offices or in the private clinics used by some middle-class persons. The original act even provided that the optional nature of the two eligibility classes that states could elect to include or exclude from their programs—those persons who were not on federally matched cash grant assistance (see Chapter 10)—was to be only a temporary transitional arrangement. By 1975 all states were to be required to include in their Medicaid programs all persons without access to medical care and thus, in effect, the United States would have had universal access to medical care. But after first advancing this target date to 1977 the proviso was entirely repealed in 1972 (see p. 302). And even for those on its rolls, Medicaid provided only a partial solution of the access problem. The program was never willing to pay physicians the going rates they demanded and were getting from privately insured patients and those on Medicare. The costs of meeting these prices were considered prohibitive. The proportion of physicians who accepted Medicaid patients freely was never very large and dwindled further with time. Those who did accept and actually see large numbers of Medicaid beneficiaries often tried to equal the total income of physicians who did not by seeing a large number of patients, each for a short time, leading to public exposés of "Medicaid mills."

The downward turn of the U.S. economy in the 1970s, with the attendant drive toward cost containment, led the federal government to view the growth of Medicaid expenditures with increasing alarm. What continued to remain in place after the federal government entirely reneged in 1972 on its 1965 promise that Medicaid would become the vehicle of universal entitlement within a decade, was a legal entitlement for only some poor people and actual access to a smaller number still.

Many poor persons were indeed helped by Medicaid. Increases in utilization and improvements in health status were recorded for poor persons after 1965, and much of this was attributed to Medicaid (Davis and Schoen, 1978, 66). But many poor persons, including some entitled ones, received few or no benefits, which were unequally available among the states and between rural and urban areas. As Davis and Schoen remarked in *Health and the War on Poverty,* "benefit patterns bear no obvious relation either to the level of need or to health care costs" (1978:69).

The need to increase resources for providing actual access to services—clinics and personnel and not just payment programs with heavily circumscribed eligibility—had been evident to some policymakers in government as well as commentators and analysts for some time as they watched the attrition of public general hospitals and the severe eligibility restrictions of publicly supported medical programs for the poor before Medicaid. But the the need for the federal government to expand sources of locally available primary care in the middle 1960s rapidly became more widely perceived as an outgrowth of the development of the federal antipoverty program. It resulted in the launching of a program of federally financed neighborhood health centers (NHC) in 1965, the same year that Medicaid was passed. Thus, a system of federally supported neighborhood health centers for providing health care directly to the poor was established in the same year that the system for federal-state fee-for-service reimbursement of providers was substantially expanded. This chapter is mainly concerned with these NHCs, their historical roots, goals, development, significance, and fate.

The Neighborhood Health Center (later called Community Health Center) was managed by a privately organized local community board and financed by federal grants given to local government or private not-for-profit entities. Its services were free and accessible to all within its catchment area. Therefore, persons living in areas where an NHC was readily reached had access to the range of services the center supplied. For them, a source of specially designed appropriate care was actually available and eligibility was universal.

ANTECEDENTS OF THE NEIGHBORHOOD HEALTH CENTERS

The aims and scope of function of the OEO (see p. 342) NHCs derived from three different historical roots: the neighborhood health center sponsored by the public health department and/or private philanthropy; the prepaid group practice movement; and the "War on Poverty" program. The public health/philanthropic neighborhood health center and the prepaid group practice movement were initiated in the first half of the 1900s when their ways of delivering primary care were new and differed from the usual patterns of organizing medical practice. Their early manifestations were, by the very nature of their newness, crusading in spirit, with their founders and leaders often bent on demonstrating the feasibility of reformist theories of how health care should be organized. Overlaying the ideas of the two older historical developments were those of the Kennedy-Johnson War on Poverty, to which I shall return later.

The prime goal of the War on Poverty was to use the NHC as one of the programs to help eliminate—not just ameliorate—poverty. Beyond this, a number of notions about how the neighborhood health centers should be structured to meet the needs of their target populations were embodied in the program's design. These ideas were a mixture of those underlying the programs that were the progenitors of the NHC program. Some of the conceptual strands that were woven into the fabric of the NHC program were: (1) delivering primary care in the client's neighborhood; (2) using health teams with different types of practitioners to provide an integrated package of diagnostic, health education and promotion, disease prevention, and home health services; (3) providing health care to an enrolled population through a prepaid group practice working on salary; (4) eliminating poverty, since much poverty was related to poor health and poor health was a leading cause of disqualification for getting a job; and (5) giving poor persons opportunities for exercising initiative to learn how to use "the system" to get out of poverty. It was hoped that the NHCs would finally plug the remaining access loopholes in the health care system.

These ideas and visions of the 1960s neighborhood health center "movement" represent some of the main thoughts held by the leadership of this movement about changes needed in the organization of health care delivery to achieve equity, effectiveness, and efficiency and further the goals of the War on Poverty. They are helpful in understanding the ideas behind the federal program. In the following sections the three main roots of these ideas are considered historically.

The Public Health Department and the Philanthropically Sponsored Neighborhood Health Center

The first historical antecedent of the War on Poverty neighborhood health center, the public health/philanthropic neighborhood health center, or briefly, the public health neighborhood center, was a neighborhood branch of a local public health department (Hiscock, 1935). It evolved from the privately supported settlement house movement, which came to the United States from England in the late 1880s. Living in these settlement houses in the immigrant ghettos, reformers like Stanton Cort, Jane Addams, and Lillian Wald established neighborhood social services that were available at the settlement house and were also given in clients' homes. All sorts of troubles were brought to the settlement house workers by the local residents, involving problems with housing, jobs, health, and education. Because the health problems were important, health education, prevention, and first aid soon became major functions of the private settlements. The settlement workers lived in their clients' neighborhoods and aimed to become part of the community, with their services delivered "on terms most considerate of dignity and independence of patients" (Hiscock, 1935). One of these centers, the Henry Street Settlement of New York, was described by a professor of public health at Yale in these terms: "The local office soon became the neighborhood center, with mothers' clubs, behavior classes, and a milk station. Preschool and maternity clinics ... were associated with the nursing center while 'first-aid room' care was associated with the tuberculosis service" (Hiscock, 1935). A way of organizing primary care medical practice (albeit with only a rudimentary scope of medical services) to include both preventive services and close integration with family support services was demonstrated in these centers and left a lasting imprint on the development of ideas about how medical care should be organized. The notions of close personal relationship between settlement workers ("providers") and neighborhood clients, emphasis on prevention and health education, and integration of health and social support services in a one-stop service center were to become important goals of urban local public health departments in the period 1890 to 1940. The influence of these ideas is clearly seen in the early aims of the War on Poverty centers, aims that were formulated by persons some of whom were steeped in the history and spirit of the settlement house movement.

Coincident with the privately organized settlement house service centers established mostly in the 1890s other philanthropically sponsored neighborhood health service centers also developed, most of them focusing on mother and child welfare or on tuberculosis prevention and control. Much of this work was directed toward reducing the high infant mortality rate, and at first it was heavily concerned with infant feeding. Some sponsors of these centers took their lead from the work of Henry Koplik in New York and Francois-Joseph Herrgott and Pierre Budin in France, emphasizing the importance of breast feeding, while others followed Gaston Variot of France and stressed the distribution of safe cow's milk. One of the better-known philanthropic efforts establishing distribution centers for uncontaminated, pasteurized milk was the chain of milk stations opened across the country by Nathan Straus in 1893. The impressive results of the experience with these philanthropically supported stations in New York City led to their offical adoption by the city of Rochester in 1897. Gradually, mothers' education as a whole came to be stressed, especially instruction in sanitation and hygiene in the home (Hiscock, 1935). These and other philanthropic developments led to the evolution of a network of infant welfare stations in a number of large cities, notably New York, Cleveland, Philadelphia, and Boston. The service scope of the infant welfare stations were soon enlarged to encompass provision of prenatal and obstetrical care, exemplified by the Irene Kaufmann Settlement Health Center in Pittsburgh.

These disparate developments gradually coalesced into a health center "movement" with two main goals. One was to establish a widespread network of neighborhood health centers, each of which would be responsible for providing health services to a designated local population. This would combine the epidemiologic goal of enabling the collection of population-based local rates of disease incidence and prevalence with that of improving neighborhood access to health services. The other goal was to have the health center operate in an integrated, cooperative way with social-support services, especially social work.

While the earlier health centers were mostly under philanthropic sponsorship, local public health departments began to establish such centers in a number of cities between 1910 and 1935. In some cases the centers were built and some even initially operated under philanthropic auspices and later turned over to the city health department. In Boston the Department of Health established a neighborhood health and welfare center in 1916 (the Blossom Street Health Unit), and a chain of seven health centers was built by the philanthropist George Robert White and turned over to the city of Boston during the years 1924 through 1935. Each of these housed both a neighborhood health center of the Boston Department of Health as well as city welfare and private philanthropic service offices. In New York, several neighborhood health centers were established by the City Department of Health between 1914 and 1917, and a Division of Health Districts was formally established in 1917. In 1934 the New York City Health Department officially assumed control over a complex of health and welfare agencies that had been established in a central building in Harlem by twenty-one public and voluntary agencies. By that time a Bureau of District Health Administration had been established with a full-time director and seven full-time district health officers. Also in 1934, the federal Public Works Administration granted funds to construct seven health center buildings. Other major developments had taken place in Los Angeles county beginning in 1915 (see Chapter 7), with the first large health center completed in San Fernando in 1926 (Hiscock, 1935).

By 1930 there were 1,511 major and minor neighborhood health centers throughout the country, with 80 percent of them established after 1910. Of these about half (725) were directed by private agencies and 729 by local public health departments. The remaining 57 were operated by the American Red Cross, hospitals, child health organizations, social work agencies, tuberculosis associations, and the like.

One can readily see the similarity between the practices and programs of these neighborhood health centers and their predecessors to some of the initial goals of the later War on Poverty health centers: location in poor areas; one-stop service accessible to neighborhood residents, accessible being defined both in terms of short travel distances and affordability; emphasis on preventive services and health education; integration with support services; and close empathy between providers and clients. The adoption of the neighborhood health center organization, functions, and structure as part of the standard functions of local public health departments, often by direct absorption of existing neighborhood centers, was seen by some public health leaders as a modernizing development in what they called "public health administration." As Hiscock (1935) put it:

The problem of disease prevention is closely linked with social service, especially among families of low economic level, and the health and welfare workers may aid each other in the solution of their inter-related tasks. A health center of this type may be regarded as the latest development of the original infant welfare or milk stations . . . [and] is the focal point of modern *district* health administration. . . . The modern [in 1935] conception of a health center visualizes a community agency engaged primarily in *preventive* medicine and public *health education,* centering in an organization of physicians, nurses, and other health and social workers, and *volunteers.* It aims to reach all people within a *district* who need the services, and to coordinate the health, and sometimes the medical, recreation, and social service activities. Such an institution is sometimes called a major health center, in contrast with the so-called minor health center, which may be a well-child health conference or a small district headquarters for one or more specialized health services. In either case the program is designed *to supplement the services of the private physician.* [Emphasis added.]

As may be surmised from the last sentence of this quotation, the early health center movement of 1910–1935 did not usually provide *general* medical primary care. What made the public health department (and the philanthropically sponsored) neighborhood health center of this period "modern" was its location in needy neighborhoods and its increased, but still limited, emphasis on some personal health care: maternal and child health, venereal disease control, and tuberculosis control. Before 1910 the typical local health department in large cities had done local environmental control (sanitation), collected and kept vital statistics, and aided private physicians with laboratory support. These did not involve much contact with patients, especially not in their own neighborhoods, and the department facilities generally comprised only or mainly its central administrative quarters (see Chapter 2).

The Prepaid Group Practice

The Prepaid Group Practice has been an alternative way of organizing the practice of medicine in the United States in contrast to the mainstream form of solo private office practitioner who is paid fee-for-service by patients.[2] The pioneers of this form of practice organization argued that it was a better way to practice medicine from many points of view, but mainly that it produced superior medical practice because it conformed better to the conditions needed to apply modern biomedical knowledge than did solo, fee-for-service practice. Conceptually, the PGP would provide the patient with a comprehensive array of different medical specialists assisted by an appropriate complement of auxiliary staff with access to adequate equipment for diagnosis and treatment. Working as a group, the physicians could easily consult as needed, and informal peer review was constantly taking place. The prepaid features meant that there would be no economic incentives to prescribe unneeded services, on the one hand, nor would a physician have to hesitate to prescribe treatment because the patient perhaps could not afford it, on the other. Similarly, the economic basis for physician resistance to delegating tasks to allied health personnel would be greatly diminished.

Thus the principles of the Prepaid Group Practice movement called for a form of practice organization that was said to provide better medical care in a technical sense as well as guaranteeing better access. These points had been discussed in the medical care literature for many years, and the federal neighborhood health centers that were established in the 1960s showed the influence of these ideas.

The War on Poverty

The Great Society programs, begun under John Kennedy and implemented mostly under Lyndon Johnson, were meant to further the realization of the visions for America of Franklin D. Roosevelt's New Deal and Harry Truman's Fair Deal. They "included numerous services and benefits for those who were not poor" (Aaron, 1978). The War on Poverty was the component of the Great Society programs that concentrated on poor persons with the Office of Economic Opportunity (OEO) as its administrative agency. What distinguished the OEO programs from the others targeting the poor was their particularly strong emphasis on equipping the poor for jobs that paid enough for self-sufficiency. The overriding goal was to turn dependent persons into economically self-sufficient ones. Participants in OEO programs were to be the cutting edge in demonstrating how this might be done. The War on Poverty was a commitment to end poverty in the United States, not, as previously enacted antipoverty measures had intended, merely to alleviate it. It was meant to strike at the *causes* of poverty and eliminate them. The causes were assumed to lie not so much in the workings of an economic structure that was producing too few jobs as in the social structure that was producing people who were not equipped to compete in the job market. Specifically, the causes were primarily lack of education, work skills, and job experience. The situation could be remedied by programs designed to correct these lacks. Not only did the use of assistance in cash and kind as permanent solutions fail to remedy the causes of poverty, it actually helped to perpetuate it. "'Opportunity is our middle name,' the poverty warriors were fond of saying, 'We don't give handouts,' [OEO] Director Sargent Shriver said on many occasions" (Kershaw, 1970). It was not that assistance in cash and kind was entirely shunned, but the earlier programs, like cash assistance and publicly reimbursed medical care, were seen as income transfer programs that only provided needed sustenance for poor persons but did nothing to help them get out of poverty.

There would always be a need for such programs for a part of the poor population who could not be made employable. But for those poor persons who could be made employable the OEO programs were directed at making them so rather than merely providing them "relief" assistance. Welfare assistance was for permanently or temporarily disabled persons or for others going through temporary misfortune, the old "worthy poor," and temporarily unemployed groups. All who could work among the chronically nonemployed, the old "able-bodied poor," were to be rehabilitated to economic self-sufficiency.

The "war" was formally declared by President Johnson in his State of the Union Address of January 1964, barely two months after the assassination of President Kennedy. Calling for an "unconditional War on Poverty," he followed up with the appointment of a task force charged with drafting legislation to carry it out. The resulting law, the Economic Opportunity Act of 1964 (P.L. 88-452) set up the Office of Economic Opportunity (OEO) to administer the program. Nine specific programs made up the overall program, three to be administered directly by the newly created OEO and six delegated to existing government agencies.[3] In addition, programs like the later-enacted Elementary and Secondary Education Act of 1965 and Medicaid were also considered part of the War on Poverty, as were portions of certain programs that mainly helped other than poor persons, such as Social Security, veterans' benefits, urban renewal, and Medicare as well as previously enacted aids to the poor like public housing, public cash assistance, and the Manpower Development and Training Act of 1962.

The programs administered by the OEO itself, the core of the War on Poverty, were, as has been noted, looked upon as fundamentally different from earlier assistance programs for the poor in that their major task was seen to be making the unemployable employable. They consisted of three programs: the Job Corps for training youth in work skills; the Community Action Program (CAP) to encourage local participation in and control of the War on Poverty programs; and Volunteers in Service to America (VISTA), the "domestic Peace Corps" (Kershaw, 1970) to allow middle-class America to work in the poverty programs and to establish "a bridge between middle-class America and the poor" (Kershaw, 1970).

The emphasis on helping the poor by making them employable through education, training, and work experience rather than through direct financial support led to a policy that rejected public work job creation after a heated disagreement on this question in the Johnson task force. The underlying assumption was that the jobs would be available because of the expected growth in the economy. All that was needed was to render the physically eligible (i.e., able-bodied) poor competent to compete successfully in the job market. The OEO's emphasis on making poor persons employable through education and training was to have important effects on the future of the OEO programs. It meant that the effectiveness of programs, including the health centers, were to be judged against two goals. Not only were the health, education, and training programs to be judged on accomplishing their immediate objectives, providing good services and improving health, education, and skill status, but also on whether they increased the ability of the poor to compete for jobs in the marketplace based on actual employment figures (Aaron, 1978).

The OEO Health Centers

The subsequent entry of the OEO into health programs has been characterized as "inevitable" by a well-known chronicler and analyst of proverty programs (Levitan, 1969, 191). A correlation between poverty and ill health had been well established over the years (Davis and Schoen, 1978), and the question was now being raised whether improved health services for the poor would increase their employability. A priori it seemed reasonable that they would, for, if nothing else, "[E]ntry into training and employment programs normally included at least a diagnostic medical check-up and frequently remedial treatment was needed to help the poor bridge the gap from poverty to gainful employment" (Levitan, 1969).

Thus, although some of the goals of the OEO neighborhood health centers of the 1960s were those of the local health department neighborhood centers—the two held in common the aims of stressing prevention, health education, and neighborhood orientation—there were also important areas in which the aims of the OEO NHCs differed from those of their public health department and philanthropic antecedents. The main difference lay in the OEO centers' aim to provide *general* medical care, "personalized, high-quality care given by a 'professional staff of the highest caliber,'" and in the implied aim of obtaining at first at least a "registered" if not an "enrolled" population whose members would see the NHC as their major source of primary medical care. Indeed, as will be noted later, for a time some centers even tried to obtain an enrolled population.[4] The OEO centers, then, were attempting to combine the prepaid group practice concepts of *comprehensive* medical care provided in a group practice setting to a specified population with the earlier neighborhood health center ideas of emphasizing preventive services, health education, and supportive services and making them available to all who needed them. They represented the confluence of two major longstanding movements to reform the delivery of personal health care in the United States. Superimposed on these goals were those of the War on Poverty. These were to focus on the poor, to improve their clients' health in order to make them employable, and to operate the health centers in such a way as to give practical work experience to the neighborhood poor as well as community participation skills through directing the health center. A tall order.

The Economic Opportunity Act provided for the formation of local community action agencies (CAA), consisting of residents of poverty areas, their leaders, and local public officials. Under the administration of the Community Action Program (CAP) these local agencies were to mobilize the community to upgrade the economic conditions of the poor in their areas by a combination of local organization and participation in educational and training programs in all of which there would be, in the language of the act as amended in 1967, "maximum feasible participation of the areas and the members of the group served."

Many of the early health centers were closely allied, either structurally or by leadership outlook, to the community action agency (CAA), the local branch of the national Community Action Program (CAP) of the OEO. The CAP focus was on the eradication of poverty due to unequal employment opportunities, and the NHC had become a component of the CAP program mainly because poor health was considered an important barrier to employment. In 1965 the neighborhood health center (NHC) program was informally initiated by the Office of Program Planning of OEO. At first it provided grant support for ambulatory care programs in low-income communities on a ''research and demonstration'' basis. After eight health-care projects were funded in this manner, support for neighborhood health centers was formally established by legislation. A specific appropriation designated for this purpose was made in November 1966 with a special Comprehensive Health Services (CHS) program being set up within the OEO (Marcus, 1981). In 1967 the mandate of the Comprehensive Health Services program was expanded to include health personnel development and its scope of service to include family planning, alcoholism, and drug addiction. The Office of Health Affairs (OHA) was also established at this time within OEO and the Comprehensive Health Services program with its neighborhood health centers embedded in it. The OHA offered project grants to qualified local groups for establishing health centers that would offer primary care, largely with their own personnel. The NHC would be accessible, free, and governed by a board controlled by users of the services. An important corollary aim would be to employ local residents as community health workers for doing outreach work and facilitating communication between users and professional staff.

The OEO neighborhood health center was, then, a federally supported program providing direct ambulatory services under local government or private nonprofit auspices. The local NHC governing structure was intended to be consumer-dominated, and the grantee could be a government health department, a medical school, or a local association of activist-led laypeople. The forms of organization of the grantee organization were varied, but these were the main types.[5] Table 11–1 gives the distribution of NHC sponsorship by type of sponsoring organization for 1966 and 1971. As Roemer points out, this table indicates that the earlier grants

Table 11–1. Percentage of NHC Grants by Type of Center Sponsorship 1966 and 1971

NHC grant receipient	Percentage	
	1966	1971
Hospitals	50	10
Medical schools	37	7
Health departments	13	—
Private group practices	—	3
New organizations	—	59
Other	—	21
All sponsors:	100	100

Source: Zwick (1972), as adapted by Roemer (1981)

were largely to professional health organizations, while by 1971 they were going mainly to consumer organizations. The principal features of the OEO neighborhood health centers were declared to be: (1) a focus on the needs of the poor; (2) a one-door facility readily accessible with almost all primary and some secondary care ambulatory health services available; (3) ''intensive participation by and involvement of'' the target population both in policy making and as employees; (4) full integration with other existing sources of services and funds; (5) personalized, high-quality care given by a ''professional staff of the highest caliber''; (6) close coordination with other community resources; and (7) a wide variety of public and private sponsorship (Schorr and English, 1968).

By June 1968 30 primary-care ''projects'' (not all were formally organized as neighborhood health centers) were in operation and 44 more had been approved. They employed 700 physicians on a full- or part-time basis and were involved with one-quarter of the nation's medical schools. Some of the policy issues that had come to the fore were: (1) the working out of ''totally'' new relationships between consumers and providers and making policy more responsive to consumer wishes; (2) the development of new health personnel roles and careers with new methods of training; (3) the degree of participation by the NHC in community action to improve social support services such as welfare, housing, and education; (4) the degree to which the NHC itself should offer nonhealth services and day care; and (5) how to adapt the typical ''mainstream'' health service delivery system to offer more personalized and family centered care and still conform sufficiently to accepted high technical medical quality to attract "professional personnel of high caliber" (Schorr and English, 1968).

Many of the early health centers, were closely allied, either structurally or by leadership outlook to the Community Action Agency (CAA), the local branch of the national Community Action Program (CAP) of the OEO. Those NHCs whose structure or leadership outlook were most strongly motivated by the CAP goals laid special emphasis on achieving community outreach, encouraging client input into program operations, and employing neighborhood poor people at the center. There was always a conflict between the persons stressing these goals and those wishing to concentrate more on the technical medical excellence of the centers because they had a more restricted view of the goals of the health center. They saw these goals as being more confined to achieving medical excellence in delivering primary and "some secondary" health care to the target population.

Undertaking to provide "comprehensive" and "high quality" primary medical care to their target populations implied the employment of highly trained primary physicians, the availability of up-to-date equipment and facilities, and a referral system to specialist consultation and inpatient care. In this area the experiences of the earlier public health neighborhood health centers was of limited value as a guide. At their best, those were devoted to performing the "basic six" public health functions well and in depth. They offered, for the most part, only those personal medical services included in these six and typically might have readily available specialist consultation and inpatient facility liaison for tuberculosis, maternal and child health, and venereal disease cases, but all other medical problems were referred to the local public hospital or a nonprofit philanthropic private hospital if one was available. The OEO centers were proposing to treat or manage all types of cases including following them through consultation with recommended specialists or perhaps even seeing them in the hospital, as private physicians do.

The attempt to be medically sophisticated ("high-quality care given by a 'professional staff of the highest caliber'") while also carrying out the social and behavioral goals—emphasizing health education and prevention, closer empathy between clients and employees of the center, use of local volunteers, assigning a high degree of responsibility to nurses, and having a large home-visiting component—created a dilemma. Maintaining good networking relationships with referral specialists and hospitals meant employing NHC physicians with good credentials in formal advanced training. Having such physicians at the center tended to encourage a great degree of overall decision making about policy and priorities by highly expert physicians and less by clients, social workers, and even nurses. The contradiction between the needs and priorities of the social rehabilitation and support functions and the technical medical functions of the NHCs remained unsolved and led to a great deal of controversy and confrontation at many of the centers and in their governing boards.

There were repercussions in Congress from these issues, and the OEO, wishing to show that neither medical excellence, cost-efficiency nor effectiveness were suffering, commissioned a series of evaluations of the operations of the NHCs. It was also expected that these evaluations would serve as research guides to indicate which approaches worked and which did not in building a network of local population-based primary care centers. The general tenor of the findings was that "the performance of the centers is equal to and in some cases superior to that of other providers" with respect to quality of care (Morehead, Donaldson, and Seravalli, 1981) while the costs of operation of clinic service units were "comparable to private providers. Annual per capita costs of these services are competitive with those reported for major prepayment group practices. The costs of supporting services unique to NHC operation are less than 20 percent of total cost and more often under about 10 percent" (Sparer and Johnson, 1971). Other evaluations carried out under other auspices reached similar conclusions. A policy review in 1972 by an HEW analyst (Zwick) noted that: "The capability of health centers to reduce needs for costly inpatient care has been documented in a number of cases. . . . The health center program has tended to place increasing control and responsibility in consumers. . . . [and] The annual per capita costs attributable to outreach, transportation and such special items as in-service education appear to be less than the costs of a half day of inpatient care.''

A 1982 study by independent academic researchers reviewed survey data collected by the OEO during two periods: 1968–1971 and 1975 (Freeman, Kiecolt, and Allen, 1982). These surveys had covered five communities across the country that had NHCs in the planning stage during 1968–1971 and that had centers in operation by 1975 (by which time they were called Community Health Centers). The study found that (1) CHCs served low-income and minority areas with the same frequency of ambulatory visits and ''probably'' with the same costs as private physicians' care; (2) they ''considerably'' lowered use of hospital outpatient departments (OPDs) and emergency rooms (ERs); (3) their target population experienced ''measurably'' lower hospital inpatient utilization, even after controlling for differences in population characteristics.

Despite these favorable reviews, opposition to the OEO health center program mounted in Congress and was clearly evident in the White House during the Nixon and Ford administrations. The germ of this opposition had been there from the first, but the onrushing tide of support for the War on Poverty emanating from the Johnson White House and the liberal Congress had muted it. With time, as the government, the media, and academia became more conservative and conservatively oriented research institutes grew, opposition to the NHCs mounted. This occurred despite the fact that the opposition from two important professional sources—local medical societies whose members had been apprehensive about possible competition and academic medical quarters that had expressed misgivings about the technical quality of the medicine practiced in the centers—had been largely neutralized by the Office of Health Affairs (OHA) of the OEO.[6] It was chiefly the fact that the NHCs were part of the War on Poverty program with its proactivist and community organizing philosophy that raised obstacles to their being judged simply as demonstrations of how to provide community-oriented primary care to poor persons effectively and efficiently. The opposition from ideological opponents of the social programs encompassed by the War on Pov-

erty was politically much more powerful and sustained than any professional fears of competition or low quality, and eventually it prevailed in diluting many of the innovatory features of the OEO neighborhood health centers.

In addition to blaming the OEO programs for contributing to the unrest in ghetto areas, the campaign to eliminate the OEO was buttressed by research showing that these programs were not perceptibly eliminating poverty. There was a ''collapse of the intellectual consensus about the nature of and solution to poverty and unemployment, about how to improve education and training. . . .'' (Aaron, 1978, 155). In his perceptive analysis of the effect of this research on national thinking and why it was so derogatory of the results of the War on Poverty programs, Brookings scholar Henry Aaron noted the circumstances that made this research ''an intellectually conservative force in debates about public policy'' (1978, 158). After listing a number of well-known caveats about uncritically accepting results of this type of social research,[7] he stresses a critique that proved to be particularly harmful to the cause of the OEO centers in the debate over their accomplishments because it lay beyond effective defense by argument pertaining to the centers' activities. One frequent criticism was that although a War on Poverty program was operating well in terms of its own objectives (such as providing useful services at acceptable costs to target populations that had previously not received these services) it was not demonstrably contributing to the result that proponents of the program had predicted for the War on Poverty as a whole: more jobs, fewer people on welfare, less (almost no) poverty. Many of the programs were dubbed unsuccessful by outside evaluators because they could not be shown to have directly contributed to returning many unemployed poor persons to the ranks of the economically self-sufficient. Aaron argues that the reason they could not was due to the original misconception of the causes of unemployment and poverty rather than demonstrable operating faults of the OEO programs. Much of the failure to obtain jobs was due to discrimination against the poor because of race or cultural attitudes. Perhaps even more important, the unemployment rate had always varied more according to the stage of the business cycle the economy was in than the educational and training level of the poor. But the studies making the "poor employment record" critique did not look in these directions; they merely asked whether the programs had substantially increased employability (as proved by actual employment), as the legislation demanded, and found that they had not.

All this was very much true of the OEO health center program. The audits and other surveys of its operation, as noted above, found the centers to be useful, economically run, and providing care of high quality, but their effects on eliminating the causes of poverty were not provable. Also, the conflicting goals set for the centers often made it impossible to satisfy all of them at the same time. An example of how conflicting goals laid down by Congress affected the program is provided by a report of a GAO investigation in 1978 as to whether the NHCs were "providing services efficiently and to the most needy." Among other things, the report stated that some centers were making conscious efforts to extend their market into areas that would yield more patients who could pay or who were covered by a third party and were thereby serving clients from areas that were not designated as underserved. But by 1978, although federal goverment policy was still demanding that the centers concentrate on reaching uncovered populations, it was at the same time insisting that they also become increasingly self-sufficient financially through obtaining increased user payment. Similarly, many centers were found to devote too little of their effort to preventive services, yet the federal government was cutting its grant support for preventive services, and its third-party payment programs (including Medicare and Medicaid) did not, in general, reimburse for such services.

The opposition to the Neighborhood Health Centers was first reflected in moves to transfer the program away from the OEO to HEW. Along with the transfer came changes in emphasis in the management and service content. We recall that in 1966 (see Chapter 4) the Public Health Service Act had been amended to include a new section, Section 314e, providing for special project grants to public health departments. The Partnership for Health Amendments of 1967 had provided grants for community health projects to be administered by HEW. When Nixon assumed the presidency in 1969 he used the appropriations for section 314e to award grants establishing new HEW health centers, which were to be administered by the Bureau of Community Health Services (BCHS) of Health Services Administration (HSA). Between 1970 and 1973 control over many of the existing OEO centers was shifted in stages to the Department of Health, Education and Welfare, and in 1973 OEO was abolished, with all its remaining Neighborhood Health Centers turned over to HEW. HEW administration was seen to be more strictly medically oriented, and with OEO gone the centers would presumably be free of the War on Poverty orientation with its emphasis on social activism.

However, there was also an attempt to sharply reduce the size of the health center program. The Community Health Center Act of 1974 repealed section 314e of the Public Health Service Act and added a new section 330 dealing with the neighborhood health centers, defining their mandated services and the criteria for determining the medically underserved areas (MUAs) of the United States. In 1976 all Neighborhood Health Centers, Family Health Centers and Networks of various health providers were reclassified by HEW as community health centers (CHCs) (Davis and Schoen, 1978, 170). The Nixon and Ford administration made repeated attempts to cut the number of centers and reduce the level of funding but could not prevail on Congress to do so (see Chapter 4). President Ford made several attempts to give the states the option of funding the CHCs but these also were not successful (Davis and Schoen, 1978). However, the centers received no increase in funding despite the substantial inflation prevailing at the time. Thus what had originally been envisioned as a program of 1,000 centers serving 25 million persons funded at $3.35 billion would up in 1976 with 125 centers serving 1.5 million persons funded at $197 million. The program content also changed substantially in response to attacks, becoming more technically medical.[8]

The demand by Congress that the centers increase their fee collection was a particullary erosive development. In the initial years of the program, services were free of any requirement for out-of-pocket payment by the patient. It was anticipated that Medicare and Medicaid would meet a substantial portion of the NHCs' costs, perhaps as much as 80 percent. But opposition from local providers had caused Congress to change the law in 1967 to restrict care at the centers largely to very low-income patients, limiting paying or partially paying patients to 20 percent of all registrants. This federal stance was reversed by later amendments that "encouraged the centers to admit patients who were not poor, to charge a sliding fee schedule based on patients' incomes, and to recoup, where possible, revenues from third parties. Pressure on the centers to become, or at least to behave like, financially self-supporting medical practice intensified" (Davis and Schoen, 1978).

But the patient income simply was not there. The criteria for a federally supported Community Health Center demanded that it serve a Medically Underserved Area. It was very unlikely that persons using these centers in such areas could contribute anything substantial, even on a "sliding scale" fee schedule. In addition, the expected income from Medicaid and Medicare did not materialize, reaching only 10 to 20 percent of the operating costs by 1975. For one thing, most third-party payers, including Medicaid, did not reimburse many of the supportive and preventive services offered by the centers. Basically, third-party payers covered strictly medical services. Many state Medicaid programs did not then cover services provided in clinics, and an attempt to get the federal government to cover such services under Medicaid with only 5 percent state matching was defeated in 1972. And Medicare usually did not pay for services rendered by nurse practitioners and physician's assistants (Davis and Schoen, 1978). "Consequently, the program had to rely on annual appropriations and federal grants for its continued survival" (Davis and Schoen, 1978). Also, by 1978 the HEW centers were no longer funded for training personnel, and funds for environmental and other nonmedical activities were reduced.

In its efforts to adapt to the changing Congressional climate and unfriendly federal administrations, the national health center program had sought to develop new structural forms that would tap additional sources of income. In the early 1970s the national administrative agency

of the HEW neighborhood health centers, the Bureau of Community Health Services (BCHS), adopted a policy of encouraging voluntary enrollment by Medicaid clients as HMO members in a health center with the state Medicaid program paying the premiums. Non-Medicaid low-income families might enroll on their own. Health centers using this mechanism were called Family Health Centers, and they involved 35,000 persons. The term family health center was subsequently discontinued but the practice continued. Also in the 1970s the "health network" was adopted by BCHS. Groups of existing ambulatory care facilities in selected metropolitan areas were linked together as a system to supply care to poor people. The network was supported by a consolidated grant, and as of 1976 there were ten such networks involving 25,000 users. By 1980 this term, too, had been discontinued. By that time only one such network still existed—in Rochester, New York (Roemer, 1981).

With the advent of the Reagan administration the federal government attempted to transfer responsibility for the Community Health Centers to the states as part of the devolution of federal grants for health. At first there was an attempt to fold them into one of the other block grants, but this was defeated in Congress. Instead, the Omnibus Budget Reconciliation Act of 1981 (OBRA), P.L. 97–35, treated the CHCs as a single block grant, the Primary Care block, thus keeping the federal funding earmarked for CHCs. (see Chapter 4). Since OBRA did not permit states to begin taking over the CHCs until the beginning of FY 1983, the fact that the federal money that came with it would not be in a catchall block grant like the Preventive Health and Health Services block, would, for the time being at least, serve as some protection for the centers against hostile state administrations.

OTHER TYPES OF GOVERNMENT-SPONSORED COMMUNITY HEALTH CENTERS

Although the community health center program was the main source of sponsorship for this form of health services delivery, other federal programs in the 1960s and 1970s also sponsored neighborhood health centers providing medical care with federal funds and featuring private and local government administration.[9]

In 1962 Congress passed the Migrant Health Act, which provided grants to states and localities to establish or help support existing clinics for migrant agricultural workers and their dependents. By 1979 there were 112 clinics in 35 states serving an estimated 557,000 migrants and supported by $34.5 million in federal grants. These clinics comprised a wide assortment of facilities offering services ranging from full-time and comprehensive to intermittent and categorical and operating in various types of facilities ranging from standing clinic facilities to those that only referred patients to private physicians or offered essentially only consultative services. The Rural Health Clinic Services Act of December 1977 permitted Medicare and Medicaid to reimburse these clinics for the services of physician extenders "even though a physician was not permanently at hand" (Roemer, 1981). These migrant workers clinics did not, in general, have the formal structure of the Community Health Centers or their progenitor OEO Neighborhood Health Centers. They were more modest in scope, being established to fill a local gap in service for a special transient population and their goals did not include demonstrating a "new" model of comprehensive primary care. They were, however, a step forward in providing a solution to a rural health service problem that the original OEO center had not addressed.

Other forms of more modest clinics were established in rural areas and in central-city ghetto areas. The Applachia Regional Commission, organized in the mid-1960s as part of the War on Poverty, helped local communities start and operate small primary care clinics, some of which were no more than a private physician's office. In 1978, 101 such rural clinics were operating supported by $10.1 million in grant support from the Commission.

In 1975 the Bureau of Community Health Services established the Rural Health Initiative by administrative action. Existing authority for health center funds was used in a flexible way to expand existing nonprofit health facilities in rural areas as well as to establish new ones. In a book coauthored by Karen Davis, a former Assistant Undersecretary for Health of HEW in the Carter Administration, the promotion of this form of center is considered evidence of the "stagnating" of the neighborhood health center program after HEW took it over.

The Nixon and Ford Administration downplayed the neighborhood health center model and supported less comprehensive approaches such as the rural health initiative projects, which use National Health Service Corps personnel and are usually sponsored by county governments, and family health centers, which emphasize a more traditional range of medical services for family health care. In part the programs were added to reduce the OEO centers' original emphasis on urban poverty and relative neglect of rural problems; the new projects, being smaller, are better able to survive in areas of low population density (Davis and Schoen, 1978, 171–172).

In 1979 this type of grant was extended to underserved inner-city areas under an "Urban Health Iniative" program. Also in the late 1960s, the Department of Housing and Urban Development (HUD) included in its Model Cities program of urban development funds for establishing or expanding clinics "for children, drug abusers, or others" (Roemer, 1981). Some HUD funds were used to help support CHC and Urban Health Initiative clinics.

The Maternal and Infant Comprehensive Care (MIC) and the Children and Youth (C&Y) clinics discussed in Chapter 4 should also be recognized as part of the neighborhood health center development. The MIC clinic programs were administered by state health departments, but the clinics were again operated by an assorted group of different nonprofit health service providers. In 1975 the federal grants for C&Y clinics were folded into the Maternal and Child Health (MCH) money given to states under Title V of the Social Security Act (see Chapter 4). The inconsistencies in various sources of official data on the number of local health centers make it difficult to accurately estimate the size of this phenomenon.[10] It would seem that there were in 1979 over nine hundred federally supported centers under the various classifications shown in Table 11–2. According to a 1976 survey that counted 872 centers, they were serving 4.2 million persons of whom 71 percent were poor, 80 percent minority, 49 percent had no employed family members and 41 percent were under 18

Table 11–2. Comprehensive Health Centers Supported by Federal Grants: Unduplicated Count, 1979

Type of health center	Number
Community health center[a]	158
Rural health initiative clinic (RHI)	356
Health underserved rural area clinic[b]	41
Migrant health clinic[c]	39
Urban health initiative clinic	77
Appalachian health clinic[d]	80
Maternity and infant care (MIC) clinic	88
Children and youth (C & Y) clinic	98
All health centers[e]	937

Source: Roemer, 1981.

[a]These include the original neighborhood health centers of the OEO, plus the equivalent health centers initiated by the HEW. They also include health centers partially supported by prepayment, formerly termed "family health centers" or "health networks."

[b]These HURA clinics were originally funded by the SSA Medicaid program but later transferred to the BCHS of the PHS, where they are now regarded as equivalent to RHI clinics.

[c]Beyond these 39 migrant health clinics, there are an additional 73 projects receiving migrant health project grants, thus totaling 112 clinics serving migrants. These 73 are, however, included in other categories (such as RHI clinics), and therefore excluded here to avoid double counting.

[d]These 80 clinics are the facilities, among the 101 mentioned in the text, that meet qualifications entitling them to grants from the BCHS.

[e]Dr. Roemer's text explains that there is a probable understatement of this total.

(Davis, Gold, and MaKuc, 1981). These comprised "in sum, the population that has the highest health risks; the greatest burden of illness, disability, and preventable death; the least access to primary care; and the highest rates of hospitalization" (Geiger, 1983).

The "Community-Oriented Primary Care" (COPC) Concept

Although the notions of making primary care available at the neighborhood level and of providing ambulatory care by a salaried group of physicians and other health professionals to a specified target population had been known and tried for many years, the development of the OEO Neighborhood Health Centers in the 1960s gained a currency for these ideas on a scale previously unknown. Because the Neighborhood Health Centers were part of the OEO's War on Poverty program, some of their initiators and promoters at the national level presented them to Congress primarily as important levers for reducing poverty because they would help improve employability. A part of this argument was that they would help poor communities organize themselves to take better advantage of government programs for improving the health of the poor as a means for getting themselves out of poverty. As such they were the health adjuncts of the OEO Job Corps and Community Action Programs.

As has been noted, other elements in the national leadership of the NHC administration were primarily interested in demonstrating a better way to delivery primary care. They concentrated more on assuring that the technical level of medical care was good, that access was actual instead of merely declared, and that support services needed to make the medical care effectual were available. They were strongly interested in advancing the art of evaluating the quality of medical care and furthered its application to medical practice. The year 1983 (when the states began taking over the Community Health Centers under the OBRA-81 block grant provisions) saw some of these people staying on to operate surviving Community Health Centers and others having become involved in academic teaching and training programs dealing with community health centers. Using the experience with the Neighborhood Health Centers/Community Health Centers and looking at experiences abroad to adjust and expand their arguments in support of this type of primary care delivery, some propounded an idea of what they called Community Oriented Primary Care (COPC). Their ideas were set forth in a number of papers presented at a conference held by the national Institute of Medicine in 1982 (Geiger, 1983). In one of these papers, Dr. H. Jack Geiger generalized the COPC ideas in a formulation that clearly showed some of its Community Health Center origins. A COPC system of medical practice would ideally include the following basic features: (1) complementary use of epidemiologic and clinical skills; (2) a defined population; (3) programs designed to deal with the health problems of the community or its subgroups in the primary care framework; (4) community involvement in both governance and implementation of the practice; (5) geographic, fiscal, and cultural accessibility; and (6) integration of curative, rehabilitative, preventive, and promotive health care (1983). The important "new" point claimed for this thinking is *"the insistence that all these elements of community orientation, demographic study, epidemiologic investigation, personal medical services, environmental intervention, community organization and health education be performed by the same practice or team,* or at least by a small number of practices and health agencies *working as a single system* (not just 'coordinated')." Geiger particularly stressed that COPC should use a model of primary care delivery that fused epidemiological and other public health approaches with the clinical practice of medicine and use managerial, administrative, and organizational methods that would bring this type of medical practice to a defined population.

The idea of tying medical practice closely to epidemiological studies of the target population and emphasizing preventive and health promotive measures based on the findings of the epidemiological studies is, as Dr. Geiger notes, an old one. It is the basis of public-health-oriented health planning and it was envisioned as one of the benefits that might be expected from the public health neighborhood health center (1983). But to be able to do this one needs an organization of practice that has a target population on which denominators can be obtained for health indicator rates[11] and a financing system that pays for the extraclinical activities and provides access for the entire target population.

CLOSING REMARKS

This chapter is the last of Part III, which deals with government outlays for health care of specified populations. Programs that have been passed to fill the void in medical care coverage for large numbers of the U.S. population, mostly the poor and near poor, have been described. From the Social Security Act of 1935 through the War on Poverty legislation the development and provisions of MCH, crippled children programs, Medicare, Medicaid, and other have been surveyed. The neighborhood health center described here completes the major programs. It should be noted that the concepts that have been added by advocates and organizers of the health

center movement are community control, neighborhood availability, and the special importance of the integration of medical with social services for disadvantaged populations.

All these programs have been gap-fillers in the face of the failure to enact universal entitlement to medical care. They have all followed similar paths. Typically, they were initiated during times of relative economic prosperity and their early history was one of expanding resources accompanied by a rising trend of support among intellectuals and commentators. When the economy took a downturn the trend of opinion turned negative and a period of reductions in support for the programs began, culminating in their sharp attrition or even complete elimination.

It is not surprising, of course, that in times of retrenchment health care for the poor and near poor should be so vulnerable. This is perhaps one of the principal reasons for advocating a single system in any national health insurance proposal. While there is not, and perhaps never will be, any inbuilt structural feature that will guarantee that the poor and near poor will not be the first to suffer cuts in health service access, a single system of eligibility to equal benefits will still be a strong deterrent against harsh victimization of the poor in times of economic hardship. This has been shown by the national health insurance systems of the other developed countries.

NOTES

1. In terms of the more general formulation throughout this book, this constituted a greater public acknowledgment that enunciated policy, or even de jure policy, should not be confused with de facto policy.

2. "Solo" here includes the small-group single-specialty practice.

3. These were the Department of Labor, the Office of Education in HEW (two programs), the Farmers Home Administration in the Department of Agriculture, the Small Business Administration and Welfare Administration in HEW (Levine, 1970, 52).

4. An enrolled population is one whose members "sign up" with a particular provider agreeing to use that provider for all their health care entailing specified services. It usually involves a capitation periodic flat fee. A registered population is one whose mem-

bers have used a particular provider at least once during a specified period, usually one year. These aims were more akin to those of the prepaid group practice movement than the public health neighborhood health center.

5. Milton I. Roemer (1981) has summarized the experience of some of the better known and larger centers that were organized in the early years of the program.

6. The earlier traumatizing experience with the provision of general medical care by public health departments, like that of Los Angeles County in 1934 (see Chapter 2), had influenced the earlier public health neighborhood health centers to avoid clashes with local medical societies that might result from their being perceived as threats to the practices of local private physicians. The core group of health professionals and program analysts who drafted the plans and obtained support for the first OEO health centers were well aware of this problem: "potential opposition from the AMA to reformist ideas of prepaid group-practice-type medicine had been neutralized by the senior staff within the OEO who had made it clear to the AMA that the project would not interfere with existing private practices of AMA members" (Marcus, 1981, 15).

7. Chief among these were the ambiguous and often contradictory goals set forth for War on Poverty programs; the drive of young academics to achieve status by challenging the conclusions of the dominant academics who had helped formulate the programs; the masking of a priori held values under cloaks of technical neutrality; and the methodological weaknesses of social science in proving causality in a multivariate world.

8. By 1978 the mandated services of a CHC under section 330 were:

1. Diagnostic, treatment, consultative, referral, and other services rendered by a physician or a "physician extender" (nurse practitioner or physician assistant).
2. Diagnostic laboratory and X-ray services.
3. Preventive health services, including nutritional assessment, medical-social services, well child care, immunizations, etc.
4. Emergency medical services.
5. Transportation, as required for patient care.
6. Preventive dental services.
7. Pharmaceutical services (drugs).

The "high priority supplemental services" that HEW could refuse to fund if it could be demonstrated that they were not needed were:

8. Home health services.
9. Dental services.
10. Health education.
11. Bilingual and outreach services.

The criteria for defining an area as medically underserved were derived from a formula combining variables that measure the following four features:

1. Poverty level, defined by local per capita incomes.
2. An excessive infant mortality rate.
3. A shortage of primary care physicians (including general practitioners, pediatricians, internists, and family practice specialists).
4. A certain proportion of people over sixty-five year of age.

This description of services and medically underserved area designation is from Roemer, 1981.

9. Most of the information in this section is based on Roemer, 1981, chap 9.

10. These inconsistencies are explored by Dr. M. Roemer (1981).

11. Geiger's paper offers suggestions on how this might be approached even by existing group practices that operate on a fee-for-service basis. In essence, he proposed that such a group use the "registration" system for determining denominators, that is, consider the patients that use the practice as the target population (see note 4 above). Depending on the stability of the clientele the method can produce results, but it is not the same as actually having an *enrolled* population or a geographic areawide target population.

There is an aspect of these ideas that lay at the core of the conception that Herman Biggs brought to the work of the New York City Health Department in the 1880s (see Chapter 2). In establishing the first local public health laboratory Biggs envisioned that prevention would be enhanced by a liaison between the public health department and private practitioners in the community. By providing needed immunizing biologics and laboratory diagnosis based on analysis of specimens provided by private practitioners, the local public health department would encourage the introduction of more preventive care into the private practice of medicine. And the health department would take advantage of the close liaisons thus formed between it and private medical practitioners to guide the emphases of private practice in directions indicated by the department's epidemiological monitoring of the community's health status. Public health departments attempted to further this aim by requiring reporting of the incidence of certain ("reportable") diseases and by informing practitioners of current developments in preventive techniques and the status of epidemics.

Biggs's approach never became a prominent factor in much of private practice because of the lack of strong enforceability and became even weaker with the advent of private laboratories for medical diagnoses. The post-Flexner medical school complex, rather than the public health department, became the central guiding influence on the content and orientation of private medical practice. The emphasis became the subspecialty and the acute technological component of care rather than the shaping of primary care to meet needs indicated by community health status indicators.

12. Of course, if there is a multitude of jobs that pay a living wage for which qualified workers cannot be found in the face of existing large numbers of potentially physically able employables, then improved health services or education might be the answer. But even then, such factors as affordable housing and child care may be the main factors, i.e., the wage offered may not really be a living wage.

IV

Government Roles in Developing Health Services Resources, Promoting Research, and Fostering Coordination and Planning of the Health Delivery System

12

Government Support for Expanding the Supply of Health Facilities

THE HILL-BURTON LEGISLATION

The adequacy of the national stock of medical care facilities and personnel was under continuing scrutiny by federal administistrators and by writers in the field of medical care organization during the years of national debate over health insurance after World War II. If we were to have universal entitlement to medical care, surely the demand for services would increase and the existing supply of resources would be inadequate. Just how many facilities and medical personnel would then be needed? It would not do to wait until demand increased, for medical care resources are not produced overnight. And although universal entitlement was never legislated in the United States, the various gap-filling programs that were established did increase demand substantially during the postwar years. Increasing the national supply of resources turned out to have been an example of justifiable anticipatory planning.

Determining the actual number of facilities that would be needed, however, presented many problems. The question most often raised was, "How many hospital beds are needed?" The earliest attempts to answer this question were based on a combination of extrapolating empirical data and applying theoretically derived formulas that gave answers in terms of total number of beds per population: a certain number of general acute beds and a certain number of specialty types such as tuberculosis beds. However, it was soon found that estimates of the required number of beds derived from the application of a fixed national beds-to-population ratio (e.g., 4.5 general acute care beds per 1,000 persons) to the

population of every state or local region did not give accurate, and sometimes not even sensible, estimates for many areas. The required number was found to be dependent on corollary questions. How should beds be geographically distributed within the local area, that is, where should the hospitals be located and how many beds should be in each hospital[1]? What should the composition of total beds be in terms of the types of patients they were intended to serve, i.e., long-term, short-term, general, special, high-intensity care, nursing care, and the like? Should these various facilities with different types of beds be linked in regional networks, and if so how should this be done?

Even for a small, relatively closed community with only a single hospital, the answer to the question, "How many hospital beds are required?" could not be definitively answered. A determination of "proper" level of hospital utilization also eluded investigators, depending as it did on what services were offered by ambulatory facilities as well as on prevailing styles of medical practice that differed substantially from place to place in the customary hospitalization rate for the same illness. And when one tried to estimate this quantity for more populous areas with numerous hospitals available to the population, the problems were correspondingly multiplied.

But perhaps the greatest obstacle to properly determining need was the absence of universal entitlement to hospital service. A fundamental planning assumption used (usually implicitly) in making most estimates of need for hospital beds was that all persons would use the medically appropriate hospital within the shortest distance of their dwelling. This assumption was in fact widely inapplicable because so many persons would only be served at special hospitals set up for special populations (e.g. Veterans Administration, local government).

Before 1946 there had been a number of studies of this question. Three of the main ones were:

1. The Lee-Jones Report of 1933, *The Fundamentals of Good Medical Care*, one of the component volumes of the study by the Committee on the Costs of Medical Care.
2. The report of the Commission on Hospital Care, *Hospital Care in the United States* (the Bachmeyer Report). It was not actually published until 1947, but the research went on during the years 1944–1946 and its contents substantially influenced the Hill-Burton legislation despite its official publication one year after the Hill-Burton Act was passed.
3. The 1945 Public Health Report of Joseph W. Mountin and associates, "Requirements for General Hospitals and Health Centers." It used much of the material of the Commission on Hospital Care, and recommended a nationwide regionalized hospital system.

The Lee-Jones Report was a landmark investigation. Its approach, scope, and techniques will be discussed more completely in Chapters 13 and 15 from the viewpoint of their importance to health planning methodology. Here the important point is that the study laid out national facilities and personnel requirements for a system of medical care to meet the medical care *needs*[2] of the population. The report found the supply of physicians adequate but hospital beds in short supply. This finding (and many of the data that underlay it) was used as the basis for the postwar federal effort to increase the number of hospital beds.

The other two studies also materially influenced the content of this legislation. For example, the Commission on Hospital Care developed the concept of requisite local bed supply per population being in part a function of population density, and the Public Health Service (or Mountin) Report raised lawmakers' consciousness about the virtues of regionalization. But the numbers of acute beds required per thousand population recommended by the Lee-Jones Report had the strongest effect on the guidelines

laid down in the legislation. And while the opposition of the AMA might have prevented consideration of expanding the numbers of physicians after World War II anyway, the fact that the Lee-Jones Report found the supply of physicians to be sufficient to meet the *need* for medical care undoubtedly helped steer national attention to hospital bed expansion before turning to medical personnel.

In 1946 Congress had before it the then-current version of a Murray-Wagner-Dingell bill providing for national health insurance. Included in this bill were sections establishing federal aid to the states for hospital construction to assure that the increased demand for hospitalization anticipated from the increased access to be provided by the *proposed* national health insurance legislation could be accommodated. Partly to block the health insurance portions of this bill, which were vigorously opposed by the AMA, and partly to satisfy some of the demands of its pro-national health insurance supporters, the Congress extracted the section calling for support of hospital construction almost bodily and passed it in the form of the *Hospital Survey and Construction Act of 1946* (P.L.79–725, the Hill-Burton Act). Thus, the first major entry of the federal government into supporting the general medical care system was to provide capital for building hospitals and was passed without assuring that payment for increased services would be available. This was to have far-reaching effects on the U.S. health care system.

The Hill-Burton Act of 1946

The law itself, an amendment appending a new Title VI to the Public Health Service Act, declared two broad purposes:

1. To assist states in inventorying existing hospitals and public health centers and making surveys leading to formulation of statewide plans for the development of adequate, coordinated hospital systems and required public health centers; and
2. To assist the states in their support of local organizations that wish to *construct* hospitals "in accordance with such programs. . . ."

This was the first federal grant program aimed

at developing statewide systems of health *planning* for medical care services. In the words of the legislation, the state plans were to look toward creating a hospital *system* "as will, in conjunction with existing facilities, afford the necessary physical facilities for furnishing adequate hospital, clinic, and similar services for all their people. . . ." Again, the planning aspects of the Hill-Burton legislation are treated in some detail in Chapter 15. Here, the focus is mainly on the federal role in expanding the supply of health facilities. For almost thirty years, until about 1975, the Hill-Burton legislation (the original act and many subsequent amendments) was the major instrument used by the federal government to shape the contours as well as determine the size of the United States system of health facilities. The activities under Hill-Burton were, therefore, a major determinant[3] of the shape and size of the health services system that was in place by 1980.

Although most of the detailed provisions of this act were designed to meet the need for additional hospital beds reported in the Lee-Jones report, they also aimed at improvements to meet some of the criteria developed in the other two studies previously cited, especially that of establishing a system of regionalization. The Surgeon General was instructed to "prescribe" the number of hospital beds required in each state to "provide adequate hospital service." The upper limits of the prescribed requirements were set at 4.5 general acute beds per 1000 population (except in sparsely settled states, where 5.0 per 1000 were permitted). Separate standards were prescribed for tuberculosis beds and for chronic disease (long-term care) beds. The methods of determining the appropriate number of beds were to be prescribed by regions within the state, as well as the priority ordering for construction grants to meet the desired goals.

In actual practice there developed a system in which the Surgeon General accepted any set of methods included within the "State plan" which was consistent with the *objectives* of the law. These objectives[4] proved to be important in subsequent developments. The requirement for establishing "general standards" led to a very large increase in the number of states requiring licensing of hospitals and in setting standards for such licensing. The requirements prohibiting ra-

cial and religious discrimination, mandating provision for hospitalization for poor persons, and favoring rural and poor sites for construction grants were later used by activist advocates of these aims to enforce compliance through court action as well as lobbying in Congress.

Funds were also made available to construct public health centers. The standard of adequacy was set at 1.0 per 30,000 population (per 20,000 in sparsely settled states). This too was a recommendation of the Mountin study, although the foundations had been laid by the work of the Committee on Administrative Practice (CAP) of the APHA, especially the Emerson commission (see Chapter 2).

In order to receive federal funds for the required initial survey, a state was required to designate a single state agency to administer the program and a state advisory council to include representatives from state agencies, nongovernment groups, experts, and consumers. Each state was required to submit a state plan that provided an inventory of all nonfederal inpatient and outpatient facilities exclusive of mental health facilities, institutions furnishing domiciliary care, and institutions not providing a community service. Inpatient facilities were reported by general, long-term care (chronic disease and skilled nursing home beds), and tuberculosis categories. Outpatient facilities were reported by public health centers, diagnostic or treatment centers, and rehabilitation facilities categories.

Congress appropriated $75 million per annum for each of the next five years for actual *construction* of hospital and other facilities covered by the legislation. The allocation of funds among the states of the total $3 million appropriated for *surveys* was based on population, with federal monies making up one-third of the total. This had to be matched two-thirds by the state with a minimum of $10,000.

The allocation of the total amount for *construction* grants to each state was inversely proportional to its per capita income. Federal monies met one-third of the cost of any approved project, the state had to meet one-third, and the local group or organization that was sponsoring the project had to meet one-third. Construction grants were limited to public and nonprofit hospitals.

A consultative federal hospital council was

established with eight members appointed by the Federal Security Administrator—three members were to be experts, four were to be consumers, and there was to be one other. The Surgeon General was ex officio chairman.

Provisions for numerous quality and program controls, such as minimum standards of maintenance and operation, use of the merit system in the state agency, and inclusion of a computation of relative need for each section of the state were stipulated as requirements for a state plan to be acceptable.

Major Amendments

As the implementation of the original Hill-Burton legislation progressed, it soon became evident that some of its provisions encouraged undesirable trends or discouraged desirable ones. These criticisms formed the substance of a battle cry that was to be heard often in the next three decades, that the law provided "perverse incentives." Medical care organization scholars and writers were by now quite generally advocating a system that not only offered good access to care for all, but also operated efficiently because its hospitals were regionalized, emphasized primary care, and delivered services of high medical caliber because it was subject to quality control either by group modes of practice or by government bodies or both. The Hill-Burton Act provisions, and especially its administration, coincided only minimally with these aims. The advocates of universal access to good quality care supported the Hill-Burton Act because it was politically feasible, but now that it had been passed they consistently pointed to its weaknesses and urged its amendment. These advocates were politically prominent during the Truman administrations (1944–1951) and had strong voices in Congress, the White House, federal agencies, among intellectuals, and in organized labor. The original act and the series of correcting amendments to it became known collectively as the Hill-Burton legislation and its implementation as the Hill-Burton Program.

The main objection to the design of the original act raised by advocates emphasizing access shortcomings was that while it was a welcome commitment to needed health resource development, it was starting at the wrong end. The

correct order was to first empower persons to receive needed care, that is, to pass national health insurance, and then (or concomitantly) concentrate on resource development to meet resulting increases in utilization demand. As described in Chapters 9 and 10, all through a period ending in 1980 with the election of President Reagan, these "equity" advocates introduced bills for comprehensive national health insurance that often included resource development sections meant to *accompany* expanding access to the entire population. Although they failed to achieve their main objective, several of their criticisms were acted on by a series of amendments that slowly changed the focus of the Hill-Burton program. The more important of these objections were that requiring a local sponsoring body to meet one-third of the construction cost caused high-need poor areas to be passed over for grants and discriminated against local public hospitals receiving grants because they could not raise the required local one-third of the cost; requiring grants for construction of ambulatory medical facilities to be given only to hospital-affiliated outpatient departments neglected the growing need for freestanding accessible ambulatory facilities for those who lacked good access to ambulatory care; and restricting grants to *new* construction overlooked the growing and more serious need of old facilities in the inner cities and other poor areas for renovation and upgrading. It was further argued that because of the way grant priorities within states were being established, the legislation was producing an excess of beds ("overbedding") in many areas while others continued to have shortages; the shortage of nursing and trained administrative personnel was making it difficult to operate newly built hospitals effectively and efficiently; and the heavy support available for hospital bed expansion in economically comfortable areas coupled with the emphasis on hospital insurance by private insurance was distorting utilization toward hospital use, with a good deal of it being arguably unnecessary or even harmful.

The policies embodied in the major amendments to Title VI (the Hill-Burton program) of the Public Health Service Act, which are further described in Chapter 15, are briefly considered here as attempts to meet the objections noted above, objections that revealed problems that were coming to light in the program's operations.

1949 The main policy adjustment was to change the federal contribution to construction grants from a fixed one-third to a variable proportion ranging from one-third to two-thirds, the calculation of the exact proportion to be based on "economic status of areas, relative need as between areas . . . and other relevant factors." This amendment was aimed at decreasing or even eliminating the need to raise one-third of the cost locally and thereby enable low-income areas to get full construction support if the state would pay its usual one-third. It was meant to remedy the fact that many poor areas with need for a local hospital were receiving high initial priorities for Hill-Burton grants in the state plans based on need, but then were passed over because of their inability to raise the requisite locally provided third of the cost. Although this change permitted more hospitals to be built in poor areas, the operating costs of the new hospitals often could not be met because the financing for the needed utilization was inadequate. (This recalls the similar problem of the community mental health center program of Chapter 6.)

The 1949 amendments also provided for grants-in-aid to states, their political subdivisions, universities, hospitals, and other public and nonprofit institutions and organizations for research and demonstrations dealing with "utilization, and coordination of hospital services, facilities, and resources." This was specified as an additional "purpose" of the program and reflected the growing demand in medical care circles for inclusion of some controls on the operational efficiency of the hospital system instead of merely paying for construction. It was hoped that the results of this research would spur adoption of more efficient operating techniques. The research component was not funded until 1956, but it thereafter became one of the main sources of federal grants for health services research, which were later consolidated in the National Health Services Research Center[5] in 1968 (see p. 433).

1954 A special appropriation of $2 million

was provided for inventorying (1) diagnostic or treatment centers; (2) chronic disease hospitals (or those "for the impaired"); (3) rehabilitation facilities; (4) nursing homes. The federal government was to pay 50 percent of the cost. Funds earmarked for the *construction* of these special types of facilities were appropriated for each of the following four fiscal years. Under the terms of the original act, grants to help finance the construction of these types of facilities had been permissible, but the money had to come out of the total amount appropriated for facility construction. Thus if a state plan were to have provided loans for constructing these nonacute types of facilities before 1954, available federal building funds for acute hospital construction in that state would have been that much less. Now specially sequestered additional funds were set up just for these types of facilities.

These amendments addressed the objection that there had been an undue emphasis on subsidizing the construction of acute short-term facilities, and an ill-advised neglect of ambulatory and less expensively operated chronic and extended-care facilities. This lack of balance had fostered inefficiency by contributing to overutilization of the more expensive segment of the health care network, the short-term general acute-care hospital. The equity advocates also favored these amendments because of their concern about quality of care. Many had long asserted that the general acute-care hospital is not the best place for long-term care and also that ambulatory specialized diagnostics and treatment needed to be expanded.

1956 Traineeships for graduate training of health professionals, mostly nurses, were established. They provided for the establishment of an advisory committee on health "manpower" and provided grants for developing nursing education, including reasearch, training, and education. These provisions were subsequently moved from the Hill-Burton legislation when administration of these grants was transferred to special offices in HEW that administered health personnel training grants. However, at the time these provisions were passed, they were seen as a valid part of the Hill-Burton program, reflecting a growing recognition that building facilities in the face of a shortage of health workers was again a one-sided approach. I shall postpone further detailed discussion of these amendments to Chapter 13, which is devoted to health personnel development questions.

Also provided for in 1956 were special grants for mental health research and demonstration projects. The mental health amendments were part of the attempt (described in Chapter 6) to aid the development of programs that would relieve the load the state mental hospitals were carrying by transferring part of it to community-based services. They also reflected a growing recognition of the importance of mental health care.

1958   Amendments passed in this year provided the option of receiving loans in addition to the outright grants that were previously the only option available for hospital construction.

1961   Money was appropriated annually for the following five years for "studies, experiments, and demonstrations looking toward development of new or improved methods of providing health services *outside the hospital*, particularly for chronically ill or aged persons." Again, these amendments represented a perception that the general acute-care hospital was often inappropriately used because more suitable and less expensive facilities were not available.

1963[6]   These amendments contained the text of the Community Mental Health Centers and Retardation Facilities Construction Act of 1963 described in Chapter 6. They provided for aid to construct research centers and facilities for the mentally retarded and to construct community health centers. The federal, state and local planning for mental health care facility construction required under this community mental health system produced a national network of planners and facilities operating distinctly from the hospital system network.

After 1966, inventories of mental hospitals were included in the state plans developed under the Community Mental Health Centers Act program rather than under Hill-Burton planning data, and grants for comprehensive regional mental health service planning were later transferred from the Hill-Burton program to the Comprehensive Health Planning and Public

Health Services Amendments (P.L. 89–749) of 1966.

1964   These amendments (P.L. 88–443) were of particular importance, incorporating a number of changes introduced in previous amendments and adding new ones. It constituted a major overhaul and expansion of the Hill-Burton program, altering its directions in important ways. Some of the main changes were

"Special Projects Grants for Assisting in the Areawide Planning of Health and Related Facilities"[7] were authorized. The federal government matched 50 percent of the costs of these projects "for developing . . . and . . . carrying out of comprehensive regional, metropolitan area, or other local area plans for coordination of existing and planned health facilities . . . and services provided by such facilities." This first appearance of federal grants for local areawide planning for facilities reflected the growing recognition that the Hill-Burton program had succeeded very well in realizing its purpose of constructing more hospitals and other facilities but not at all well in realizing its purpose of welding them into a coordinated, regionalized, efficient system. It presaged the later health planning legislation of 1966 and 1975, which is discussed in Chapter 15.

Beginning with fiscal year 1966, funds exclusively for facility modernization were to be set aside for the first time. Of the total funds, the proportion used for new hospital construction was 78 percent in 1948; by 1971 it was down to 48 percent. This was a particularly important provision that recognized the need for refurbishing the obsolete and dilapidated plant and equipment in the inner cities and other poor areas.

The suggested formulas for calculating need for beds used in determining the allocation of grant awards within states were changed to more nearly reflect the internal population and geographic differences within the states. Although states had been free to devise their own formulas for determining the need for beds among the specified subareas within the state (the so-called Hill-Burton hospital planning areas), they in fact had nearly all been following the suggested PHS guideline of "4.5 beds per thousand population" as a criterion for acute beds, an approach widely criticized on both theoretical and empirical grounds as not being suitable for small-area planning. Under this amendment fixed national bed/population ratios were discontinued and instead the state plan was required to use criteria calculated on "the basis of a Statewide inventory of existing facilities, a survey of need, and ... [taking into consideration] community, area, or regional plans." The surveys were to obtain the number of long-term hospital beds as well as the number of acute short-term hospital beds needed and take account of such factors as (1) their distribution throughout the state; (2) the number of public health centers, diagnostic or treatment centers, and rehabilitation facilities needed and what their geographic distribution should be; and (3) the extent to which existing facilities needed modernizing. These provisions were precursors of the regulations and guidelines later put out under the national health planning acts of 1966 and 1975.[8]

An important feature of the 1964 amendments was a reaffirmation that a purpose of the program was "to assist the several states in the carrying out of their programs ... as may be necessary, in conjunction with existing facilities, to furnish adequate hospital, clinic, or similar services to all their people. The Surgeon General ... shall by general regulations prescribe ... that the State plan shall provide for adequate hospitals, and other facilities for which aid under this [law] is available ... to *furnish needed services for persons unable to pay therefor*" [emphasis added].

Thus, the Hill-Harris amendments of 1964, as they came to be called, attempted to meet three of the major objections to the way the program had been operating:

Objection 1: The legislation had not markedly succeeded in rationalizing the distribution of health facilities. Incorporating encouragement of areawide facility planning (voluntary) for such coordination and improved rationalization into the granting mechanisms was expected to help remedy this.

Objection 2: The public hospitals in inner-city and poor rural areas were in a state of decrepitude, and the modernization of these facilities was a greater need than building new hospitals, except in some very poor and rural areas. Grants for modernization would address this condition.

Objection 3: The fixed bed/population ratios for distributing federal grants within a state were inappropriate in many areas. Flexible allocations of beds based on local and regional need were now encouraged.

1970   The major trends observable in earlier amendments to the program were continued: a greater emphasis on ambulatory facilities, in favoring poor urban areas (while continuing to aid poor rural areas also), and on encouraging cooperative coordination among elements of the facilities system. Specifically, grants were provided for constructing or modernizing emergency rooms in general hospitals, constructing neighborhood health centers, constructing outpatient facilities in poverty areas, constructing facilities "providing comprehensive health care, training in health or allied health professions, and facilities which provide treatment for alcoholism," and for "equipment-only" projects if such equipment were needed to provide a service lacking in the community. And in all these, states were to accord priority in awarding grants to local areas with relatively meager financial resources.

The continued federal emphasis on channeling aid to poor areas was evident not only in calling for special grant priority consideration for such areas but also in now permitting the federal share of the costs of such projects to be as high as 90 percent. The federal share could also be as high as 90% for the cost of those "projects offering potential for reducing health care costs through shared services, inter-facility cooperation or through free-standing outpatient facilities."

As has been noted, construction loans were introduced in 1958 as an option for the applicant. The 1970 provisions not only continued to provide for loans, but also made available loan guarantees and interest subsidies.[9]

In 1972 President Nixon vetoed the congressional extension of the Hill-Burton program, saying that it had served its purpose, but Congress overrode the veto. By 1975, however, the prevailing sentiment in legislative, administrative, and health care circles was that there were now too many hospital beds and that whatever the shortage had been in 1946, it had been more than rectified. The watchword was now cost containment, especially reduction of excess hospital utilization. Whatever support was needed in some localities for expanding or remodeling facilities was now seen as mostly due to maldistribution rather than overall shortage.

The national Health Planning and Resources Development Act of 1974 (P.L. 93–641) incorporated the Hill-Burton legislation with some further amendment into a new Title XVI of the Public Health Service Act—"Health Resources Development." This law which became effective on January 1, 1975, provided for continued grants along the lines of the amendments of 1964 and later. The act continued to provide formula grants to states, which would distribute them within the state as project grants to applicants wishing to modernize medical facilities, construct new outpatient facilities, or convert existing medical facilities to specified new services. Federal aid for constructing new inpatient facilities was thenceforth available only to areas experiencing rapid population growth, and this aid could be in the form of loans, loan guarantees, or interest subsidies, as well as outright grants with the federal share being two-thirds. It was to be 90 percent for loans and loan guarantees and 100 percent for either in poverty areas.

The program remained on a greatly reduced scale, targeted only on demonstrably underserved areas and emphasizing primary-care facilities. The declared policy after 1974 was to stress local area health planning and thereby coordinate and rationalize the health system's resources, especially hospitals. The de facto policy largely ignored rectifying the distribution of resources and became focused almost entirely on reducing the number of acute hospital beds.

Overview and Summary of the Hill-Burton Program

By 1975, the date of the implementation of the new national health planning act that was to focus on containment of new health facility construction, the Hill-Burton program had achieved an impressive record of health facility expansion. The following is an excerpt from a 1973 HEW report of the cumulative accomplishments of the Hill-Burton Program:

As of June 30, 1971, a total of 10,748 projects had been approved under the Hill-Burton Program for the construction of various types of health facilities—particularly hospitals and nursing homes. Since the award of the first Hill-Burton grant in 1947, more than 470,000 inpatient care beds have been provided. Of the total number of grants, nearly 30 percent, or 3,083 projects, were for outpatient and other health care facilities such as public health centers, rehabilitation facilities, and State health laboratories.

More than 3,800 communities throughout the country have been aided during this period, and 6,265 public and voluntary nonprofit facilities have been provided construction funds. These projects involved:

Total costs	$12.8 billion
Hill-Burton funds	3.7 billion
State and local funds	9.1 billion

From July 1, 1947 through June 30, 1971, a total of $3.7 billion in Hill-Burton funds was spent on constructing and equipping inpatient and outpatient care facilities. The following types of facilities have been aided:

Type of Facility	Inpatient Care Beds	Hill-Burton Funds (in millions)
Inpatient care facilities	470,329	$3,264.8
General hospitals	344,453	2,635.5
Long-term care facilities	97,358[1]	523.1
Units of hospitals	51,983	312.5
Nursing homes	37,884	171.6
Chronic disease hospitals	7,491	39.0
Mental hospitals	21,034	78.5
Tuberculosis hospitals	7,484	27.7
Outpatient and other health care facility projects		453.2
1,078 Outpatient facilities[2]		204.1
552 Rehabilitation facilities		135.0
1,281 Public health centers[3]		99.7
41 State health laboratories		14.4

[1]Exludes 7,209 long-term care beds built in conjunction with general and other hospital projects, for which funds cannot be separated from the total project costs. These beds are reported in the following categories of facilities: general hospitals, 7,113 beds; mental hospitals, 60 beds; tuberculosis hospitals, 36 beds.

[2]Previously designated "diagnostic or treatment centers."

[3]Excludes 131 public health centers built in combination with general hospitals.

This chapter has dealt with governmental policy for altering the supply of health service facilities to achieve the volume, type, and location of facilities appropriate to perceived health service *needs* of the population. As the chapter title implies, most of the Hill-Burton program activities were directed at implementing a policy for *expanding* the supply; activities directed to controlling the expansion or even contracting the supply began to appear late in the program's history and have accordingly been only peripherily treated here.

During the twenty-five year expansion period from 1947 through about 1971, attempts to change the composition of the facility supply by type of service and location were made by changing the priorities with which additions or modifications were funded in conformance with perceived changes in need. The main trends were an initial emphasis almost solely on new acute-care hospital construction, giving way to emphasizing outpatient hospital-based and long-term facility construction, followed by an emphasis on inner-city needs for freestanding ambulatory facilities and modernization of old hospitals, with grant priorities for medically underserved areas and specially favorable federal matching for poverty areas.

Beginning in the early 1960s there was a growing perception that the implementation of general policy objectives—such as more emphasis on facilities for ambulatory care in the states and local areas within them—was far from a straighforward administrative task. Earmarked support for specially designated local planning agencies began to be legislated in the Hill-Burton amendments of 1964, to be followed by the Comprehensive Health Planning Legislation of 1966–67 and finally the Health Planning Act of 1974. The health planning program became an essential part of the federal governments's efforts to alter the mix of the supply of facilities to provide a better fit to population needs. There were many differences between the way the Hill-Burton program and the later federal health planning programs went about the task of rationalizing the supply of health facilities. As we have seen, the Hill-Burton program used grants for construction as its lever and operated primarily under the direction of federal and state agencies. The planning program had no grants to distribute to cooperating providers and local boards of directors and so needed other types of leverage to induce conformance with planning

objectives. Furthermore, the planning program was primarily under the direction of volunteer local health planning agencies. The outcome of these arrangements will be discussed in Chapter 15, but first we turn to a consideration of the federal program for developing an adequate and rational supply of health *personnel* through the use of grants and loans for education and training. This program paralleled the efforts to develop an adequate and rational system of health *facilities* by the use of grants and loans for construction.

NOTES

1. These questions viewed as problems for health planners are discussed in Chapter 15. Only the aspects of these problems needed to understand the course of government policy in supporting resource expansion are touched here.

2. That is, based on health status indicators and assuming financial access to care judged appropriate by medical professionals.

3. Others were the way the private health insurance system developed, the federal health "manpower" legislation (dealt with in Chapter 13), the way the federal government chose to support biomedical research, and the passage of Medicare and Medicaid. Some of these have already been discussed and others are discussed in subsequent chapters. They are all discussed together in Chapter 16.

4. These objectives included:

a. Setting general standards of construction and equipment for hospitals;

b. Prohibiting discrimination on account of race, creed, or color ("separate but equal" was acceptable, however);

c. Providing for "adequate hospital facilities for persons unable to pay therefor";

d. Giving priority to rural and poorer areas of the state.

5. Now the Agency for Health Policy Research and Development (AHPRD).

6. There was also a 1962 amendment to the Act but it did not deal directly with the basic content of the Hill-Burton program. This amendment seems merely to have been entered in the Hill-Burton legislation for special reasons that made it convenient to use Title VI of the Public Health Service Act as a temporary repository within the United States Code for legislation that established Institutes of Maternal Health, Child Health, and Human Development and provided funds for supporting research and training in these fields. Also established was the Institute of General Medical Sciences. This amendment will be discussed further in Chapter 14, where health research and the various National Institutes of Health are treated.

7. $2.5 million, for fiscal year ending 1965, and $5.0 million for each of the following four fiscal years.

8. In fact, most states then adopted a formula suggested by the PHS that called for estimating future short-term hospital utilization as a direct projection of the previous year's utilization, with some adjustment for population changes. This created a new set of problems of inaccurate estimation that were perhaps equally serious because of the implicit assumption that existing hospital utilization was appropriate. Again, this is discussed further in Chapter 15, where the effects of health planning methodology on policy formulation are treated.

9. The Housing and Urban Development Act of 1968 (P.L. 90–48) authorized the Department of Housing and Urban Development (HUD) to administer a program of mortgage insurance under the National Housing Act for constructing, modernizing, and equipping nonprofit hospitals. In 1969, a Memorandum of Agreement between HUD and HEW established joint administration of this program. In 1970 for-profit hospitals were made eligible for mortgage insurance under this program. As of June 1971 a total of thirty-four projects had been insured for $286.6 million; $143 million through the FHA alone, $143.6 million through the joint Hill-Burton/FHS program, and $25.2 million through Hill-Burton funds alone. Certificate of need (see Chapter 15) approval was needed for the proposed construction or modernization to be eligible for mortgage loan insurance (HEW).

13

Government Support for Expanding the Supply of Health Personnel

STATE AND FEDERAL ROLES BEFORE 1965

Two dominant features characterized the medical care personnel picture during the early development of modern medical practice in the United States, approximately 1870 to 1930. The first was that medical care was provided predominantly by physicians and nurses and mostly outside the hospital. The second was that the vast majority of physicians were general practitioners. Furthermore, certainly through 1920, doctors and nurses worked in an epidemiological milieu in which communicable diseases of childhood were the chief causes of acute illness and mortality.

The physician, carrying much of his total equipment in his fabled black bag, saw private patients in his office or in their own homes, and diagnosis was largely symptom-based. Fewer than two other persons were involved in medical care for every practicing physician.

Before 1920 the hospital was mostly used to care for the indigent sick, and general nursing duties in the hospital were performed virtually entirely by student nurses who received very little, if any, compensation other than their room and board at the hospital. Nurses were educated in hospital nursing schools, and graduate nurses typically served as private-duty nurses caring for patients in their own homes. These nurses worked as assistants for private physicians with whom they were informally affiliated (Brown, 1966). It was not until after about 1930 that hospital nursing began to be performed to any considerable degree by graduate rather than student nurses. The scientific content of medical education before 1920, with the exception of a few

extraordinary medical schools, was very weak.

After 1920 the picture began to change. Advances in medical science and technology, resulting from the incorporation (''transfer'') of the rapidly developing scientific knowledge, are widely credited with having reduced infant mortality and increased life expectancy.[1] The age distribution of the population was shifting toward a larger proportion of older persons, and with this shift a corresponding change developed in the composition of the medical services demanded. The prevalence of chronic diseases was increasing and that of acute communicable diseases declining. Along with important social and demographic developments, all these changes combined to bring with them an increased use of the hospital as a locus of medical practice for private nonindigent patients. They also brought a tendency to encourage physician specialization, which changed much of the organizational structure and task definition of medical practice (Stevens, 1971).

Although these trends were perceptible soon after 1920, they developed slowly at first. Even as late as 1930, about 86 percent of physicians were in private practice, with 71 percent in general practice and only about 14 percent engaged in a full-time specialty. At that time, about 40 percent of encounters between private patients and doctors still took place in the patient's home, and the average physician saw about fifty patients per week.

Another important feature of medical care in the United States, especially in the years before World War II, was the predominant location of government regulation of medical care practice at the state level. Legislation regulating medical practice focused almost exclusively on the credentialed competence of physicians and nurses, and occasionally also dentists. Under state licensure laws, all persons other than licensed physicians were prohibited from engaging in general[2] medical practice, although they might be licensed under other state laws to engage in the practice of a limited set of medical functions, such as those involved in nursing or optometry.

It is instructive to compare the stance of the states on quality assurance of and population access to personal therapeutic medicine with their stance on "classical" public health or law enforcement. In the latter areas states saw the protection of the health, safety, and welfare of their residents—the "public"—as entailing a concern with whether the population was indeed being served and with whether sufficient resources were available to deliver the required services as established by monitoring of outcomes—crime statistics, vital statistics, and the like. Chapter 3 described the preoccupation of state public health departments with monitoring local public health services, their population coverage (access), quality, and scope of function.

Consistent with the notion that personal medical care was a commodity rather than a public service available as a "right," however, the states limited themselves to guaranteeing only that persons claiming to be physicians had met certain educational and training qualifications as judged by their peers. Requirements were also set for registered nurses, but the credentialing (not licensing) granted permission for nurses to perform certain medical tasks only under physician supervision, and the credentialing boards were dominated by physicians, not by nurse "peers." The states did not concern themselves with whether the supply of medical personnel was adequate to meet the health service needs of their populations nor whether the population was well "covered" by the services of licensed physicians.

After 1930 suggestions that the federal government enter the picture began to be voiced with the gradual spread of the idea that medical care should be available and accessible to all citizens as a matter of right. Advocacy of this position began to appear in print with increasing frequency beginning with the 27 studies of the Commission on Costs of Medical Care circa 1930. One of these studies, the volume by Lee and Jones (1933), concerned itself with estimating the existing numbers, types, and distribution of medical personnel and facilities compared with the required numbers, types and distribution of these resources. Another volume (Comm. on Costs of Medical Care, 1932) dealt with the organizational and political actions needed to help bring the existing demand into congruence with the medical need for services. This approach is clearly quite different from one that confines the governmental role to facilitation, requirement, and oversight of self-regulation by the medical profession via state licensing. It represents a "public health" way of looking at universal service requirements, basing them on estimates of the health service needs of populations, not only on the economic demand for services, and taking it as a governmental responsibility to see that these needs are met, i.e., that the population's health is "covered" for medical care. (Chapter 15 contains a fuller discussion of this subject.)

The notion of regarding access to reasonably adequate medical care as a right is a view of the public interest that received a powerful impetus from public statements made during World War II. The Beveridge Report in Britain and the report of the National Resources Planning Board in the United States both declared one of the four freedoms the Allies were fighting for to be "freedom from want." Implied in this was a complete social security system that would assure basic economic security "from the cradle to the grave" for all persons. Access to medical care was generally seen to be a fundamental part of such security, and indeed the British began to work on upgrading their National Health Service system when the war ended. It comes as no surprise, therefore, that the earliest federal law intervening in the medical care delivery system, the Hill-Burton legislation of 1946, should reflect a "public health" attitude in its avowed aim of increasing the supply of medical care facilities in a manner that accorded with population need and would correct imbalances in the distribution of such facilities as determined by federally financed surveys. The same approach was used when federal laws and administrative actions were later directed toward extending the supply of medical care personnel and rectifying its distribution using geographic, specialty mix and relative need as criteria.

The earliest federal efforts to improve the supply of health service personnel were made in the 1950s and early 1960s. They were largely explorative being directed toward sponsoring research and surveys of the activities of the states and voluntary organizations with respect to credentialing of personnel (SASHEP, 1972(a); HEW, 1971). Support for such activities grew in the following years. Governmental concern centered on finding out how many health workers there were and of what kinds, where they worked, and how well their distribution served the needs of the population.

Credentialing

There was some state licensing of physicians through the early 1800s, but many of these laws were repealed during the period 1820–1870. The reaction against licensing seems to have been part of the revolt against professional monopoly and elitism stemming from the Jacksonian period as well as the decline in public esteem for the medical profession stemming from the fratricidal strife among the many schools of medical theory that were busy denouncing each other as "quacks." Many of the state licensing procedures in effect before 1820 had consisted of a state delegating the right to confer a license to a medical school or a medical society, and as the quality of many schools deteriorated in the face of competition for students, so did the public perception of the value of such a license as an affirmation of competency. State-enforced medical licensure laws began to be enacted again in the early 1870s, but the big drive by state medical societies for such licensure took place around 1900, and by 1915 the practice of medicine was effectively licensed in each state (Carlson, 1970; Friedman, 1965; Shryock, 1967).

State credentialing of health professions took different forms for different professions in different states, and various writers and analysts have set forth typologies of these forms for analytic purposes that I shall use only selectively here. The weakest form of credentialing was the registration statute under which all persons per-

forming functions specified in the registration act must have their names listed in a public registry. A stronger form of credentialing was certification, sometimes called permissive licensing. Under this procedure, persons could not publicly use a specified title (e.g., "registered nurse") unless certified to do so by the appropriate state agency. They could, however, perform many of the functions of this position even if not credentialed unless a function were specifically forbidden to nonlicensed personnel.[3] The strongest form of credentialing is licensing, sometimes referred to as "mandatory licensing." Under this form of credentialing, no unlicensed person may perform *all* the duties of a licensed person and is also forbidden from advertising himself or herself under the "licensed" title. Other professions may perform *some* of the functions of, say, the licensed Doctor of Medicine but only if they are specifically permitted to do so under other and more limiting credentialing legislation for nurses, optometrists, and so forth. This classification is provided by Milton Friedman as cited in Carlson, 1970.[4]

Licensing for the practice of medicine is now of the mandatory type in all states and has been essentially controlled by the state medical societies since at least 1920. This control has been exercised in numerous ways but two factors by themselves sufficed to assure effective control. First, all states have required graduation from an approved medical school, and the medical licensing boards were empowered to specify approved medical schools; and second, the state licensing agencies, generally known as state boards of medical examiners, have been composed preponderantly of physicians. In 1967 physicians constituted "the entire board in 29 States and a large majority in others. . . . In the great majority of States, the Governor appoints the Board of Medical Examiners or its equivalent from a list of licensed physicians recommended by the State's medical society" (Forgotson, Roemer, and Newman, 1967).

State licensing of medical practitioners can serve at least two disparate functions. On the one hand, licensing laws can help assure the public of a physician's qualifications, but on the other they can also serve to restrict the number of physicians, including the exclusion of qualified persons from practice and indirectly the exclusion of qualified medical applicants from receiving a medical education. Licensing acts can enable the organized medical profession to control the number of licensed physicians if the licensing boards are composed overwhelmingly of physicians, if they can specify the type of medical school whose graduates will be acceptable to them, and if the medical profession can control the number of places available in acceptable medical schools.

In addition to arguing that licensing is necessary to prevent incompetent physicians from practicing, the medical societies have often asserted that the very act of restricting the volume of licenses to the number of physicians needed to serve the expected demand is a quality-assurance measure. The argument essentially states that even if all applicants for licenses or for admission to medical school were technically and intellectually qualified, too large a number of physicians could lead to unethical competition to attract patients via recommending medically unnecessary services or charging fees too low to permit adequate services.

On the other hand, critics of the licensing laws have pointed out that they do not protect the public well (Roemer, 1973). Their arguments have asserted that a license permits the licensee to perform an unlimited range of medical functions; that the license is conferred for a lifetime often with little or no requirements for reexamination in the face of changing medical knowledge; and that licenses have been used to restrict the number of physicians, thus artificially raising the price of physician services to the public (Friedman, 1965). Furthermore, in addition to the opportunities for racial, ethnic, and economic discrimination that licensing controlled by the medical profession has provided, the power to limit enrollments in medical schools is a form of national health planning with the decision making placed in private hands with little public input. As medical care came to be more widely regarded as a public benefit or right, professional control over a crucial national health planning question came increasingly into question and actions were taken to meet some of these objections.

Licensing and the Control of Medical Education

The publication of the Flexner report in 1910 gave a strong impetus to the rapid spread of (mandatory) licensing tied to graduation from schools approved by medical societies. Abraham Flexner, working under the auspices of the Carnegie Foundation for the Advancement of Teaching, spent a year and a half investigating all 155 medical schools in the United States and Canada, most of them proprietary institutions, and turned the floodlight of publicity on what he termed to be their flagrant inadequacies. In the ensuing crusade to improve the quality of medical education, undertaken with the support of the American Medical Association, more than half the schools were forced out of business and many of the survivors were completely transformed. From Flexner's recommendations, implemented with the aid of grants totaling $80 million from the Rockefeller Foundation and other sources, emerged the model for today's medical schools. Its underlying principles were that medical education should be under university control and should be pursued full-time for four years. Many of the faculty members should be full-time employees who had given up their private practices and who divided their time among teaching, research, and treating patients in university hospitals. The curricular reforms spurred by the Flexner report brought teaching hospitals and laboratories into the medical schools, integrating clinical medicine with the basic physical and biological sciences and turning academic medicine into an expanding, ever-changing discipline based on observation and experiment, including scientifically conducted clinical trials.

Although the main announced aim of the Flexner report recommendations was to close the gap then existing between biological knowledge and what was transmitted in medical education, two approaches to accomplishing this could have been taken. One might have been to bring all or nearly all of the existing substandard schools up to standard. This approach would have implied an intent to avoid reducing the number of physicians being produced. The other approach would entail bringing only those schools that were not too far below par up to standard as quickly as possible and closing substandard schools. Action in this direction necessarily involved a sharp reduction in the output of physicians. The latter course was adopted.

The curriculum of one of the leading research-oriented medical schools then in existence, Johns Hopkins University, was taken as the criterion model for determining whether a school was "grade A" (Kessel, 1970). Only graduates from "grade A" schools were to be permitted to take licensing examinations, so that even if a graduate from an unapproved school might have been able to pass the examination, he or she would not be permitted to demonstrate it. Since state medical societies were empowered to designate "approved" schools, this decision effectively placed control of the number of physicians educated with the state medical societies. Coincidentally, but importantly, it also gave control of the medical school curriculum to these societies. The curricula, as a result, subsequently became "as alike as peas in a pod" (Kessel, 1970). The adoption of this educational model as the only one has been cited as one of the factors that subsequently led to overspecialization and to a dearth of black physicians (Kessel, 1970). Black physicians could not make their voices heard in the councils of the AMA because they were excluded from membership. (Black physicians had organized their own National Medical Association in 1870.) There had been considerable discrimination against Jews and Catholics in admissions to medical schools but that against blacks was most severe. (In 1940 this discrimination was said by liberals to have been increasing (Shryock, 1967).)

The immediate result was a sharp reduction in medical school places following the closing of nonconforming schools. The data in Table 13–1 show this reduction. Not until 1950 did the annual number of graduates return to almost the 1904 level despite the great increase in population during the intervening years. The number of physicians per 100,000 population only reached the 1910 level in 1967 and had not attained the 1904 level even by 1970. Virtually every year after 1935 saw from 40 to 60 percent of the applicants for medical school rejected. That a great many of those rejected were well qualified, especially in the later years, is suggested by the fact that "the average non-accepted applicant for 1971–72 achieved higher verbal and quantitative scores [on the Medical College Admissions Test—MCAT] than the average accepted applicant for 1954–55" (AAMC, 1973).

Some twenty years after the issuance of the Flexner report, the organized medical profession was again faced with a critical choice between reducing physician output or seeking alternative solutions. By 1932 the Great Depression had reduced demand for physician services to a very low point. Between 1929 and 1932, physicians' incomes "fell almost 40 percent" (Rayack, 1967). During these years the Weiskolten survey, which has been called a "little" Flexner report, "found that some schools had become lax in their standards and admitted too many students" (Carlson, 1970). In 1932 the *Journal of the American Medical Association* (JAMA) stated editorially that "Perhaps there is a need for professional birth control" because "it is evident that an oversupply of physicians threatens, with an inevitable lowering of the standards of the profession." (Vol. 99, No. 9, Aug. 27). Moving to carry out this suggestion, the AMA Council on Medical Education and Hospitals in 1933 publicly invited the cooperation of the Association of American Medical Colleges "in bringing about a substantial reduction of their enrollment." In a speech at the association's annual meeting that year, Dr. William D. Cutler, the AMA Council's secretary, deplored the practice of making up medical school classes "without any regard to the needs of the profession or of the country as a whole." A year later, the Council reported that "seven schools have definitely stated that their enrollment will be decreased and others have indicated adherence to the council's principles." Between 1934 and 1939, the number of freshmen accepted by the medical schools was reduced by 1,355, or 18 percent, despite the fact that the number of applicants was virtually the same in both years.

It is true that general college enrollment also went down during the depression years, but the decline was neither as sharp nor as prolonged as medical school enrollment and more important, it was not due to closing down college capacity. "It was appallingly shortsighted," one medical writer has commented, "to take the bottom of the Depression as a guide for the country's fu-

Table 13–1. Physician Supply and Education—Selected Years, 1904–1991

Academic year ending	No. of medical schools	No. of osteopathic schools	Total number of schools	Active M.D.s per 100,000 population	Active D.O.s per 100,000 population	Total active physicians per 100,000 population	No. of M.D. graduates	No. of D.O. graduates	Total no. of graduates	No. of applicants to medical school	% of applicants accepted
1904	160	—	—	157	—	—	5,747	—	—	—	—
1910	131	—	—	146	—	—	3,165	—	—	—	—
1920	88	—	—	136	—	—	3,047	—	—	—	—
1925	80	—	—	127	—	—	3,974	—	—	—	—
1930	76	—	—	125	—	—	4,565	—	—	—	51.9
1935	77	—	—	129	—	—	5,101	—	—	—	52.6
1940	77	—	—	133	—	—	5,097	—	—	—	—
1945	77	—	—	134	—	—	5,145	—	—	—	28.3
1950	79	9	88	134	7.1	141	5,553	373	5,926	—	55.6
1955	81	6	87	134	7.0	141	6,997	459	7,456	—	55.6
1960	85	6	91	133	6.6	140	7,081	427	7,508	—	58.8
1961	86	6	92	—	—	—	6,994	506	7,500	—	58.8
1962	87	5	92	135	—	—	7,168	363	7,531	14,381	56.5
1963	87	5	92	137	—	—	7,264	367	7,631	—	51.3
1964	87	5	92	137	—	—	7,336	355	7,691	—	47.2
1965	88	5	93	139	5.7	145	7,409	475	7,884	—	48.2
1966	88	5	93	142	—	—	7,574	360	7,934	—	

Year											
1967	90	5	95	146	—	—	7,743	405	8,148	—	50.0
1968	95	5	100	144	5.0	149	7,973	427	8,400	18,724	51.8
1969	99	5	104	146	6.0	152	8,059	427	8,486	21,118	47.9
1970	101	7	108	150	6.0	156	8,367	432	8,799	24,465	43.1
1971	103	6	109	—	—	161	8,974	472	9,446	24,987	46.0
1972	108	6	114	—	—	164	9,551	485	10,036	29,172	42.3
1973	112	—	—	—	—	164	10,391	649	11,040	36,135	—
1974	114	—	—	—	—	169	11,588	594	12,182	40,506	—
1975	114	9	—	169	6.5	176	12,714	702	13,416	42,624	—
1976	114	9	123	172	6.6	179	13,561	809	14,370	42,303	—
1977	116	—	—	173	6.8	180	14,469	908	15,377	42,155	—
1978	122	—	—	179	7.0	186	14,393	971	15,364	40,569	—
1979	125	—	—	184	7.2	191	14,966	1,004	15,970	36,636	45.2
1980	126	14	140	190	7.5	198	15,135	1,059	16,194	36,141	47.5
1981	126	15	141	191	7.8	199	15,667	1,151	16,818	36,100	47.5
1982	126	15	141	197	8.0	205	15,985	1,017	17,002	36,127	47.1
1983	127	15	142	203	8.3	211	15,824	1,317	17,141	36,730	47.1
1984	127	15	142	—	8.8	—	16,327	1,287	17,614	35,200	48.9
1985	127	15	142	211	9.1	220	16,319	1,474	17,793	35,944	47.8
1986	127	15	142	212	9.6	222	16,125	1,560	17,685	32,893	52.4
1987	127	15	142	—	—	226	15,836	1,587	17,423	31,323	54.6
1988	127	15	142	—	—	233	15,887	1,572	17,459	28,123	60.5
1989	127	15	142	—	—	—	15,620	1,617	17,237	26,721	
1990	127	—	—	233	—	—	15,336			26,915	
1991	126	—	—	—	—	—	15,499			29,243	

Sources: Rayack, 1967; HEW, 1971, 1981, 1990; AAMC, 1971, 1973; JAMA, 1989, 1991, Pestana, 1884; Schofield, 1984

374 GOVERNMENT ROLES IN HEALTH SERVICES

ture health needs'' (Greenberg, 1965). It was not until 1951–52 that acceptances to medical schools reached 1933–34 levels. (Even then, the 1952 acceptances represented 38 percent of applications compared with 62 percent in 1934 (AAMC, 1972, 1973). So much for the notion that the output of physicians has traditionally been centrally unplanned and was only responding to ''free'' market forces.

At both of these decision-demanding junctures, 1910 and 1932, the American Medical Association and its associated organizations could have opted for increasing medical school capacity so that all qualified applicants could be accepted, a position they came to adopt publicly only in 1968. In order to avoid having this result in underemployed physicians, they could have decided to support measures to help increase effective demand. However, as noted in chapters dealing with national health insurance legislation, such measures were actively and even vigorously opposed by the AMA. At both of these decision points, 1910 and 1932, the response was to reduce the number of places in medical schools. The general argument of the organized medical profession was that effective demand really represented true need, because philanthropic and public sources, as well as physicians' contributed services, ensured the delivery of all the medical care the population was prepared to seek out.

The AMA's positions favoring restriction of access to medical education were frequently subjected to public criticism that became more insistent as the issues they raised became more prominent after World War II. With increased public interest in national health insurance and the growth of private health insurance coverage it became evident that the demand for more health services would grow in the future. An important federal policy question developed over whether the United States would have enough health personnel, especially physicians, to meet the increasing demand. Did the government have to take measures then, in the 1950s or 1960s, to ensure an adequate supply of physicians and other health personnel by the 1960s and 1970s?

Some estimate was needed of the expected future adequacy of the supply of health personnel and the first problem addressed was the proper determination of the number of personnel, especially physicians, that would be required by specified future dates, say 1960, 1970, and 1975.[5] A prolonged public debate over what ''true needs'' are took place accompanied by a series of studies by individual scholars and various commissions during the 1950s and 1960s. Most of the findings issuing from these studies determined that federal action of various sorts would be required if the future supply was to be adequate and the actions recommended followed suit.

How Many Health Personnel Does the Nation "Require"?: 1950s and 1960s Studies of Future Health Personnel Needs

Thirteen studies published during the years 1938–1966 made varying assessments of the future adequacy of the national supply of health care personnel.[6] Because a long lead time is involved in training some health personnel, particularly physicians, if the federal government were to intervene in a timely manner to alter the supply of such personnel, it needed estimates of conditions likely to prevail eight to ten years ahead. The various studies attempting to provide these estimates were faced with formidable methodological obstacles (Butter, 1967) both in determining what the numbers and mix of health personnel should ideally be some years into the future as well as in estimating what they were likely to actually be if no government action were taken.

If one could estimate health personnel requirements under conditions of complete information on future population and medical knowledge trends and general agreement on using a ''population needs'' (i.e., public health) approach, the result would be a rational procedure for deriving an ideal (''normative'') configuration of the needed future health service personnel supply. It would entail a series of steps beginning with estimating the future health status of a population and ending with normative estimates of future resources ideally required to adequately service a population with the health problems yielded by the estimates.[7] But the data collection that such algorithms require was not possible under the funding, and even more important, the time restrictions faced by the ''manpower" studies of the 1950s and 1960s. Consequently there was the usual reliance on "reasonable" criteria and assumptions and "quick and dirty" arbitrary procedures to produce recommendations in time to affect current policy formation.

It is also clearly not possible to retroactively determine definitively how accurate the estimates of the actual numbers of practising physicians at some future date "if nothing were done" were. For example, the data from a study of some of these projections (Butter, 1967) show that most of the forecasts for 1970 and 1975 were underestimates. But the first major health "manpower" legislation was passed in 1963, and the actual data for 1970 and 1975 therefore already included increases brought about by the legislation in response to the estimates of future shortages. Since the projections for 1970 and 1975 were made in years ranging from 1958 through 1967, the actual physician supply in 1970 and 1975 was clearly not the result of "nothing being done" by the government.

Although whether the projections for 1970 and especially for 1975 would have proved accurate had there been no federal intervention with health personnel legislation remains a moot point, the underestimates of forecasts of future numbers of physicians shown for 1960, a year predating the first year that effects from legislation could have been felt by about seven years, obviously cannot be explained in this manner. In this case the likely reasons for the misreading of the existing trends are that the estimators did not sufficiently take into account the effect of an increasing number of foreign medical school graduates, perhaps they also overestimated the rate of attrition from death and retirement of physicians, and underestimated the effect of early efforts by medical schools to produce more graduates, as well as some increase in the number of medical schools between 1950 and 1960, as shown in Table 13–1. Thus, the estimates of future *requirements* for physicians depended heavily on methodological assumptions whose validity has not been amenable to objective verification, while the estimates of the number of physicians that would be available if no intervention were made has been shown to be too low, where verifiable (by relative amounts ranging from 11 percent to 15 percent). These un-

certainties would continue to becloud the discussion of the adequacy of physician supply in later years.

Economists arguing from a theoretical market point of view, however, had no difficulty justifying the need for more medical school places. They largely ignored the question of whether the expected future supply of physicians would be sufficient to meet population demands, and certainly needs. Their focus was on the clearcut violation of market principles by government's interference with the market for medical education. As long as large numbers of qualified applicants to medical school were not admitted because of lack of places, it was clear that the market supply was being artificially restricted and that the price of physician services would continue to be above free market levels, thus lowering demand below free market levels and thereby restricting access to care.

Early Government Responses to the Studies: Federal Legislation in 1963–1964 to Stimulate Expansion of the Supply of Physicians, Dentists, and Nurses

While the numerical estimates of requirements and actual supply projected for 1970 and 1975 differed from report to report, they all projected a "need" for more personnel than were expected to be available. This led to federal legislation to bring the expected future supply into congruence with the estimated requirements. The political factors that led to federal attempts in the 1960s to provide more personal health care resources to inner-city populations (see Chapter 7) were also operating to induce this type of legislative response.

One of the reports whose projections influenced federal health personnel legislation was that of the Surgeon General's Consultant Group on Medical Education (the Bane Committee), which had been requested to answer the question "How shall the nation be supplied with adequate numbers of well-qualified physicians?" The 1959 Report examined factors affecting the need for physicians such as geographic distribution, changing patterns of medical practice, growth of specialization, urbanization, and the problems brought on by aging and chronic illness. The observed trends in these factors indicated increasing need for medical service and if access were properly funded would lead to increasing demand. Maintenance of the 1959 ratio of 141 physicians per 100,000 population (one physician per 709 persons) was set as a minimum goal for 1975. This implied an increase of almost 50 percent in the graduating output of medical schools by the end of the period. Existing schools would need to be expanded and twenty to twenty-four new schools established.[8] Obstacles to the desired expansion of medical schools were found to include the high cost of constructing new teaching facilities, the heavy expense to the student of a medical education, and the rapidly rising operating costs of the schools.

The Consultant Group recommended that the federal government help overcome these obstacles by providing, among other forms of assistance, matching grants for the construction of teaching facilities, educational grants-in-aid to medical students, and specified contributions toward the basic operating expenses of medical schools. Although the Consultant Group was charged with considering needs only in the field of medical education, it recognized that physicians could not carry out their growing responsibilities without the help of an increased number of associates with a variety of skills and educational preparations. A summary statement on dentists was prepared, pointing to the need for an approximate 75 percent increase by 1975 in the number of dental school graduates just to maintain the existing inadequate ratio of dentists to population. The group also saw urgent need for expansion of the educational capacity for nursing and other health professions (1959).

This report, along with a 1961 report of the Commission on the Survey of Dentistry in the United States, was followed by the passage of the *Health Professions Education Assistance Act of 1963* (P.L. 88–129), which defined itself as "an act to increase the opportunities for training of physicians, dentists, and professional public health personnel." Federal funds were made available for construction of teaching facilities to train medical, dental, and other health personnel, and for loans both to students and to the professional schools. The act was amended in 1965 to extend and improve the construction loan programs and also to provide funds for direct to the student scholarships. Several features of the act are worth noting. (1) No funds were voted for direct use by the schools for supporting their educational operations, the third major recommendation of the Bane Committee. (2) Although the major focus of this act was on increasing the output of physicians and dentists, it did provide for expanding other classifications of health personnel. It was therefore of the omnibus type in terms of classification of personnel provided for. Other later acts were narrower in scope, focusing on only one classification, and were therefore of the single-profession type. (3) The student loan funds granted under these earlier acts did not provide loans directly from the federal government to students. The loan funds were granted to the medical schools, which then dispensed them to the student who was thereby made dependent on being accepted by a school that had money to lend and would choose to give him or her a loan. These grants were thus institutionally administered loan funds rather than individual loans to students.

A consultant group similar to the Bane Committee, the Surgeon General's Consultant Group on Nursing (Eurich Committee), was appointed in 1963 and given the assignment of advising the Surgeon General on the appropriate role of the federal government in ensuring adequate nursing personnel. Though this Consultant Group estimated that 850,000 professional nurses would be required to fully meet the needs of the nation in 1970, it set 680,000 professional nurses as a realistic objective. To meet this goal would have required a 75 percent increase in the number of nursing school graduates in 1969 over 1961. The Eurich group indicated areas in which federal assistance could be of particular help and significance (recruitment, expansion and improvement of educational programs, advanced training, and research), and stressed the need for a well-organized educational structure for the training of nurses.

The *Nurse Training Act of 1964* (P.L. 88–581) appropriated funds "to increase opportunities for training professional nursing personnel." Funds were made available under this legislation for construction grants, grants for improvement and expansion of training programs, student loans, and traineeships for advanced training.

The several governmental study commissions

appointed over the 1950s and 1960s were repeatedly arriving at the same conclusions: that it would require a substantial increase in physicians, dentists, and nurses merely to keep up with the anticipated growth of the population and with technology. If greater utilization rates were also to be anticipated because of greater third-party coverage or population shifts to higher income brackets, then even more personnel would be required to meet the demand. Though it was a long time coming, legislation finally began to be enacted in response to repeated calls for federal assistance.

It is interesting to note that the federal legislation of the 1960s and 1970s increasing the supply of physicians, dentists, nurses, and some classes of public health personnel first began to be passed in the two years just before passage of Medicare and Medicaid in 1965. It is not entirely or even largely true, as some critics have charged, that this 1965 legislation to increase the demand for medical care was passed by Congress in utter disregard of the necessity to increase the supply of medical personnel concomitantly or beforehand. The provision for increased demand was nearly always accompanied and sometimes preceded by provision for increased supply. In 1946 this took the form of major help for facility construction and reliance on the growth of private health insurance to increase demand.[9] In 1963–1965, the form used was to provide help for personnel enhancement. What often did happen was quite the opposite. Supply was increased in anticipation of increases in demand that then failed to materialize, leading some commentators to cavalierly proclaim the existence of a surplus of resources.

STATE AND FEDERAL ROLES DURING AND AFTER 1965

Health Personnel in 1965

Physicians

With the passage of Medicare and Medicaid in 1965 and the attendant anticipation of increased demand for medical services, government agencies and health organization scholars turned even more energetically to surveying the prospects for an adequate future supply of health personnel.

By 1965 the United States had over 300,000 active physicians, but the ratio of physicians available for initial visits when people were sick or perceived that they had a medical problem (i.e., primary care physicians) was smaller than the gross pool of medical personnel would indicate. The increase in the number of physicians going into administration, teaching, research, industrial health, and public health and other governmental employment was increasing. The result was that although the number of active physicians per 10,000 population had increased slightly, from 14.1 in 1950 (1 physician per 709 persons) to about 15.0 in 1965 (1 per 700 persons), well over half of these were not in patient care or were specialists who were not always available for the initial diagnosis and treatment of disease. There had been a rapid decline in the proportion of doctors who were general practitioners. By 1970, 71,260 physicians, only 27 percent of the 278,535 active medical doctors in patient care, were listed as general practitioners. By contrast, 74 percent were in specialty patient care. (The remaining 35,000 of the 311,000 active physicians were not in patient care.)[10] In addition, all through this period heavy reliance continued to be placed on the services of foreign-educated physicians.

Foreign-trained Physicians in the United States Medical Care System From about 1950 on, the American medical care system came to depend increasingly on the services of physicians whose medical education had been obtained outside the United States or Canada. In 1950 23 percent of filled hospital residencies were held by foreign medical graduates; in 1970 the figure was 33 percent. The corresponding figures for hospital internships were 10 percent in 1950 and 29 percent in 1970 (AMA, 1972, Table 25). Indeed, the increase in the M.D. population from 145 per 100,000 persons in 1950 to 164 per 100,000 in 1970 was due entirely to the influx of foreign-trained physicians. "Without this immigration of foreign medical graduates to the United States, the ratio of U.S. trained M.D.s to population would be virtually the same in 1970 as it was in 1930" (AAMC, 1972). As of December 31, 1970, there were approximately 57,200 for-

Table 13–2. Type of Practice and Primary Specialty of Active Federal and Non-Federal Physicians: 1967 and 1970

Primary specialty	Total active[1]	Office-based practice[2]	Training programs	Full-time physician staff	Other professional activity[3]	D.O.'s (Dec. 31, 1967)
			M.D.'s (Dec. 31, 1970)			
			Patient care			
			Hospital-based practice			
Total	310,845	192,439	51,228	34,868	32,310	[4]11,381
General Practice[5]	77,363	54,914	10,400	5,946	6,103	[6]8,651
Specialty practice	233,482	137,525	40,828	28,922	26,207	1,416
Medical specialties	77,214	44,428	14,139	8,646	10,001	1,416

Sources: AMA Center for Health Services Research and Development: *Distribution of Physicians in the United States, 1970*, Regional, State, County, Metropolitan Areas. J.N. Haug, G.A. Roback and B.C. Martin. Chicago, American Medical Association, 1971. AOA Membership and Statistics Department: *A Statistical Study of the Osteopathic Profession, December 31, 1967*. Chicago, American Osteopathic Association, June 1968.

Adapted from:(HEW-1972, Table 86)

[1]Excludes 3,204 M.D.'s with addresses unknown, and 358 unclassified M.D.'s.

[2]Previously called solo, partnership, group, or other practice.

[3]Includes medical teaching, administration, research, and other.

[4]Includes 1,314 D.O.'s (775 in training programs, 181 in full-time hospital staff positions, 186 in other professional activities, and 172 Federal D.O.'s) for whom data are not available on specialties.

[5]Includes no specialty reported and other specialites not listed.

[6]Includes 827 with practice limited to manipulative therapy.

eign medical graduates in the United States, 48,200 of whom were providing patient care (HEW, 1971). A journalist writing often on medical matters noted, ''In no other field does the United States draw to the same extent on personnel trained abroad as it does in medicine'' (Greenberg, 1965). By 1965 the foreign medical graduate (FMG) was clearly an important part of the pool of physicians practicing in the United States.

The participation of foreign medical graduates in U.S. medicine was of two types. First, many of these physicians became licensed in the United States and thus part of the regular pool of licensed physicians. And second, many foreign medical graduates worked as house staff in United States hospitals, with some of them going on later to join the first group by becoming licensed to practice in the United States. The proportion of newly licensed foreign medical graduates of the total of new MDs licensed was 5 percent in 1950 and rose to almost 20 percent in 1959. After that it fluctuated from year to year, and by 1970 it had stabilized at between 15 and 20 percent each year. The foreign graduates licensed each year during 1957–71 included some American citizens who had received their degrees in foreign medical schools, but the proportion of the newly licensed FMGs

who were American citizens decreased over these years.

Furthermore, the number of American citizens receiving medical degrees in foreign countries did not fully reveal the extent of foreign education of United States physicians. In 1970–71, for example, an estimated 3,922 Americans were enrolled in foreign medical schools (AMA, 1972). A number of these transferred to American medical schools each year with advanced standing for two to four years education received in a foreign medical school and thus appeared in the statistics as U.S. medical school graduates. In 1970 the Association of American Medical Colleges (AAMC) instituted a special program to facilitate the transfer of U.S. citizens from foreign to U.S. medical schools. During its first three years of operation, the number of transfers it effectuated rose from 82 (1970) to 214 (1972) (AAMC, 1973). Known as the Coordinated Transfer Application System (CO-TRANS), this program was operated jointly by the American Association of Medical Colleges and the National Board of Medical Examiners. Applicants for COTRANS's services were admitted to Part I of the National Board of Medical Examiner's (NBME) examination if their credentials met stipulated requirements. For those who passed the examination, a record of their credentials and their NBME grades was circulated among the medical schools to which they applied.

The role of foreign-trained physicians became a particularly important public issue with respect to the staffing of the house officer positions in U.S. hospitals. The data revealed the following salient facts (AMA, 1972).

1. Between 1941 and 1971[11] the total number of hospital internships offered in the United States increased from 8,182 to 15,422 (88 percent), while residencies offered rose almost tenfold, from 5,256 to 50,193. These rises are indicative of the great increase in hospital requests for house staff officers during these years resulting in large part from the growth of private hospital insurance and the rapid expansion of hospital beds after 1946 under the Hill-Burton program. The figures also indicate the changing emphasis from internships to residencies reflecting the growth of specialization in response to the development of technology. The journal of the Association of Medical Colleges announced that "by June 30, 1975, all internships are to be coordinated with residency programs. . . ." (AMA, 1972).

2. The proportion of "offered" intern positions that remained vacant rose from 25 percent in 1950–51 to 27 percent in 1960–61 and fell to 22 percent in 1971–72. For these same years the comparable vacancy rates for resident positions were 25 percent, 13 percent, and 15 percent respectively.

3. The percentages of filled positions whose incumbents were foreign medical graduates were:

Year	Internships	Residencies
1950–51	10.3 percent	9.3 percent
1960–61	14.0 percent	28.8 percent
1971–72	32.7 percent	31.9 percent

Clearly, the actual operating experience of the hospital system was indicating a shortage in the production of physicians by U.S. medical schools, particularly for house officer staffing. Hospitals were proclaiming shortages in these positions (i.e., "unfilled" positions) all during the years following World War II, and the holding of about one-third of the filled residencies

by foreign-trained physicians lent credence to the assertion that the U.S. medical schools were not meeting the demand for physicians.

The qualifications of the foreign-trained house staff physician had become a subject of widespread public discussion in the early 1950s, with concern expressed by medical care professionals, hospitals, and lay commentators. In response to this uneasiness, the Educational Council for Foreign Medical Graduates (ECFMG) was formed in 1957, sponsored by the American Hospital Association, the American Medical Association, the Association of American Medical Colleges, the Association for Hospital Medical Education, and the Federation of State Medical Boards of the United States. The main function of the ECFMG was to examine foreign medical school graduates both in medical knowledge and in English proficiency to determine their fitness to work effectively on the house staffs of U.S. hospitals. However, by 1961 many hospitals were reportedly employing foreign medical graduates who had not passed the ECFMG examination claiming that they could not otherwise fill their house staff vacancies (Rayack, 1967).

Federal legislation was eventually enacted with the apparent aim of encouraging foreign medical graduates to stay on in the United States. In 1970 an amendment to the Immigration and Nationality Act (P.L. 91–225) left to the discretion of the Secretary of State whether a foreign medical graduate had to leave the United States. Only physicians from countries that the Secretary determined needed them for their own medical services were required to leave the United States at the completion of their training programs.

Dentists

In 1930 there were 59 dentists for every 100,000 Americans. In 1967 the ratio was 56.3/100,000[12] (HEW, 1969, 1972), and it was expected to be down to 50 by 1975 unless dental school capacity was expanded. Just to maintain the 1967 ratio would require an increase from the 3,400 dental graduates of 1967 to more than 6,000 a year by 1975. Unless at least twenty new dental schools were established within the next decade, it was estimated that there would be about 15,000 fewer dentists by 1975 than the number needed merely to maintain the totally inadequate dentist-population ratio of 1967.

As in medicine, the ratio of dental specialists to general practitioners had been steadily rising (HEW, 1972, Tables 39, 41, 43) and the number of persons graduating as dental hygienists and dental assistants had also been increasing relative to the number of dental graduates. However, although projected future trends were for increased specialization and increased output of allied dental personnel, the degree to which additional non-dentist personnel were being used in conjunction with increased specialty work on relatively few persons, as opposed to being used to increase the number of persons seen by general dentists, was not known.

Nurses

Despite the passage of the Nurse Training Act of 1964 and the increased pace of federal aid to schools of nursing, a serious shortage of nurses was proclaimed by the hospitals throughout the nation. This was in face of the fact that there were 621,000 employed registered nurses in the United States in 1966, almost one and one-half times the comparable number for 1956, and more than double the 280,500 said to have been active in 1948. Furthermore, the number of nurses per 100,000 population had been rising steadily from 259 in 1956 to 319 in 1966. A 1970 count showed almost 70 percent to be working in hospitals and nursing homes (HEW, 1972, Tables 93, 94). The shortage of the mid-1960s seemed to be essentially a continuation of a chronic problem that had been gradually worsening.

The nursing supply situation had become highly complex and was rapidly changing in response to a variety of factors and trends. In an attempt to identify these trends affecting nursing personnel, the Division of Nursing of the National Institutes of Health supported numerous studies on topics relating to nursing, including the questions subsumed under the amusing frequently used heading, "health manpower in nursing." During the period 1955–1968, at least 175 such projects were supported (Abdellah,

1970). These and other research (Davis, 1966; Etzioni, 1969) were identifying some of the main problems in determining the number of nurses required, as well as investigating the hospitals' complaint of a shortage of nurses. The major problems identified were:

1. *Economic* Hospitals were saying that they needed more professional ("registered") nurses, but they were unwilling or unable to pay a competitive market price for them. Economists were characterizing the hospitals as monopsonists or oligopsonists who colluded to fix the price of nurses at levels that were insufficient to attract and keep promising personnel in the face of competition from other professions or home-making (Yett, 1965, 1968, 1970; Archibald, 1971). It was argued that the lifetime expected earnings of a professional nurse compared with the true cost of her training (actual costs plus earnings foregone during training) were too low compared with those of other professions (Yett, 1968; Archibald, 1917). Empirical comparisons of earnings and fringe benefits of nurses with other workers showed nurses to be at a disadvantage (Moses, 1965).

2. *Social* The supply of professional nurses was seen to be particularly affected by the changing status of women and the generally high level of the economy. Opportunities other than in the "women's" professions (Davis, 1966; Etzioni, 1969) were opening up, and they paid more with better working conditions and benefits. Furthermore, a large number of qualified nurses were not practicing. Presumably the rewards of working, both personal and financial, were not sufficient to induce them to work as opposed to being full-time homemakers. As early as 1951, the U.S. President's Commission on the Health Needs of the Nation had found that on average only about 45 percent of registered nurses were active. This proportion ranged from 53 percent for those under 30 to 30 percent for those in the 50 to 59 age category (Johnson, 1957). Many published articles reported research on causes for withdrawal of nurses from the labor force after marriage, with the principal ones being the dead-end nature of the job; frustration on the job; lack of available child care at fees making it worthwhile to work; perception of women's role as full time homemakers and mothers; lack of flexible work schedules to per-

mit part-time work; need to care for dependents; and ill health.

3. *Organizational* The main organizational components discouraging expansion of the supply of nurses were found to be: lack of status on the job, particularly vis-à-vis the physician; lack of job security; and the failure to use highly trained baccalaureate nurses (i.e., graduates of a four-year college program awarding a bachelor's degree in nursing) in tasks utilizing their university training.

In a move to improve the professional status of baccalaureate nurses, leaders of the nursing profession were urging increased allocation of educational resources for broader curricula for professional nurses and less for vocational training (ANA, 1965). The gradual but steady decline in participation by the student nurse in the day-to-day regular service tasks of hospitals reflected this approach of the university-based nursing schools.

In the hospitals, meanwhile, the licensed practical nurse (LPN), alternatively called a licensed vocational nurse (LVN), was doing most of the actual bedside patient care assisted by nurse's aides. The LPN typically was a graduate of a twelve- to eighteen-month program of training in a trade, technical, or vocational school operated by a public school system or a private school controlled by a hospital, health agency, or college. She (most LPNs were women) had completed two to four years of high school. The nurse's aide, orderly, or attendant was generally a product of several months of on-the-job training in a hospital (HEW, 1972, pp 174-75). The registered nurse, on the other hand, was increasingly moving away from the bedside and into an administrative role. In an attempt to fill more vacancies with registered nurses, hospitals had been increasingly staffing these positions with part-time personnel (Testoff, Levine, and Siegel, 1963). Part-time nurses per 1,000 full-time nurses went from 189 in 1948 to 591 in 1962 (Testoff, Levine, and Siegel, 1963).

By the 1960s the organizational picture had become quite confusing as two-year junior colleges began to produce registered (professional) nurses that worked side by side with four-year baccalaureate registered nurses and three-year diploma-program hospital-trained practical (vocational) nurses. Some investigators cited this incoherent organizational structure as contributing to the frustration of the baccalaureate nurses, lowering their morale and encouraging them to stop practicing.

In summary, along with teachers, librarians, and social workers, nurses have been part of the traditionally women's professions that have been sharply underpaid for the training and responsibility required of their practitioners. With the continued expansion of opportunities for women in better-paid professions, the continued low pay for professional nurses and their unsatisfactory work environment resulted in a continuing shortage of nurses. It was doubtful whether increasing the output of new nurses could, taken alone, be expected to remedy the situation.

Allied Health Personnel

The continued perception that shortages of doctors and nurses were persisting, the long lead time involved in producing more physicians, the sharp rise in the cost of a medical education, and the seemingly intractable persistence of the inactive nurse problem contributed to a change in focus in the recommendations of governmental studies of health personnel resources undertaken during the 1960s. They were increasingly adopting a premise that requirements for highly trained medical personnel under existing modes of organizing medical practice were so great, and likely to continue growing so fast, as to be unattainable, perhaps not even desirable. Their emphasis was shifting toward finding alternatives. More efficient use of allied health personnel[13] by upgrading education and task definition was seen as an alternative, perhaps the only realistic one. To guarantee an adequate supply of allied health personnel, educational assistance was legislated largely following the recommendations of these studies. Their nature and tone may be inferred from some of the main studies whose recommendations are outlined below:

1. The President's Commission on Heart Disease, Cancer, and Stroke in 1964 viewed personnel needs for the prevention and control of heart disease, cancer, and stroke as inseparable from personnel needs for medical care generally and concluded that a full-scale attack on these three diseases would require expansion of all

components of the entire health services work force. The commission accordingly recommended that efforts be made to use existing personnel in the most effective way possible and that the nation immediately begin a massive program for the training of additional physicians, dentists, nurses, and a large variety of other health personnel. Prominent among the specific suggestions for strengthening personnel resources was the recommendation of a greater federal investment in recruitment and training of various types of health technicians and other paramedical personnel. A Public Health Service "health manpower" unit for continuous assessment of the changing personnel requirements for health services was to be formed. The effects of these recommendations were immediately evident in the 1965 amendments to the Health Professions Educational Assistance Act (P.L. 89–190). The report of this commission cut across a number of different major features of the health services system and it will be discussed again in Chapter 14 on research and in Chapter 15 dealing with health planning.

2. In 1965 a committee headed by Lowell Coggeshall (the Coggeshall Committee) was formed to provide guidelines for the future development of the Association of American Medical Colleges. Basing its recommendations on a broad view of health in the United States, it defined the emerging trends in both society and health care, including scientific advances, population changes, increasing individual health expectations and demand, greater specialization in medical practice, increased use of technological advances and equipment, increasing institutionalization of health care, need for larger numbers of physicians and other health personnel, the expanding role of government, and the ever-increasing costs of health care. The committee concluded that enough physicians would never be produced to satisfy growing national requirements. Therefore, it was "essential that physician productivity be increased through delegation of specific tasks to others." To achieve this end, the committee noted greater need for more health personnel to support the physician acting as a team leader, and a need to improve the organization of the practice of medical care so that it could be effectively and efficiently delivered. Two main conclusions were that the

general university (i.e., not its medical school) should assume increasing responsibility for education in the basic health and medical sciences, a theme that was to reverberate through subsequent studies and reports; and a warning that unless the medical colleges, through the American Association of Medical Colleges, took aggressive action to provide broader and more positive leadership in medical education, "the initiative may be seized by others—organizations less qualified to make the decisions and to take action required to meet the needs and preserve the standards of medical education in the future" (AAMC, 1965).

3. A Task Force on Health Manpower appointed by the National Commission on Community Health Services,[14] which was sponsored by the American Public Health Association and the National Health Council (a national organization of voluntary health organizations), recommended a series of actions in 1966 for all levels of government—local, state, and regional—but mostly for the federal level. These recommendations were a proposed response to the vast increases it foresaw in the need for qualified health personnel at all levels of skill. The report was particularly concerned with ensuring adequate numbers of competent allied and auxiliary personnel, listing many recommendations on how to achieve these goals. It concluded that although financing for education in health professions should remain the responsibility of both government and nongovernment sources, government support at all levels was essential for producing adequate numbers of high-quality health personnel, and federal government support had to be the main source.

The new focus in commission policy pronouncements on greater delegation of the physician's functions to allied health personnel was soon to manifest itself in de facto policy attempts to implement various physician's assistant training programs.

Measures to Accelerate the Output of Medical Care Personnel after 1965

Allied Health Personnel

Partly in response to the recommendations of these studies dealing with the potential of allied health personnel for helping increase physician productivity, the Allied Health Professions Personnel Training Act of 1966 (P.L. 89–751) was enacted. It amended the Public Health Service Act "to increase the opportunities for training of medical technologists and personnel in other allied health professions, to improve the educational quality of schools training such allied health professions personnel. . . ."[15]

The Surgeon General charged the Allied Health Professions Educational Subcommittee of the National Advisory Health Council with developing policy recommendations for implementing the new legislation with respect to determining the needs for allied health professions personnel and services, the development of new kinds of health workers, and the education of allied health personnel. The subcommittee defined the allied health occupations to include a broad range, virtually every group beyond medicine and dentistry, although other definitions exclude nursing from the "allied" occupations (see note 18). It embarked on its assignment with an a priori acceptance of the premise that making comprehensive health services available to all people would require not only more physicians, dentists, and other highly trained professionals, but also more and new kinds of technicians and assistants as well. Achievement of this goal would require an appropriate educational structure large enough to produce adequate numbers of well-prepared personnel as well as an organizational structure of the health services delivery system that promoted the development of smooth-functioning, practicing health teams. The subcommittee found that neither existed. It judged the current output of schools for the allied health occupations to be grossly inadequate and the institutional placement of educational programs badly fragmented. There were 2.8 million persons in health occupations in 1966, when the subcommittee reviewed these statistics. This number was expected to increase to 3.8 million persons by 1975. Population growth, especially in the older age groups, was projected to require increased numbers of health personnel. As has been noted, there were approximately 12 health workers for each physician in 1966, and the ratio of nonphysician health workers to physicians was already increasing rapidly, but apparently this rate of increase was judged to be too slow

for the future that the subcommittee envisioned.

The Allied Health Subcommittee's report, issued in 1967, presented both a survey of existing allied health personnel and a set of recommendations that may be viewed as an overall planning document for implementing the Allied Health Professional Personnel Training Act of 1966. The task of defining the roles and functions of an expanding group of new health professions was and has remained an area of contentious turmoil, that made it difficult to achieve consensus on even the boundaries of the problem, let alone the solution. The subcommittee found ambiguity in general definitions and substantial diversity in the specific functions and the educational requirements they implied assigned to positions with the same or similar job titles. Conversely, in other cases different job titles were used for positions with essentially the same functions. These problems arose in trying to answer such general questions as: What is a health profession? What is a health occupation? Are they usefully differentiated? And with respect to job titles, in some fields, the word "technologist" was used to denote a person with baccalaureate preparation and "technician" a person with one or two years' preparation. In similar fashion, the word "therapist" could denote a wide range of educational levels. A physical therapist had a baccalaureate degree; an inhalation therapist often received only one year of technical preparation. "Assistant" is yet another word that in some fields required one or two years of post–high school preparation and in others a baccalaureate degree. In some cases a "physician's assistant" with twenty-four months' training was being proposed as qualified to do general tasks under a physician's supervision that were usually not assigned to registered nurses (see Table 13–3). Clearly any recommendations for appropriate curriculum development would depend heavily on how job titles were defined.

The subcommittee found that for many of the occupations involved in the provision of health services, educational patterns were already undergoing substantial change both in length and in locus of training. There was a growing emphasis on the complementary roles of educational and clinical experiences. Programs were already being developed in 1965[16] and imme-

Table 13–3. Examples of Allied Health Professional and Technical Occupations for which Educatioin Was Provided in 4-Year Colleges, Junior Colleges, and Technical Schools by Level of Education and Major Orientation—as of 1966

Level of education	Patient-oriented	Laboratory-oriented	Administration-oriented	Community-oriented	Other
Primarily postbaccalaureate	Audiologist Clinical psychologist Medical social worker Rehabilitation counselor Speech pathologist	Pharmacist Radiobiologist	Hospital administrator Biostatistician	Public health administrator Health educator Nutritionist Engineering specialties	Biomedical engineering Medical economist Medical sociologist
Primarily baccalaureate (some with postbaccalaureate clinical training)	Dietitian Occupational therapist Physical therapist	Medical technologist	Medical records librarian	Sanitarian Radiological health technologist	Medical illustrator Science writer
Baccalaureate and prebaccalaureate	Dental hygienist Nurse Orthoptic technologist	Prosthetist Radiologic technologist			
Associate degree and other prebaccalaureate	Dental assistant Dispensing optician Food service supervisor Occupational therapy assistant Orthoptic technician Psychiatric aide	Cytotechnologist* Dental laboratory technician Medical laboratory assistant X-ray assistant	Medical records technician		
One year	Practical nurse Inhalation therapist Operating room assistant Surgical technician	Certified laboratory assistant	Medical assistant Medical office assistant Medical secretary Nursing unit management assistant		

Source: Allied Health Submcommittee (1967).
*There is also one baccalaureate program.

diately thereafter to train new health workers to perform a variety of duties supportive of and complementary to existing health occupations. The subcommittee felt it to be important that some of these training programs also offer further training to workers who were in "dead-end" jobs, individuals who had had previous training or experience at health delivery sites but who had been prevented by circumstances from further professional development.

Particular interest centered on the new curricula that were training individuals to be assistants to physicians, dentists, and optometrists. For some, the training was fairly short; for others it required a college degree plus additional education. Referred to under the generic name of "physician's assistant," these positions were seen by some to be different from other allied health jobs (Sadler, 1972). Many of the existing allied health personnel were performing fairly restricted and narrowly defined technical tasks such as administering routine laboratory tests and taking the simpler kinds of x-rays. The physicians' assistant was perceived to be something else, a direct assistant to the physician, helping him or her handle patients over a broader spectrum of functions but limited to tasks requiring less than a full medical training. Thus, although the concept was that of a health professional who was a *general* assistant to the physician, rather than narrowly restricted to a set of routine, largely repetitive tasks, it was not oriented toward developing independent practitioners and required all work to be done under the supervision of a physician (Sadler, 1972). The health profession whose work boundaries the physician's assistant most often crossed was the professional nurse, and a lack of agreement on what these boundaries were led to frictions. The position of "nurse practitioner," essentially a nurse trained to be a "physician's assistant," developed in an attempt to bridge this difference.[17]

Taking cognizance of these facts and considerations, the subcommittee proposed doubling the output of educational programs for professional and technical workers for the allied health services, with particular attention to achieving a better balance of opportunity for training among the geographic regions of the United States. To assure a high quality of preparation, the subcom-

mittee report made major recommendations[18] dealing with the education and training of allied health personnel and calling for studies of appropriate methods for credentialing them.

And indeed, one of the first problems posed by the changes in the allied health personnel field was that of credentialing. Once the implementation of the Allied Health Professions Personnel Training Act got into full operation some time after 1966 a large number of new educational programs for training allied health personnel, many with new titles and functions, including physician's assistants, were instituted. Each of these occupations was forming its own body for accrediting graduates of these programs and many were seeking state licensing.[19] The accrediting bodies operated with varying standards of thoroughness and frequency of reviews. The number of such accredited programs grew by 28 percent between 1956 and 1970, with some 2,000 programs being reported in the latter year by the American Association of Junior Colleges alone. Many other programs were accredited by joint bodies representing some arm of the AMA and the occupation being accredited. The accrediting bodies were themselves accredited by two national organizations, a governmental body—the U.S. Office of Education—and a voluntary body—the National Commission on Accrediting, comprising representatives of some 1,500 colleges and universities. The rapid proliferation of accredited programs led to an attempt to coordinate their quality and perhaps reduce their number. In 1969, a study of the situation was jointly commissioned by the AMA Council on Medical Education, the National Commission on Accrediting, and the Association of Schools of the Allied Health Professions. This *Study of Accreditation of Selected Health Educational Programs* (SASHEP), published in 1972, presented a detailed analysis of the health personnel situation both past and present.

One of the main recommendations of the SASHEP report was that accrediting bodies be held accountable to the host educational institution of the program, potential employers, federal and state governments, students, and "ultimately to the public-at-large." This recommendation spoke to the fact that the accrediting bodies were found to be composed of health professionals and therefore tended to be responsible mainly and often only to these professionals.

Another important recommendation was that reforms in accrediting procedures be tied to reforms in licensure and certification procedures, since private and state certifying agencies and some state licensing agencies required graduation from accredited programs as a prerequisite for taking an examination. Other recommendations dealt with the composition of their boards, methods of financing the costs of accreditation, and the need for a body that would coordinate and perhaps integrate new accrediting programs.

There was also a trend in state licensing laws that had the potential for legally expanding the scope of the physician's assistant functions in a new way. "In the 1960s four States, Arizona, Colorado, Kansas, and Oklahoma, enacted legislation that exempted from the medical practice acts certain delegations of functions" (Roemer, 1973). These "general delegation" statutes, as they are called, specified a broadly defined general permission for physicians to delegate some of their functions to physician's assistants working under their supervision. The innovative feature of this legislation was that it specified only the appropriate degrees of supervision that physicians must exercise in delegating tasks to others without enumerating specific delegatable tasks as such. (By 1973 eleven other states had legislated specific tasks that a physician could delegate, and still others had enacted legislation allowing for expanded functions of existing health care personnel, especially dental hygienists and professional nurses.)

However, these programs, as implemented, had only limited success in achieving the desired outcome, an increase in the use of allied personnel working under the supervision of physicians that would produce a substantial abatement of the perceived shortage of physicians. A 1969 editorial in the *New England Journal of Medicine* stated that the basic difficulty in the education and use of allied health personnel (especially new types) was that the nation's physicians (both in community and academic practice) and hospitals had yet to commit themselves to changing their patterns of providing patient care sufficiently to use increasing numbers and categories of allied health personnel. Along with

more adequate records and communication it was hoped that this would contribute to more personalized comprehensive care, especially preventive and rehabilitative but also diagnostic and curative, and that it would make medical care more readily available to all people. Major progress in this direction was needed because the urgency for such changes was becoming increasingly apparent. The author of the editorial, Ward Darley, asserted that the federal government would have to provide more funds for comprehensive health planning and health professions education than it had up through 1969.

With the approach of 1970, federal officials reiterated even more strongly their continued interest in the development of allied medical personnel. Goaded by the mounting pressures for better service and the rising costs stemming in large part from the implementation of Medicare and Medicaid, HEW Secretary Robert Finch and HEW Undersecretary for Health Roger Egeberg, with President Nixon's support, drew attention in 1969 to what they termed an "impending breakdown in the delivery of health care," and called for "immediate action" on the part of both the government and private sectors of the nation. The immediate fiscal problems that were attributed to Medicare and Medicaid were accorded top priority, and among causes and remedies considered were the growing shortage of health personnel and the need to alleviate it. They announced the establishment of an Office of New Careers whose top priority was to develop programs for returning Vietnam medical corpsmen, stating that there must be "a major commitment by the varied segments in the private health care industry to drastic changes." Among other items, Finch and Egeberg asked that training be oriented toward the immediate needs of the country, particularly toward comprehensive care of the poor and the near poor; that a review be mounted of the requirements for licensing and certification which they deemed to be standing in the way of the proper use of scarce personnel resources (see "SASHEP" p. 385), and finally, that new and competitive forms of organization for the delivery of comprehensive health services on a large scale be developed. (The latter was one of the earliest intimations of the Nixon administration's subsequent support of the HMO movement and of the "competition" strategy later to be prominently advocated during the period 1975–1982. The HMO organization, especially the prepaid group practice, is particularly amenable to use of allied personnel to do some of the tasks usually done by physicians in fee-for-service solo or specialty group practice.)

Thus by the end of the 1960s federal legislation had been passed to stimulate the education of larger numbers of physicians, dentists, nurses, and allied health personnel; expanded use of allied personnel in a special physician's assistant role was being strongly advocated by government officials and nongovernment scholars, writers, and health administrators; and pilot programs to develop such personnel under academic and professional society auspices were in operation and growing in number with federal support. Yet there were no signs of a substantial abatement of the perceived shortage of physicians. As the Ward Darley editorial intimated, one of the main difficulties was the slow pace with which physicians, hospitals, and reimbursement agencies proceeded to accept substantial delegation of physician's tasks to allied health personnel. Despite this, rejection rates of qualified students for medical schools continued to rise, physicians' incomes and prices continued to climb in the face of the resultant "shortage," and hospitals continued to report high vacancy rates for house staff. In view of these facts, it is not surprising that government attention returned to the physician shortage with an acceleration of efforts to increase the output of physicians.

Developments Contributing to Continued Efforts to Increase the Output of Physicians

It had been widely taken for granted that the proliferation of allied health personnel would reduce the pressure for a greater output of physicians. Apparently it did not, unless one wishes to argue that this pressure would have been even greater had there not been such an expansion. As noted above, there were those who argued that this shortfall in expectation was mostly due to the failure of physicians, hospitals, and reimbursing agencies to accept the integration of newly trained allied health personnel into med-

ical practice quickly and fully enough. However, an equally important question was whether most of the expanded allied health work force was performing some of the tasks that had previously been performed only by physicians but were now being delegated to physicians' assistants or whether it was for the most part merely performing entirely new tasks for technicians and technologists brought about by the growth of new medical knowledge and technologies. If the latter were the case, then clearly increased numbers of allied health workers should not be taken as evidence of a decreased need for physicians. The technician-technologist (medical technologist[20]) nature of many of the new and expanded allied health professions lends credence to the conclusion that this expansion did not by 1970 constitute, only, or perhaps even mainly, a delegation of tasks that had traditionally been performed only by physicians. Indeed, if this is true, then an increased number of allied health personnel performing newly developed repetitive technical tasks could reasonably be supposed to increase the required number of physicians because of the need for specialists to supervise the "teams" performing these tasks. Thus, more allied health personnel were needed, but not because they would necessarily decrease the need for more physicians. In fact, national attention had never turned away from the question of physician supply while measures to increase the supply of allied personnel were being implemented. The question, "How many physicians did the country need?" remained open, or rather was refined to: "How is it that we have so many physicians and hospitals, on average, and yet hear so many widespread accounts of lack of access to care?"

The analyses of medical care organization and patterns of health service utilization by the population were becoming more sophisticated during the 1960s. They were looking at variables representing a wider band of medical and societal interrelationships. At the same time, other variables were being considered that delved beneath overly broad generalities in which reasonably acceptable national averages obscured regional and local trouble spots. Many of these newer studies that were examining and analyzing changes in the physician supply ratio (number of physicians per population) were considering both the numerator and the denominator of this ratio in greater detail (Knowles, 1969).

They were pointing to the necessity, when studying physician supply (the numerator of the ratio), of looking at specialty distribution, physician worksite (practice, research, teaching, administration), geographic location, and other variables. Similarly, in studying population needs or demand (the denominator of the ratio), scholars were increasingly looking at variables such as age, sex, ethnicity, geographic distribution, income distribution, and cultural values (Knowles, 1969). Social and behavioral scientists as well as analysts in government agencies, practitioners, and medical care writers who were looking into some of these factors after the passage of the Health Professions Education Assistance Act of 1963 with its 1965 amendments, continued to foresee sharply increasing demand with physician supply, of the right type (i.e., whose distribution and mix were a good match for the population distribution and mix), falling increasingly behind requirements.

For example, in a study published in 1967, the economist Rashi Fein stratified the population by such variables as income and race, and by projecting future population shifts among the strata and taking into consideration differential demand for services by the various population strata he derived an estimate of a 22 to 26 percent growth in the demand for physicians' services by 1975 and a 35 to 40 percent growth by 1980. Although the estimated 19 percent growth in the number of physicians by 1975 exceeded the expected growth of only 13 percent in population, he noted that the demand for physician visits would outstrip the improvement in physician/population ratio because the number of visits per person would rise in response to the upward shifts in the distribution of income that were expected to occur. Thus, even without assuming any worsening of the physician to population ratio, a shortage of physicians was forecast as the ability to pay for more services increased both because of higher earnings and the introduction of government programs.

Another example of these newer analyses was one by John H. Knowles, a well known physician administrator and policy analyst, who at the time he issued his analysis in 1969 was director of Massachusetts General Hospital. He noted

that the 22 percent increase in the number of active physicians between 1955 and 1965 exceeded a 17 percent growth in population. However, the number of patient *services supervised* by the physician had increased much more rapidly, at an average annual rate of 4 percent, *due to greater use of auxiliary health personnel*, diagnostic medical technology, and special facilities. This increase in patient services supervised meant that physicians were spending less time with patients. Services had greatly increased in number while personal contact between physician and patient had decreased. Over the thirty years 1940–1970 the average number of contacts by a white person with a physician had doubled to over five per year, and the proportion of the population that failed to see a doctor during a year had fallen from one-half to less than one-third. During the same period the number of patients that the physician saw per year increased markedly, as much as 300 percent in the case of general practitioners. Yet the proportion of medical services delivered *directly* by the physician himself or herself had gone down sharply. Thus, if one valued the time spent by a physician with a patient, it could be inferred that a growing shortage of physicians was to be expected if technology were to continue to develop and the tasks that physicians needed to supervise continued to proliferate. This was inevitable if allied personnel continued to multiply in the form of medical technologists without compensatory growth in physician assistant type personnel.

The Latent Demand among the Poor Perhaps the most important factor in these new estimates that were paying greater attention to differentiating need and utilization rates (demand) among specified population strata was the large latent demand found to exist among the poor, leading to estimates of large future demand. It was estimated that there existed a population of some 40 million, or 20 percent, of the people of the United States, that had serious but unvoiced needs and were as yet exercising little or no demand. There were, in 1969, some 45 million people in the United States who were classified as poor following the Social Security Administration's definition at that time. (The poverty line for an urban family of four was estimated as annual income below $4,345.) As has been noted, the question of how many poor people there were in the United States, who they were, and why they were poor had been an ongoing matter for sharp public debate. For the purposes of looking at the federal government's policy on health personnel development, perhaps the most cogent consideration is the relationship of poverty to ill health and the need for health services. A 1967 government analysis projected only slight declines in the number of poor people, to 44 million for 1969 and 41 million for 1973. This analysis, contained in a report issued by the Department of Health, Education and Welfare in 1967, noted a number of cogent facts:[21]

1. Twenty-nine per cent of the people with a family annual income of less than $2,000 have chronic conditions limiting their activity as contrasted with less than 7.5 percent of those in families with an annual income of $7,000 or more. Heart disease, arthritis, mental disease, high blood pressure, and visual and orthopedic impairments are all more common among the poor. Between the ages of seventeen and forty-four, the poor suffer twice the rate of such conditions in the aggregate as the nonpoor; and between the ages of forty-five and sixty-four, the rate is 5.5 times greater. For "mental and nervous conditions," 26.4 per 1,000 population is the rate for those with an family annual income under $2,000 as contrasted with 4.2 per 1,000 for those with a family income greater than $7,000 a year; and the lowest class seems to have more severe diseases.

2. Males in the age group forty-five to sixty-four, in the $2,000 annual-income group, have 3.5 times as many "disability days" (forty-nine and a half days per year) as the over $7,000 annual-income group (fourteen and three-tenths days per year).

3. Low-income families have more multiple hospital admissions, are more often hospitalized for non-surgical conditions, and stay longer in the hospital (ten and a half days per hospital stay for under $2,000 and seven and a half days for over $7,000).

4. Using color as a surrogate measure of economic position (nonwhite people experience poverty at 3 times the rate of white people), life expectancy at the time of birth is sixty-three and six-tenths years for nonwhite people and seventy and two-tenths years for the white population. This reflects largely the disadvantageous position of the black population, which is proportionally more poverty stricken than the white population. Thus, reduction in life expectancy may be a reflection of poverty per se.

5. Maternal mortality rates in 1965 were 90.2 per 100,000 live births among nonwhites as contrasted with 22.4 among white mothers.

6. Death rates due to tuberculosis, syphilis, influenza and pneumonia, vascular lesions of the central nervous system, and homicide are 2 times higher for nonwhites than whites. Cancer of the cervix, a curable lesion if diagnosed early, results in a higher nonwhite mortality.

7. The children of "under $2,000 income" families average 2 physician visits per year as contrasted with 4.4 visits in the "above $7,000 income" families.

8. Of nonwhite children, ages one to four, 22.5 percent have not been immunized with DPT as compared with 8.6 percent of white children.

9. Twenty-two percent of "under $4,000 income" families have never seen a dentist as compared with 7.2 percent of "over $10,000 income" families.

10. The oft-quoted figures relating to infant mortality and life expectancy in the United States as contrasted with the other countries of the world bear repeating here if only to make final the plea that we stop proclaiming our superiority in medicine to the world. In 1965 the United States ranked 18th among the countries of the world in infant mortality (11th in 1959); 22nd in male life expectancy (13th in 1959); and 10th in female life expectancy (7th in 1959).

The reasons attributed by this report for these conditions included inaccessible facilities in terms of travel time and location, lack of education as to health service needs (therefore inadequately voiced needs), distrust of the medical establishment, inability to pay for services despite recent legislation (therefore inadequately expressed demand), and most pertinent to our purposes here, large health personnel scarcities in areas where they were needed the most. Effective demand, and complaints, were still coming mainly from the middle and upper classes, where the economic and political power resided. However, the Medicaid, Medicare, and other programs such as those of the OEO were expected to continue to increase the demand by the poor with the passing years, which magnified the urgency for rectifying health personnel shortages and maldistribution.

The Problem of Primary-care Physicians In the meantime, the trend since at least 1940 in the change of the worksite and specialty mix of physicians entering the profession was continuing unchanged with decreasing proportions going into full-time, direct medical practice and even smaller percentages into general practice (see Table 13–4). The increase in proportions of medical school graduates entering teaching, research, and administrative and institutional ca-

Table 13–4. Full-time Specialists and General Practitioners in Private Practice as a Percentage of Total Physicians in Private Practice, Selected Years, 1940–1970

Year	Full-time specialists as a percentage of total physicians	General practitioners[a] as a percentage of total physicians
1940	23.5	76.5
1949	36.5	63.5
1957	47.8	52.2
1963	61.8	39.2
1970	74.4	26.6

[a]General practioners include part-time specialists. Part-time specialists were 15 and 8 percent of the total physicians in private practice in 1949 and 1960, respectively. *Medical Economics*, April 24, 1961. *Source*: Percentages calculated from data in U.S. Department of Health, Education, and Welfare, Public Health Service, *Health Manpower Source Book*, Sec. 10, 1959, p. 2, and *Health Manpower Source Book*, Sec. 18, 1964, p. 28. Reproduced from: Rayack, 1967, Table 26, except for year 1970 which is calculated from HEW, 1972, Table 86. Denominator comprises all active physicians in patient care.

reers continued at an accelerated pace, as did the increase in numbers preferring specialty to general practice. Therefore, even the projections of future physician shortages "if nothing were done" were held to be understated in terms of being able to meet future demand for service. The potential shortage of primary-care physicians was sufficiently severe by 1964 for the Council on Medical Education of the American Medical Association to appoint an Ad Hoc Committee on Education for Family Practice, consisting of representatives from the Council on Medical Education, the American Academy of General Practice, the AMA Section on General Practice, and the Association of American Medical Colleges. The Ad Hoc Committee's 1966 report emphasized the need for developing and enlarging a class of physicians that could provide, through their own direct services as well as through "case management," comprehensive personal health services of high quality for the American people. The Committee recommended that medical schools develop departments of comprehensive medical care or family practice. It further concluded that family practice should have specialty certification similar to that granted by other specialty boards. The report of this committee, along with those of other similar groups (AAGP; National Commission on Community Health Services, 1967; AAMC, 1966), represented the most recent, detailed, and methodologically sophisticated at-

tempt to date attempting to show how the disappearing general practitioner could be replaced in the future by the much-needed specialist in family medicine.

It will be recalled that the Coggeshall Report of 1965 (see page 382) indicated the need for a specially trained coordinating leader for the medical care team. The emphasis on the team concept of comprehensive medicine was not intended to minimize the importance of specialization but rather "to show that the specially trained family physician and his cadre of specially trained helpers, properly related to other specialty areas, is essential if we are ever to equate the performance of our medical establishment with its potential" (Darley and Somers, 1967). In its report issued one year later, this ad hoc committee was asserting that such a leader needed to be not only "specially trained" but accredited for the task. The authors of articles on the subject of medical personnel seemed to be at least implicitly concurring in the view expressed by some that the time had come for another Flexner report, another careful assessment of the capacity of medical education to turn out the numbers and types of physicians that had been shown to be needed. If in 1910 medical school curricula needed to be attuned to the potential of applying the new discoveries of natural science, the task in 1970 was to further attune these curricula to be concordant with the findings of social investigations with respect to new biotechnical, social, and economic configurations of medical practice organizations, population changes, and the new configuration of health problems.

President Johnson had created a National Advisory Commission on Health Manpower in May 1966 to plan strategies for eliminating or at least mitigating both existing and projected shortages of health personnel. The report of the Commission was presented in two volumes (1967).[22] Its recommendations brought together most of the suggestions that had appeared piecemeal in numerous writings on physician, dental, nursing, and other health service personnel, as well as other special problems, such as closing the gap in access to health care for the poor and the availability of primary ambulatory care. Much of the federal and legislative activity that resulted, as well as that of professional and academic organizations in the health personnel training arena, followed along the lines outlined in these recommendations, which appeared in summary form in volume I of the commission's report.

Concomitant with the appointment of this government-sponsored commission, the board of trustees of the American Medical Association appointed a Committee on Health Manpower in 1966. This body issued a statement on medical personnel in June 1967 asserting that a "critical need for more physicians, for a better distribution of physician resources, and for allied health personnel in all categories" existed. It recommended expansion of existing medical schools as well as recognizing the need for additional schools. Continuing ongoing study of the "effect of new roles for health personnel and new interrelationships and interdependencies between health professions, as well as the impact of innovative concepts on the organizational structure evolving in the general system of health care delivery" (Glaser, 1970) was also recommended. While concurring with most of the recommendations of the National Advisory Commission on Health Manpower report, the AMA committee disagreed with the concept of using federal funds as an incentive for increasing the numbers of medical students.

Joint AMA-AAMC Action Differences had been developing between the Council on Medical Education of the AMA and the American Association of Medical Colleges (AAMC) over government policy on intervening to increase the output of physicians. Apparently the weakening effect on lobbying that could be wrought by such divisions concerned both organizations, and in 1968 representatives of the AMA Board of Trustees and Council on Medical Education met with representatives of the AAMC Executive Council to consider the problem of the national shortage of physicians. The issuance of a joint AMA-AAMC statement on health manpower on March 5, 1968, was a historic occasion. The document emphasized "the urgent and critical need for more physicians" and declared that "[B]oth associations endorse the position that all medical schools should now accept as a goal the expansion of their collective enrollments to a level *that permits all qualified applicants to be*

admitted" (emphasis added). Taken at face value, the position implied that all academically qualified persons who wanted a medical education should be admitted to a medical school and that the number of physicians in the United States should be allowed to be determined by market forces (with medical schools constituting the supply and qualified applicants the demand) instead of controlled by restricting the number of medical school places. This open market condition had not been in effect in American medical education since the disappearance of the proprietary medical schools in the post–Flexner era. In addition to encouraging an increase in enrollment across the board, the statement called for curricular innovations and "other changes in the educational programs which would shorten the time required for medical education and minimize the costs." Furthermore, "the development of schools of quality whose primary mission is the preparation of able physicians for clinical practice as economically and rapidly as possible is to be encouraged. Such schools may have less emphasis on fundamental biological research than is appropriate for a number of other schools," a sharp departure from the view that had been held by medical educators since 1910. Finally, support through public as well as private financing was recommended.

This statement was amplified and expanded in a second joint statement issued three months later, in June 1968, urging that "increased emphasis be given to support of the educational component of academic medical center activities with the intent that the production of physicians and other health personnel by such centers be assigned the highest possible priority" (AMA/AAMC, 1968). This second statement contained an additional significant departure from previous AMA policy with regard to federal aid to medical students. Opposition to federal loans given directly to medical students was discontinued.

During 1969, the AMA and the Association of American Medical Colleges continued their series of joint meetings to consider the national shortage of physicians and issued yet a third joint statement in September 1969, "Financial Support of Medical Schools by the Federal Government." Earlier joint statements issued in March and June 1968 had only called for a substantial increase in enrollments of existing U.S.

medical schools (despite AMA concurrence in the previously described report of the National Advisory Commission on Health Manpower that additional schools be opened). The third joint statement, however, accepted President Nixon's challenge to the medical schools to expand the number of physicians being trained, with the added assertion that such plans could not be implemented without a marked increase in federal financial support for medical education. The federal government responded to these three statements.

Health Manpower Act of 1968 A number of federal laws of importance to medical education were due to expire during 1968, including the Nurse Training Act of 1964, the Health Professions Educational Assistance Amendments of 1965, the Allied Health Professions Personnel Training Act of 1966, and the Health Research Facilities Amendments of 1965. These four pieces of legislation, as well as additional legislation dealing with the construction of medical libraries, were consolidated into the Health Manpower Act of 1968 and passed as P.L. 90–490 on August 17, 1968. Many of the recommendations of the National Advisory Commission and the joint AMA-AAMC statements as well as the studies on allied health manpower personnel were incorporated into this codification of health personnel legislation. In addition to bringing together under one statute most of the many federal programs for financing education in the health professions, the administration of those programs was centralized in one agency, the Bureau of Health Manpower in HEW.

The federal aid that had gone to the medical schools thus far was earmarked for expansion of their research, construction, and medical education capacities. It was assumed that a gratuitous by-product of this aid would be expanded enrollment of new medical students through some trickle-down mechanism. Like most trickle-down devices, it produced some effect on enrollment but the expansion was small for the money expended. It was being argued by some that grants that were more directly aimed at increased enrollment would be more effective in expanding enrollment than relying only on the indirect effect of money granted for general program expansion. Following passage of this act, the Department of Health, Education and Welfare announced a new Physician Augmentation Program in 1969 to help medical and osteopathic schools increase their first-year enrollment by a national total of 4,000 over the next four years, with a target initial increase in enrollment of 1,000 students for the fall of 1970, over and above any increases to which the schools were already committed in fulfilling participation requirements for other federal programs. When the Act came due for legislative renewal in 1972, grants specifically targeted to increasing the size of entering classes in medical schools featured prominently in the provisions.

Early Effects of Increased Federal Funding Some early results of the expanded support programs and conclusions that were drawn from them were:

1. During the years 1967–1972, the number of medical schools increased from 90 to 108, the number of annual graduates from 7,743 to 9,551, the students enrolled in medical school from 34,538 to 43,399, first-year students from 9,479 to 12,361, and the number of physicians[23] per 100,000 population from 146 to 160. The percentage of medical school applicants accepted, however, fell from 51.8 to 42.3 (Table 13–1 and Figs. 13–1 and 13–2).

2. The percentage of black students enrolled rose in the fiscal years 1969 through 1972 from 2.3 to 4.8 percent (AMA, 1972).

3. Although medical student loans continued to come primarily from federal sources, the percentage declined from 73 percent in fiscal year 1969 to 53 percent in 1972 (AMA, 1972, Table 26).

4. The sources of support for regular operating programs were slowly shifting, with ever-heavier proportions coming from state and federal sources (AMA, Council on Medical Education, 1972, Table 34).

5. Federal obligations to medical schools increased from 688 million dollars in fiscal 1967 to an estimated 832 million dollars in 1971. However, as of 1971, 51.1 percent of all federal funds to medical schools were still being granted for research, 19.8 percent for

graduate research training, with only 9.0 percent for construction of teaching facilities and 11.7 percent for undergraduate medical education (AAMC, Vol. 46 #10, Table 2, p. 907).

The general conclusion seemed to be that while the output of physicians had been increased, very largely due to federal and state funds, the increased enrollment in medical schools had not kept up with applicant demand.

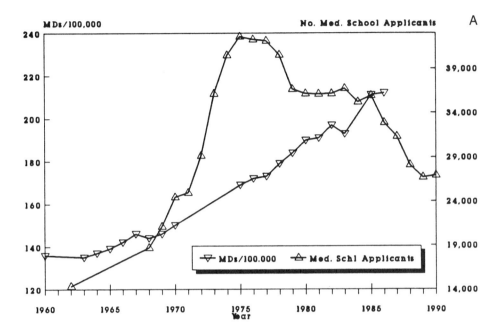

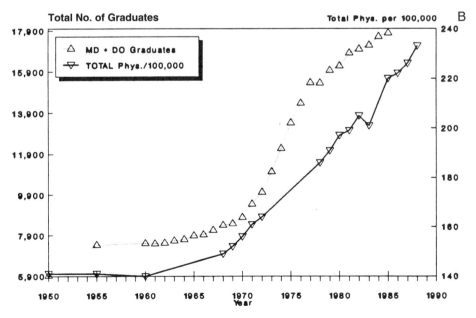

Fig. 13–1. (a) Number of MDs per 100,000 and number of applications to medical schools. (b) Active physicians (MDs and DOs) per 100,000 population and total number of graduates. *Note*: The markers on the lines indicate actual data points. *Source*: Table 13–1.

Nor had the output of graduates gotten substantially ahead of the population increase. Whether the geographical and specialty disparities had been even partially equalized and rationalized was not clear.

The Comprehensive Health Manpower Training Act of 1971 (P.L. 92–157) With the Health Manpower Act of 1968 scheduled to expire in 1972, the legislation extending the functions of this act took account of the observed shortfalls of the program in reaching federal goals during 1968–72. Its scope was substantially expanded and the emphasis on grants that more directly targeted enrollment increases was increased. Capitation (based on numbers of students) grants to health-professions schools that met certain legislative standards were provided for, as were special project grants for curricular improvement, start-up grants for new schools of medicine, osteopathy, and dentistry, conversion grants to change existing two-year medical schools to degree-granting institutions, incentives to increase the enrollment of minority group students, and incentives for training of family physicians and physician's assistants. In its summary of this legislation, the staff of the AMA Council on Education stated:

This was easily the most important federal legislation ever enacted for the support of medical education. It was based on the principle that federal financing is necessary for the regular operational support of schools of medicine, osteopathy, dentistry, optometry, podiatry, pharmacy, and veterinary medicine. While basic institutional grants and special project grants had been provided under previous health professions educational assistance acts, *this marked the first time that funds were provided on a specific capitation basis*—i.e., with a certain number of dollars provided for each student enrolled. [Emphasis added.]

The legislation also marked the first time that federal support had been tied specifically to requirements that certain activities be carried out by the institutions receiving the funds. Accordingly, it marked the first time that there has been intervention by federal agencies in the internal program decisions of the educational institutions.

According to the provisions of the capitation grants, the grants may not be received unless an institution presents a plan to carry out projects in at least three of nine categories described in the law. These include such things as shortening the length of training; establishing interdisciplinary training and the use of the team approach to the provision of health services; training new types of health personnel including physician's assistants; offering innovative educational programs including those in the organization, provision, financing, or evaluation of health care; increasing the enrollment; increasing the enrollment of disadvantaged students; training primary-care health professionals; and establishing programs in clinical pharmacology, drug use and abuse, and in the science of nutrition.

Specific provisions are contained in the legislation for incentives to increase the enrollment of students and to increase the number of graduating students. Expansion of enrollment is required for every school that receives a capitation grant, but special bonuses are provided for enrollment increases over the required minimum. Special project grants and health manpower education initiative awards[24] [my note] are available for many of the categorical purposes listed above as well as certain others. A special section is provided for grants to initiate, expand, or improve professional training programs in family medicine. Student loan and scholarship provisions are expanded and extended under the new legislation.

When fully implemented, the new comprehensive Health Manpower Training Act will provide a substantial portion of the operating support of virtually all educational institutions in the health professions field. Initial appropriation and expenditure of funds has been at a level substantially below that authorized by the legislation, but these amounts may be expected to be greater in subsequent years (1972).

Thus, the three fiscal years ending in 1972, 1973, and 1974 saw the launching of a large-scale amended federal program to increase the output of physicians using a wide spectrum of types of support and regulation.

The National Health Service Corps The provisions of the Health Manpower Act of 1968 and their amendments in the 1971 Act were mainly directed at increasing the global total of health personnel by raising the output of the various training schools, with some provisions directed at attempting to change the specialty mix and other features of the additions to the medical personnel pool. Other legislation and proposals were focusing more strongly on rectifying the distribution of physicians by geography, cross-stratified by specialty, work setting, and availability to low-income persons.

As has been noted, geographic maldistribution of physicians has long been recognized as a shortcoming of the U.S. medical care delivery system. Indeed, during the years when AMA spokesmen were vehemently denying that the

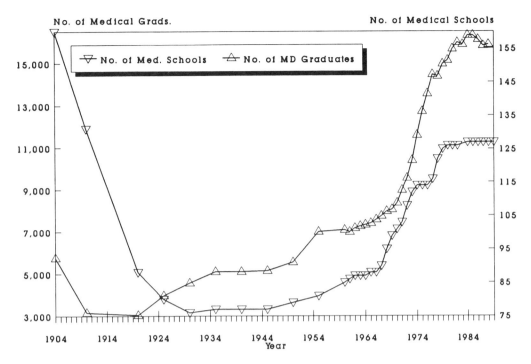

Fig. 13–2. Number of medical schools and number of graduates from medical schools. *Note*: The markers on the lines indicate actual data points. *Source*: Table 13–1.

total numbers of physicians practicing and being produced were inadequate to the tasks society wished performed, one of their rejoinders was that it was entirely a matter of maldistribution. They noted that more sparsely settled areas of the United States were seriously underdoctored, and that urban centers were if anything over-supplied with physicians. Yet even in the urban centers access to primary care for the poor and near-poor was unsatisfactory and growing worse. The main source of such care, the local public general hospital, was having trouble recruiting physicians, as the earlier discussion on the foreign medical graduate pointed out. Even after Medicaid was passed in 1965, many physicians did not accept Medicaid beneficiaries. The new neighborhood health centers also were in need of medical personnel. The need for medical personnel to serve the primary-care needs of the poor and near-poor was therefore apparent both in rural and in inner-city areas. Thus, it may have been true that maldistribution of physicians was to blame for a lack of physicians rather than an overall "shortage," but rurality alone was clearly not the only cause of the maldistribution.

Federal health "manpower" legislation had taken some cognizance of the geographic maldistribution problem before 1970. The Health Professions Educational Assistance Amendments[25] of 1965 (P.L. 89–190) provided for partial cancelation of indebtedness on federally financed student loans that had been advanced to medical, dental, and optometry students if they practiced in medically underserved areas. This privilege was later extended to pharmacy and podiatry students. The Allied Health Professions Personnel Training Act of 1966 (P.L. 89–751) increased the loan cancelation proportion.

The formation of the National Health Service Corps was an attempt by the federal government to accelerate the alleviation of physician maldistribution through a more formally organized special program dedicated to this purpose. The Emergency Health Personnel Act of 1970 (P.L. 91–623) authorized assignment of Public Health Service personnel to areas designated as having a critical shortage of health personnel. The designation of an area as "underserved" was to be made by the Secretary of HEW upon application from organizational entities of the area involved with the determination based on such criteria as need (population composition, ratio of physicians to population, and numbers and types of other health personnel and facilities and their accessibility) and receptivity of the community to having PHS personnel provide medical care. Also required for PHS personnel to be assigned were the recommendation of the local health planning agency and, interestingly enough, the local professional society. The last item was meant to allay fears of professional—especially medical—societies of government-subsidized competition. (Although the organizational framework of the National Health Service Corps was created by this legislation, there was sufficient nervousness in Congress about professional society opposition and possible labeling of the enterprise as "socialized medicine" that the language of the original act provided that the program be administered by an "identifiable administrative entity" within HEW. The National Health Service Corps was never referred to by name.) The Comprehensive Health Manpower Training Act of 1971 (see page 394) further increased the portion of the health professional student loans that could be canceled (to 85 percent) for specified years of postgraduate practice in medically underserved areas, and an additionally funded loan forgiveness program was established for medical students who agreed to practice primary care in a physician shortage or migratory health worker area.

The Emergency Health Personnel Act Amendments of 1972, P.L. 92–585, extending the authority of the 1970 legislation, clearly identified the program by name as the National Health Service Corps and authorized a new program of scholarships for students in specified health services professions. Students assumed an obligation to serve in assigned medically underserved areas after graduation for specified periods in return for each year of scholarship.

It is important to note the difference between the nature of the incentives for medical graduates to serve in medically underserved areas for specified periods provided under the NHSC *scholarship* program and those offered under the *loan cancellation* programs of prior Health Professions Assistance legislation such as those of 1965, 1966, and 1971. The earlier incentives had been based on retroactive cancelation of indebtedness by health professionals for loans they had received to pay their way through a health pro-

fessional school. The loans had been obtained with no promise by the student to serve in medically underserved areas after graduation, let alone in areas *assigned* by HEW. If, after graduation, the new physician or other health professional did choose to serve in an identified shortage area, he or she was then entitled to cancelation of a specified percentage of the indebtedness. There was no implied advance obligation per se to serve in an underserved area. Under the NHSC program the medical[26] student received a scholarship, not a loan, to cover the costs of his or her medical education and undertook to serve in an *assigned* medically underserved area after graduation, one year for each year of scholarship granted. If the graduating medical student did not serve as promised, he or she was required to reimburse the federal government for the cost of the scholarship plus interest, but the obligation to serve was clearly implied in the granting of the scholarship.

By February 1972, 28 physicians, 10 dentists, 18 nurses and 12 supporting professionals had been assigned to 18 communities. . . . Recruitment . . . has been difficult . . . the major incentive for doctors to join has been fulfillment of military obligation (Sadler, 1972).

This comment on the inappropriate motivation of some physicians who joined the NHSC scholarship program anticipated the concern that was later to arise over the fact that for physicians, paying the default penalty on a scholarship loan could be more financially rewarding than serving the obligated term in an underserved area. The default penalty was increased in 1976 to three times the scholarship loan plus interest in the Health Professions Educational Assistance Act of 1976, P.L. 94–484, which also added other new provisions to the existing legislative mandate of the NHSC and recodified all the appurtenant legislation into a more coherent body of law. After the passage of the Act on October 12, 1976, the main outlines of the program were:

1. The National Health Service Corps consisted of physicians, dentists, nurses, and other "health-related" specialists such as optometrists, podiatrists, and nurse practitioners. The personnel consisted both of Public Health Service commissioned corps and "ci-

vilian" members who were not part of the commissioned corps and they were assigned to serve in medically underserved areas. Members received salaries whether or not they were serving to pay off loan obligations.

2. The National Health Service Corps Scholarship Program granted professional school scholarships for medical and related personnel students who agreed to serve in an assigned medically underserved area upon graduation. There were separate and distinct appropriations for running the NHSC and for the scholarship program. In 1977/78, for example, the appropriations were $24.6 million for the NHSC operations and $40.0 million for the scholarship program (HEW, 1979).

3. The Health Services Administration of HEW determined what areas of the country were to be designated as medically underserved according to a formula and these were listed in priority order. One of the criteria was that each county should have at least one physician. Other criteria were based on health status and on measures of health personnel availability. HEW could place physicians in areas without local medical society approval if this approval had been "arbitrarily and capriciously" withheld. Acceptable NHSC sites were community health centers, outpatient departments of public and nonprofit hospitals, and clinics of all sorts serving persons with inadequate access to medical care. Also included as placement sites were private practices offering primary care in medically underserved areas.

4. "Reasonable effort" had to be made by NHSC sites to collect fees for services. This requirement could be waived by HEW if meeting it would seriously diminish outcomes of the program.

5. Grants were available to local communities to establish NHSC service sites, but the community had to share in the cost of the salaries of providers, the scholarships the providers had received, and the repayment of any loans that had been used to establish the site. This requirement also could be waived.

6. A revised loan forgiveness program was established (in 1976) to be part of the NHSC program operating alongside the scholarship program.

7. Hospitals that refused staff privileges to NHSC physicians could be denied participation in Medicare and Medicaid.

During the period 1973–79, the federal government spent $170 million on this program. Each year the appropriation rose both for operations and scholarships until 1980–81. Thereafter the amounts appropriated for scholarships declined but the amounts for operating costs did not. By 1978 there were 1,281 health professionals serving in 643 communities with NHSC sites, 410 of them having gone through professional schools with NHSC scholarships. Two hundred of the scholarship recipients were serving in the Indian Health Service or providing care to federal prisoners. In 1978 1.3 million persons utilized NHSC services and 9,061 students in ten disciplines received scholarships obligating a total of 16,254 man-years of service over the period 1973–1979. In 1978–79 almost 6 percent of all U.S. medical students and 13 percent of osteopathic students were scholarship recipients. Among the scholarship students, blacks, Hispanics, Indians, and women were "overrepresented" (HEW, 1980).

Despite this measurable progress, the 643 NHSC sites in operation should be compared with the total of 1,233 areas designated as underserved. Although the number of placements rose in subsequent years (e.g., 1,834 NHSC field personnel at 820 sites in 1979), the progress still fell far short of supplying all the designated underserved areas.

Report of the Carnegie Commission on Higher Education We have been looking at the federal government's efforts to increase the output of physicians and other medical care personnel in the 1960s and 1970s. Thus far the measures described have involved increasing the size of professional school enrollment and in the case of the loan forgiveness programs and the NHSC scholarship programs, inducing a change in the geographic distribution of medical personnel to improve access in underserved areas. Some of these efforts had also attempted to alter the medical care provider mix by increasing the number and types of allied health personnel and the production of primary care physicians. By the end of the 1960s the question was also being raised whether it was not time to do more to alter the curricula of medical schools to better meet the needs of the population for health personnel with respect to both geographic distribution and specialty mix. Was the very nature of the Flexner model curriculum itself still appropriate?

This question was addressed in 1970, sixty years after the issuance of the Flexner report, by another study dealing with medical education in the United States, again financed by the Carnegie Foundation for the Advancement of Teaching. This time the work was done by a staff working under the guidance of a broadly chosen committee chaired by Clark Kerr, with advisory input from educators, economists, and other professionals. Summarizing much of the thinking that had been expressed in the reports and writings of the preceding twenty years (including the joint AMA-AAMC statement discussed on pp. 391–392), this report squarely asserted a need to move away from considering the Flexner model as the *sole* model for medical education. The arguments of the Carnegie Commission are succinctly expressed by some salient excerpts from its own words:

The Flexner model and new models. The Flexner model, based on Johns Hopkins, Harvard, and, before them, German medical education, called for emphasis on biological research. Science was to be at the base of medical education. The Flexner model has been the sole fully accepted model in the United States since 1910. Some schools have fulfilled its promise brilliantly; others have been pale imitations; but all have tried to follow it. It has led to great strides forward in the quality of research and the quality of individual medical practitioners. The Flexner, or *research* model, however, looked inward to science in the medical school itself. It is a self-contained approach. Consequently, it has two weaknesses in modern times: (1) it largely ignores health care delivery outside the medical school and its own hospital, and (2) it sets science in the medical school apart from science on the general campus with resulting duplication of effort. . . . The self-contained Flexner model thus leads to expensive duplication and can lead to some loss in quality.

Two new models are arising: (1) the *health care delivery* model, where the medical school, in addition to training, does research in health care delivery, advises local hospitals and health authorities, works with community colleges and comprehensive colleges on the training of allied health personnel, carries on continuing education for health personnel, and generally orients itself to external services; and (2) the *integrated science* model, where most or all the basic science (and social science) instruction is carried on within the main campus (or other general campuses) and not duplicated in the medical school which provides mainly clinical instruction. In this model (as in England), the medical school may be, essentially, a teaching hospital; but this is not necessary—it may, rather, carry on all its "Flexner" functions except the traditional first one or two years of science education.

Mixtures are of course possible and are occurring among these "pure" types. . . .

We believe that the new interests in health care delivery and in the integration of science and other disciplinary efforts are wise. The simple Flexner research model is no longer adequate as the sole model. A few schools, and many parts of schools, will, and should, stay with the Flexner model, but we believe that the nation will be better served as many schools move in different directions.

Pacesetter schools . . . are moving toward health care delivery, or the integration of science, or both. We support these directions of movement. The nation has a sufficiency of the pure research model type of school. New developments should be toward greater integration with social needs, or toward greater integration with the general campus, or both (1970).

The data on basic science instruction carried on in the medical schools during 1967–1972 show that not only did they have full faculties of their own teaching basic science to medical students during their preclinical years, but they were also granting their own graduate degrees (M.A., Ph.D. and postdoctorate) in these sciences (AMA, 1972, Tables 8, 11). In fact, six of the 108 medical schools operational in 1972–73 were two-year schools teaching only the basic medical sciences (AMA, 1972, Table 2). Their graduates then had to gain admission to four-year medical schools to do their clinical work.

The Commission took at face value the oft-stated assertions that many more physicians and dentists than were being turned out by the existing schools would be needed and that much of the projected shortage (if "nothing were done") would be due to a mismatch of the specialty mix and geographic distribution of physicians with the needs of the population rather than a shortfall in the absolute number of physicians and dentists.

To remedy the existing inadequacies in health personnel and avoid their getting worse, the Commission report made a number of recommendations on changes in medical school education, principal among which were:

1. Development of nine new university health science centers and 126 Area Health Education Centers (AHECs).

   The university centers would contain full-blown medical schools and other health personnel training schools or programs (dentistry, nursing, allied health personnel, and others), while the AHECs would be located at local community hospitals that would operate health personnel training programs administered by the university health science centers. They would be located in relatively sparsely populated areas or in poor, densely populated, and medically underserved urban areas. The function of the AHECs would be to provide major, medically upgraded health care centers in areas where they were needed but where full-fledged medical schools were not likely to locate, as well as clinical experience for health personnel in training. The settings of such training would inculcate in the trainees an appreciation for working among persons at these locations and strengthen the attraction of general and family practice as a choice for future graduates. Even for those who later chose the standard subspecialties, the experience of perhaps just a rotation through a family practice non-Flexner type of program would leave a lasting imprint with respect to the patient care aspects of practice.

2. Curriculum reform.
   a. Shorten the medical training period (after the baccalaureate) from eight to six years by using a three-year medical school program and a three-year residency period.
   b. Provide an interim stopping point in health care training by awarding some sort of master's degree in biomedical studies. This point could be a node in a student's decision tree, with available branches being stop, continue to Ph.D., continue to M.D.
   c. Greatly increase the number of allied personnel being trained.
   d. Combine all science work on the university campus.
   e. Convert all two-year medical schools that do not have automatic transfer to four-year schools to full-fledged four-year schools.

3. Financing.
   a. Establish a revolving loan fund—"Educational Opportunity Bank"—for medical and dental students.
   b. Provide a larger federal share to meet the operating costs of medical and dental schools.
   c. Provide state support for private as well as state schools.
   d. Hold federal research expenditures to a constant percentage of the GNP.

As of 1971–72, some of these recommendations were being tried, but some of these trials were so small that they could fairly be called only pilot or experimental applications (HEW, 1972 pp. 976, 977). Eight of the 108 medical schools were operating programs that could be completed in thirty-six successive calendar months or less, often entailing attending school during summer. An additional twenty schools had some students on an individual accelerated track. Also, as noted previously, the general rotating internship was to be discontinued after 1975, so that it was expected that the previous one-year internship and three-year residency would in many cases be reduced to a single three-year residency.

FEDERAL SUPPORT FOR AHECS. One aspect of this report, the recommendation for the establishment of Areawide Health Education Centers (AHECs), was almost immediately translated into legislation as part of the well-named Comprehensive Health Manpower Training Act of 1971, which provided for "health manpower initiative awards" among its far ranging provisions. These initiative awards were to be available for developing centers that were similar to the AHECs of the Carnegie Commission report. Their purpose was to establish health personnel training sites with a public or nonprofit community hospital providing a patient care nucleus although they were to be relatively far from a medical center (i.e., school of medicine or osteopathy or a university health science center). Each AHEC was to be formally affiliated with a medical center that would be responsible for supervising the training of health care personnel at the AHEC site. The AHEC would run continuing education for physicians, residency training programs stressing primary care, and clinical instruction of undergraduate medical[27] students. An initiative award could also be obtained for conducting continuing education and clinical undergraduate instruction for nonphysician medical personnel. The Bureau of Health Manpower Education (now the Bureau of Health Professions), which operated the national program, defined these centers in the following terms:

An AHEC is therefore a new institutional arrangement developed through a medical center to supply manpower and leadership resources to meet community health service needs. It is designed to link the educational institutions and health care facilities and resources so that these total resources can be related in a way that best meets the health service needs of the defined community or area.[28]

The principal expectations for these centers were that they would supply continuing education and state of the art expertise to remote areas, increase access to allied health professions for women and minorities, reduce the pressure for opening more new medical schools than were needed or in areas that were inappropriate, and induce a larger proportion of medical students and young physicians to enter primary care. The first request for proposal (RFP) issued in June 1972 resulted in eighty-five institutions expressing interest, twenty-seven being asked to apply and eleven being chosen. Those chosen were awarded five-year contracts and most of these program activities began on October 1, 1972 (Gregorieff and Kell, 1976).

The program was renewed in 1976 as part of the Health Professions Educational Assistance Act of that year (P.L. 94–484), discussed above in connection with the renewal of the NHSC. By this time the federal objectives for the program had been further spelled out. Correcting the geographic and specialty maldistributions of physicians were established goals of the program and were being enunciated in Congressional reports (Gregorieff and Kell, 1976). This included emphasis on training primary-care specialists. The extension spelled out details of operations only vaguely referred to or implied in the original law. (For one thing, section 781 of the law now referred to the centers specifically as AHECs instead of "health manpower education initiatives.") It also specified more defin-

itively that some undergraduate medical student as well as graduate residency training of the supervising medical center was to take place at the AHEC site and required at least 25 percent of the operating funds of an AHEC to be met by the program itself. Each AHEC would now have to have an advisory board consisting at least 75 percent of residents of the service area, providers and consumers alike. Funding was guaranteed to an AHEC for three years and available for five upon satisfactory progress in development. Four additional AHECS were funded in 1977, five in 1978, and three in 1979 under the 1976 act. AHECs could now be of three types; urban, rural, and statewide but the establishment of AHEC sites in the inner city was now pronounced a priority of the program. After the initial five years of federal funding with local matching, the AHECs were expected to continue operating with state and local funds.[29]

Although the federal AHEC program has been the largest and most easily identified program of this type, other similar programs had been formed under other auspices. A report of a review by the Carnegie Council on Policy Studies in Higher Education, *Progress and Problems in Medical and Dental Education*, published in 1976, identified eight under VA sponsorship, "a far larger number" under the Regional Medical Programs (RMP, discussed in Chapter 5) but which were not "really fully developed, comprehensive AHECs," and some "community-based AHEC types." The same report noted:

There were a number of antecedents involving elements of the AHEC concept or system, although not called by this name. It made reference to residency programs in Cooperstown, New York, and the impact of the Mayo Clinic on medical care in Southeastern Minnesota, of the Duke Foundation on rural care in North and South Carolina, and of the Bingham Associates on hospital care in Maine. It called attention to the efforts of individual states in recent years to encourage decentralized medical education programs, noticed that by 1974 nine states had significant developments of this type and three others had them under serious consideration.

Despite the efforts of the Reagan administration to discontinue the program, a "third generation" version went into effect in 1984 and seventeen additional projects had been funded by 1988.

The 1970 Carnegie Commission Report and the federal AHEC program initiated in 1972 were based on a growing perception that continued proliferation of physicians would not alone remove the shortages of medical personnel. It was more likely, this view held, to lead to surpluses in the well-supplied areas and continued (perhaps worsened) shortages in the medically underserved areas. The concentration should be on righting the imbalances in geographic and specialty distribution. The Carnegie Commission Report had recommended a different curriculum for some medical schools that would be based more on primary care practice and shortened periods of university training. The AHEC centers were seen as a potent instrumentality for achieving these ends. The requirements in some of the federal AHEC legislation that the participating medical center's students rotate for a specified period through the AHEC site was meant to help attract some of them to later practice at these sites. The requirements for allied health personnel training at the centers, with emphasis on women and minority recruitment, were intended to both expand the inadequate pool of allied health personnel and widen opportunities for underrepresented groups to achieve valuable training. The evaluations of the AHEC program carried out by the Carnegie Council on Policy Studies in Higher Education and by various Congressional committees and independent investigators (Odegaard, 1979) indicated some advances along these lines, but substantial and clearly visible results were not expected for many years.

The AHEC centers were mostly in areas with a poor and inadequately insured target population. Whether one can expect to make a major dent in the redistribution problem without first raising the demand for health services in the shortage areas is a moot point. Is it actually feasible to rationalize the supply of health care resources to provide for access to all who need care without first effectively entitling them to care? Again, access is a function of both consumer entitlement and provider availability. Those who advocate relying only or almost entirely on market forces to increase access joined in supporting increased medical school enrollment because it would increase availability, thus increasing competition. This would increase access by lowering prices and it would then be easier to make care available to all. As we look at program after program that concentrated only or predominantly on increasing output (availability) of providers we find that the results were at best an exacerbated surplus of resources in well-supplied areas and a trickle-down overflow of some of the surplus to shortage areas. The AHEC program has been judged useful and successful in producing more women and minority allied health personnel, more primary care physicians, and a small increase in physicians who chose to practice in medically underserved areas. These are in and of themselves highly desirable outcomes, but there is as yet no conclusive evidence that the program has as yet made a big difference in altering the shortage of physicians in underserved areas. The NHSC program had a much more immediate and direct effect during the years it was well supported, perhaps because it focused almost entirely on directly providing service for which the program paid in addition to its outlays for education of physicians.

Public Health and Health Administration Personnel The federal efforts to increase the supply of health workers discussed thus far have considered clinical personnel working in medical care settings. Legislation was also enacted that reflected growing Congressional interest in developing training programs for health administration and planning personnel, including those skilled in program evaluation and health services research. As we have seen, many observers saw the remedy for the shortage of health personnel as lying largely in rationalizing the health service system to be more efficient, that is, to make better use of fewer resources. We have also noted a growing emphasis on prevention and health promotion as a means of controlling the rising cost of health care. If the health service system was to be rationalized and health promotion and prevention made a more important part of health care, then more persons trained in health planning, administration, epidemiology, health education and promotion, and allied disciplines would be needed.

Some of the earliest health "manpower" legislation dealt with public health personnel. The Health Amendments Act of 1956 (P.L. 84–911) provided traineeships for professional public health personnel, and in 1958 P.L. 85–544 established formula grants to schools of public health. In 1960 P.L. 86–720 added project grants for schools of public health as well as for nursing or engineering schools that offered graduate or specialized training in public health. The Graduate Public Health Training Amendments of 1964 (P.L. 88–497) extended these granting programs to other types of institutions, and the Health Professions Education Assistance Act of 1963 included schools for training professional public health personnel in its construction grant program (see p. 854). The Comprehensive Health Planning and Public Health Service Amendments of 1966 (P.L. 89–749) provided grants to a wide variety of organizations for training health planners (see Chap. 15). The *Health Professions Educational Assistance Act of 1976* (P I, 94–484) included training programs in occupational health in its grants or contracts for area health education center (AHEC) programs. It also established special project grants for schools of public health and graduate programs in health administration, introducing or expanding programs in biostatistics and epidemiology, health administration, health planning or health policy analysis, environmental or occupational health, and dietetics and nutrition. Some institutional grants were authorized for graduate programs in health administration, hospital administration and health planning for which schools of public health were not eligible.[30]

In 1978 21 schools of public health had 7,722 enrolled students, about 25 percent in health services administration programs and another 13 percent in public health practice programs. In 1961 a total of 1,631 students were enrolled in 14 schools, and even this is an overstated figure for comparison purposes because it included Canadian schools that are excluded from the 1978 figure (Hall, Rudolph, and Parsons, 1980). By 1985 there were 23 schools of public health. A similar proliferation took place over the period 1960–1980 in graduate programs of health administration, exclusive of those offered in schools of public health.

Summary and Remarks In 1910, The Flexner Report was precipitated by the failure of the de-

veloping body of scientific medical knowledge to be appropriately transmitted to medical students under the existing system of physician education. Fifty years later, during the 1960s, a gap was again perceived, but this time not so much between the state of biomedical scientific knowledge and the curricula of medical schools as between the type of medical care potentially achievable with the existing scientific medicine being taught in the medical schools and the medical care actually being received by wide sections of the American people. In 1910, the major problem was seen to be improving the qualifications of the graduating physician, with a view toward improving the scientific quality of clinical practice. In the 1960s, it was seen to be ensuring that this technically good clinical practice was widely available. In 1910, "improvers" looked mainly inward to what was going on inside the medical school and the degree to which state-of-the-art medical knowledge was being transmitted to medical students. In the 1960s, the improvers were largely looking outward to how the state-of-the-art medicine now being taught in the medical schools was being delivered to the population. They were asking how many persons of what type from what neighborhoods were receiving how much medical care, delivered by whom, and of what quality. Access to existing state-of-the-art medical care had become as important an arguments about the comparative merits of different therapies and diagnostic techniques; for disadvantaged populations it was perhaps even more important. Some investigators and commentators were even suggesting that the goals of improved access to medical care on the one hand and the relentless and overwhelming emphasis on research and introduction of ever more complex technology on the other hand might not be entirely compatible. As the previously quoted section from the 1970 Carnegie Commission report (page 398) implied, too heavy and singleminded a concentration on scientific research and producing scientist-physicians was even being viewed by some as detrimental to the quality of the health care delivered to the population as a whole and in particular to the care given underserved populations. The social and political evolution of the country after the victory of the scientific approach, around 1920, had caused the emphasis of many reformers and critics to gradually shift from a laboratory-clinic-hospital focus to a public health population-based social focus. The medical establishment, as represented by its official organizations, was ill at ease with such considerations. Both the AMA, and to a lesser degree the medical colleges, found population-based public health considerations to be outside their accustomed purview of concerns.[31] Their notion of public health was a local public health department restricted to a scope of function that was even narrower than the "basic six" of the standard public health department defined in the Emerson report. (See p. 32 for a 1962 AMA definition of this scope.) Organized medicine had been much more at home with the 1910 challenges. Flexner's challenge was exclusively to the education of physicians, whereas that of the 1960s was also to the education of the nurse and all the new health professions and occupations that had developed since the Flexner era and that make up the preponderant cadre of current health and medical personnel. The new challenges were not, except at the fringes, Luddite in character. They continued to support the scientific basis of medicine and indeed one of their major concerns was the extension of scientific education to these new professions. But they were also concerned with the adjustment of all health personnel to new social institutions and changed working relationships in new institutional settings. These institutions and settings, in turn, had arisen in answer to new technology, new levels of popular expectation, new forms of social organization, and new economic relationships.

Governmental responses to the 1910 and the 1960s challenges were also quite different. The consequences of the Flexner Report included the use of state licensing laws to improve the technical quality of medical education mainly by reducing the number of medical schools and consequently the number of medical school student places. Its implementation was heavily directed and financed by a few large corporate foundations (Brown, 1979), and although its emphasis was on upgrading scientific quality it also contracted the supply of physicians. In the 1960s the government response was largely federal, and it took the form of subsidizing expansion of the supply of physicians and supporting personnel along with efforts to increase the number of black physicians, which had been curtailed with special severity by the post–Flexner school closings.

The actions of the state medical societies after 1910, backed by state licensing apparatuses and corporate foundation financing, were based on the Flexner report, which itself was financed by corporate foundation money. The federal government's actions in the post–World War II era, on the other hand, were based on the findings of numerous commissions and individual scholars, most of them funded by the government rather than corporate foundations, and many of them mainly concerned with questions of equity and access. Although there was some federal legislation before 1960, the major laws focusing on questions of primary care and health personnel availability were the Health Professions Educational Assistance Act of 1963 with its 1965 amendments, the Nurse Training Act of 1964, the Allied Health Professions Act of 1966, the Health Manpower Act of 1968, and especially its extension and renewal in 1971, and the 1976 amendments to the Professions Educational Assistance Act. These acts made federal funds available for the construction of facilities for health personnel education, for expenditures for health personnel education programs, for capitation grants for medical students, and for direct student loans, scholarships, and educational program improvement grants for virtually all categories of health personnel—physicians, dentists, nurses, public health workers, specialists in mental health, retardation, rehabilitation, and a good many others. At the same time, programs administered by the United States Office of Education, the Department of Labor, and the National Welfare Administration were making financial assistance available for both academic and on-the-job training of nurses' aides, practical nurses, technicians of all sorts, home health aides, and many other categories of health occupations. With respect to physicians, the data clearly indicate the beginning of a sharp increase in medical school graduates and physicians per population beginning in 1963, as well as growth in the number of medical schools (see Figs. 13–1, 13–2).

Along with these programs oriented toward increasing the supply of health service personnel, other federal legislation was supplying funds to transform perceived health care needs into demands and thereby help assure that a substantial portion of the increased output of health personnel would indeed be used to improve service to some of the previously underserved. Medicare and Medicaid were operating to increase the demand, and as initially passed were designed to foreswear any attempt to introduce changes in the organization of medical care. The antipoverty program and later HEW with its Community Health Center programs influenced not only the overall demand for medical care but also the mix and nature of the supply of health care personnel, as discussed in Chapter 12. Although these demand- inducing programs differed widely in their emphasis and focus, they all relied primarily on nonfederal and especially on nongovernment institutions and agencies— state, local, and voluntary—for their actual operation. Thus, they continued and even added to the complexity of the American health care scene with its three levels of governmental involvement, its programs for special classes of eligibles, and the interaction of public and private organizations. Furthermore, private operation of publicly financed services, albeit with government regulation, was continuing to be the dominant mode of federal support for services. It was greatly expanded with the establishment of the community health centers, the passage of Medicare and Medicaid, much of the operations of the National Health Service Corps program as well as the manner in which the expansion of medical education was supported.

Despite all these programs to increase access to medical care, many people continued to have little or no access to needed medical care. They were not entitled to available sources of care and many of those they were entitled to use were still not available either for geographic or provider rejection reasons.

Cost Containment and Retrenchment in the 1970s

While federal funds had substantially improved physician/population ratios, helped open new medical schools, increased the number of nurses and allied health personnel, and helped increase effective demand for health care among the aged

and poor, a large part of the major recommendations of the many study commissions that had helped to spark the federal programs remained unfulfilled in 1975. The percentage of rejected applicants for medical school continued to be high, as did the number of foreign-trained physicians practicing in the United States. Physicians' incomes were still very much higher than those of other professions with comparable training, the use of physician's assistants had not become widespread, the percentage of professional nurses who were inactive remained high, state licensing laws continued to inhibit innovative use of health teams, and only in a few schools—and then generally only for some students—had medical school curricula been redesigned to shorten the training period or integrate basic science instruction within the university.

There seemed to be a consensus that the demand for health services would continue to rise sharply. The two main views about the best way to gird for this demand continued to be debated. One held that the health care system should be reorganized to permit greater delegation of duties being performed by physicians, with social control of quality of care being achieved through institutional supervision (Carlson, 1970). The other view was that even if restructuring were desirable, it was a long way off. The only answer for affecting the near future was to continue to turn out more physicians. But the cost of supplying these in sufficient quantity, without system restructuring, had been estimated to be about $430 million per year above the then-current operating costs, in addition to about $4 billion for the capital costs of building about forty-three additional medical schools and university-affiliated hospitals (Gerber, 1973). Actual government policy was to attempt working toward both goals. Measures like the HMO Act and the Community Health Centers program attempted to restructure the way medical care practice was organized, while the Hill-Burton and Health Manpower legislation attempted to correct perceived shortages in facilities and personnel resources as well as altering the mix within both.

As has been previously noted, with the decline of the United States economy that set in during the 1970s and the concomitant mounting interest in controlling the rise of expenditures, the movement of opinion toward containing the cost of social, especially medical, services accelerated within federal policy-making circles. Top industry circles led the demands to lower health service expenditures. As the Congress became more conservative, and under the administrative leadership of four presidents, Nixon, Ford, Carter, and Reagan, who were all conservatives with respect to advancing the social welfare state's agenda in the area of universal access to medical care, the voice of the corporate boardroom came to influence government health policy increasingly toward contraction of all health services, government-sponsored services in the first instance, but privately sponsored ones also. We have seen how this affected funding for the public health services, Medicare and Medicaid. We now look at the influence of this trend on the program to increase the number of physicians.

Concerns over a Physician Surplus: The GMENAC Report

As the notion that additional physicians increase medical care expenditures[32] became more firmly ensconced in the conventional wisdom, the disadvantage of having perhaps too many physicians came increasingly to be a subject of public scrutiny. By 1975 some analysts and public leaders were beginning to express concern over whether continuing the programs for expanding health personnel would not in ten or fifteen years produce a surplus, especially of physicians. In addition to the "cost-containment" contingent, the professional medical groups and societies were once again beginning to worry about a surplus of physicians, but from a guild-protectionist perspective. In 1976 yet another federal commission was established, this one to investigate the adequacy of the supply of physicians with respect to number, specialty mix, and geographic distribution. The charge to the commission was very familiar—"to advise the Secretary [of HEW] on five national health planning objectives": (1) a correct number of physicians to meet the health care needs of the nation; (2) an appropriate specialty distribution of physicians; (3) an appropriate geographic distribution of physicians; (4) appropriate ways to finance

intern and residency training ("graduate" medical education); and (5) a determination of ways of achieving these goals.

Appointed and sponsored by HEW, the Graduate Medical Education National Advisory Committee (GMENAC) issued a seven-volume report in late 1980. The committee concluded that the situation likely to prevail in 1990 "if nothing were done" was an overall surplus of 70,000 physicians; most specialties would have surpluses, but a few would have shortages; primary care would be "in balance," while psychiatry, physical medicine and rehabilitation, and emergency medicine would experience shortages. Factors contributing to the impending surplus in 1990 were said to be an increase in entering class size in United States medical schools from 8,000 to 19,000 over the 14 years before release of the report, an annual influx into practice of 3,000 to 4,000 graduates of foreign medical schools, and a steady increase in numbers of visits to physician extenders, nurse practitioners, physician's assistants, and nurse-midwives. By the year 2000 a surplus of some 145,000 physicians was predicted (Vol I, p. 99).

To forestall or mitigate the projected disparities between requirements and supply with respect to total numbers, practice mix, and geographic distribution, the main recommendations were:

1. A 17 percent decrease in U.S. medical school enrollment and "sharp restrictions" of entry into the United States of students from foreign medical schools.
2. No further increase in the number of nonphysician health care personnel being trained.
3. "Prompt adjustments" in the number of residencies in the various specialties to "bring supply into balance with the requirements in the 1990s."
4. An increase in the number of minorities in medical school.
5. Improvements in the geographic distribution of physicians.

The report pleaded unavoidable ambiguity about the specifics of what should be done about the last point, because "systems of data collection necessary for creditable geographic manpower planning do not exist," and urged that a major effort should be made to "develop criteria for assessing the adequacy of health services in small geographic areas." In the meantime, this by now familiar recommendation seemed to call on those responsible for planning and financing physician training to note that unequal geographic distribution of physicians continued to be an increasingly significant problem whose urgency demanded that steps be taken to correct it even before precise means of measuring its extent were available. These steps included tax credits and differential reimbursement schedules as incentives to choose certain practice locations, and continuance of direct incentives to serve in underserved rural and urban areas, even though "underserved" was still being defined by criteria judged inadequate by GMENAC.

The questions posed by the HEW charge to GMENAC had been investigated all through the period 1958–1975 by academic scholars doing individual studies as well as by numerous commissions, Congressional staffs and a variety of consultants. Some of the individual scholars' undertakings had attempted to stand on the shoulders of the pioneering work of the Lee-Jones study and the model of public-health-oriented research for health planning it established. The concepts and methodology of that research model are discussed more fully in Chapter 15, which deals with health planning. It needs only to be noted here that the sequence of steps in doing research for planning under that approach begins with determining the health status of a population, proceeds to determine the types and quantities of health services that these needs imply, and ends up with a determination of resources (personnel, in this case) required to provide the indicated needed services in a consumer-sensitive and cost-efficient manner. The various health "manpower" study commissions as well as most individual analysts, on the other hand, had nearly all made their prognostications of future medical personnel requirements by extrapolation of physician per population ratios from existing baseline utilization data translated into personnel requirements. While this produces a quick result it is also very "dirty." It never stops to evaluate the adequacy of the existing ratios. If they are grossly inadequate, this inadequacy is embedded in all the extrapolations

to the future. (See also the discussion on pp. 374–375 and note 6.)

The GMENAC project, however, did use a Lee-Jones, public-health-oriented approach, and more than any other recent U.S. study, it attempted to also use more recent refinements in methodology. It began with examination of health status data on incidence and prevalence of health conditions that could be helped by medical attention, proceeded to estimate the required volume and type of services these conditions implied, and concluded with estimates of the numbers and types of health personnel that would be required to provide these services appropriately. The method used to obtain judgments of the numbers and types of health personnel required was essentially the same as that used in the Lee-Jones report—panels of physicians and other health care personnel coming to consensus judgments. Delphi-type techniques that were formally developed only after 1932 (see Chapter 15, note 4) were used, but the basic idea was unchanged. The criterion used by the panels was a modified "need" criterion rather than the "demand" approach implied by projecting existing utilization and physician/utilization ratios in "well-served" areas.

Reactions to the GMENAC Report

Despite the similarities in methodological approach, however, there was an important underlying difference between the problems faced by the Lee-Jones and GMENAC studies. The former was estimating *existing* conditions while the latter was attempting to *forecast* ten and twenty years into the future, introducing a host of new sources of possible error in estimating future trends in health status, need, medical practice, and medical technology changes. Furthermore, these forecasts were being made during a period of accelerating rates of change in all these factors. Quite different forecasts would be obtained by altering any of the assumptions about the direction or magnitude of expected changes in any of them. Thus, while the [health status → needed utilization → required resources] (→ = implies) algorithm would greatly improve an evaluation of current needs for health personnel, the errors involved in projecting health status, needed utilization, and required resources into the future could produce estimates of future physician need that were just as far off the mark as would projecting present utilization and physician/utilization ratios.[33]

It was no surprise, therefore, that the findings of the GMENAC report were met with a storm of protest and counterstorms of support. Medical schools and some consumer groups attacked the findings as based on spurious methodology and reasoning and warned that if the recommendations were followed it would nip in the bud the slowly expanding access to underserved persons. The projected ''surpluses,'' they argued, reflected mainly the imbalance among the specialties and geographic regions. Supporters of the report were the medical societies, who had found the leverage of their seventy-five-year guild-controlled ''shortage'' reduced; the ''cost containers'' who pointed to research findings that each physician generated several hundred thousand dollars of utilization regardless of the shortage or overage of physicians in his or her area; the neoclassical economists who objected to nonmarket control of physician supply; and some health planners who rejected the notion that disparities in specialty mix and geographic distribution of physicians would be rectified by the overage in the surplus sectors spilling over or trickling down to the shortage sectors.

NOTES ON THE REAGAN ADMINISTRATION

With the advent of the Reagan administration in 1981, soon after the GMENAC report was issued, questions about the implementation of the report's recommendations became part of the Washington turmoil accompanying the push to reorder national priorities under the new administration. On the one hand there were battles between President Reagan and much of Congress over the extent of the overhaul of social welfare legislation; on the other hand there was confusion in administration circles between the President's strongly held ideological tenets and what seemed to some as unavoidable imperatives of the economy and political reality for stronger government regulation in some areas. Many of

the ideological formulations of the Reagan administration contradicted each other and led to confusion among the civil servants and political appointees charged with implementing them. Not least among these was the contradiction between the aim of regulating to achieve cost containment and the expressed devotion to the free market. We have already seen in Chapter 10 how this led to the inability of David Stockman, director of the President's Office of Management and Budget, to move on a ''competition''-based national health plan. In the case of health personnel legislative policy, the same sort of dichotomy appeared.

The administration's desire to cut health service costs implied a reduction in physicians at least as great as that recommended by GMENAC. On the other hand, the professed ideology of the administration seemed to imply facilitating the production of a large number of physicians who would compete in the market and lower the price of medical care. The problem, again, was defining what market was being talked about, the neoclassical economist's normative market or the actually existing health services one. The normative market, postulated by the predominant general economic theory taught in the United States, had as one of its underlying assumptions that a greater supply of physicians should result in increased competition and therefore lower prices provided monopoly pricing could be controlled. Many health economists (Herbert Klarman for one) had found, however, that because of strong guild control of medical practice, physicians were more likely to respond to the increased ''competition'' of a larger supply of physicians by raising their prices and generating more services—i.e., that monopoly pricing had not been controlled. It was estimated that an additional physician generated some $300,000 of annual public expenditure irrespective of the existing physician/population ratio.[34] Other studies questioned this result noting that there were signs of greater use of competitive devices by physicians in the 1980s such as advertising and formation of preferred provider organizations, ''emergicenters,'' and ambulatory surgery centers. That the net result of all these activities were lower costs has not been established, but it should be noted that these compet-

itive alternative forms of medical practice organizations may have been due as much to
private corporations moving toward self-insurance as to a surplus of physicians *independently*
competing for patients on the open market by
lowering their prices. (See Chapter 10.)

In 1983 and 1984 signs were appearing that
the increased number of medical school graduates was producing a shortage of residency
places to accommodate them. "Medical schools
have been advised not only to refrain from increasing the size of their entering classes but to
consider decreasing it" (Stimmel & Graettinger,
1984). If the output of physicians were to be
reduced, the methods used to accomplish the reduction represented fundamental policy choices.
Restricting the number of foreign medical graduates who could fill U.S. residencies was opposed by some because it violated the "free
market" approach of open competition based on
competence and by others because these graduates were found to practice in underserved areas more often than graduates of U.S. medical
schools. Restricting admissions to U.S. medical
schools might work to the disadvantage of minority applicants and reducing scholarships and
loan support would hurt lower-income applicants. More rigorous accreditation standards for
medical schools would affect smaller and less
powerful schools, leaving only the larger, more
prestigious, and most strongly Flexner-type ones
to monopolize the field. In any case, 1983 saw
a decline in enrollment in medical schools for
the first time in seventeen years (see Fig. 13–2),
reflecting declines both in applications and admissions. Whether this was due to the concern
over physician surpluses or the fact that private
medical school tuition averaged $10,700 with
some schools charging $25,000 at a time when
the federal and state governments were cutting
aid, is not known (Washington Report on Med-
icine/Perspectives, February 27, 1984). The outcome of all this ambiguity was the failure of a
definitive federal policy to appear.

The question of whether the geographic distribution of physicians was appropriate, and if
inappropriate by how much, continued to remain
without a definitive answer because the criteria
for defining underserved small areas continued
to escape definitive formulation. The Health
Manpower Amendments of 1981, appearing as

Title 27 of the Omnibus Budget Reconciliation
Act of 1981 (OBRA) reduced the number of new
NHSC scholarships (actually, none were offered
for 1981/82) and encouraged use of the private
practice placement site to discharge scholarship
obligations. In 1981 the Reagan administration
tried to decertify several subareas as "underserved" based on global county-wide data, despite
all the caveats contained in the literature about
the fallacies that can arise from the tyranny of
averages. Harlem, with less than one physician
per 4,500 population, was to be decertified because it was in the "county" of Manhattan,
whose overall ratio of physicians was a very
high 1 per 164 persons (Washington Report on
Medicine, 1984). Some studies were predicting
that the number of counties with a federally designated physician shortage would be halved in
1994 and that the competition would make physicians more willing to practice in the remaining
underserved areas. Two Rand studies came to
similar conclusions.

The 1981 amendments also eliminated the requirement for maintenance of increased student
enrollment and the program of capitation grants
for schools of nursing. Emphasis was shifted to
improving education in family medicine and
preventive medicine by making residencies in
these fields eligible for grant support. Authorization for health professions assistance, nurse
training programs, and the National Health Service Corps (NHSC) was due to expire at the end
of FY 1984 with reauthorization in FY 1985 required for continuance. The Reagan administration's fiscal 1985 budget request called for eliminating all NHSC scholarships and decreasing
the FY 1984 $180 million for health professions
education assistance to $100 million in FY 1985.
Cuts were also proposed for Area Health Education Centers (AHECs), nurse training, and
training in primary care/family medicine. An increase of $11 million for helping medical
schools recruit and retain more minority students was called for. These cuts had been proposed in the prior year's budget (FY 1984) but
were ignored by Congress and the struggle between Congress and the Reagan Administration
over reducing federal assistance to medical students and redirecting the geographic placement
of graduates was settling into a pattern.

As the middle of the 1980s decade approached, the notion that there was a surplus of physicians was becoming more widespread. Phrases like "doctors quickly are becoming a surplus item in America" (Washington Report on Medicine, April 25, 1983) were often seen in health newsletters and other publications. And, as has been noted there was a proliferation of new forms of practice organization, such as free-standing primary care centers, "emergicenters," freestanding ambulatory surgery centers, birthing centers, retail shopping-center dentistry offices, and preferred provider plans. Some researchers and analysts credited this surplus with making more physicians amenable to participating in these new forms and thus aiding the trend toward self insurance. Others were asserting that the surplus was making it easier to get specialist physicians to locate in rural areas (Newhouse et al., 1982)[35] as well as agreeing to be part of vertically integrated health plans like HMOs and some PPOs.

There continued to be strong disagreement in 1983 about whether there really was a surplus and whether one was actually in the offing for 1990 or 2000. Professional groups, especially the AMA, and health planners were continuing to argue that there was a surplus or would soon be. The contrary view was being put forth primarily by persons basing their arguments on free market competition assumptions. They noted that there was no market "surplus" (see Jeffers, Bognano, and Bartlett, 1971; Shonick, 1976, pp 8–9 for discussions of neoclassical economists' concepts of "surplus" in supply) because physicians were not unemployed or without income. They were simply having to go to places where a demand existed, as in rural areas, but where they preferred not to practice if they did not have to. Similarly, they were having to work during hours and in settings consumers wanted. Such a view, for example, was expressed in a *Wall Street Journal* article late in 1983 and reinforced by the research and analysis of the study cited above. This article and a rebuttal were published in a newsletter by the state Health Planning Office of California and sent out free of charge to its mailing list. The rebuttal contended that California experience showed that an unacceptably large increase in the total number of physicians was necessary to get even a small number to practice in underserved areas. For example, of

the 19,000 increase in California physicians between 1970 and 1980, 2,950 went to decrease the shortage of physicians in underserved counties but 8,900 went to increase the surplus in already overserved counties. Thus some three physicians had to be added to overserved counties for every one added to an underserved county (Breining, 1984; Meeks and Merwin, 1984). The argument that simply letting the number of physicians grow would eliminate lack of access by a trickle-down process was opposed by some because only a small trickle resulted and the cost included an unacceptable increase in oversupply in overserved areas. If the diffusion of physicians to areas of unmet demand were to be accomplished, direct forms of incentives would be needed rather than relying on an overflow of urban surpluses to rural areas.

Some of the most determined opponents of the trickle-down argument were advocates of areawide planning as the better way to target supply to geographical areas with unmet demand and into specialties in short supply. This is treated in the consideration of health planning in Chapter 15.

New analyses were appearing. Some purported to show that the GMENAC forecast of a physician surplus by the year 2000 was based on erroneous methodology and that supply was likely to be in balance with need; it was even likely that there would be a shortage. Other analysts using different methodology thought the GMENAC forecast of surplus was if anything too conservative. They forecast a much larger surplus of physicians. Much of the difference in methodology had to do with differing estimates of the size of future HMO utilization.

The concern with a future overall surplus of physicians had abated by 1990. In that year the Department of Health and Human Services was reporting that although the ratio of physicians/ 100,000 population had risen from 155 in 1980 to 233 in 1988, medical school applications had declined 27.2 percent, from 36,727 to 26,721 (Medicine and Health). However, the Department of HHS returned to expressing the earlier concern "about whether the supply of health personnel will be adequate to meet the nation's requirements" in a report issued "under a mandate from Congress to advise the nation on the supply, distribution, and training of health professionals, as well as estimate what will be needed to maintain adequate care" (Medicine and Health Perspectives, Vol 44, No. 17, Apr. 30, 1990). Characteristically, although the rate of expansion of the physician supply is expected to be more than adequate by 2020, shortages continue to be forecast in "some urban and rural settings and in some specialties, such as primary care" (Medicine and Health).

The fact remains that despite the substantial increases in numbers of physicians (and other health personnel) per population since the large and effective government health personnel expansion programs were first introduced in 1963, scarcely a dent has been made in reducing the numbers of people who are denied access to medical care because of cost. The efforts to fill the gaps in medical care coverage through financial incentives for medical graduates to practice in underserved areas was helpful because they actually put physicians where the need was and provided for free access to them. But the NHSC physicians had only temporary assignments, and in any case the program was gutted. Turning out more generalists has produced more physicians better qualified to meet the needs of rural persons, but doctors could only serve in areas where means of paying them were available. In an era of curtailment of public programs like Medicaid, public hospitals, and community health centers, it could not help fill the gap for uncovered poor persons. The entire enterprise of training more generalist and practice-oriented physicians could not succeed in reaching such people until they were legislatively entitled to access to medical care.

Failing such entitlement, increasing the numbers of physicians, even if the mix were less research- and subspecialty-oriented, could only serve to produce and then increase a surplus of physicians for well-insured persons while maintaining a dearth for the uncovered. If the 35 to 40 million uninsured are to be served, then either all the gap-filling programs for paying physicians must be restored to full strength, expensive as such a system must necessarily be, or a national universal-coverage medical care program must be enacted with its possibilities for also being cost-effective. With payment for every U.S. resident assured, it is likely that most of the

efforts to expand and restructure the supply of health personnel of the past thirty years can be channeled to meet the objective of producing a sufficient number of health personnel, properly distributed by specialty and geography, to make good health care available for all persons.

NOTES

1. "Widely" credited but not universally. See Crawford, 1977 and McKinlay and McKinlay, 1977.
2. A state license permitted a physician to perform all aspects of medical practice, including those generally associated with specialists, such as complicated surgery. Specialists were not licensed as such. See the section on credentialing beginning with page 369.
3. While this classification is useful for analysis and enhancing our understanding of the medical personnel landscape, credentialing statutes themselves use terms like "licensed" and "registered" quite loosely. For example, California law provides for a "licensed clinical social worker" (LCSW) but only defines schooling and experience as requirements for the "license." While no person can announce himself or herself to be a LCSW if the state has not awarded the required credential, anyone can go into private practice or be employed to do what a clinical social worker does without a license. A "registered" nurse, on the other hand, has a limited license to perform certain functions which no one else except a physician may perform.
4. Other definitions of these terms have been given in HEW, 1971 and are cited in Roemer, 1973.
5. These dates suggest themselves after a reading of Butter, 1967.
6. These are summarized in National Advisory Committee on Health Manpower, 1967, Appendix VI. I focus on the studies of the 1950s and 1960s as the more important ones in affecting federal policy.
7. Such proposals for an "ideal" way of projecting future requirements were indeed being put forth and represented a growing value orientation that saw medical care as a right and a societal obligation. But the time to do it was never found, and the "Lee-Jones" approach was never again used.
8. These estimates were based on the assumption that there would be a continued influx of foreign-trained physicians to fill hospital staff positions, a trend that had started about 1950 (discussed later in the text).
9. Federal and state tax exemptions were used to encourage greater use of private health insurance, and out-of-pocket medical payments also received limited income tax exemption.
10. These figures do not include the 12,300 Doctors of Osteopathy (DOs) shown on Table 3.2. These physicians are discussed later.

11. These are academic years defined by: 1941 = 1941–1942 in the cited source.

12. These ratios include *all* dentists and the entire population. The number of active dentists per civilian population was 46.4 in 1967.

13. The term "allied health personnel" is used in different senses. Unless otherwise noted I shall use this term to include all persons other than physicians, dentists, and nurses performing medical tasks.

14. The recommendations of this Commission on Public Health questions are discussed in Chapter 2.

15. Here I discuss only the provisions dealing with allied health personnel but provision was also made "to strengthen and improve the existing loan programs for medical, osteopathic, dental, pharmacy, optometric, and nursing students."

16. For example, the Duke University physician's assistant (associate) program (established 1965) provided twenty-four-month training in primary or specialty care, and the pediatric nurse practitioner program established in 1965 at the University of Colorado for baccalaureate nurses and offering four months of training. Some well-known programs that were established a few years after 1966 were the Medex program, established in 1969 at the University of Washington for returning military medical corpsmen and offering three months' university education and twelve months' preceptorship with a practicing physician; the Child Health Associate program, a two-year college and three-year sequence of professional studies including a year of internship established in 1969; the Department of Defense–operated Project Transition, a program for ex-corpsmen, and Project REMED, a similar program run by the Department of Health, Education, and Welfare.

17. The development of educational programs to turn out physician's assistants had originally been directed toward two main pools of prospective applicants, returning Vietnam medical corpsmen, who would work under the actual title of "physician's assistant" (PA), and professional nurses, who would work as "nurse-practitioners." The PA programs ranged from four months to five years in length. The nurse practitioners' (or clinician) programs encompassed "areas traditionally reserved only for the physician . . . . Nurse clinicians are trained in one to two years to acquire 'physician-like' skills and work under physician supervision and control" (Sadler, 1972). As of 1972, eighty of the PA programs and fifty of the nurse practitioners (NP) programs were in "various stages of development" (Sadler, 1972). About 200 physician's assistants had been graduated and other programs were being operated by the armed services.

18. These may be found in Allied Health Subcommittee, 1967.

19. Most of the information on accrediting programs is from Roemer, 1973.

20. The term "medical technologist" has some-times been used to represent the general category of technician-technologist.

21. These are cited here in some detail because they pithily present fundamental health conditions among the poor that have been with us since the relevant health statistics were first collected and continue unabated.

22. Volume I, containing the summary of the commission's findings and its recommendations, was released in 1967; Volume II, containing the detailed findings and reports of its seven subpanels, appeared in 1968.

23. Active physicians excluding doctors of osteopathy.

24. These "health manpower initiative awards" were for establishing entities similar to the Areawide Education Centers (AHECs) recommended by the Carnegie Commission on Higher Education in its 1970 report described later in this chapter. (My note.)

25. These amendments were to the 1963 Act (see p. 376).

26. Throughout this discussion references to medical students apply to the other specified health professions eligible for the NHSC program unless otherwise noted.

27. In all of this discussion of AHEC, the term "medical students" includes osteopathic school students.

28. Much of the material about the development of AHECs follows Odegaard, 1979. This quotation is from p. 17.

29. Some projects received small AHEC "special initiative" federal funds after the federal funding phase (National AHEC Bulletin, Spring 1989).

30. Much of this compendium of legislation follows Wilson and Neuhauser, 1985 Ed. closely.

31. While the attitude of organized medicine toward population-based criteria may be directly inferred from public statements and documents, that of the medical schools are evident by the content of their curricula and the hierarchical ordering of their faculties within the schools.

32. Again, a blanket statement of this sort ignores the question of whether the added expenditures reflect needed medical services that had not been available before. After all, the purpose of increasing physician supply is to enable the system to serve persons previously underserved. The implied assumption that most of the added services provided by the additional physicians are unnecessary is similar to the assumption that cost sharing in health insurance reduces only, or even mainly, unneeded utilization.

33. The presentation of both sides of a planning argument is not meant to imply that good planning could not greatly increase the accuracy of the estimates. The idea is only to indicate the nature of the problem. There are many ways of improving the estimates if the will to provide an accessible and efficient system exists.

34. Much of this description on questions about

the adequacy of physician supply in the period following the issuance of the GMENAC report follows the Washington Report on Medicine and Health, 2/27/84.

35. This study showed that the number of small towns with populations over 2,500 with some form of specialist physician increased between 1970 and 1979 and that the degree of dispersion of specialists among such places depended on how many specialists of that type existed nationally. The study covered twenty-three states clustered in four regions. The authors attributed this to the impact of "competitive forces."

14

Government Support for Research Related to Personal Health Care

In tracing the development of federal policy for promoting a nationwide system of personal health services, I have thus far discussed programs that built networks of preventive services, of medical services directly operated by the government, of government payment systems to private providers for the delivery of medical services to special populations, and of government-sponsored health insurance for some populations. Programs promoting the construction of health facilities and the education and training of health personnel have also been described. All these activities were directed using current knowledge about interventions that enhance the health status of a population to build an effective, accessible, and efficient health service delivery system.

The health status of a population may be viewed as resulting from a combination of genetic factors, environmental influences, and the efficacy of personal health care. The efficacy of personal health care, in turn, depends on the state of biomedical knowledge and the effectiveness of the health delivery system in providing services that embody this knowledge to people who need them. It was not lost on federal policymakers that a delivery system can improve health status only to the extent that it has an effective product to deliver. The appropriate use of the armamentarium of known effective interventions represents, after all, the upper limit of what a personal health care delivery system can do.

There has been some federal support for biomedical research since about 1900, but it accelerated after World War II. As the expenditures for biomedical research grew, many questions were raised about the directions that the support

should take. If the federal government were to subsidize such research more heavily, then it could excercise greater control over which areas would be more intensively investigated than others and choices had to be made as to which areas should receive research priority. Some observers began to note that the development of new techniques and products—as in radiology, surgery, and pharmacology—was sharply accelerating the rate of increase of medical costs and paradoxically thereby arguably threatening to diminish the overall efficacy and efficiency of the delivery system. With successive administrations expressing a desire to limit health care cost increases, there arose a growing competition for budgetary allotments between research and delivery system improvement, and research usually won. The biomedical research advocates were led by highly placed social figures including famous physicians who invoked the formidable aura of hard science. Some of them argued that expanding research was or should be synergistic to increasing access rather than antagonistic. The greater number of federally subsidized research physicians in the medical schools would make more physicians available for teaching and supervising residents and interns in delivering patient service. The advocates of improvements in the delivery system counted socially prestigious personages among them but their aura was tinged with the softness of social concerns about access for those who could not pay market prices. In times of economic prosperity and public generosity of spirit on social welfare issues, these advocates wielded considerable influence, but never as much as the advocates of biomedical research.

During periods of economic decline and

growing social Darwinism, the service advocates were inundated by the budgetary cost-cutting deluge but the biomedical research advocates continued to ride high and dry. Attempts to cut health care costs were accompanied by assertions that no reduction in access to medically valuable services was intended. The argument was that the health care delivery mechanism was inefficient largely because much utilization was not only unnecessary for optimal medical care but was also so excessive as to be detrimental to health. It consisted in large part of interventions of scientifically unproven value. Expanded biomedical research would help establish which interventions were of little or no use and thus make possible containment of medical costs without diminishing the delivery of useful services.

In addition to the earlier support for biomedical research directed toward differentiating between effective and ineffective interventions, the federal government later also undertook to support health services research. A major aim of this research was to identify methods of reducing inefficiency in administrative practice, as well as identifying ineffective medical procedures through various methods of outcomes research such as "technology assessment."

BIOMEDICAL RESEARCH

Early Development: Through World War II

The federal government entered the biomedical research arena as early as 1887 with the establishment of the Laboratory of Hygiene at the Marine Hospital on Staten Island, New York. This modest one-room installation was a bacteriological laboratory whose purpose was to do research on cholera and other infectious diseases. Renamed the Hygienic Laboratory in 1891, its early status was well described by John J. Hanlon:

[F]rom the start it was developed with such skill, imgination, and foresight that it soon became one of the world's leading centers of public health and medical research. Originally organized in three divisions of chemistry, zoology, and pharmacology, its functions were expanded in 1912 by an act authorizing the laboratory to "study and investigate the diseases of man and conditions influencing the origin and spread

thereof including sanitation and sewage, and the pollution directly or indirectly of navigable streams and lakes of the Untied States and may from time to time issue information in the form of publications for the use of the public." Under consistently able direction the Hygienic Laboratory, which was later to become the National Institute of Health, attracted and developed a steady stream of outstanding investigators, including Carter, Sternberg, Rosenau, Goldberger, Frost, Leake, Armstrong, Stiles, Lumsden, Francis, Spencer, Maxcy, and Dyer, to name but a few. The contributions of these men and their co-workers caused Dr. William H. Welch to state publicly that there was no research institute in the world which was making such distinguished contributions to basic research in public health (1969).

When the Hygienic Laboratory was renamed the National Institute of Health in 1930, $750,000 was appropriated to construct new quarters and set up a system of fellowships. During these early years the Public Health Service staff itself also studied certain diseases. For example in 1899 the Public Health Service's predecessor, the Marine Hospital Service, (see Chapter 4) was directed by Congress to investigate leprosy in the United States, and in 1902 the "earliest studies of Rocky Mountain spotted fever took place in Montana." In 1921 the Rocky Mountain Spotted Fever Laboratory was established in Hamilton, Montana, as a field station of the Public Health Service (HEW, 1921).

In addition to research of this type carried on by the agency's own staff, there are some early examples of grants given by the U.S. Public Health Service[1] to nongovernment scientists for research, the so-called extramural research that was to become so prominent in later years. For example, the Chamberlain-Kahn Act of 1918 for venereal disease control included grants to twenty-five institutions whose scientists were to aid the federal government in research on venereal disease, and in 1922, a Special Cancer Investigations Laboratory was established by the Public Health Service investigators at Harvard Medical School.

The first specialized disease-oriented research institutes, the National Cancer Institute (NCI), was established by Congress in 1937, and it began awarding fellowships for cancer research shortly thereafter. When the Public Health Service was finally moved from its original berth in the Treasury Department to the newly created Federal Security Agency in 1939, it was organized into eight divisions. One of these, the Division of Scientific Research, included the National Institute of Health and the National Cancer Intitute. At this time the National Institute of Health still retained many state control functions, such as setting public health laboratory standards, that were for the most part transferred to other portions of the Public Health Service during later years.

During the period from 1935 through 1945, the Public Health Service's efforts were primarily directed toward the establishment of a national network of local health departments, regionally coordinated by state health departments (see Chapter 4). The writings of Joseph W. Mountin and the Haven Emerson study reflect the national attention being given to controlling environmental and epidemiological threats to the health of people. The early National Institute of Health was therefore primarily a *public health* laboratory concentrating on finding the cause and method of prevention of the acute diseases with which public health was then mostly concerned. It focused on finding and diseminating better ways in which local health departments could abate the death, morbidity, and debility caused by these diseases.

With acute infectious disease control being relatively stabilized by 1945, communicable and childhood diseases were supplanted as the major causes of death and disability by the chronic, degenerative, and debilitative diseases. As far as was known, these were not transmitted by infected carriers, and although they were suspected by some to be related to pollutants in the environment, the basic factor associated with their incidence was advancing age. Not only public health but also medical practice was affected by these changes in the patterns of debility and disease. With so little known about the etiology of the degenerative diseases associated with aging, often the best that could be done by physicians and other health workers, was to help the patient "manage" the illness so as to optimize his or her daily functioning and minimize discomfort and disability. The changing nature of the illnesses that physicians were being called upon to treat has been one of the fundamental causes of dissatisfaction with the curative health service system that began to appear about 1946.

In 1900, 11 percent of all deaths were from tuberculosis and 12 percent were from influenza and pneumonia. In 1967 these diseases combined accounted for only 3.5 percent of all deaths. By contrast, cancer and cardiovascular-renal diseases, which accounted for 24 percent of the death rate in 1900, were responsible for over 70 percent of all deaths in 1967. This was accompanied by a change from 19 percent of the population being 45 years of age or over in 1900 to 31 percent in 1968 (U.S. Bureau of the Census, 1980).

Post–World War II Development

One reaction to these phenomena was an increased interest in support for biomedical research after 1945. The etiology of the chronic and degenerative diseases was little known as were specific methods for preventing or curing them. Palliative measures were often not very effective and many were not firmly based on science. It was increasingly being argued that further progress in ameliorating the effects of these diseases required more basic research into their fundamental causes. This thinking dovetailed well with the post-Sputnik (1957) national sense of urgency about rapid scientific advancement and helped to foster a climate in which prestige was attached mainly to scientific and technical, rather than to societal and humanistic, research.

Growth of the National Institutes of Health

The principal vehicle for the postwar expansion of support for biomedical research was the National Institutes of Health (NIH), name adopted in 1948. From the two original institutes, the National Institute of Health and the National Cancer Institute, existing in 1945 with a total appropriation of $2.8 million, it had grown by 1980 to twelve institutes and two general and administrative offices with a total appropriation of $3.4 billion, an increase in appropriation by a factor of about 1200. It is worth noting that in 1945, $2.7 million of the $2.8 million appropriation (95%) was for direct NIH operations, while in 1908 only 1.1 billion of the total $3.4 billion (32%) appropriation was for direct NIH operations. In 1980, $2.4 billion, or almost 70 percent of the total appropriation, was for extramural

Table 14–1. NIH Obligations of Appropriations:*
Totals and Amounts Obligated for Grants and for
Direct Operations, 1939–1988 (Amounts in
thousands of dollars)

Fiscal year	Total appropriations*	Grants	Direct operations	Percent direct operations of total
1938	464	140	324	69.8
1939	464	171	293	63.1
1940	707	277	430	60.8
1941	711	237	474	66.7
1942	700	230	470	67.1
1943	1,278	181	1,097	85.8
1944	2,555	182	2,373	92.9
1945	2,835	142	2,693	95.0
1946	3,415	850	2,565	75.1
1947	8,076	4,004	4,072	50.4
1948	28,876	12,475	16,401	56.8
1949	43,484	30,469	13,015	29.9
1950	59,235	43,823	15,412	26.0
1951	45,561	29,626	15,935	35.0
1952	52,010	34,863	17,147	33.0
1953	56,227	38,205	18,022	32.1
1954	69,444	48,196	21,248	30.6
1955	80,963	54,214	26,749	33.0
1956	98,099	63,243	34,856	35.5
1957	169,855	123,111	46,744	27.5
1958	210,261	147,187	63,074	30.0
1959	285,210	208,407	76,803	26.9
1960	381,317	292,910	88,407	23.2
1961	521,647	417,690	103,957	19.9
1962	638,657	518,823	119,834	18.8
1963	751,442	607,137	144,305	19.2
1964	876,969	715,152	161,817	18.5
1965	958,267	774,520	183,747	19.2
1966	1,099,161	887,521	211,640	19.3
1967	1,061,581	798,923	262,658	24.7
1968	1,082,861	804,230	278,631	25.7
1969	1,483,143	813,052	670,091	45.2
1970	1,443,977	771,259	672,718	46.6
1971	1,596,314	848,292	748,022	46.9
1972	2,081,580	978,744	1,102,836	53.0
1973	1,523,101	967,529	555,572	36.5
1974	1,994,432	1,120,828	873,604	43.8
1975	2,108,886	1,306,475	802,411	38.0
1976	2,238,410	1,398,556	839,854	37.5
1977	2,581,988	1,566,451	1,015,537	39.3
1978	2,828,014	1,785,435	1,042,579	36.9
1979	3,184,641	2,096,031	1,088,610	34.2
1980	3,428,842	2,343,220	1,085,622	31.7
1981	3,572,506	2,514,010	1,058,496	29.6
1982	3,643,461	2,566,068	1,077,393	29.6
1983	4,013,135	2,874,673	1,138,462	28.4
1984	4,493,553	3,262,598	1,230,955	27.4
1985	5,121,557	3,811,120	1,310,437	25.6
1986	5,296,977	3,920,848	1,376,129	26.0
1987	6,175,038	4,644,400	1,530,638	24.8
1988	6,610,430	4,930,061	1,680,369	25.4

Source: USDHHS, 1989, Part 3

*The data represent "amounts obligated" out of appropriations and
differ somewhat from the actual appropriations that appear in NIH,
1991. Because these data on obligations are presented annually by
the NIH as a historical time series, revised wherever possible for
accuracy and year-to-year comparability, and because they differ
only slightly from the actual appropriations, I use the entries of this
table and the graphs based on them as the basic data for discussing
NIH appropriations.

grants—those given to "outside" investigators
and universities. The trend for an increasing proportion of the NIH funds to be appropriated and
spent for extramural support has continued. In
1988, 75 percent of the NIH appropriation of
$6.6 billion consisted of grants for research, re-
search training and some other minor expenditures (See Table 14–1 and Fig. 14–1A,B).

In the early 1960s, almost as much was being
appropriated by the federal government to sup-
potr biomedical research through the NIH as for
AFDC medical care and state health services and
construction combined; in 1962 the NIH appropriation actually exceeded the total for these
items (HEW-S, 1966) (HHS, 1983).

Total federal support (expenditures obligated)
for health research and development rose from
$448 million in 1960 to $4.7 billion in 1980, and
federal percentage of total U.S. health research
and development grew form 51 percent to 60
percent during those years. Over the same period
NIH research and development support grew
from $281 million to $3.2 billion, from 63 percent of federal support in 1960 to 67% percent
in 1980 (see Table 14–2 and Fig 14–2A,B).
Equally dramatic was the growth in the proportion of total U.S. research and development
funds that went for health research. It was 6.4
percent in 1960 and 12.4 percent in 1980, a 94
percent increase. It was estimated to be 15.5 percent in 1990 (NIH, 1991). Thus the NIH has
been directing a significant part of the total U.S.
expenditures for health research and development and its expenditures constituted a substan-
cial portion of all federal government expenditures for research and development.

Method of Operation of the National Institutes of Health

What the institutes do and how they do it stems
both from new legislation passed after 1950 and
from a legacy inherited from the past. Many aspects of the Institutes' operation have of course,
changed over the years, but their main structural
features were already in place by the 1960s.
They have remained recognizable over the years
despite the changes made to accomodate criticism and to reflect political, epidemiological,
and scientfic developments. For example, an
AIDS program was initiated, that went from

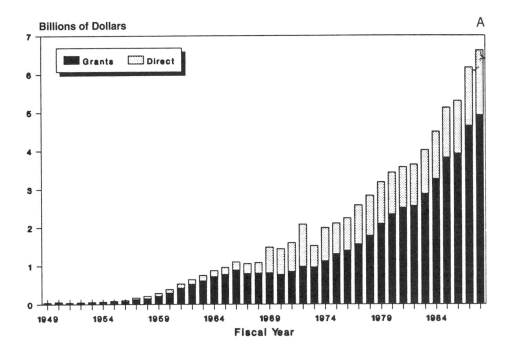

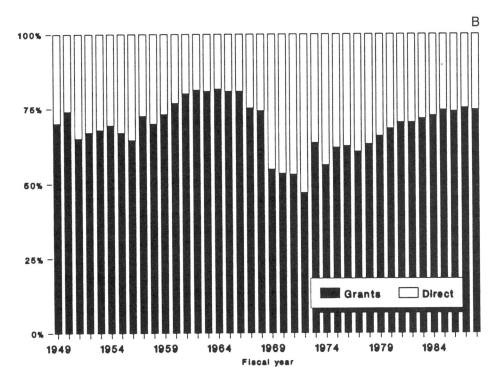

Fig. 14–1. (A) Total NIH obligations for grants and for direct operations, 1949–1988. *Source*: Table 14–1. (B) Distribution of total NIH Obligations by grants and direct operations, 1949–1988. *Source*: Table 14–1.

Table 14–2. Expenditures for Health R&D in the United States: Total, Federal, and NIH (Amounts in millions of dollars)

Year	Total health R&D in the U.S.	Federal support for health R&D	Federal as % of total health R&D in the U.S.	NIH health R&D support	NIH as % of total health R&D in the U.S.	NIH as % of federal support
1960	884	448	50.7	281	31.8	62.7
1961	1,085	574	52.9	375	34.6	65.3
1962	1,330	782	58.8	495	37.2	63.3
1963	1,523	919	60.3	566	37.2	61.6
1964	1,695	1,049	61.9	651	38.4	62.1
1965	1,890	1,174	62.1	715	37.8	60.9
1966	2,111	1,316	62.3	791	37.5	60.1
1967	2,345	1,459	62.2	812	34.6	55.7
1968	2,568	1,582	61.6	864	33.6	54.6
1969	2,785	1,674	60.1	893	32.1	53.3
1970	2,846	1,667	58.6	873	30.7	52.4
1971	3,167	1,877	59.3	1,039	32.8	55.4
1972	3,527	2,147	60.9	1,271	36.0	59.2
1973	3,735	2,225	59.6	1,323	35.4	59.5
1974	4,431	2,754	62.2	1,737	39.2	63.1
1975	4,688	2,832	60.4	1,880	40.1	66.4
1976	5,084	3,059	60.2	2,060	40.5	67.3
1977	5,594	3,396	60.7	2,280	40.8	67.1
1978	6,249	3,811	61.0	2,581	41.3	67.7
1979	7,097	4,325	60.9	2,953	41.6	68.3
1980	7,894	4,726	59.9	3,182	40.3	67.3
1981	8,723	4,848	55.6	3,333	38.2	68.8
1982	9,548	4,970	52.1	3,433	36.0	69.1
1983	10,753	5,399	50.2	3,789	35.2	70.2
1984	12,143	6,087	50.1	4,257	35.1	69.9
1985	13,512	6,791	50.3	4,828	35.7	71.1
1986	14,832	6,895	46.5	5,005	33.7	72.6
1987	16,868	7,847	46.5	5,852	34.7	74.6
1988	18,905	8,425	44.6	6,292	33.3	74.7
1989	20,900	9,230	44.2	6,778	32.4	73.4
1990	22,584	9,856	43.6	7,141	31.6	72.5
1991	24,542	10,383	42.3	7,472	30.4	72.0

Source: USDHHS, 1983; IH, 1991.

$3.4 million in 1982 to $805 million in 1991 (NIH, 1991, Table 14), and the growth of cooperative research and development agreements[2] increased from 10 in 1986 to 114 in 1990. These two developments were responding to quite different causes, and each is an example of the kinds of pressures that have affected the research content of some NIH programs while the general method of the agency's operations has remained rather constant.

The Institutes of Health as an entity have been administered by a director who at different times had reported, nominally at least, to the Surgeon General of the Public Health Service or directly to the Assistant Secretary for Health and Scientific Affairs of the Department of Health, Education and Welfare. In 1987 the director was reporting to the Assistant Secretary for Health of the Department of Health and Human Ser-

vices. Since 1966 the director had had an advisory committee. The research activities supported by the Institutes are carried on by a small intramural organization and by a large body of grant funded extramural investigators. Intramural research is conducted both at the Clinical Center in Bethesda, Maryland, which in 1990 had 470 beds, and at a complex of supporting facilities, including laboratories, computing facilities, and the like. About 400 beds are allocated among the NIH institutes, each of which selects the appropriate patients from referrals by physicians throughout the world.[3] The NIH Clinical Center is under the overall supervision of an Associate Director For Direct Research, who is in the Office of the Director of NIH.

The extramural programs had by the late 1960s become by far the dominant ones (see Table 14–1). A major study of the NIH in 1967

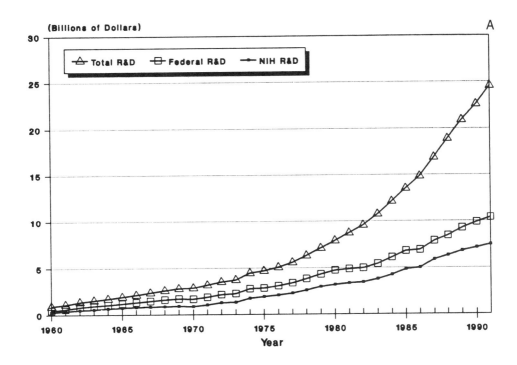

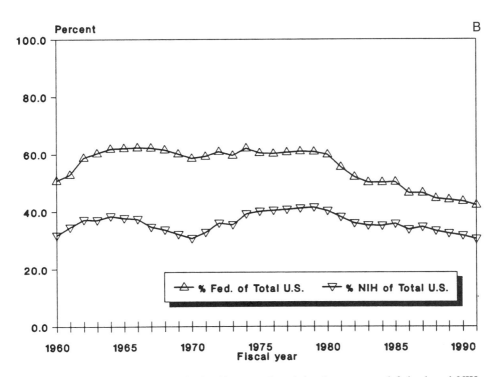

Fig. 14–2. (A) U.S. expenditures for health research and development: total federal, and NIH. *Source*: Table 14–2. (B) Percent of total health research and development in the U.S. supported by federal government and NIH, 1960–1991. *Source*: Table 14–2.

described the grant awards as falling under five classes,[4] and these classes are still recognizable (NIH, 1991). By 1990 the main classes of extramural awards were the "traditional" individual research grant, the research project grant, and the research center grant. The number of awards and the total amounts awarded under these categories are shown in Table 14–3.

The research project ("traditional") grants are almost always awarded "to an institution on behalf of a principal investigator" (Office of Technology Assessment, 1982, p. 123). The institution is expected to "provide facilities necessary to accomplish the research and will be accountable for the funds."

The review procedure set up for approval of grants, especially the traditional type, has won admiration from many quarters as a model of fairness and efficiency although it has received some criticism in recent years (Office of Technology Assessment, 1982, pp. 125–128). The NIH organizes study sections whose memberships consist of outstanding specialists in various disciplines (USDHHS, 1991, section V and IX). These study sections have titles reflecting their subjects, such as "Behavioral and Neurosciences" or "Molecular Biology." Most of them are managed by the Division of Research Grants (DRG) and consist of primarily nonfed-

Table 14–3. Number and Total Amount of NIH Awards in 1990 by Type of Award

Types of award	Number of awards	Total amount of awards (in millions)
For Research		
"Traditional" research project	15,888	$2,719
Research program project	771	692
Research centers	662	633
"Other" research	8,404	1,196
Total Research grants	25,725	$5,240
R&D contracts	1,332	715
Research training	(3,503)	(292)
Individual awards	2,046	51
Institutional awards	1,457	241
Construction grants	7	15
Grants for repair, renovation, etc.	101	11
Other		9
Total awards other than research	5,303	1,042
Total NIH awards	30,668	$6,282

Source: NIH, 1991, Tables 17, 18, 26

eral research scientists. The DRG receives the original application and assigns it to a study section. On the other hand, each Institute is disease-category oriented by its declared mission and each has an advisory council of twelve members appointed by the Surgeon General, which is mandated by law. An application is reviewed by the study section for scientific merit, and if approved, it is given a grade (the average of the members of the study section) and sent to the advisory council of the appropriate Institute where it is reviewed for the relevance it has to the disease-oriented mission of the Institute and to policy criteria formulated by NIH and the federal government. The final priority given to the proposal is a combination of the scientific merit rating by the study section and the disease-oriented public policies relevance judgement of the advisory council of the pertinent institute. Projects are then funded in order of priority assigned by the Director's office of the institute to the extent of available funds.

The program project grant is also awarded to an institution on behalf of a principal investigator, but it is for carrying out a broadly based, often multidisciplinary long-term research program with a particular major objective or theme (Office of Technology Assessment, 1982). It is typically a much larger amount ($961,000 was average in 1900) than a traditional grant ($174,000 in 1990) and involves groups of investigators who conduct research around the common theme or objective. (These proposals have been frequently encouraged or suggested by NIH staff to meet a perceived need, but this is more true of center grants, discussed below.) The proposal may be assigned for review to sections of the Public Health Service outside the institutes when these are appropriate authorities. Within the NIH, the applications are assigned to study sections (called scientific review groups— SRGs) of the appropriate institutes for review. Because these proposals entail entire programs, the review often includes site visits by committee members and NIH officals. After review by these Institute SRGs, the proposal goes to the advisory council of the institute and then to the institute director for a final decision.

Center grants, awarded to institutions on behalf of a program director and a group of collaborating investigators, provide support for long term, multi-disciplinary programs of research and development. The distinction between program project and center grants is that center grants are more likely to have a clinical orientation and are usually developed in response to announcements of specific needs and requirements of [an institute or division] (Office of Technology Assessment, 1982).

These and other miscellaneous types of program grants have dealt with topics such as efforts to alleviate personnel shortages or deficiences in facilities in various research areas and have supported health personnel training and the development of biomedical engineering and electronic computing facilities. Grants have been and are still given for developing embryonic ideas that are not yet ready to be formally presented as individual grant proposals.

In addition to these three main types of grants for research, the NIH has given resource-developing grants to establish Clinical Research and Health Education facilities, and to establish special research resources, such as computing and biomedical engineering centers to serve NIH investigators of an entire region (see Table 14–3). Various study awards have provided long-term support for well-established scholars who were free to engage in research of their own choosing. The fellowship and research career development awards have been provided for graduates in one discipline, particularly, doctors of medicine to spend time mastering additional disciplines required to do research in their fields of interest. In recent years the NIH has been awarding research training grants focusing on training of minorities and has paid increased attention to expediting the application of new research findings into everyday medical practice, an activity that has come to be known as the transfer (diffusion) of medical technology.

Problems of Administration and Definition of Mission

The rapidly expanding appropriations for the Institutes soon raised questions about the size and mission of the federal biomedical research program. As has been noted, by 1960 an impressive structure for biomedical research support had been established, costing about $380 million per year and administering $280 million of health

R&D support (Tables 14–1, 14–2). It seemed like the time had come to take stock of where the NIH was going. Questions were being asked, at first about whether these funds were being spent most advantageously. Was the total annual amount being spent a proper proportion of the nation's total resources, and was the way it was being spent a proper allocation of the total appropriation? But soon the analysts of NIH activities were emphasizing more fundamental questions of national purpose, ethical considerations, and choice of criteria for evaluating excellence in research.

A number of studies looked into these questions during and immediately before the 1960s (NIHS, 1967; B. Jones Committee), and evaluations of the NIH continued through the years that followed (Presidential Commission on Heart, Cancer, Stroke, 1965; Institute of Medicine, 1984; Office of Technology Assessment, 1982; NIH, 1980). But none provided an analysis of the basic policy questions facing the NIH both with depth of empirical description and the level of analytic generality of the Wooldridge Committee report of 1967. Most of the fundamental questions addressed by that study have remained pertinent.

The Wooldridge Report of 1965 This report was an outgrowth of a 1963 request by President Kennedy for a study of NIH operations, brought on by the rapid growth of its budget and activities and pressures for further expansion. President Johnson later reaffirmed the request and the study got under way in 1964. The resulting report, dated February 1965, arguably the most thoroughgoing analysis made to that time, relied less on oral and written opinions obtained from various top-level experts and administrators than some previous investigators did. Instead it utilized extensive field visits with study interviewers speaking to numerous investigators and administrators at their research sites. Many of the conclusions reached by the earlier Boisfeuillet Jones report were reiterated, e.g., ''[the] NIH Study Committee [again found that] the activities of the National Institute of Health are essentially sound and that its budget of approximately one billion dollars a year is, on the whole, being spent wisely and well in the public interest.'' But in addition to the aforementioned analysis, some findings and recommendations differed. Many of the basic issues of administering biomedical research supported by public funds were addressed.

Some of the administrative policy problems that were beginning to surface as federal support for biomedical research grew were identified and analyzed—the question of guidance of overall research priorities for the NIH as a whole, broadening the membership of the guidance committees of the individual Institutes, striking an appropriate balance between intramural and extramural research, the proper relationship between NIH and the universities and medical schools ("host institutions") in which extramural research was carried out, the desirability of grants for large cooperative projects compared with grants to individual investigators, and the need to restructure the central administration of the NIH and give it greater decision-making powers in dealing with the individual Institutes as well as the degree of decision-making autonomy that should be left to them. One basic issue that was addressed is worthy of special mention, the question of what is meant by excellence in the conduct of research—what are the criteria for evaluating it and who formulates them.

The central motif running through the report's recommendations for change was that the NIH had come of age. It had matured into a large and influential agency with a substantial body of operating experience, and the time had come to formalize its mission and administrative structure more definitely in the light of this past experience. The many recommendations dealt with three broad topics. These topics and some of the principal text under each of them were (pp. 46–48):

1. Issues with respect to *overall management* ("Plans and Policies") of the Institutes: The problem of program balance should be given increased emphasis by the management of NIH.

A new advisory group should be established to assist the Office of the Director of the NIH in the making of a major plans and policies, especially those related to the allocation of NIH funds and resources. Referred to as the "Policy and Planning Council," the new unit should consist of experienced and distinguished scientists together with a suitable minority of the outstanding non-scientists with the wise understanding of and dedication to fulfillment of the nation's needs.

2. Issues with respect to the *extramural* program:

The Study Section procedure utilizing scientific peer judgement is the best available method for awarding research grants. It should be perserved and strengthened by administrative devises which will lessen the load on individual Study Section Members without decreasing their opportunity to make scientific judgements. . .

NIH should modify its procedure to strengthen the authority and increase the responsibility of the grantee [host] institution for the work performed by its staff members, when the quality of institutional management merits it.

3. Issues with respect to *direct operations*[5] *and the intramural* programs:

We believe that the origination, organization and management of collaborative programs should be an important and continuing function of NIH....

With respect to collaborative programs in general, we recommend several steps to make it more likely that the projects with the highest probability of pay-off will be activiated, and that they will then be managed. These steps include:

a. Continued use by the separate Institutes of the advice of outside experts regarding the feasibility of proposed collaborative programs. . . . .

e. An inviolable rule that no large collaborative program, no matter how intrinsically promising, will be started with out the asssurance of the availability of a strong management team.

These points represented a departure in tone and viewpoint from the uniformly favorable recommendations of the earlier B. Jones report (and the De Bakey report (Pres. Committee on Heart, Cancer, Stroke, 1965) described later). While the NIH study committee[6] unhesitatingly agreed that the current procedure for awarding research grants to extramural researchers was "the best available method," its recommendations for "direct operations and the intramural programs" were hedged with caution and sprinkled with caveats and criticisms, reflecting the different viewpoints of persons working on and approving the report. It appears that some of the members of the Committee and its subcommittees had misgivings about the collaborative programs because they did not feel as assured of their scientfic excellence as they did anout the extramural programs that awarded grants to individual researchers or institutions. The excerpts from the final recommendations of the Wooldridge Committee cited above were a selection by the Committee that represented a distillation, accommodation, and homogenization of the many differing viewpoints presented to it by the various subcommittees—study groups, panels, and review groups—that were assigned to investigate and report to the committee at large on particular topics, such as biophysics, administration, or review procedures.

The different subgroups were composed of persons with various backgrounds and research experience, and the views of different groups toward certain inssues reflected the outlook and concerns of their disciplines. It is instructive to look at selective arguments and recommendations presented by some of these subgroups for the light it sheds on the relationship between disciplinary background and perceptions of scientific truth.

With respect to overall management of the Institutes, the *Report of the Panel on Administration* found that there was not enough overall planning by the central management of the NIH for allocating agency money in conformance with clearly established priorities. It was noted that the ''central planning of the total program needs more explicit attention . . . [and] the Director of NIH should have more formal authority over the management of the program, and better-defined sources of advice as to how it should be managed. (An advisory committee to the director, NIH was established May 1966 [Institute of Medicine, 1984]).

With respect to the extramural programs, the panel's report dealt mainly with research grants to individual researchers via the university or other ''host institution,'' stressing that the NIH was heavily reliant on the host institution to monitor the researcher's progress. The liason between the investigator and the granting Institute was found often to overshadow that between the faculty researcher and his or her university, causing problems for latter's academic programs. It also undermined the authority of the

host institutions to monitor the progress of NIH grantees on their faculties. The Panel on Administration recommended ''that the basic pattern or relations among the three participants in the extramural activity—the investigators, their institutions, and NIH—should be altered so as to bring the institutions into a more active and responsible role; [and] . . . that NIH should devise a more effective mechanism for continuous supervision of the extramural research grant program.'' There was little or no criticism of the scientific quality of the research of the outside scientists who were the recipients of the individual research grants; nearly all the criticism was centered on the treatment by the NIH of the universities and other research institutions in which the grant recipients worked. The Wooldridge Committee's conclusions incorporated most of this panel's (and other subcommittees') points about the host institutions being bypassed and not used as effectively to monitor the individuals' research as they might be.

The recommendations dealing with direct operations and intramural programs were a different story. Many of the subgroups addressed this area of NIH activities, some quite vigorously, with respect to the scientific excellence of the research conducted under its aegis and the adequacy of the available scientific knowledge underlying applied science projects. The report of the Collaborative Programs Review Group stated that:

The Review Group found that a substantial fraction of the *contract* [emphasis added] work on the [Cancer Chemotherapy Collaboration] program was of lower scientific quality and showed evidence of inadequate supervision. Even the work performed by essentially high-quality organizations (the majority) was less effective than it should be owing to lack of feedback, from the National Cancer Institute to the contractor, of test information he needed to do his job.

The principal collaborative projects were costing about $60 million a year in 1963 with some $34 million going to the Cancer Chemotherapy Project alone. This review group was very emphatic that such projects should not be undertaken for '' 'high risk,' speculative and exploratory activities,'' but instead should be confined to developing ideas whose basic worth had been well substantiated in ''small'' research (i.e., research done under "traditional" grants to individual extramural investigators).

It is instructive to note the different emphasis in the evaluation of these collaborative projects in the report of the Review Procedures Panel. While agreeing with The Collaborative Programs Review Group (CPRG) that "It seems to be generally agreed that the quality of the various activities conducted as collaborative projects is considerably more variable than that of the traditional extramural research grants and that the average is lower," this panel points to factors that make the then standard way of judging quality in the case of traditional research grants not entirely feasible and perhaps not even appropriate for evaluating collaborative projects. The Review Procedures Panel quotes from the National Cancer Institute description of the difficulties involved in applying "small grant" criteria to collaborative projects:

In any applied and developmental program, many essential tasks such as routine testing, quality control, pilot plant operation, and the like, though essential, do not impress reviewers as being high quality research. Outside advisers reviewing such projects have great difficulty in separating them from research grant applications and subconsciously place them in scientific competition with basic research. Additional difficulties arise as collaborative research program expands and becomes well established. Most of the more competent advisers become contractors themselves or become paid consultants to contractors, particularly industrial contractors. As time goes on, the advisers come to have vested interests in certain portions of the program and resist evaluation and change.

Other subcommittee reports also differed with respect to the relative worth of individual research grants, program-project research grants, collaborative programs, and clinical research centers. The Biochemistry Panel, for example, was "not very favorable" to program project grants, "strongly against" collaborative projects and saw "real advantage" in clinical research centers. The Behavioral Sciences Panel, on the other hand, found that the "clinical centers we know have given us a cause for concern," and that collaborative programs are often neccessary even though "extra care needs to be excercised" in dealing with them. The Biophysics Panel found that the clinical research centers varied in quality—some "seemed very

good" and others "should be discontinued or dramatically improved," but found that in general "The idea of 'Program Project' grants seemed good," though it recommended changes in method of administration.

These examples illustrate the differences in perceptions typical within the various disciplines about what excellence in biomedical research means and how it should be evaluated. The subcommittees generally agreed that the most rigorous quality review from the strictly scientific viewpoint could and was being given to the individual research grant and that large program grants or collaborative projects were more difficult to evaluate and were more amenable to misuse and abuse. But the fact remained that the leading causes of death and morbidity presented many pressing research questions that could not wait for the ideal answers more likely to be provided by laboratory studies followed by impeccably conducted clinical (and field) trials. The need for tradeoffs between the pressure to produce new (interventions) more expeditiously and the need to be sure of their safety and effectiveness required compromises with ideal research grant protocols. Accordingly, the perceived desirability and indeed necessity for having large program grants and collaborative programs directly initiated and managed by an Institute (including contracts) varied from panel to panel.

The disparity of viewpoint reflected not only the differing priorities accorded to the short-term social imperatives to expedite useful interventions and the political imperatives to show results, as against protecting and nurturing what is seen by some to be the pure scientific spirit. It also reflected the differences among investigators from different disciplines as to what is meant by "truth," "scientific rigor," and investigator "bias" (Kuhn, 1970; Myrdal, 1969).

Thomas Kuhn's much-discussed formulation of the evolution of scientific paradigms (1970) was not to appear until a few years later, but articles—some by Kuhn himself—on the subject of scientific paradigms and their influence on what gets investigated were appearing with increasing frequency before then. They showed the way a particular set of assumptions, often based on interpretations or findings of prior research, determines what types of questions are asked in proposed future research, and of equal importance, determines the methods used to answer to the questions. These methods and these questions are what the accredited researchers in any field are taught in their training to be "the" question of interest and "the" way to conduct research. Much of the difference in approach amoung medical researchers seems to stem from whether they seek their guidance for research directions from within the problem agendas of their own disciplines or specialites or from the priorities suggested by public health problems, with the political, social and economic factors they involve.

Applied vs. Basic Research: The Question of Medical Technology Transfer An underlying policy question for government-supported biomedical research, therefore, has been the appropriate balance between basic research and applied research. What proportion of total health resources should be allocated to bringing the existing body of basic research to a form in which it can be brought to bear on improving the health of the population? This latter process is what is meant by the term "transfer of medical technology." The NIH has defined medical technology transfer as "[involving] the transfer of research findings to the healthcare delivery system (Office of Technology Assessment, 1982). Because the mission of the NIH is to conduct and fund biomedical research and related activities to improve the health of the nation (NIH, 1980 forword), the question of medical technology transfer has been an important one in its planning and activities.

A medical technology may consist of drugs, devices, medical and surgical procedures used in medical care, and the organizational and supportive system within which such care is provided (Office of Technology Assessment, 1982, 10). The development of new technology has greatly accelerated in the last dozen years or so and the speed with which some of it has proliferated has caused concern even though many of the technologies have been widely beneficial. There are risks attached to the use of many of them that often have not been adequately considered or perhaps even adequately known, as well as questions about the great cost of some of them when compared with the benefits derived. The particular drawback that is of interest here is that "[m]any technologies have been widely diffused before their *efficacy* has been established. Concerns . . . are raised when a new technology is introduced without proof of its efficacy (e.g., electronic fetal monitoring . . .), . . . or when the relative efficacy of alternative therapies is compared (e.g., the radical mastectomy)" (Office of Technology Assessment, 1982, 29).

The major weakness indentified by the Office of Technology Assessment (OTA) study of technology transfer at NIH in 1982 were: "(1) inadequate attention as to whether technologies being considered for transfer rest on sufficient knowledge to justify the transfer,[7] and (2) insufficient attention to the scientific evaluation of emerging technologies to determine their potential benefits, risks, costs, and conditions for appropriate use" (1982).

Returning to the findings of the various subcommittees of the Wooldridge Committee, one can readily understand, in light of the foregoing discussion of technology transfer, the discomfigure expressed with the evidence of scientific looseness is such an undertaking as the cancer chemotherapy collaborative project and in other projects of this type. It must have been particularly vexatious to the "traditional" investigators. Whether the clinical trials used to develop the chemotherapy technology were not being run with the kind of supervision that could assure validity of the results or whether the basic scientific knowledge about the chemical agents and their effects was not sufficiently understood to proceed to technology development, the findings of the OTA study in 1982 corroborated aspects of the Wooldridge findings in 1965, that the "applied science" activities using large collaborative studies needed more careful attention.

When NIH first took off in its modern form about 1944, its policy was at first almost singlemindedly oriented toward sponsoring "basic bioscience research organized around categories of disease" (Office of Technology Assessment, 1982, 37). By 1965 its policy orientation was changing to include more applied science and technology transfer, and by 1978 it had established the Office for Medical Applications of Reseach (OMAR), whose main role was to oversee and promote technology transfer. Its primary activity was the development of consensus among "scientists, practitioners, consumers, and others in an effort to reach agreement on the safety and efficacy of medical technologies (Office of Technology Assessment, 1982, 45). Other technology transfer activities of the NIH also operational by the late 1970s were demonstration and control programs and information dissemination, including dissemination to scientists (e.g., the National Library of Medicine), health professionals, and the public. In the 1980s NIH increased its technology transfer to industry, such as drug and medical device companies, who complete the technology development and market the product under license or patent. The OTA analysis of 1982 stated that "relationships with industry are growing due to the clear commercial value in applications from basic science fields where there has been no precedent for profit (e.g., genetic engineering). Industry patents and licenses are very important aspects in this regard, with approximately 370 patents li censed to industry" (1982, 52).

Research Under Other Paradigms: Social/ Behavioral Research and the Question of Validity Another area of health-related research for which federal support eventually appeared was that of social/behavioral disorders—alcohol abuse, drug abuse, and mental health. A significant body of thinking in this area saw such disorders as basically biomedical, and it led to attempts to generalize the causal agent/remedy/ clinical trials research paradigm to the social and behavioral sciences. Others in the field postulated that because many of the suspected contributory causes ("risk factors") of chronic and debilitative disease were thought to lie in the social environment and in personal behavioral patterns, whatever the underlying biological pathogenic process might be, effective short-term remedies would involve changes in social environmental factors and in personal behaviors. To test such hypotheses, social and behavioral disciplines began to enter the health-related research picture and to study the role of behavioral and social environmental factors in disease incidence or prevalence. However, the standard biomedical research paradigms often did not complement the disciplinary paradigm of the social and behavioral scholars in a simple, straightforward manner. Experimental variables that represented mental contructs rather than per-

ceived physical entities posed a particular problem in designing measurable variables and determining how to interpret the results. For example, feelings of anger, love, hatred, frustration, and feeling sick without apparent physiological cause could not be measured in the same way as blood pressure level, vital functions, or potassium intake. Attempts to measure a phenomenon like patient anxiety by methods are approximating those used in the physical and biological sciences produced putatively objective measuring instruments, but these measures— tests, questionnaires, and structured interview techniques—were not uniformly accepted by the "hard" scientists as truly objective. They were seen as partially or even largely subjective systems constructed by the investigators. Questions thus arose about the objectivity of social and behavioral research.

It is true that the estimates derived form biomedical research using sampling techniques are also open to uncertainty. Three questions about the outcomes are fundamental. How wide is the range of the estimated efficacy (precision)? If we repeated the experiment with additional samples how often would we get similar results (reliability)? And how representative is the sample of the population to which it is being generalized (generalizability)? However, in social and behavioral research an additional question arises: How valid are the results? That is, does a measurement on a surrogate variable, like blood pressure, adequately measure "anxiety"? To what degree do the measurement results really address the research question? This additional uncertainty arises because the hypothesized remedy to some form of ill health is often a general factor that is not directly measurable, such as patient rapport with the physician. To test the proposition that better rapport will mean better health status, some measurable variables have to be assumed to be good surrogates for the conceptualized factor "rapport." One such variable may be taken to be "physician speaks the patient's language fluently." A correlation between health status and this variable may be found, but usually the correlation of any one of these variables with health status is small. And a question might also arise about the validity of the variable "physician speaks patient's language" as a true surrogate for the experimental factor "rapport." For example, does "speak the patient's language" say much about "rapport" if the physician is arrogantly elitist and the patient timid and retiring? Many of these underlying issues were thoughtfully treated in the Woolridge report, and a number of its recommendations were implemented.

The fact that research into social and behavioral factors in disease etiology is not easily designed under paradigms originally formulated for biomedical research does not alter the importance of this research. Many sociologists and psychologists devoted their efforts to refining the quantitive tools of their professions, often paying scant attention to or even simply ignoring the special problems of validity posed by using surrogate measurable variables to draw conclusions about the immeasurable factors that were the focus of interest in attempts to make their research methods resemble more closely those of the paradigms of biomedical disciplines. Some techniques that received special attention by such persons were Factor Analysis and Path Analysis. A minority of voices among the social and behavioral scientists began to argue that other paradigms based more on in-depth case studies were more appropriate. Later thought suggested that establishing generalizability through some form of integrative literature review covering the reports of many case studies would be a rewarding technique. Some argued that an attempt to cast most social and behavioral research in the biomedical paradigm mode was a Procrustean undertaking and would usually lead to false results. Among these possible false results were overlooking important factors and variables that must be obtained from direct observation even to the point of the investigator's immersion, perhaps even participation, in the details of the events he or she is studying. It is easy to see that panels consisting of researchers who had been wrestling with these matters would differ substantially from those made up of biomedical scientists in their views of the value of different types of research. The NIH and other agencies, like the Alcohol and Drug Abuse and Mental Health Agency (ADMHA), have constantly struggled with these questions. This area of research seems to lie somewhere between the domains of biomedical and health services research because the disorders it addresses stretch across the ranges of medicine. caretaking, and the elusive but undeniable existence of a state of well-being.

The DeBakey Report of 1965 The DeBakey Commission Report was different in character from other reports and studies accompanying the development of the National Institutes of Health. It was a bold proposal to combine basic and applied research on a breathtaking scale—large enough to cover the entire country. The B. Jones and Wooldridge studies arose from the demands of Congress and the President for reviews of the growing federal research support system to guide them in making desirable course corrections for future development. The DeBakey Commission was established in large part as a result of persuasive lobbying by members of the medical, political, and foundation elites. As opposed to its broad geographic scope, it had a relatively narrow categorical disease emphasis not found in other studies of the federal biomedical research support structure. Although by 1964 the (obligated) appropriation for NIH had grown to $1,994 million from the $381 million of 1960, with most of the dollar recommendations of the B. Jones Committee having been realized, spectacular results in terms of new methods of treating or better still preventing or postponing the onset of the most serious diseases associated with advancing age were not at hand. The Wooldridge Committee recommendations had dealt with improving NIH-sponsored research across the board, covering many topics and aspects, both administrative and biomedically theoretical. The DeBakey report was different not only in its focus on a restricted group of diseases but also in its call for establishing a system of government-directed special biomedical research institutes that would tie biomedical research on these diseases more closely to the medical care delivery system. Not only would such a tie greatly improve the diffusion of state-of-the-art knowledge on these diseases among practicing physicians, it would also improve consumer access to medical care. The crash programs during World War II that led to dramatic developments in armaments, in particular the Manhattan Project and its successful development of an atomic bomb, led to thinking in some quarters that similar all-out approaches could be productive in the health research field—that the development of effective technology for the prevention and cure of disease could be accelerated by brute force, as it were.

President Johnson's health message to Congress early in 1964 singled out cancer, heart disease, and stroke as the leading causes of death in the United States. This was so he stated, because of both a lack of sufficient biomedical knowledge to prevent and treat many cases effectively and a failure of much of the benefits of already available knowledge to reach the public. He appointed the President's Commission on Heart Disease, Cancer, and Stroke (DeBakey Commission) in 1964 to formulate a plan for a massive attack on these three diseases featuring a concentrated attempt at breakthroughs in acquiring new knowledge of the etiology, prevention, and treatment of these conditions; improved dissemination of existing knowledge among providers; and more widespread application of this knowledge to benefit the entire population through improved access to the requisite medical care. The Commission justified the concentration on heart disease, cancer, and stroke by noting that in 1963 about 70 percent of all deaths in the U.S. had been due to these diseases.

The existing research programs of the NIH were evaluated by the Commission and found to have many advantages and a few disadvantages. The good points were considered to be permitting large-scale use of federal funds for research without direct federal control, and leaving the initiative with the individual scientist with proposals judged by peers. The disadvantages were seen as certain cost and administrative burdens to the host institutions,[8] proliferation of individual grants creating "tremendous administrative problems," especially in the cost of the pool of scientists whose time is used in the review process, and the dependence of project continuation on support that is unstable from year to year, which resulted in an undue amount of research being channeled into short-term projects at the cost of neglecting long-term investigations.

The Report's proposals fell into two categories. One called for major increase in support for the existing research activities and structure. The other called for the establishment of an additional program of "mission-oriented" institutes dedicated to research on a specific problem, such as heart disease or cancer, in which research is more directly programmed. Accompanying this would be a "National Network for Patient Care, Research and Teaching in Heart Disease, Cancer, and Stroke." It would consist of heart, cancer, and stroke regional centers for clinical research combining research with patient care: twenty-five for heart disease, twenty for cancer, and fifteen for stroke. Within each of these regions there would be a number of local diagnostic and treatment stations for screening and emergency care services, each of which would refer appropriate cases to their regional center to become part of the clinincal research pool of cases. Other programs to support the operation of the "National Network" would entail aid to medical complexes associated with university medical schools, hospitals, and "other research agencies and institutions" for their development, support for less affluent medical schools to become additional "centers of excellence," and establishment of a National Stroke Program in the U.S. Public Health Service. The Report was vague on how the new networks of regional categorical centers and their affiliated local treatment stations were meant to fit into the existing noncategorical health care delivery system, either with respect to allocation of patient load, distribution of health personnel, or facility support.

The appropriations suggested to implement the entire program entailed a total of almost $140 million in new expenditures for the first year of operation with substantial increases for each of the next four years (1965). Even in retrospect, it is difficult to understand or to be sure about all the motivations behind the recommendations for so huge an expenditure for a program with so categorical a focus, notwithstanding the serious nature of the diseases targeted. In particular it is difficult to understand how the politically sophisticated sponsors of this legislation would have judged the proposal to be politically viable, especially since its centerpiece, the regional centers research program, looked very much like a collaborative project, one of the more controversial areas within the NIH. It may be that the framers of the report wished to avoid alarming the existing university-based research establishment when it asserted that these institutes were not to supplant it but would constitute an additional structure. Perhaps they had in mind that this would be a temporary transition to a federal research program that would more strongly stress targeted research in federally subsidized facilities and function as an integral part of the total health delivery system.

The expanded support for existing research activities, and the creation of new facilities along "traditional" lines, were partially effectuated. The creation of an additional and entirely new national system of regional and local centers esentially was not. The regional centers that were funded were a far cry from those envisioned in the report. The Medical Library Assistance Act (P.L. 89–291), passed in 1965, authorized the establishment of the National Library of Medicine's (NLM) Extramural Programs; a Toxicology Information Program was established at NLM in 1967, and in 1968 the Lister Hill National Center for Biomedical Communications was authorized by P.L. 90–456. But the Wooldridge report had also recomended these kinds of expansions, and it is not immediately apparent that their establishment was primarily the outcome of the DeBakey report.

The main legislation stemming from the DeBakey Report, the Heart Disease, Cancer and Stroke Amendments of 1965 (P.L. 89–239), did deal with establishing new national networks of "Regional Medical Programs", but it was very much more modest in the amounts and scope of its authorizations than the Report's recommendations. These authorized networks contained no local centers, and the regional centers that were funded were quite different in structure and function from those proposed in the Report. (The Regional Medical Programs will be more fully discussed in Chapter 15.)

Still, this Report introduced a note into NIH program evaluation different from that of the B. Jones or Wooldridge reports. It called for a new program of greatly increased federal support of biomedical research conducted in institutions fully dedicated to federal objectives and structurally tied to clinincal research and medical care provision. It proposed widening the existing scope of NIH grants beyond (not instead of) the emphasis on independent university researchers operating in the conventional university environment investigating topics often largely of

their own choosing. The Report attached great importance to the integration of federal biomedical research support program concerns with health service access concerns.

Although the inclusion of health access concerns lent a new dimension to a report on biomedical research, it must be noted that the political infeasibility of the recommendations did not rest only on consideration of their extraordinary research costs. While there was some mention of providing the same services for the medically indigent and indigent as for the rest of the population, the report provided no serious discussion of methods of financing such care. Since this had all along been one of the main roadblocks to providing universal access to medical care, it would certainly seem that a mere recommendation that health services be available to all, and in fact conveniently accessible to all, was by itself not entirely to the point.

The overriding fact was that the originial recommendations in their entirety looked very much like an expensive plan for altering the health delivery system without giving the nation a truly universal comprehensive national health insurance system, on the one hand, while running counter to the strongly prevailing preference among the existing NIH leadership for grants to individual researchers in academic institutions on the other. Thus the act that was passed bore scant resemblances to the Debakey Commission recommendations.

The Heart Disease, Cancer and Stroke Amendments of 1965, creating the "regional medical programs," largely ignored the grand master plan of the report and established a limited program of support for a vaguely defined program of disseminating current biomedical and medical technology research results from existing regional medical centers to peripheral institutions and local practitioners.

Although this program never became very large and was rather short-lived, its existence was evidence of changing trends in NIH policy. As an OTA evaluation of NIH policy put it:

Until 1965, NIH was oriented as a supporter of basic bioscience research organized around categories of diseases . . . . However, in 1965, Congress authorized the Regional Medical Program to be administered by NIH. The program was designed specifically to facilitate the application of medical advances by using regional medical centers as a focus of technology diffusion and information dissemination (Behney, April 1, 1978). According to Tilson et al. (Tilson, Reader, and Morison, 1975), this legislation "epitomizes the emerging congressional interests in making the NIH responsible for the practical application of new knowledge as well as its development."

While not generally considered successful, the Regional Medical Program signaled the start of new trends in congressional interests and action for NIH . . . The President's [Biomedical Research] Panel research and report began to focus on the overall appropriate role and effectiveness of NIH as a "transfer agent" in the continuum from fundamental research to accepted medical practice. . . . (Sherman, 1977)[9]

HEALTH SERVICES RESEARCH

Until recently, it was common for public health policy writers to attribute improvements in health status almost entirely to advances in biomedical science. In particular, the decline of infant and child mortality and the decline in morbidity from causes such as postoperative infections, poliomyelitis, and tuberculosis were attributed solely to advances in the medical knowledge of these diseases. Notwithstanding some dissenting voices (see Chapter 4), there is little question that advances in medical knowledge were indeed an important cause of the decline of morbidity and morality, particularly those attributable to certain types of illness. As long as the main causes of death and morbidity were the acute, contagious diseases, the campaign to extend the areas reached by the state-of-the-art public health services was the principal government effort to bring the applications of biomedical knowledge to bear on the health of the entire population.[10] The development of the federal network of local, state and federal public health departments was the nation's answer, as described in Chapters 2–4.

But with the shift of the main burden of illness mortality to the chronic long-term diseases and the growth of private practice—fueled by the expansion of health insurance and increased support for biomedical research—the question of optimizing the effect of current biomedical knowledge upon the health of the population became one of diffusing state-of-the-art research knowledge among medical practitioners and assuring access of all persons to them. We recall the discussion on page 413 in which health status is considered as a function of inborn genetic factors, environmental factors, and the efficacy of the personal health care system. The latter in turn is a function of the state of biomedical knowledge and the efficacy of the health delivery mechanism (this includes the diffusion of new medical knowledge, especially medical technologies, to practitioners).

Earlier, Primarily Privately Sponsored, Research in Health Services

The Committee on the Costs of Medical Care (CCMC), in its study of what was required to deliver appropriate medical care to people in the early 1930s (see pp. 597-600) fully appreciated the necessity of including consideration of a plan for implementing the alterations found to be required by the existing personal health care system. It became increasingly accepted after 1945 that support for research on the operational and structural aspects of the delivery system was a necessary component of the federal effort to support the quest for knowledge that would improve it. Early health services research consisted primarily of data gathering and rather rudimentary descriptive analysis to determine the health status of the population and the utilization of the health care system—globally as well as by specified population strata. Few attempts were made to assess either the quality of the personal health care being delivered in terms of adherence to standards dictated by the current level of biomedical knowledge or the validity of much currently accepted dicta about "good" methods of medical practice organization in terms of the effects on the health of the population.

Important work had been done under government auspices on assembling population statistics during earlier years (1900–1930) that laid the methodological foundations for later more analytical work. The federal government was first concerned with the development of uniform statewide systems of data collection in reportable and communicable diseases, and the Census Bureau, in cooperation with many of the states, had begun by developing and refining the reporting of vital statistics.[11] In 1907 the first Model Vital Statistics Act was proposed to the states, and close conformity of a state's law to the Model Law was a requirement for admission to one of the national registration areas that had been set up in the national reporting system. Also at about this time, the first standard birth and death certificates were issued (HEW, 1968).

The annual collection of mortality statistics for the earliest national death registration area had been started in 1900. It covered ten states, the District of Columbia, and a number of small cities in states outside the registration states. The Bureau of the Census, when it was organized in 1902 as a full-time agency of the federal government, was given the authority to define birth as well as death registration areas. However, birth registration areas were not established until 1915. After 1933, all forty-eight states and the District of Columbia were included in birth and death registration areas; in 1959 Alaska was added and in 1960, Hawaii.

Shortly after 1920 the United States Public Health Service began operating a population "laboratory" at Hagerstown, Maryland, for research on morbidity in the general population and its use of health services. One of its researchers, Edgar Sydenstricker later a member of the CCMC, "visualized the possibility of utilizing data on morbidity [for Hagerstown] to measure the need for health services." The Children's Bureau sponsored a series of studies on the "relationship between economic factors and infant mortality . . . and in the early 1920a published a monograph."

Early major studies during the period immediately after 1930 dealing with the distribution of population health status and the need for and adequacy of health service resources were for the most part privately financed, usually by philanthropic foundations.[12]

The study of the Committee on the Costs of Medical Care was the largest one that had ever been undertaken up to that time. Its twenty-eight reports contained a large amount of data on the distribution of health status, health service resources, and utilization across the population, stratified both geographically and demographically. The committee had delineated the following areas for intensive research:

1. Incidence of disease and disability in the population;
2. Existing facilities;

3. Family expenditures for services;
4. Incomes of providers of services; and
5. Organized facilities for medical care serving particular groups of the population.

The work started in 1927 and the last report (constisting of recommendations) was issued in 1932.

The federal government in 1935–36 augmented and widened the findings of the Committee with the *National Health Survey*,[13] covering over 7 million urban households in eighteen states and 37,000 more households in three additional states. For the next fifteen to twenty years, the data collected by these two studies "provided the basic data on health and medical care in the United States" (Anderson, 1967). This data was collected by investigators—generally biostatisticians, economists, and public health workers—and the results repeatedly pointed to an uneven distribution, both geographically and by population economic stratum of morbidity as well as the utilization of health services. The conclusions were generally that the poor and disadvantaged were sick more often and with more serious illnesses than more affluent people, while their utilization of health services was lower.

Despite these findings, government-sponsored National Health Insurance (NHI) had not been included in the Social Security Act of 1935 (Chapters 8 and 9), but its advocates were partially mollified by the establishment in the Social Security Board of the Division of Research and Statistics, headed by I. S. Falk, who had been a leading economist on the Committee on the Costs of Medical Care. During the 1935–52 period most of the energies of health services scholars were absorbed in the debate over the desirability of legislating government sponsored national health insurance as against promoting the development of private health insurance with the Division of Research and Statistics leading the way in formulating pro-national health insurance arguments and collaborating supportive data. It was prominent in helping organize the 1938 and 1948 national health conferences sponsored by the federal government to help popularize national health insurance (Anderson, 1967, Note 24). The Division continued to assemble and publish national data on health service utilization and health expenditures during this entire period and its data collection efforts culminated in a five-volume report by the 1953 President's Commission on the Health Needs of the Nation, a compendium of the data of most of the studies to that date dealing with the health status of the American people and the quantity and distribution of resources and utilization of the American health care system.

There had been many good books and studies during the 1935-1952 period focussing on the organization of the existing health care system and private health insurance, and these topics became the main thrust of a health service research after 1952.[14]

But a "change in the direction of developments began in 1951. A stalemate in disputes about national health insurance, which had been proposed in a succession of bills in Congress, led to a proposal for paid-up health insurance benefits for aged and other social-security benficiaries. This was a tactical retreat from proposals on health insurance for all persons covered under the national social insurance system. In the next 14 years, this newer but more limited proposals was a major focal point of debate" (Falk, 1970). After 1952 the emphasis of health care services research on the study of population health status, and health resources available to and used by populations, and the need for government-sponsored national health insurance subsided. Anderson attributed this phenomenon to "the election of Eisenhower as the first Republican president in 20 years, [which] ushered in a new period of consensus." The gist of this consensus, according to Anderson, was the widespread view among policymakers that voluntary health insurance was here to stay and the main tasks of health services research were now to "evaluate the benefit structure of voluntary health insurance," and "[investigate] the operational and organizational problems of the system. . . . The types of research, compilations of data which had characterized the period from 1932 to 1952, had now spent its force" (Anderson, 1967).[15] The focus was moving toward the internal operational and organizational problems of the system—financing and management. While most of the earlier health services research was sponsored by nongovernmental sources, government now increasingly became more important sponsor.[16]

Government-Sponsored Health Services Research

The morbidy studies, data collection, and publication activities of the Public Health Service, the Bureau of the Census, and the Social Security Board have already been mentioned. These provided much of the underlying data base for the analytical and imperative studies carried out before 1950 in the research sponsored by private sources, mainly the foundations. Beginning shortly after 1950, programs with formal grant procedures for health services research began to appear within the United States Health Service. The 1950 Amendments to the Hill-Burton legislation included a section authorizing grants for the "conduct of research, experiments, and demonstrations relating to the effective development of hospitals or other medical facilities . . . including projects for the construction of experimental or demonstration hospitals or other medical facilities and projects for acquisition of experimental or demonstration equipment for use in connection with hospitals or other medical facilities." (Flook, 1969). Although $1.2 million annually was authorized for this purpose, no funds were made available until 1956, when money was appropriated for a program of grant and contract support for hospital research and demonstrations, administered by the Division of Hospital and Medical Facilities of the Public Health Service. The 1961 Hill-Burton amendments increased authorization to $10 million annually, but again, it was not until 1968 that the full annual authorized amount was being appropriated (Flook, 1969). It should be noted that this program linked research with development (i.e., "R&D") and demonstration from the very start.

By 1967 the federal government was operating grant programs for research and development projects dealing with health services in many different sections of the governmental structure,[17] including seven divisions in the Public Health Service alone[18] as well as in some agencies other than the Public Health Service.[19]

This dispersal of the functions of supporting research and development in health services led to a proposal by President Johnson in his Health Message to Congress in February 1967 that a

National Center for Health Services Research and Development be established along the general lines of the National Institutes for Health. The 1967 Amendments to the Comprehensive Health Planning Act, P.L. 90–174, provided that the research support programs of the Division of Hospital and Medical Facilities and many of those be combined under the authority of a new National Center for Health Services Research and Development (NCHSR), which was established in May 1968.[20]

The National Center for Health Services Research and Development was set up to fund six types of research grants configured with readily recognizable similarity to the NIH classifications (Flook, 1969):

1. Research project grants analogous to the individual grants of NIH. Applications for these were to be reviewed by the type of dual-review system used by the NIH, with four study sections set up to review scientific and technical merit and two advisory councils to review "relevance to mission." These advisory councils were the Federal Hospital Council and the National Advisory Council.
2. Research program grants for well-known investigators and researchers for supporting a core staff to investigate a number of questions in a particular study area.
3. Exploratory research grants as seed money to establish the feasibility of large studies on a specified subject.
4. Grants to provide long-term support for well-established research teams to concentrate on one particular aspect of health services with respect to health systems and methods research.
5. Development and demonstration project grants.
6. Research training grants and fellowships. These were to be available to institutions "to train investigators from various fields so that they may conduct independent research in health services."

The original two priorities that the Center established for research areas to be funded were disparities in health care delivery between the relatively affluent and disadvantaged sections of the population, and methods of evaluating the worth of a system of health care delivery in terms of results (outcomes), both social and biological. The question of "distributive justice" lay at the center of these health services research goals in 1970, as it had generally for much such research since 1932.[21] In fiscal year 1969, the Center funded $41 million in projects, of which $4 million was for direct operation and $22.3 million was for research grants. These figures compare with a total of $1.5 billion obligated out of appropriations by the NIH in 1969.

Thus by 1970 administration of some of the federal government health services research support that had been slowly emerging in different agencies since about 1950 had been centralized. Federal support for health services research and development was also beginning to be institutionalized, organized along the lines of the National Institutes of Health in the area of biomedical research. The amounts appropriated were still miniscule compared with those available for biomedical research, however.

Before much bigger investments could readily be justified, not only would the need for health services research have to become more widely appreciated, but the internal structure of the research field—its content, methodology, and training pathways—would have to be further defined and institutionalized. The degree of analogy between the two types of research remained open to question since the acquisition of sufficient data of reliable quality in the health services involves problems that are quite different from those encountered in collecting biomedical data. The areas to be researched are more deeply enmeshed in politically controversial areas, and the directions of needed research are therefore more determined by social and political developments than in the case of biomedical research. It remained problematic whether the answers to these questions were best sought in a research framework borrowed from the biomedical sciences. If they were not, the question was: What is health services research and how should it be conducted?

There was disagreement also about the degree to which health services research should be carried out by a freestanding general research agency and the degree to which each operating agency should autonomously manage its own health services research. Should almost all federal government health service research be short-term program-oriented, or was there also room for long-term study of basic issues in health services delivery? If the latter question were answered in the affirmative, who should decide what a "basic" issue is? The Institute of Medicine was asked to investigate these and other issues under a contract from the office of Science and Technology in the Executive Office of the President.

The Institute of Medicine Report of 1979

Completed late in 1978 and issued in 1979, this report systematically laid out the background and existing issues of the government sponsorship of health services research and presented recommendations with accompanying rationales. The four major questions addressed by the report were:

1. What is health services research?
2. What is the nature of the research community that does health service research, or as the report put it, "What is the nature of the field of health services research?"
3. How is health services research organized within the federal government? How should it be?
4. What is the role of the National Center for Health Services Research and Development?

Some of the major findings and recommendations with respect to these questions were:

1. Health services research sponsorship whould be coordinated within the federal government, but its administration should not be all centralized in a single agency. Operating agencies should be equipped to do their own program-oriented research, and the NCHSR should "be maintained as a general-purpose health services research agency within the federal government . . . to conduct and sponsor synthesizing research aimed at filling gaps in research and knowledge . . . [Its] purview must not be limited to particular types of questions."
2. It was recommended that "a significant portion of all monies . . . go to support investigator-inititated extramural research"; that "in view of the limited funds available . . .

the requirement that the Center support [outside] centers for health services research [be discontinued] . . . " and that the existing provisions in the legislation mandating a minimum percentage of funds to be used for intramural research be eliminated. All extramural studies should be required to use "peer review by nongovernmental personnel of all projects involving appreciable expenditures."
3. Health services research was defined by two criteria:

It deals with some features of the structure, processes, or effects of the *personal* health services. At least one of the features is related to a conceptual framework *other than* that of contemporary biomedical science [emphasis added].

The report notes that "this definition is similar to that proposed by the National Research Council Committee on National Needs for Biomedical Personnel," but adds, "the boundaries of health services research are neither fixed nor sharply distinct," and "research in this area draws upon concepts and methods from various fields of inquiry. . . ." The subject matter of health services research was divided into clinically oriented and environmentally oriented with these orientations ranging from the most micro interests of clinical practice to the most macro concerns of environmental management and population effects. What makes them part of health services research is their adherence to the two criteria cited above. Health services research was also cross-classified by methodology, which was dichotomized as descriptive or analytic.
4. A warning emphatically expressed about the dangers of too cavalierly using biomedical research paradigms in the design of health services research.

The classical experimental design remains the ideal foundation on which to conduct research, With few exceptions, however, studies in health services research are based on nonexperimental designs. As a consequence, it is seldom possible to draw strong conclusions regarding cause and effect, such as those drawn in the laboratory sciences. The practical and ethical obstacles that prevent investigators from controlling events and circumstances that are extraneous to their principal research problems introduce errors into analytic studies where magnitudes often cannot be estimated. Because of these problems, analyitcally-oriented health services research relies heavily opon the comparative approaches of studying so-called natural experiments and of applying complex statistical procedures to historical data to adjust for characteristics of cases and situations that are known or presumed to be related to the question under investigation. . . . [Although] there is unmistakeable evidence of progress within the field [there is also] need for further improvement. [T]hose who sponsor health services research should recognize the limitations of current theoretical and methodological approaches and encourage replications to validate and extend findings of the studies.

In 1978 a National Center for Health Care Technology was established as part of the National Center for Health Statistics in the Public Health Service. The function was later transferred to the National Center for Health Services Research[22] which was then called the National Center for Health Services Research and Health Care Technology Assessment (NCHSR). In December, 1989 the name was changed again to the Agency for Health Care Policy and Research (AHCPR). It is the eighth and newest agency of the Public Health Service (HHS, 1992).

It is also important to note that with all the development of broader health services research support by the federal government, the long-standing and vital primary functions of data collection and analysis of data collection methodology were not overlooked. They were formally centralized in the formation of the National Center for Health Statistics. (NCHS), organized in 1960 through a merger of the National Center of Vital Statistics with the National Health Survey. The NCHS became part of the Centers for Disease control in 1987 (USDHHS, 1992).

The National Center for Health Statistics collects data from state agencies and issues the official U.S. vital statistics. It carries out a program of studies, data evaluation, and methods research relating to the collection and analysis of health data. This includes special periodic surveys such as:

The National Health Interview Survey—a national household interview study of illness, disability, and health service utlilization.[23]
The National Health and Nutrition Examination

Survey—a program of examination and testing of national population samples.
The National Hospital Discharge Survey[24]—surveys of patient utilization of short-stay hospitals.
The National Survey of Family Growth—surveys changes in childbearing practices and measures of reproductive health.
The National Ambulatory Medical Care Survey,[24] begun in 1973—collection of data from a sample of practicing physicians.
The National Nursing Home Survey[24]—surveys of nursing homes and their residents and staff.
The National Master Facility Inventory[24]—a listing of all U.S. inpatient health facilities, periodically updated.

The center is responsible for the Nation's official vital statistics and cooperates with the states in collecting them on a uniform basis; has an active statistical research program in survey and statistical methods; and leads or participates in a number of office activities (Wilson and Neuhanser, 1985, USDHHS, 1992).

SOME SUMMARY REMARKS

With the national shift in emphasis away from access and equity concerns and toward cost containment in the 1970s, an increasing amount of health services research began to focus on cost questions, and the principal investigators were more often economists and operation research experts than sociologists, social psychologists, and medical care scholar physicians. Accordingly, the priorities of the renamed National Center for Health Services Research (NCHSR) were increasingly oriented toward cost saving objectives, and the research awards increasingly went to proposed studies dealing with cost containment questions. The economists doing this new health services research in the 1970s were of a different school than those who had carried out the CCMC research and written much of the interpretive and expository material during 1932–1952. Those of the older school were largely empirically oriented, and if they adhered to an economic "school" it was likey to be loosely Keynesian rather than Marshallian or even Friedmanite. They generally believed that the state should ensure economic security in some way and had basically used the data of the CCMC, as enhanced by the National Health Survey, to argue and prove the need for improving access to medical care through extending health insurance. The new economists coming to the fore after 1950 were increasingly trained and operated under a quite different paradigm. The essence of this paradigm is an axiomatic assumption that the society that depends most the "free" economic market to distribute almost every good or service possible is the best society because it is based on maximum freedom of choice by the consumer. This *ispo facto* guarantees the most efficient production of goods and services and their optimum distribution distribution to match consumer tastes and preferences. If society wishes to provide for some "deserving" human casualties of the operation of untrammeled competition, then it should do so by income transfers, that is, giving these people money to buy needed services in the open market. Government should rarely and reluctantly intervene in the health services and delivery system, either to directly provide service or to pay for it under special arrangements, because this distorts the operation of the free market and causes more harm than good.

The apposite point here is that this paradigm leads natrually to a certain type of research in the health services. If the free market is overwhelmingly the most important motor that runs or should run the health care system, the investigation of questions of cost reduction should focus on identifying those forces that impede normal market functioning rather than on methods of regulating utilization or prices.

While this paradigm could be made to include hypothesized determinants representing patient access and satisfaction, in practice it infrequently did so. This is because the calculation of values to describe them numerically is a complex procedure with important subjective components involving evaluation of such items as responses to interviews and questionnaires as well as techniques such as case observation— procedures that are foreign and unsettling to the neoclassically trained economist.

In the 1980s, a realization of the shortcomings of over-dependence on so-called econometric research results alone began surfacing and

"qualitative" research slowly come to be recognized as a necessary adjunct of strictly qualitative research. During the Reagan administration this type of research was not given significant support by the NCHSR because the issues of cost contaminant were paramount.

The issue of defining the boundary between biomedical and health services research also deserves further mention. We have seen that the Institute of Medicine Report considered the boundaries between the two to be neither fixed nor even sharply distinct. For "pure" examples the differences between these two are clear, as is usual in this type of dichotomy. Testing a new cancer drug on mice is biomedical research; seeing if dividing one seven hundred-bed hospital into two smaller hospitals will reduce patient travel time enough to compensate for a possible reduction in percent occupancy is a health services research question. But what about evaluating the cost/benefit ratio of heart bypass surgery? Presumably, biomedical research has judged this to be an effective procedure (i.e., a statistically significant difference has been found between the average value of the criterion used to measure effectiveness for those who had surgery than for those who did not), for it is so accepted at medical centers and major private and government insurers. This would imply that further evaluation is now a health services research question. What do health services decision makers want from this research? A simple reply is that the procedure is biomedically effective, and if we can afford it we should finance it. However additional questions arise. How effective is it? In what sense is it effective--does it prolong life? Ameliorate pain? Increase the ability to be normally active? What degree of unanimity is there in biomedical research about the degree of effectiveness? In fact, some well-conducted biomedical research may have come up with the results declaring the procedure effective but health service research may find it effective only at a very low level of cost/benefit ratio.

These questions are the concern of technology assessment. Both the Congressional Office of Technology Assessment (OTA) and the Public Health Service's Office of Health Technology Assessment (part of the AHCPR) are dedicated to this type of research. The result is very important to the consumer and to health services decision makers because it works to assure the effectiveness of the technology and enable evaluation of the cost of its benefits compared with the extent of these benefits. But the consumer may be more interested in knowing about its effectiveness and decision makers more interested in the ratio of benefits to cost.

As an example,

OHTA evaluates the risks, benefits and clinical effectiveness of new or unestablished medical technologies that are being considered for coverage under Medicare ... at the request of the Health Care Financing Administration (HCFA). They are the basis for recommendations to HCFA regarding coverage policy decisions under Medicare.

Questions about Medicare coverage for certain health care technologies are directed to HCFA by such interested parties as insurers, manufacturers, Medicare contractors, and practitioners. Those questions of medical, scientific, or technical nature are formally referred to OHTA for assessment (Agency for Health Care Policy, 1991).

But HCFA must still make the decision, and its independence from administration influence will depend heavily on the nature and independence of its advisory bodies.

Furthermore, many biomedical research results that have been approved as a technology are based on follow-up studies of the clinical trials type. Patients who have received a treatment are compared with persons who have approximately the same symptoms and are in the same age and sex (and perhaps other strata-defining variables) groups but who did not get the treatment. Health services research, on the other hand, often takes a public health approach and looks at the entire population of two regions to see if the effectiveness as measured by health status levels is correlated with the extent to which a particular procedure has been used in each region on persons having the same medical diagnosis. Of course, this approach is only available if different areas can be found where the use of a particular treatment for a similar diagnosis varies substantially, but there has been considerable evidence that such variations exist (Wennberg and Gittelson, 1982). The results can be quite different under these two approaches. For one thing, the medical research center

matching is often quite restricted in the populations available to be sampled from by the center. In addition, the medical center research is usually carried out when the procedure is new or experimental. Once it is pronounced effective, further research cannot ethically be carried out by denying the procedure to a selected control group with similar symptoms. If, once the procedure becomes commonly used, it is no longer as effective as when it was tested by a highly trained and specially motivated research team, this hypothesis can scarcely be tested by medical-center-oriented research. The biomedical research establishes the efficacy of the treatment when given under ideal conditions; the areawide health service research establishes a result that indicates the degree to which it is actually *effective* in improving the health of populations.[25]

The main point here is that health technology assessment research may be carried out by either biomedical research oriented personnel or health-services-research personnel. A useful approach may be to consider it biomedical research if its main aim is to inform medical practitioners about what procedures have been found by R&D methods to be medically effective for a given condition. The same research could be considered health services research if its main aim is to determine whether a particular procedure makes a suffucient difference in health status or quality of life to warrant public support for ᵢ application given its cost; or whether a proᵤᵤ dure of well-established biomedical worth is being applied appropriately to a specified population. The health services research experimental design will not always attempt to follow in the footsteps of the biomedical research model, with its ''cases'' and ''controls.'' It will often focus on reviewing the published accounts of the biomedical research to attempt arriving at consensus about the benefits of the procedure based on the experience of previous investigations (and often these experiences disagree) with respect to vital statistics, statistics of morbidity, and indicators of health status.[26]

The federal government has been very active in supporting both biomedical and health service research more in the case of biomedical than in health services. If, as I shall argue in Chapter 16, one can clearly discern, in retrospect, a federal health policy, both enunciated and actual that commits it to providing a health services system that will make state-of-the-art medical care available to all who need it, then support for improving the biomedical and administrative content of that care through research is a well-established fact. The support has not been consistent. A graph depicting it would show jiggles up and down, largely reflecting different administrations but also reacting to differences in Congressional composition. But the trend has been unmistakably a rising one.

NOTES

1. This new name was given to the Marine Hospital Service in 1912.

2. The NIH defines such an agreement as one between a federal laboratory and one or more collaborators (usually private corporations), who work on a joint project in which the collaborating party is granted, in advance, an exclusive right to license any resulting invention.

3. The remaining beds are allocated to the National Institute of Mental Health and the National Institute on Alcohol, Drug Abuse, and Mental Health Administration (ADAMHA) rather than NIH.

4. (a) The traditional or individual research grant; (b) the research program grant; (c) the collaborative project; (d) grants to develop supporting resources for research; (e) fellowships, research development awards, and career research rewards. (See also Table 14–3).

5. Funds for "direct operation," as shown in Table 14–1, include intramural research, research and development contracts, the National Library of Medicine, and funds necessary for administrative and program management of NIH. (Intramural research followed R&D contracts are by far the main items) (USDHHS, 1989; NIH, 1991, Table 9).

6. The Wooldridge study committee was formally known as the NIH Study Committee. Wooldridge was the chair.

7. Cf. the allusion to the remarks on this matter by the subgroup on direct operations and intramural programs in the Wooldridge report noted on page 423.

8. We recall that both the B. Jones and the Wooldridge reports, especially the latter, had also identified the treatment of the host institutions as a major problem.

9. The works referenced in this quotation are cited in the source of the quotation: Office of Technology Assessment 1982, pp. 37–38.

10. Still, wide sections of the United States and other populations continued to be afflicted by these

very diseases to an unnecessary degree due to the failure of the health care system to reach them. Such unnecessary disease incidence is now on the rise again.

11. "Vital statistics . . . describe events related to individuals entering or leaving life or changing their civil status. They come from records of live births, deaths, fetal deaths, marriages, divorces, adoptions, legitimations, annulments and separations. They provide information on the number and characteristics of vital events that take place in designated populations during given periods of time." (HEW, 1968).

12. Much of the material on the early studues in the following sections is based on Odin W. Anderson's review of 1967. The 1979 study of health services research by the Institute of Medicine also discusses this background material, both private and government sponsored, and includes some studies not mentioned here.

13. This was a one-time survey and should not be confused with the *National Health Survey* started in 1956 by the National Center for Health Statistics, which has continued to conduct it as a systematic ongoing activity (See also note 23.)

14. Most of these examples come from O. W. Anderson's seminal review of health services research through 1965 (1967). The Committee on Medicine and the Changing Order of the New York Academy of Medicine sponsored a notable series of books on these subjects dealing with medical education, medical services provided by government, medical research, health insurance in the United States, new works on rural populations (Hoffer and Schuler, 1948; Hoffer et al., 1950; Mott and Roemer, 1948), and other topics. The school of Public Health of the University of Michigan pioneered in introducing the beginnings of medical care studies into universities, starting in the 1940s. The next big national study was that of the Commission on Hospital Care (privately financed by the Commonwealth Fund, W. K. Kellog foundation, National Foundation for Infantile paralysis).

15. It should be noted that O. W. Anderson described these developments with apparent relief, for he seems to have decided that the controversy over private versus public health insurance led the field of health services astray from its true path of focusing on operational and managerial matters, including structure of private health insurance benefits. After noting the establishment of health service research and teaching units in six universities in the years after 1940, he added:

But the bitterness and rancor which attended research in the controversial area of health care inhibited their development to a variable degree [sic]. In the early 1950's, as the immediate possibility of the enactment of some form of government-sponsored health insurance subsided, a new framwork of policy decision emerged. Social research in this type of framework was possible on an accelerating basis (1967, p. 26).

16. It is ironic that this trend of the sponsorship of health services research to turn toward government sources should have coincided with the trend of the subject matter of health services research to turn towards private health insurance for its content.

17. Many of these programs and some others are discussed in the seminal article by Evelyn Flook (1969).

18. These were:

a. The National Institute of Mental Health support of research in community mental health services.

b. The Bureau of State services support for service-oriented research in community health services.

c. The Division of Nursing administering research grants in the field of nursing and patient care.

d. The Division of Hospital and Medical Facilities grants for investigating community planning for hospital facilities, hospital design, problems of hospital organization and administration, and other topics relating to hospitals.

e. The Office of Comprehensove Health Planning (established by P.L. 89–749 and discussed in Chapter 15) grants for studies, demonstrations, or training to improve existing methods of providing health services. "These were administered largely through the regional office structure."

f. The Division of Regional Medical Programs support of research, including some health services components.

g. The Division of Physician Manpower, Bureau of Health Manpower, support of research in the education and use of physicians.

19. Such as:

a. The Children's Bureau grants for studying health services for mothers and children.

b. The Social Security Administration grants to study aspects of medical care economics, particularly those that would help improve administration of Medicare.

c. The 1967 Social Security Amendments had given the Medical Services Administration of the Social Rehabilitation Service (the "welfare" component of HEW) authority to award grants for research and demonstration projects dealing with the provision and financing of health services. These authorizations were aimed at improving administration of Medicaid.

20. The programs previously assigned to the Divisions of Community Health Services and Medical Care Administration, and the National Center for Chronic Disease Control, as well as the Division of Hospital and Medical Facilities and the Partnership for Health, were also transferred to this new center. The programs in the Social Security Administration Children's Bureau, Division of Physician Manpower, Regional Medical Programs, and Nursing remained where they were. The NCHSR was housed in the Health Services and Mental Health Administration.

21. See O. W. Anderson's remarks in note 15 for the basic focus of most privately funded research, especially after 1952.

22. It will be recalled that the original name was the Health Services Research and Development Center. After 1973, there were two other name changes before this name was adopted but they were in force for very brief periods. The development of the NCHSR is described in greater detail in Institute of Medicine, 1979.

23. This was the first system for the regular collection of health-related data by the Public Health Service. (Wilson and Neuhauser, 1985). It was developed under the National Health Survey Act of 1956. It should not be confused with the one-time National Health Survey of 1934. Findings are published in series 10 of *Vital and Health Statistics* series (See also note 13.)

24. Work is in process to merge and expand these four surveys to form a National Health Care Survey that will be an integrated survey of health care.

25. The technology assessment literature recognizes the difference between these two measures and labels them "efficacy" and "effectiveness": "Efficacy refers to the probability of benefit to individuals . . . under ideal conditions of use. Effectiveness, a term used interchangeably with efficacy by some, refers to the benefits of a technology under average conditions of use"(Office of Technology Assessment, 1982).

26. Evaluating the worth of new biomedical procedures, mainly through literature review and analysis techniques (such as meta-analysis, critical literature analysis, or the integrative research review), has been a major function of the Office of Technology Assessment (OTA), established by Congress in 1972 to advise it on questions of cost effectiveness and the cost/benefit ratio of biomedical procedures.

15

Health Planning: Governmental Efforts to Promote Coordination and Rationalization of the Health Services System

CONCEPTS OF HEALTH PLANNING

There are two broad types of planning for health services—institutional and community-wide. Institutional health planning is the internal planning done by health providers and is similar to general corporate business planning.[1] The need for this type of planning has never been in question. Community-wide planning for health services has been done by voluntary associations of nonprofit social service agencies and health service providers and is similar to planning for other social services. Its desirability and the form it should take have been the subject of frequent controversy. Institutional health planning is basically done from the point of view of strengthening and promoting the survival of the institution; community-wide health planning is fundamentally interested in the receipt of health services by a defined population. The main lines of disagreement over the structuring of this type of health planning have been whether it should be done by private or by government organizations and the extent to which planning decisions should be optional or compulsory for health providers. This chapter deals almost entirely with community-wide health planning. It also concentrates on hospital services because that is where the planning "action" was.

The two main dimensions of health planning are shown by the matrix in Figure 15–1. The sharpest differences have existed between those whose views fell in cells 1 or 4. The adherents of the "cell 1" view have generally held that before 1946, with its Hill-Burton Act, the U.S. health services system developed out of felt *local* needs. These were responded to by local citizens who erected facilities as needed and by health personnel, mainly physicians, who settled and practiced in areas also individually chosen by them in response to local needs. We know the needs were genuine because they were expressed through the free market; people were willing to pay for the services directly or fiscally responsible private philanthropy was ready to support them. Whatever joint action was undertaken among private providers was voluntary "cooperation" and not compulsory "planning." After 1946, and especially after 1960, this free-market-oriented system was gravely distorted by the intrusion of government health planning, which artificially pumped up supply or demand to meet supposedly "proper" levels that centralized bureaucratic planners in Washington concocted out of faulty abstractions.

If health planning is arbitrarily defined as what the federal government does or proposes to do under this set of constructs, one can then readily see why one would prefer "nonplanning" to "health planning." And for the most part, publicly expressed antipathy to "health planning" was based on some variant of this set of assumptions.

Actually, the United States health system as of 1945 was not as much a product of pure market forces as the antiplanners made it out to be; many features of the system were already largely planned. The number, race and gender characteristics of physicians were largely the result of state (compulsory) licensing laws passed at the behest and administered under the aegis of

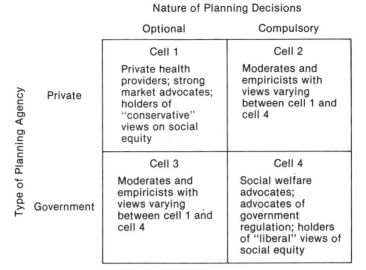

Fig. 15–1. The two main dimensions of health planning.

medical societies; the content of medical practice was largely the result of post–Flexner medical school education (''forced'' on the medical schools under a plan implied by the Flexner report) and by state laws determining which type of training was acceptable for licensing. Hospitals were developing in conformance with what their medical staffs, reflecting the positions of the medical associations and medical schools, thought a hospital should be, and the form of organization of medical practice was strictly regulated by states to conform to the economic organization ''planned'' by local medical societies. All of these developments converged to a national uniformity and were clearly planned— not by the federal government, it is true, but by provider organizations, wealthy business people, corporations who worked with them to help finance the resources they needed, and state legislatures who put the force of law behind implementing many of these plans. The planning structure was formally organized into local medical societies who sent representatives to state societies who in turn sent representatives to the national AMA. In addition, various commissions of the AMA and separate accrediting bodies issued formal edicts about what a medical school should be, who would be professionally regarded as a specialist, what sort of training sites in hospitals would be deemed appropriate

to produce an accredited specialist, and what ways of organizing physicians into practice units would be acceptable and which would not.

Provider groups and libertarian theorists deplored health planning most vociferously when it involved the federal government's estimating what the configuration of the health services system should be to serve the estimated medical needs of the entire population. Actually, because most of these opponents were defending the status quo they could not really have been opposed to the concept of health planning or even centralized planning, for a health services system as complex and as tightly controlled as the U.S. system has been could not but have been the result of planning. Most of the actual planning, however, has been invisible to the general public, because the important decisions and their enforcement have been carried out in professional and trade councils. The real question has not been planning versus nonplanning but rather: ''Who makes the planning decisions?'' It is need-based, publicly conducted and enforced health planning that has been attacked by most antiplanning advocates rather then planning itself, and this applies even to large-scale centralized planning. Corporate planning, for example, is an entirely acceptable form of planning.[2] As will be further described in this chapter, many liberal, progressive, humanitarian, radical, activist, and similarly designated "people" advocates have been slow to recognize the real issues in the "health planning program" in the United States. They were either only mildly interested or even antagonistic to the major federal health planning program at the height of the public battles for its existence during 1966–1979.

Adherents of the position represented by "cell 4," on the other hand, have argued that the economic and social structure of the United States became incomparably more complicated after 1945, and this applies a fortiori to the health services systems. Considerable data collection and analytic technique are required if the health care system is to be made more efficient and access to quality care simultaneously improved. A national system of community-based health planning is the only way to find out what is required and what is surplus. Society as a whole will have to decide how many of the changes indicated by the planning process it wishes to implement. That is a matter to be democratically determined in the political arena. Community-based health planning is simply the process by which planning entities determine optimal ways and means of getting from here to there—from what is to what we want it to be.

This process of needs-based health planning may be conceptualized in a diagram like that shown in Figure 15–2. The first task is to obtain good estimates of existing health services resources, health services utilization, and population health status. The existing health services resources are here presumed to be approximately appropriate for providing the existing volume and mix of health services, and the existing health services being provided are assumed to be a major determinant of existing health status. This part of the process is represented by the boxes A, B, and C in Figure 15–2.

The second task is to analyze the health problems revealed by the data on health status and formulate a goal of mitigating these health problems to achieve an improved health status, expressed in specific objectives that designate numbers (e.g., infant mortality rate) to be achieved by a specified effective date. This part of the process is represented by boxes D and E in Figure 15–2. A specified improved health status (E) implies access to an improved volume and mix of health services (F) which in turn implies an improved volume and mix of health services resources (G).

Having arrived at required resources and required health services (measured in utilization units such as patient days), the final step is to plan for the transformation of present resources and health services utilization to the required ones. This process is represented by box A-G (which represents the plan for implementing the resources change), and box B-F (which represents the plan for implementing the utilization change). Whether the action plans (A-G) to improve resources to the recommended level and utilization (B-F) to its recommended level are actually implemented depends on societal action, particularly legislative appropriations.

As we shall see, all forms of health planning implied by the four cells of Figure 15–1 were used at some time in the United States. It started with cell 1, progressed through cells 2 or 3 to cell 4, and is now on its way back to cell 2 or 3.

NATIONAL GLOBAL HEALTH PLANNING

Committee on Costs of Medical Care Report as Nationally Global Health Planning

Previous chapters referred to the Committee on the Costs of Medical Care (CCMC) which first enunciated national requirements for appropriate health care for the United States population in 1933, after five years of work. The Lee-Jones report (AHA, 1965), one of twenty eight volumes issued by the committee, established a methodology for estimating utilization and resource requirements that remains the prototype of many elements of population-based planning to the present day, constituting one of the best models of public health planning (i.e., based on population health needs) that has yet been formulated. As is true of much public health administration research and policy formulation, the methodology used to derive estimates strongly implied the public policy and philosophy that undergirded it, a question I have discussed in considerable detail elsewhere (see Chapter 14 and Shonick, 1976, 1986).

For purposes of this chapter, it suffices to note that the methodological essence of the public

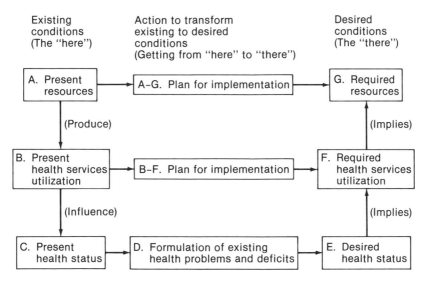

Existing
conditions
(The "here")

Action to transform
existing to desired
conditions
(Getting from "here" to "there")

Desired
conditions
(The "there")

A. Present
resources

A–G. Plan for implementation

G. Required
resources

(Produce)

(Implies)

B. Present
health services
utilization

B–F. Plan for implementation

F. Required
health services
utilization

(Influence)

(Implies)

C. Present
health status

D. Formulation of existing
health problems and deficits

E. Desired
health status

Fig. 15–2. Schema of the population-based community health planning process. *Note*: Six boxes represent the making of the "existing" estimates (A, B, C) and the requirements plan (E, F, G); boxes A–G and B–F represent the making of the implementation plans; box D represents the estimation of existing health deficits which is obtained by subtracting C from E.

health approach to health planning is the sequence of steps that begins with an assessment of the existing health status of populations by suitably small areas, determines what health services are appropriate for ("needed" by) these populations, and finally estimates the resources required to deliver these services. Any plan for implementing the recommendations of the plan would, of course, be subject to constraints determined by the prevailing economic, social, and political climate. Lee and Jones used the progression from population health status through required services to end up with needed resources (Steps E, F, and G in Figure 15–2). They did not, however, address the question of local small-area need determination, arriving only at global national estimates. In this respect, they fell short of today's concept of community-based health planning. These estimates later served to motivate legislation to raise national resource totals, especially hospital beds. The inflexible application of uniform overall formulas derived from computing national need requirements to small areas in administering programs like Hill-Burton and the later national health planning programs substantially impaired their effective implementation.

Estimates of illness incidence and prevalence rates per population by diagnostic category were derived by Lee and Jones from data of closed membership industrial health systems. Also used were studies by the United States Public Health Service and other investigators based on data from identifiable populations at risk, such as schoolchildren, military officers' families, and the then relatively isolated city of Hagerstown, Maryland. The availability of these closed systems of medical care enabled Lee and Jones to solve the fundamental problem of making health status estimates, deriving population-based *rates* for the incidence and prevalence[3] of these conditions. A panel of 125 practicing physicians submitted judgments of the quantity and types of services required on average to properly treat each unit of the prevailing conditions.[4] Multiplying these average numbers of needed services per health condition—patient days, physician visits, and other types—by the estimated national prevalence of each condition yielded estimates of aggregate services needed nationally, step F in Figure 15–2. These were then translated into national aggregate resource requirements, mainly of facilities and personnel, Step G.

The CCMC report also dealt with the underlying issue in planning to implement the recommended levels of needed utilization derived in their national requirements plan—how to get from "here" to "there," step B-F. The majority report identified the lack of access to medical care as a major barrier to implementing the required increase in utilization and recommended that effective demand for medical care be raised to the levels of utilization their planning had shown to be needed by the population. To ensure that the aggregate demand for medical services would be equal to the estimated appropriate need, the majority section of the CCMC final report[5] recommended health insurance that would cover every person. There was, however, considerable, difference of opinion, even among supporters of the majority opinion, about the relative advantages of social or government insurance as against private insurance. The majority report took no position on compulsory governmental versus "voluntary" private insurance. The minority report, voicing the AMA position, opposed all health insurance not operated by physicians, meaning at that time the medical societies.

Thus, by the time the New Deal was being put into place in the early 1930s, a private foundation-supported report had enunciated a national health plan calling, on the supply side, for specified numbers of personnel and facilities, and on the demand side, for universal health insurance of some sort to raise demand for utilization to the levels indicated as needed by the existing health status of the population. Much of the plan was actually implemented by subsequent legislation. In addition to the numbers in the CCMC recommendations being used to set goals for needed hospital beds, the general findings of the study's twenty-eight volumes set the direction of much of the federal government's health policy with respect to medical care through 1980. What was in effect a national health plan had been drafted under the private auspices of the CCMC, and many of its goals and suggestions became the long-range de facto plan of the federal government. Steps to implement the plan were taken over the forty-five years following 1935 to increase the supply of health service resources and increase the effective demand to enable all persons to use the health services they needed. Taken together, these steps comprise a national plan for a universally accessible system of comprehensive health services. To outline this national plan I

shall briefly review the most salient of these implementation steps that have been described and discussed in more detail in previous chapters.

Federal Government Health Policy 1935–1965 as Nationally Global Health Planning

The implementation of a national plan may be said to have begun in 1935, with the provision of grants for public health services (including personal services) to public health departments and other medical providers under Titles V and VI of the Social Security Act. Since these services were largely free or means tested, they were providing both supply-side and demand-side assistance to the health services system (see Chapters 2, 3, and 4). Beginning in 1946 the Hill-Burton legislation provided grants for constructing health facilities, using as objectives national estimates of need very close to the Lee-Jones recommendations; beginning in the early 1960s the health "manpower" acts provided grants that increased the numbers of health personnel, using as objectives the results of studies specially commissioned by the federal government. Starting about 1950 the federal government sought to increase the intrinsic effectiveness of medical care by launching an immense biomedical research program, which developed into the National Institutes of Health—again using as objectives the outcomes of specially commissioned studies. Around 1960 a program of research aimed at uncovering more efficient ways of administering health service was begun, first financed and directed by other programs such as Hill-Burton and nursing personnel development, and later consolidated mostly under the National Center for Health Services Research and its successor agencies.

Along with these supply-side or resource development programs there was also development of the demand side. At first, the only national assistance for paying for medical care was oblique. The federal program of sharing state costs for cash assistance "relief" payments, initiated by the Social Security Act of 1935, in addition to directly increasing demand for these services also freed some state money for use in providing better programs for the poor in those states that chose to do so. The rapid rise of private health insurance after 1945 was primarily for in-hospital coverage, and the Hill-Burton program was therefore expanding supply in an area in which demand was increasing. For persons not at all or insufficiently covered by private health insurance, a large national network of free local public hospitals and medical care programs operated by state and local public welfare agencies as well as entitlement programs like those of the Veterans Administration were there to caulk the cracks. As remaining gaps on the demand side were uncovered, more and more filler was applied. In 1956, the federal government began contributions for medical care to specially designated state and local "relief" or "welfare" medical programs (Chapter 10), and in 1965 this support was enlarged to form Medicaid. In the early 1960s federal support for what came to be called the community health centers was begun along with similar but smaller programs like the migratory health, rural initiative, and urban initiative programs (Chapter 11), and 1963 federal money was appropriated by construction of mental health centers and mental retardation facilities, and in 1965 came the Medicare program. All this time, federal and state tax policies were subsidizing the expansion of private health insurance.

VOLUNTARY LOCAL COMMUNITY-WIDE HEALTH PLANNING

While the pre–1966 planning efforts and their implementation greatly increased supply as well as access to medical services, these efforts had fallen substantially short of meeting their goals by 1965. A recurrent theme in many of the preceding chapters has been the fact that many people still had insufficient access to health services largely because of the insufficiency of the demand-increasing programs. Despite this, the health care system was inordinately expensive and rapidly becoming more so. Although more hospital beds had been made available, the distribution of physicians was uneven. Some areas were seriously underserved, perhaps worse than before 1946, and others had a surplus of providers that was an important factor in causing medical costs to rise.

Experience with programs aimed at supplying more hospital beds and health personnel was

driving home to policymakers and medical care policy scholars and writers the problem of increasing supply without attending to its distribution. Legislative interests turned to federally supported *local* areawide planning as a possible solution.

There had been a history of local, areawide health planning activity and considerable writing on this subject. It is briefly reviewed in the following pages before the more extensive treatment of the federal legislation of 1966 and 1974, which established national networks of federally supported local health planning bodies.

Early Ad Hoc Efforts at Local Areawide Planning for Hospitals Through Regionalization

Early voluntary local community service agency associations were of two types, hospitals organized into hospital associations and private nonprofit health or welfare agencies confederated into local health and welfare councils. In the health field most of the associations were among hospitals. The Hospital Review and Planning Council of Southern New York, incorporated in New York City in 1938, is reputed to have been the "earliest area-wide planning agency for health facilities" with jurisdiction comprising New York City and surrounding counties (Hilleboe and Barkhuus, 1971). Actually this type of hospital planning council was a rare and early pioneering development this far back, for in 1967 a survey found the typical council to have been in existence less than five years (Brown, 1973). The main focus of the planning by hospital councils was on inpatient services.

For many years before the formation of hospital councils, local health planning consisted of ad hoc planning for the construction and operation of individual hospitals in localities where a perception of need existed among citizens and businesses who could raise the needed construction capital and subsidize the hospital's operating costs. The trustees, board of directors, and medical staff controlled hospital policies and carried out the ongoing planning. All these bodies were formed by self-selection and were self-perpetuating. The policies of these private hospitals, especially those formulated by their medical staffs, controlled much about the medical services available in their communities. Not only did they determine what persons they accepted as patients and how they would be treated, but they also largely controlled how many physicians and of what type would be able to practice in the community through their control over granting hospitalization privileges to physicians. The result of the individual planning carried out by all the hospitals in a local area may be said to have constituted a de facto areawide plan for hospital resources. That these private efforts did not succeed in providing hospitals for every place that needed one, as a nationwide public-health-oriented planning effort might have, is indicated by the existence as late as 1976 of many hospitals that were publicly owned but served the entire community on a pay-for-service basis.[6] Various ad hoc arrangements for consultation and cooperation among hospitals arose in some localities, and some of these developed into the more formal arrangements of the hospital councils of the 1960s. Still, even the hospital council was, in general, a consultative organization for exchange of views and a place where agreements could be made for cooperative action when it was to the mutual interests of the members. Planning bodies representing the community at large with providers constituting but one interest group did not materialize under voluntary auspices. Many administrators, teachers, and writers in the hospital administration and areawide planning fields were maintaining that the existing situation was a desirable state of affairs and that such councils were what health planning was all about (Hitt, 1969; Sieverts, 1968; Sigmond, 1969).

Formal planning and cooperation among groups of hospitals began to be more widely discussed after about 1955. Two major developments were behind this: the increasing technological complexity of the hospital and the proliferation of hospital beds accompanying the development of the Hill-Burton program (discussed later in this chapter and in Chapter 12). Arising in the 1960s from these two developments were different types of voluntary local areawide hospital planning. (See the next section below.)

The technological development of the hospital within the context of the U.S. brand of capitalism had implications both for the business-managerial side of hospital operations and for its medical care organization aspects. The business-managerial aspects were strongly affected by the development of expensive capital equipment that became rapidly obsolescent as well as the increasing automation of laboratory techniques, housekeeping services, and later, information systems. These led to a growing perception that managerial economies of scale were being increasingly required and that many of these called for cooperative action among local hospitals. The hospitals' medical care organization aspects were also heavily affected by the accelerated development of medical specialization, especially of subspecialties that used complex medical technologies emerging from expanded biomedical research and development discussed in Chapter 14. Thus, increased joint action was seen to be required, not only to achieve managerial economies of scale but also to maintain state-of-the-art medical practice.

The increasing number the subspecialties, each one treating conditions that constituted but a small precentage of the diagnostic spectrum of total medical practice, required that the hospital cover a catchment area with a population large enough to yield a sufficient number of cases to adequately occupy a hospital specialty unit such as neurosurgery and to keep the specialty "team" well practiced. In very densely populated areas a relatively small geographic area might yield enough cases to fully occupy many subspecialty units as well as general medicine, general surgery, and general obstetrics, maternity, and pediatric beds. But in areas with less population density a very large catchment area is necessary to provide enough cases to keep a particular subspecialty unit fully occupied and to maintain the competence of the subspecialty staff. This area is likely to be too large to have one hospital serve the area adequately because many of its residents would then be too far away from the hospital to use it conveniently for the preponderance of general admissions and perhaps also outpatient visits. It was therefore necessary to have a number of smaller hospitals in such areas that were conveniently accessible to local residents for general medicine, surgery, obstetrics/gynecology, and pediatrics. But by the very fact of their small size and market, they were each unable to supply enough cases for efficient operation of narrowly defined subspecialties.

Leading medical care organization scholars had for many years called for a type of areawide cooperative arrangement they designated as "regionalization" to solve this problem (McNerney and Riedel, 1962). Under this concept, one (or several) large hospital(s) with subspecialties would be designated the base hospital and be the main locus of medical teaching and subspecialty care. The smaller general community (or district) hospitals would refer patients needing the technical resources of the base to that hospital, which was the center of the regionalized system. The base hospital in turn would disseminate the results of its research and some aspects of its subspecialty expertise to the community hospitals or the periphery of the system. This form of regionalization was much talked about in medical care planning circles. In 1945, the United States Public Health Service circulated a monograph written by Assistant Surgeon General Joseph Mountin and associates featuring careful explanations of this form of regionalization. Figure 15–3, excerpted from the Mountin study, illustrates the ideas that were being promoted. (It should be noted that Mountin's plan of regionalization also saw rural health centers as the "periphery" around a rural hospital.) Because the concept of regionalization involved a center and a periphery with the center having higher technological capability than the periphery, I shall call this a hierarchical (or vertical) cooperative arrangement (Shonick, 1972). Only a few instances are reported of attempts to establish such hierarchial regionalization among hospitals.

Organized in 1931, the Bingham Associates Fund used the Pratt Clinic, the New England Center Hospital, and Tufts Medical School, all in Boston, as the three components making up its center. It reached out to rural areas of Maine and other parts of New England (Garland, 1960). Formed in 1946 with support from the Commonwealth Fund, the Rochester Regional Hospital Council consisted of a group of large teaching hospitals that worked with small community hospitals to bring to them the educational and consultation advantages available in large urban hospitals. As late as 1961, the Ohio Medical Education Network of the Center of Continuing Education, Ohio State University, was formed. By 1967, is comprised fifty-four participating hospitals that were linked to the center via telephone-radio conferences (Pace and Schweikart, 1967).

A Typology of Hospital Regional Planning

The planning activities implied by the goals of the few regional cooperative arrangements discussed above were primarily directed at enhancing the effectiveness of *operations* with respect to the technical quality of medical care in existing hospitals. The cooperative activities consisted of transfers among member hospital of patients and medical technology. They were not, in the first instance, aimed at influencing the location of the hospitals themselves or the total supply of hospital beds and their allocation among the hospitals in the area.

With respect to the *managerial* aspects of hospital operation, however, an increasing trend toward voluntary cooperative arrangements among hospitals was evident, with hospitals within many areas cooperating in activities such as joint purchasing arrangements or joint use of central laundry facilities. These kinds of arrangements were much more common than the hierarchical regionalization undertakings that involved assigning patients with differing case complexity to hospitals of appropriate technological levels. Because in these managerial type joint ventures the participating hospitals were equal participants, each doing the same thing within the consortium, there was no designation of base or center hospital(s) and no community or peripheral hospitals. I shall call this kind of local cooperation associative (or horizontal) cooperation in contrast to the hierarchical (or vertical) arrangements.

In addition to hierarchical and associative types of regionalization, which describe the relationships among hospitals, regionalization arrangements may also be classified by what they were supposed to do, a functional classification. This function may entail plans either for cooperative resource allocation throughout the region or plans for a cooperative operation. Figure 15–4 generalizes the types of local areawide hospital associations cross-classified by the functions they perform and the relationships among participating hospitals. (Figure 15–5 presents the typology diagrammatically.)

Voluntary cooperative arrangements using the two different types of relationships among

COORDINATED HOSPITAL SERVICE PLAN

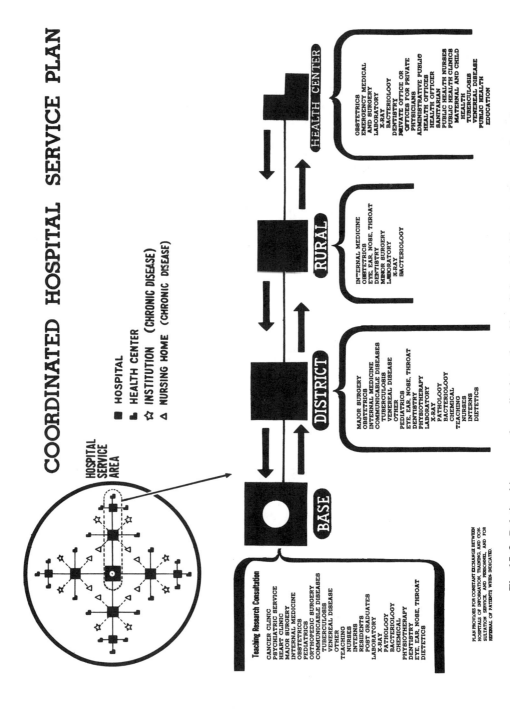

Fig. 15-3. Relationships among base, district, and rural hospitals and health centers in a coordinated service plan.

448

1. <u>Allocative</u> function. Works toward rationalizing the number and
   location of hospitals, beds, and other health care facilities in
   conformance with some sort of optimizing areawide plan for the
   community.

   a. <u>Associative</u> (lateral) relationship.
      Distributes beds and locates facilities according to geographic
      and demographic requirements only. There is an implicit
      assumption in this arrangement that all the hospitals in the
      region are of approximately equal technological sophistication
      and all the hospitals therefore have equal status. This type of
      arrangement is rarely encountered in a region in its pure form.

   b. <u>Hierarchical</u> (vertical) relationship.
      Distributes beds and locates facilities of different levels of
      technical sophistication in such a way as to facilitate
      hierarchical regionalization in operations. This arrangement
      creates base and community hospitals, or equivalently, a center
      and periphery (the Mountin model).

2. <u>Operational</u> function. Works toward rationalizing both management
   and/or patient care operations in conformance with some sort of
   criteria for optimizing managerial and/or patient care efficiency
   or effectiveness.

   a. <u>Associative</u> (lateral) relationship.
      Mainly consists of cooperative business management enterprises
      in which all participating hospitals have equal status. (They
      may be understood as trade associations within the hospital
      industry. They have been very common.)

   b. <u>Hierarchical</u> (vertical) relationship.
      Patient care and teaching duties are divided among cooperating
      hospitals based on their technological sophistication. (These
      have been few. Examples are given in the text).

Fig. 15–4. Description of two-dimensional typology of hospital regional planning. *Note*: These ideas are diagrammatically represented in Figure 15–5.

hospitals, associative and hierarchical, were responding to different impulses. The associative arrangements, being primarily business arrangements, were almost entirely provider and income-efficiency oriented. The hierarchical arrangements, being primarily medical practice arrangements, were largely directed toward providing variable levels of needed care in suitably technological facilities.

A Note on Health Personnel Planning

Before 1963 planning for medical personnel resources, especially physicians, was entirely in the hands of the national and local medical societies. By their control of the number of medical school places, the granting of hospital privileges in local hospitals, and the state licensing and quality monitoring authorities, they effectively controlled the number of physicians and the manner of their practice. The geographic distribution of physicians could be partially controlled in this way but only in a negative or prescriptive sense. A local medical society that thought it had too many physicians or who did not want any more Jewish or Italian physicians could exclude them effectively by denying them local hospital privileges. Black physicians were

Type of Relationship Among Hospitals

	Associative	Hierarchical
Allocative (allocates resources)	**(Cell 1)** Works toward distributing beds and facilities based only on geographic and demographic requirements*	**(Cell 2)** Works toward distributing beds and facilities of different technical sophistication to achieve hierarchical regionalization, i.e., creates "base" and "community hospitals" within regions
Operational (coordinates operations)	**(Cell 3)** Works to form cooperative business management enterprises or distribution of patients using agreed-upon geographic areas as only criteria	**(Cell 4)** Works toward distributing patient care and teaching duties among cooperating hospitals based on their technological sophistication**

(left axis label: Function of the cooperative agreement)

Fig. 15–5. Types of hospital regional planning classified by function and types of relationships. *This arrangement is rarely encountered in its pure form. **The hospital associations named in the text were of this type.

almost totally excluded from mainstream practice by their exclusion from white medical societies. These methods could not be used to produce positive adjustments, however. That is, they could not be used to induce physicians to practice in underserved areas because of the reliance on sanctions instead of rewards. They were proscriptive and not prescriptive methods. (This question of physician distributions by geography and specialty and the programs designed to correct them are discussed in Chapter 13.)

PLANNING ASPECTS OF THE HILL-BURTON PROGRAM

The CCMCs study of the needs for medical care had identified a shortfall in the number of hospitals as the largest immediate need. It was the first one that the Congress turned to with passage of the Hill-Burton Act. The CCMC had shown no appreciation of the importance of estimating need on a local basis and Hill-Burton was the first national health planning legislation to re-

quire use of local areawide planning in mapping the road toward expansion of national health resources based on population need. The language of the original Act indicated that its program was intended to be based on *local* areawide hospital planning and operated by the states.

The original act asserted two main purposes: (1) to provide funds for the states to "inventory their existing hospitals . . . [and] . . . to survey the *need* [emphasis added] for construction of hospitals," and (2) to provide funds for construction of facilities[7] that the surveys showed to be needed. The surveying requirements, as well as the recommended system for assigning priorities to applications for funds within a state for building new hospital beds, was an attempt by Congress to promote statewide coordinated planning for the construction of facilities based on local needs. Since the planning was to be for construction and the arrangement of hospitals was to be regionalized (along the lines of Figure 15–3), the law was calling for hierarchical-allocative planning, using the classification of Figure 15–5. The law called for the establishment of a single agency in each state to supervise the program, and a state advisory council representing state agencies, nongovernment groups, experts, and consumers[8] was prescribed for each state.

The ("single") Hill-Burton agency in each state was charged with dividing the state into hospital service (catchment) areas and establishing one or more regions within its boundaries with each region containing at least two general hospital service areas. Within each hospital service area, the hospitals were expected to cooperate to provide better-coordinated services. That the intent of the law was to regionalize services along the lines of the then-current literature can be seen in the regulations accompanying the Act, which defined hospital service areas as base, intermediate, or rural, depending on whether they contained a teaching or other large (200 beds) hospital, a fairly large (100 beds) community hospital, or neither of these. Thus the wording of the original Act not only called for regionalization of health facilities in the allocative-hierarchical sense (cell 2 in Figure 15–5), but also used the specific Mountin terminology of Figure 15–3. Neither the law nor the regulations addressed enforcing or applying any postconstruction leverage to establish a regionalized *operating* process. The general assumption, implicit throughout the provisions of the Act, was that an appropriate facility allocation resulting from construction grant policies, based on allocative-hierarchical regionalization concepts, would result in the development of an actual *operational* hierarchical regionalization process.[9] The Act contained broad guidelines for criteria to determine the number of beds a state "needed." Some features included in these guidelines were:

1. Upper limits to requirements for general beds were set at 4.5 beds per 1000 population in the more densely populated states, 5.0 per 1000 in states with population densities of only between 6 and 12 persons per square mile, and 5.5 per 1000 in states with less than 6 persons per square mile. These criteria constituted the main guidelines that determined the priority for funding of an application for Hill-Burton construction funds within a state.
2. Separate methods and numbers were to be prescribed for establishing the number of beds required for tubercular, psychiatric, and chronic disease patients. For tubercular patients upper limits on numbers of beds were based on the number of deaths annually from this disease, while for psychiatric and chronic disease patients the upper limit was again based on beds per population ratios. Both these numbers and those in "1" above were close to the CCMC report's recommendations.
3. The "general manner in which the state agency shall determine the priority of projects" was to be prescribed and was to take into account the "relative *need* [emphasis added] of different sections of the population and of different areas" and was to give special consideration to rural and poor areas.[10]
4. Standards of construction and equipment were to be set, and discrimination "on account of race, creed, or color" or *ability to pay* [emphasis added] was forbidden. But "separate but equal" was considered nondiscriminatory and the proscription of discrimination against persons who could not pay did not require all hospitals to admit all patients. Instead, the responsibility for providing "adequate" hospital facilities in each state for persons unable to pay was vaguely assigned to the states. The Surgeon General's regulations could require that states provide "a reasonable volume of hospital service to persons unable to pay therefor, but an exception shall be made if such a requirement is not feasible from a financial standpoint" (Treloar and Chill, 1961).

Many of the criteria in this landmark in the history of health facility planning legislation were based on findings built throughout the period of research and writing on this subject, especially the reports of Lee-Jones (1933), other volumes of the CCMC (Treolar and Chill, 1961) and (CCMC, 1933, pp. 219–221), Mountin and his coworkers (1945) and the Commission on Hospital Care (1946). The incorporation of some of the estimates and approaches of this research and policy literature into federal law implied the use of certain assumptions in hospital planning methodology, the main one being that a national bed-to-population ratio, like 4.5 general beds per 1000 population, could be universally a correct number for all local areas in states with population densities exceeding 12 persons per square mile. This 4.5 per 1000 figure was approximately the one derived in the Lee-Jones report (actually it was 4.62 per 1000) on the basis of an average national occupancy of 80 percent. Although the special difficulties of maintaining high occupancy in sparsely settled areas were recognized by setting higher bed limits for less densely populated states, the fact that many states with high *average* population density contained many sparsely populated areas was ignored. Furthermore, the many other important causes of variations in need for hospitalization among hospital service areas within states as well as across the country that affected the local need for hospital beds were also unaccounted for.

This assumption of the applicability of a nationwide average bed-to-population ratio to almost all individual localities contributed to formulating incorrect objectives for and therefore assigning improper priorities to many small areas (i.e., hospital service districts) within states. Despite many subsequent attempts to modify the formula and free it from the tyranny of averages, the hospital planning objectives estimates derived from federal methodology remained technically flawed throughout the period of the largest expansion of the program, generating federal support for building hospitals in some areas that did not need them and preventing aid from reaching some areas that did. In the course of developing the Hill-Burton program the question of the methodology used to evaluate an area's needs for hospital beds became an increasingly political one and an important aspect of the many amendments to the legislation over the years 1946–1970. The underlying problem was how to more closely attune estimates of bed needs to requirements specific to the local health planning area. Greater local participation in setting these objectives seemed to be a way to accomplish this. It was noted in Chapter 12, for example, that in 1964 special project grants for supporting *local* areawide planning for facilities were voted and that changes in suggested formulas for calculating bed need were legislated. With these grants the Hill-Burton program laid the groundwork for subsequent government efforts to introduce a nationwide system of local,

areawide, community-based, planning agencies instead of having all the needs assessment done at the state level using federal guidelines for their criteria.

Other features of the Hill-Burton program contributed to the development of hospital planning theory and practice for communities and had an impact on actual local and state planning for health facilities. For example:

1. A national areawide planning mechanism for localities, state-administered without systemic local planning input, was established to do allocative planning for health facility construction in every state. The state planning agencies were staffed by persons whose job included becoming knowledgeable about areawide planning technology and health facilities requirements. In a survey conducted for the American Hospital Association in 1965, it was found that 90 percent of the directors and 67 percent of other respondents felt that the "ideal role of a Hill-Burton Agency" was not only to administer the technicalities of the program but also to be a central source of knowledge on construction, operation, and planning for medical care facilities. The report stated that "The Hill-Burton program also has unique value in stimulating long range planning which contributes to both social and economic objectives."

2. The program encouraged licensure of hospitals by the states according to at least minimal standards. "Prior to Hill-Burton, fewer than a dozen States had comprehensive licensing laws. . . . Ten years after the passage of the Act, all States but three had some form of licensure laws" (1965). The existence of state licensure laid the groundwork for the state certification-of-need mechanism used by the later national planning acts.

3. Although there was a substantial increase in facilities, the geographic distribution of the increase often did not achieve its desired ends. This was partly because of the operation of the matching and priority formulas and partly because poor areas needed aid with operating costs, not just construction. Large numbers of persons continued to have little or no access to needed hospital services

even when they had some coverage for the cost.

4. Very little, if any, improvement in areawide coordination of operations was achieved by the program.

5. It is widely suspected that Hill-Burton led to overbuilding, because planning in later years was based on demand, which was suspected by many of exceeding medical need.

6. In later years, withholding of capital funds, the only weapon available to Hill-Burton for enforcing compliance with its planning priorities, exerted little leverage in stopping construction by affluent voluntary hospitals of additional beds judged to be unneeded by the state plan. With Medicare, Medicaid, and many local Blue Cross plans' reimbursement based on cost, it proved easier for well-established voluntary hospitals to borrow the needed construction funds on the capital markets and charge the debt service to reimbursable cost, or to amass it internally via funded depreciation charges that could also be charged to reimbursable cost.[12]

7. In addition to directly setting up a planning mechanism and training persons to run the Hill-Burton agencies, research on planning problems was directly supported from about 1956 on.

After 1970, the Hill-Burton program was clearly no longer needed as a primary source of capital for expanding the capacity of the acute hospital system in general, and when in 1975 it was recodified as Title XVI—"Health Resources Development"—of the Public Health Service Act by the National Health Planning and Resources Development Act of 1974 (P.L. 93–641), its remaining functions consisted of supporting the construction of selectively chosen projects that would target only underserved areas (see pp. 362–364, 462).

THE FEDERAL PROGRAM OF LOCAL COMPREHENSIVE HEALTH PLANNING

The upsurge in hospitalization insurance coverage and the Hill-Burton–assisted expansion of the hospital system that followed World War II was accompanied by an increased concern with rising hospital costs. A growing body of public opinion was expressing the suspicion that substantial portions of the increased hospital utilization was "excessive" or "unnecessary" and was being fueled by increasing third-party coverage and excess acute hospital bed capacity. Some of the features of the areawide configuration of hospital and other services coming under scrutiny were "the need for more effective utilization of services, facilities, and manpower . . . [and the] balance of the types if facilities and services, particularly between inpatient, long-term and ambulatory programs" (Lentz, 1969). Also under scrutiny were low occupancy as a determinant of increased cost (McNerney, 1962) and the assertion that under conditions of good insurance coverage, an increased supply of beds will increase utilization even in areas that by all available evidence had good access to hospitalization before the increase in bed supply (Roemer, 1960; Roemer and Shain, 1959).

By the end of the 1950s these factors and their suspected impact on costs were sparking increased support for "requiring an intensity of planning efforts at the local level" (Lentz, 1969). In response to this development, the American Hospital Association in cooperation with the Public Health Service convened a series of four regional conferences on hospital and related health facility problems in 1959, followed by the appointment of a Joint Committee of the American Hospital Association and the Public Health Service. The Joint Committee issued a report on local areawide planning (HEW, 1961) and a guide to hospital and health related facilities for the information of local areawide planning groups (HEW, 1963) that became a widely used text at a series of jointly sponsored AHA-USPHS regional workshops. This guide (henceforth referred to as the 1963 Areawide Planning Guide) recommended formulating a master plan for each area and suggested that implementation activities consist of educating, persuading, and providing technical help to member institutions to foster conformance to the master plan.

The kind of local areawide hospital planning association considered here is different from the previous examples, such as the Rochester Regional Hospital Council. Those associations, it will be recalled, were ad hoc arrangements among groups of voluntarily cooperating hospitals to participate in an operational-hierarchical scheme (Table 15–4, cell 4) of regionalization to distribute inpatient cases among hospitals according to their medical complexity and to disseminate advanced medical knowledge from teaching centers to community hospitals. What was being promoted by the Joint Committee in 1963 was an association of all or most hospitals in a geographic (i.e., "planning") area to rationalize the system, with the underlying agenda being to reduce the number of existing unneeded beds. Both operational and allocative functions could be within the scope of this concept of local areawide hospital planning association, as could both associative and hierarchical arrangements. These associations were to be concerned with total inpatient services for the entire population of a defined area, whereas the ones previously mentioned were concerned only with the proper triaging of inpatients so that they were admitted to a member hospital whose technological level matched the medical complexity of their diagnoses, and with the education of the medical staffs of these hospitals.

Voluntary Local Areawide Hospital Planning Associations During the Hill-Burton Period

Actually a number of cooperative associations, in addition to those mentioned on page 447, already existed among hospitals in various cities shortly before the formation of the Joint Committee in 1960. Most of these, but not all, were of the associative-operational (Fig. 15–5, cell 3) type with their activities directed primarily at joint management functions. J. Joel May (1967) cites the 1959 findings of a survey conducted by the Pennsylvania Economy League in seven Eastern and Midwestern cities (1959), which found three types of hospital cooperative organizations to exist: the associative-operationally regionalized association engaged mainly in cooperative business arrangements (Fig. 15–5, cell 3), which the survey called a hospital coordinating council; planning councils whose work centered on areawide planning for rationalizing the distribution of hospital beds, that is, concentrating on associative-allocative regional planning (Fig. 15–5, cell 1); and associations that combined the two functions, the integrated co-

ordinating and planning council (Fig. 15–5, cells 1 and 3).[13] In other words, the authors of the survey report considered *operational* regional cooperation to be "coordination" but regarded *allocative* regional cooperation as "planning" (see the opening discussion of this chapter). Only the hospital *planning* associations and the intergrated councils had nonhospital representatives on their boards. But in 1961 the staff of the Joint Committee found that existing planning councils were generally not really representative of the community and that "only twelve or thirteen groups are engaged in long-range planning, among the 26 staffed local organizations" (Committee on Metro Planning, 1960). The Joint Committee agreed with the Pennsylvania Economy League's conceptualization of the three types of hospital councils based on their primary activities.

The Joint Committee found that no progress had been made in forming areawide planning councils that did truly hierarchical planning, either operational or allocative— the older Rochester, Columbus, and Bingham Associates groups thus remaining the meager examples of the hierarchical-operational type. (I could find no example of private councils that did hierarchical-allocative planning for an entire area.) Associative-operational arrangements were very much in evidence, engaging in joint ventures such as wage studies, research and statistical analysis services, the collection of financial and operating statistics, state and local legislative services, public relations services, development of uniform accounting, and Blue Cross and medical staff relations. These are clearly the activities of trade and other business associations, and by 1961 the private hospitals were readily joining in activities that would improve the managerial-business practices in their institutions but not in associations that would look at a community as a whole, deduce requirements from assessed needs, and proceed to adopt binding policies that would align the total configuration of the health services market and resources to meet these needs efficiently. These functions remained in the public domain.

Following these AHA-USPHS educational and promotional activities, the federal government strove to increase the number of local hospital councils with a series of appropriations[14] providing grant incentives for more local area-wide hospital planning agencies to organize and continue operating. "From only a handful of hospital planning agencies in existence in 1961, the pioneering groups in New York City and Columbus, Ohio, [being] the only ones with much experience" (Lentz, 1969), the number was found to have grown to seventy-five by the spring of 1967 (Brown, 1973). Thirteen new councils had been formed in each of years 1962 and 1963 and by 1966 they were established in thirty-three states and were purportedly serving 84 million persons (46 percent of the population), with much higher population coverage in the largest urban centers (Lentz, 1969).

These early planning agencies were found to be following the Lindblom "muddling through" (Lindblom, 1959) model for areawide planning rather than the rational problem solving approach. In his survey of thirty of these seventy-five agencies Douglas R. Brown (1973) described the following characteristics of these organizations:

1. They were largely composed of representatives of major health care providers and "the major business and industrial interests." He saw this as an " 'affiliation between 'donors' and 'providers.' " The ongoing business of an agency was typically the responsibility of a director with varying amounts of staff support, but in practice, the direction of activities was largely determined by the staff.

2. Aside from such global aims (goals) as "conservation of resources and cost control" or "achieving rationality," the planning agencies had no clear-cut objectives in terms of what kind of services and how much might be appropriate for the area's population. The most important objective was to keep "the process" going, that is, to maintain the interest and participation of the key health care providers amd commercial and industrial representative and to proceed incrementally. The increments, moreover, were to be as small as necessary to maintain "the process," and what it was that this process was to proceed toward was not made clear. The planners eschewed master plans and dealt with problems as they arose. In fact, different "projects from the same institution were sometimes considered independently."

3. Given the makeup of the agency boards and the overriding aim to keep the voluntary process going, the types of activities that filled the major portion of the agencies' time could have been predicted. They consisted primarily of getting to be on good terms with the persons judged to be the key figures in the provider and business communities to make them "obligated . . . to return favors [by] lending further support to the planning endeavor. These kinds of exchange transactions which created social bonds among individuals appeared to be an integral part of the area-wide process." Equally important were efforts to involve the "community power structure" in council activities and the almost axiomatically held concept that areawide planning consists largely of forming a judicious amalgam of the individual institutional plans. The areawide planner's role was to encourage each institution to plan internally and to define its catchment area and the problems of its population. The planning council would then assist the institutions to "arrange cooperatively for the services that would meet the total health needs of the population in the area."

4. Given the makeup of the planning agencies and their concepts of areawide health planning, it was not surprising that when it came to actually dealing with proposals and plans submitted to the areawide agency for approval and comment,[15] the agency's work consisted largely of arranging negotiations among interested parties. Quid pro quo trading of pet projects was the main content of these negotiations, and a balancing of trade-offs was virtually the only factor that led to planning decisions. Other considerations, such as social desirability (programming in the interests of community-wide health services development) as indicated by available data, seem to have been quite irrelevant. If an institution seemed unwilling to accept the planning agency's suggestions, the agency either modified the suggestions or dropped them completely to avoid disrupting "the process."

It is clear from the above description of the areawide health planning agencies existing in 1967 that technical input for creating a community master plan was neither used nor widely demanded. Since there were no master plans and since problems were handled as they arose, with rigorous problem formulation and systematic data collection and compilation being minimal, it is safe to assume that each problem was worked on with hastily improvised procedures. Decisions were made on some sort of horse-trading basis, relying heavily on manipulation of interpersonal relationships, with data, if used at all, being cited selectively as a tactic to support the arguments of contenders—an excellent example of the disjointed incremental Lindblom approach to planning.

With the passage of the Comprehensive Health Planning Amendments[16] ("Partnership for Health," P.L. 89–947) in 1966, these area-wide hospital planning agencies were supplanted by a new type of areawide comprehensive health planning agency.

The Regional Medical Programs

By 1965, so much health legislation had been passed by the federal government that local co-ordination of all federal programs affecting the area was becoming a matter of concern (Polk, 1969). Wilbur Cohen, then Under Secretary of Health, Education and Welfare, wrote in 1965: "Never before has there been achieved in one session of Congress the volume and scope of legislation [passed by the 89th Congress, 1965–1966]" (HEW, 1965). Partly in response to the feeling that some measures were needed to help coordinate these new programs at the local level, Congress passed two major pieces of legislation in 1965 and 1966 that were meant to encourage the development of local areawide health planning.[17] These laws subsequently came to be known as the Regional Medical Programs (RMP) Act (P.L. 89–293) and the Comprehensive Health Planning (CHP) Amendments of 1966 and 1967 (P.L. 89–749 and P.L. 90–174).

Only the CHP legislation was primarily concerned with establishing a national, comprehensive health services planning network by promoting the formation and development of local federally funded areawide general health planning bodies. In contrast, the RMP legislation was an outgrowth of the major study (the DeBakey Report) on heart disease, cancer, and stroke commissioned by President Lyndon Johnson (1965). As noted in Chapter 14, almost none of the many detailed recommendations appearing in the ambitious program advocated in this report found their way into the law with the notable exception of a formal declaration of a

disease category approach: it was to focus on conquering heart disease, cancer, and stroke. In barest outline, the RMP legislation provided for grants to applicants who proposed a plan for the establishment of a Regional Medical Program providing for cooperative arrangements that would link major medical centers with other clinical research centers, local community hospitals, and practicing physicians and that would promote research, development, and biomedical technology transfer related to heart disease, cancer, and stroke. The grant applicants themselves were required to define the boundaries of the proposed region, which did not have to be coterminous with states, counties, or other local governments or existing health planning areas.

In a detailed account of the progress of the implementation of this legislation through 1969 Thomas S. Bodenheimer notes that while the law carried the vestigial categorical terminology of the DeBakey report in some of its general statements of goals, its operative text, legislative intent, and administrative history indicates that it was directed at promoting regionalization of voluntary institutions in the sense of cooperative arrangements, mainly of the operational hierarchical kind (cell 4 of Figure 15–5). The RMP program, as administered, did succeed in getting a number of regions defined with boundaries drawn around a nucleus of one or two medical schools (or centers).[18] In practice these regional centers did not proceed, as had been intended, to regionalize their activities in the sense of developing comprehensive and ongoing patterns of flow of patients on a defined basis from outlying areas (periphery) to the center and of research and education from the center to the periphery. Instead, they organized widely differing kinds of fragmentary cooperative activities, depending on the configuration of interests and forces in the medical meritocracy of the region at the time. Bodenheimer called these arrangements "weak" because they were generally limited in scope and/or because the cooperation was often only between selected special units or specialists in two hospitals with the remainder of the region having no access to the arrangements. He notes that the concepts of regionalization used to administer the RMP legislation went through two changes during the course of the first three years of implementation. The lan-

guage of the law implied an intent ''to link autonomous institutions,'' but the interpretation
used in the early period of its operation was that
''any cooperative venture, or even just conversation between institutions is sufficient'' to qualify as RMP activity. Later, any sort of planning
for the region, with or without application to operations, was taken as lying within the scope of
the program.

From the start the RMP program suffered
from the lack of clear-cut definition of its goals,
a lack that was never remedied. Reviewing the
motivation for the RMP act with the advantage
of the hindsight provided by the effect of the
program on health services development, perhaps the strongest single feature that stands out
is the duality of the original DeBakey goals and
the confusion they brought to legislative drafting
and subsequent implementation of the Act.
DeBakey's central idea had been that increased
support for biomedical research on the principal
killer diseases had to be geared up to get quicker
results. This, he argued, could be done by placing greater emphasis on clinical research, development, and technology transfer on the one
hand[19] and by improving the configuration of
health provider interrelationships through a form
of regionalization (hierarchical-operational) on
the other. The duality of research and areawide
health planning goals expressed in the DeBakey
report was not picked up in the Act that followed
it, whether by design or lack of understanding
on the part of the drafters of the legislation. The
RMP program was assigned to the NIH for national administration, and it was perhaps unavoidable that this should have been interpreted
as a message that the program's goals concerned
mainly, perhaps even only, biomedical research.
Its administration closely resembled that of yet
another research grant program, but with a regionalization ''twist'' to it.

Health services researchers and analysts,
however, perceive the main thrust of the act to
be part of the developmental stream of the ''regionalization'' idea in areawide health planning,
as Bodenheimer's article illustrates. What it proposed to establish was a widespread network
similar to the voluntary networks described earlier (see page 447). It is not surprising that the
national RMP administration and many of the
actual or potential grant applicants, most of
whom were research oriented, should have been

unclear as to what they were supposed to do
about ''regionalization.''

Beginning with an intimidating proposal for
a vast separate network of research, diagnosis,
and treatment facilities for ''heart, cancer,
stroke,'' and passed as a vague enablement of
some sort of ''regional'' cooperation among
medical centers and other hospitals, the RMP
program floundered as one attempt after another
was made to define and clarify its aims and purposes. By 1970 it had dwindled away to a residual program giving grants for miscellaneous
purposes and the Health Planning Act of 1974
called for discontinuance of any further RMP
support after June 30, 1976 (see page 462).

The mainstream of the local areawide planning movement was elsewhere. It was concerned
with costs, accessibility, and rationalizing the
delivery system rather than promoting the dissemination of biomedical research results. With
respect to regionalization of services, it was
therefore concerned more with business management (associative-operational) issues than
with matching medical diagnosis to hospital
technology level (hierarchical-operational) issues. In particular, the areawide hospital planning councils and the state health agencies were
only tangentially affected by the RMP. In fact,
one of the main concerns of the existing areawide planning councils and state agencies about
this time, the number of general hospital beds
required for a population, was scarcely ever discussed in the RMP program.

The Comprehensive Health Planning Legislation of 1966 (P.L. 89-749 and P.L. 90-174)

The CHP legislation of 1966 was responding to
two stimuli: (1) the need for cost containment
by reducing excess hospital beds; and (2) the
lessons of the Hill-Burton legislation that hospital planning for local areas had to derive local
needs from local data and be formulated by local
planning agencies.

Description of the Legislation

The Comprehensive Health Planning Act (CHP)
consisted of the Comprehensive Health Planning
and Public Health Service Amendments[20] of
1966 to the Public Health Service Act and the

1967 amendments to this law. It provided for federal grants to states to set up and administer a program of local agencies to do local comprehensive health planning.

Section A required each state to designate a single statewide comprehensive health planning agency (the "A" agency) to receive and administer the federal planning grants; to establish a state health planning council representing a broad spectrum of government and nongovernment interests, with a majority of the members representing consumers of health services; and to submit a statewide comprehensive health plan to the Surgeon General of the USPHS. Section B provided for *project* grants for local "areawide health planning" agencies (the "B" agencies) that could be awarded to "any . . . public or nonprofit private agency or organization." The state comprehensive health planning agency had to approve the formation of all local areawide health planning agencies. Section C provided for project grants "to any public or nonprofit private agency, institution, or other organization to cover all or any part of the cost of projects for training, studies or demonstrations looking toward the development of improved or more effective comprehensive health planning."

The state "A" agency was to encourage the formation of local areawide comprehensive health planning ("B") agencies. Federal grants were made available to local groups to organize these local B agencies that were approved by the state A agency with the proviso that local government health agencies have representatives on the local agency's governing body. The federal grants to operate the state agencies covered the full cost of their operation, but at least 25 percent of the total needed to operate the local agencies had to come from local private or public funds.

The Struggle over "Clout"

All the fifty states and six other jurisdictions soon formed state A agencies and local areawide B agencies. Contrary to the RMP projects, the CHP organizations, especially the state agency, were official government instrumentalities and presumably could be vested with considerable police powers if the state so wished. But although additional responsibilities involving the

making of plans and reviewing programs were constantly added to the duties and responsibilities of the agencies, the enforcement power to implement recommendations flowing from such planning was not increased accordingly and remained generally very weak. This discrepancy persisted as a major policy issue throughout the entire development of the federal local areawide health planning program.

Even before the passage of the CHP legislation, some observers and planners had been claiming all along that effective areawide planning could not be done unless the areawide planning body were given sufficient "clout" to enforce its decisions. Thus John H. Zenger of the American Hospital Council on Planning, Financing and Prepayment expressed the view in 1959 that a "fully integrated hospital system" would only be effectuated if planning agencies had enforcement power. But he thought it could not be done under a democratic governmental system (HEW, 1959). In the same year, Ray E. Brown, then a Superintendent of the University of Chicago Clinics, stated "Hospital planning has not been more effective because it has not had the necessary leverage for enforcement. . . . This can be done through the mechanism of requiring the franchising of hospitals by a state agency. . . ." However, the idea of governmental allocative controls was unacceptable to most hospital managements despite its endorsement by some high-ranking figures in hospital administration circles. To most medical practitioners controls were anathema, for they viewed a hospital's policy formation, especially with respect to the number and type of beds it supported and the policies on types of patients admitted, to be within their domain acting through the hospital's medical board (Cline, 1948). The growth of the voluntary areawide hospital planning agencies between 1961 and 1967, operating strictly in the voluntary, disjointed incrementalist mode that was described by Brown (1973), may be viewed as an attempt to ward off governmental areawide planning of a more compulsory, rational problem-solving genre. After the 1966 planning act was passed, an occasional trade association voice was heard expressing a changed attitude toward granting regulatory enforcement power to planning agencies. For example, in 1967 a statement by the American Hospital Association asserted that "local community interests take precedence over institutional autonomy," and a 1969 statement of the same association dealing with planning recommended that veto power be given to areawide planning agencies over bed expansion and acquisition of new equipment by hospitals (Hospitals, 1969; Medical World News, 1969). But for the most part, individual hospitals and their local trade associations vigorously opposed and successfully fought local planning agency decisions they did not like, and the implementation of the "veto power" was never very strong (Bodenheimer, 1969, p. 1148).

The language of the CHP Act was, in fact, explicit in its attempts to allay fears of intrusive regulation, stating that the aim of the program was "to support the marshalling of all health resources—national, state and local—to assure comprehensive health services of high quality for every person, but without *interference with existing patterns of private professionals of medicine, dentistry, and related health arts.*" [emphasis added] (P.L. 89–749, 1966). Despite the assurance of noncompulsion implied by this language, many hospital planning officials and administrators hastened to publicly reiterate their opposition to giving the newly designated local areawide comprehensive planning agencies any enforcement powers. At the Invitational Conference on Comprehensive Health Planning, convened by the American Hospital Association in 1968, David H. Hitt, then associate director of Baylor University Medical Center, expressed the concern of hospitals that "consumers and other persons external to hospital management would make decisions affecting particular hospitals." He proposed that the application of the new law "specify that [state] Comprehensive Health Planning units will depend upon voluntary [local] areawide agencies for the planning of health care services" (AHA, 1969). Even more emphatic were the comments of Steven Sieverts, then of the Hospital Planning Council of Allegheny Council, who wrote: "I must disagree . . . that the function of the [local] areawide planning agency is to do health planning for its community. . . ." He proceeded to state that "we do have something to learn from modern corporate planning . . . but a master planning role for the areawide agency is no longer the

common theme. . . . Most agencies today . . . focus their principal attention on the *planning process* of each health institution. . . . (Sieverts, 1968).

This type of publicly confrontational opposition from hospital trade leadership sources to the vesting of some sort of regulatory power in the CHP planning agencies diminished with time. Partly this was due to the discovery by the established hospitals that they could control much of the planning process as it stood especially by recourse to the appeals level, and partly it was because they found that the planning process could be used to protect established hospitals against new entrants to the industry. The opposition to strengthening the regulatory role of the A and B agencies continued to be voiced by the public commentators and especially by the academicians and theoreticians. These commentators argued that areawide planning and regulatory powers should not reside in the same agency and the nature of these arguments are discussed below in the section on state government legislation.

Despite these dissenting voices, the regulatory powers of the agencies did grow, albeit very modestly. The source of these powers lay in three legislative developments: the review and comments provisions in some federal legislation passed after the 1965 passage of Medicare; the contents of Section 1122 of the 1972 amendments to the Social Security Act; and especially the proliferation of certificate-of-need (CON) laws in the states.

The review and comment provisions of some federal laws required the local areawide planning agency to review and supply written comments on requests arising within its jurisdiction for grants under specified federal programs (Curran, 1973).

Section 1122 of the 1972 amendments to the Social Security Act provided that specified capital expenditures by hospitals be denied as an admissible item in the calculation of reimbursable costs for specified federal programs[21] if the expenditures had not received approval from the state's "Designated Planning Agency" (DPA). Proposals had to be submitted initially to the local areawide CHP agency in whose jurisdiction the capital expenditure would be made (USDHHS, 1973) and the local agency would generally first review and comment upon them before the DPA acted.

The CON state laws prohibited construction, expansion, or alteration of any health facility or its equipment without state approval. The relationship of these laws to the B agencies is discussed later.

The federal Comprehensive Health Planning Service was designated by the Secretary of HEW to administer the program nationally, and most governors nominated their state CHP agencies as their DPA for administering Section 1122. Where the CHP agency was not chosen as the DPA, the 1972 amendments provided that the DPA must consult it.

The National Health Planning and Resources Development Act of 1974 (P.L. 93–641)

Signed into law on January 4, 1975, this act continued and amended both the CHP legislation of 1966 and the Hill-Burton legislation. The first part, entitled "National Health Planning and Development," was added to the Public Health Service Act as a new Title XV and consisted of the amended continuation of the original Comprehensive Health Planning Act. The second part, entitled "Health Resources Development," added as a new Title XVI, was the amended continuation of what was left of the Hill-Burton program. The planning portion of the Act (Title XV) provided for a major reorganization of the federally supported network of statewide and local areawide planning agencies created in 1966. Many of the shortcomings raised by health planning and other health services policy commentators with respect to the Hill-Burton and 1966 CHS planning procedures were addressed by the 1974 amended version.

Goals and Objectives

The wording of the new Title XV affirmed its adherence to public health, population-based health planning principles and its provisions did in fact follow them. A "findings and purpose" preamble stated the general goals of the act and cited data in empirical justification of them. Furthermore, the Secretary of HEW was directed to provide guidelines for the measurable objectives

(subgoals) "which . . . to the maximum extent practicable, shall be expressed in quantitative terms."

The forthright proclamation of adherence to the population-based planning model using health status data to determine health service needs, as established by the Lee-Jones Report of 1933 but amended to incude *local* areawide planning, was an unusually explicit and detailed enunciation of federal policy, asserting adherence to the principle of public-health-oriented health service planning. It represents an infrequent instance of explicit legislative declaration of what Congress and the president affirmed to be federal health planning policy at the beginning of 1975 when the plan was to go into effect.

Operations and Structure

The National Council A National Council on Health Planning and Development consisting of fifteen members was established, with three non-voting ex officio federal officials and twelve voting members. At least five of the twelve were to be nonproviders and the rest were to be federal government employees, representatives of local planning agencies (HSAs), and members of state coordinating health councils.

State and local health planning agencies At the state level, federal support was provided for a statewide policymaking body, the State Health Coordinating Council (SHCC), and an operating agency, the "State Agency." The SHCC was to advise the State Agency and generally supervise its activities. It was to consist of sixteen or more representatives appointed by the Governor from persons nominated by the local areawide agencies; other appointees of the Governor, not to exceed 40 percent of the total SHCC membership; and a VA ex officio representative in states containing at least two VA facilities.

The State Agency was to be designated for one year by agreement with HEW and had to be the sole statewide health planning agency. It was charged with formulating an annual state plan for approval by the SHCC and conducting the health planning activities of the state, including administration of a statewide certificate-of-need (con) program whose decisions would be based on recommendations from the local areawide planning agencies. Thus a direct link between the federal program of support for local (and state) areawide planning agencies and the State certificate-of-need legislation was formally established. The nature of the operating links between the two types of programs is discussed later in this chapter where the CON legislation is treated at greater length.

The federally supported local areawide planning agency was now called a Health Systems Agency (HSA). The state was to be divided into health services areas, each of which would have its HSA, which could be a nonprofit private agency or a public regional body. If they were public bodies a majority of the governing board had to consist of elected local government officials, or have been authorized to carry out the functions described in the Health Planning Act by a state law passed before passage of the Act. They could also be a single unit of local government (for example, a health department), if the boundaries of its jurisdiction were the same as those of the health services area.

The governing board of an HSA was to consist of from ten to thirty members, with an additional twenty-five members permitted to serve as an executive committee. All members had to be residents of the health service area, and 50 to 60 percent had to be nonproviders. The remainder were to consist of representatives of health professionals, health care institutions, health insurers, health professional schools, and allied health professions. Elected local public officials, as well as local public and private health agencies, had to be represented.

The operating staff of the HSA was to consist of one staff member for every 100,000 population, up to a maximum of twenty-five staff members, and no HSA staff was to have less than five persons. The staff members had to include persons with expertise in administration, data gathering and analysis, health planning and development, and use of resources.

The function of the HSA was to assemble and analyze pertinent data on health status, health care delivery, and environmental conditions affecting health; establish and annually review a health systems plan (HSP) for the area; establish and annually review an annual implementation plan (AIP); review and approve all use of federal funds for development or support of health re-

sources—specifically mentioned were health resources development funds under Title XVI of the PHS Act (the remnants of the Hill-Burton program), the Community Mental Health Act, and alcohol abuse program funds—and to conduct a review and recommend action to the state health planning agency on all proposals for changes in medical facility resources in its health services area.

The state and local agencies were funded somewhat differently. The state agency's operating costs were met by federal grants covering only 75 percent of its outlays, while the local agencies received *formula* grants that required no matching. (It will be recalled (p. 458) that this is the reverse of the federal funding in the predecessor Comprehensive Health Planning Act of 1966–1967. In that law the local agency received 75 percent and the state agency the full amount.) Each HSA was to receive annually 50 cents per person in its planning area, with a maximum of $3,750,000 per annum and a minimum of $175,000. The HSA was permitted to raise a limited amount of additional operating funds under specified conditions that pointedly prohibited contributions from providers or payment for services performed by the agency.

In addition to the grants given by the federal government to the HSAs to cover their own operations, additional funds (Area Health Services Development Funds) were to have been made available to these local health planning agencies for giving short-term grants to local health agencies to do their own planning, but this pass-through provision of the Act was never implemented.

HEW guidelines were to be drawn up to establish procedures under which HSAs were to review proposed local use of federal health funds (PUFF review) and installation of new health services, facilities, or equipment. Existing institutional health services were to be reviewed at least once every five years. All such review activities were to be fully open to public scrutiny and carried out with reference to the area's HSP and AIP; the manner in which the existing health care system was meeting the needs of the population; the special needs of HMOs and certain specialty institutions; and the existence of other less costly or more effective alternatives (in addition to HMOs).

HEW was to assist state and local agencies in developing and applying planning technology with HEW providing technical assistance, both directly and through grants and contracts. A national health planning information center was to be established within HEW, and at least five centers for health planning methodology development throughout the country were to be funded.

Former CHP B agencies (as well as RMP projects) were to receive priority consideration for being designated as HSAs in the process of transition from the planning agency structure under the 1966 CHP legislation to the structure specified under this act, and the states had until June 30, 1976, to sign a State Agency designation agreement with HEW. After that date, federal health funds were to be discontinued for any noncomplying state until such an agreement was signed. No old B agencies and RMP centers would be supported beyond June 30, 1976.

The Act required HEW to have established by January 4, 1976, uniform accounting and reporting systems for: aggregate and unit costs and utilization rates for health service institutions; calculating per diem costs to be charged to third-party payers; and classifying types of institutions by bed complement, geographic location, teaching program involvement, and complexity of services provided. Some of these tasks were accomplished only to a minimal extent and only in some areas; most were never done at all.[22] Thus, a complete and apparently powerful regulating program was blueprinted (i.e., enunciated as policy) that would use the data bases emerging from these accounting and reporting systems to guide the operation of a large network of federally supported local planning agencies toward achieving a coordinated health services system, sensitive to local consumer input, available to all on the basis of need and efficiently run. Its implementation (i.e., de facto policy) fell far short of the blueprint.

Health Resources Development The health resources development portion of the Act provided for some continued federal support for health services facilities construction, modernization, and conversion—largely along the lines emphasized by the later of the Hill-Burton amendments outlined in Chapter 13. Formula grants were provided to the states for distribu-

tion to applicants wishing to modernize medical facilities, construct new outpatient facilities, or convert existing medical facilities to new services. Federal money for constructing new inpatient facilities was to be available only for areas that had experienced recent rapid population growth. This support could be in the form of outright grants, loans, or loan guarantees, including interest-reducing subsidies. The maximum federal share of outright grants was two-thirds of the total grant; for loans or loan guarantees, the portion of the total cost for which a loan could be made or guaranteed was 90 percent. In poverty areas the federal share was 100 percent for both grants and loans. States, local governmental bodies, and nonprofit organizations were eligible for grants under these provisions. In addition to the grants, loans, loan guarantees, and interest subsidies funneled through the state agency, project grants were to be available directly from HEW only to governmental units for the purpose of eliminating fire and other safety hazards and removal of noncompliance barriers to accreditation or licensure.

For a state health planning agency to qualify for dispensing these development funds it had to formulate a State Medical Facilities Plan approved by its SHCC including a survey of state needs. The SMF plan had to be in accordance with the overall state plan and the HSPs of the HSAs within the state. The priorities assigned to the needs of the local areas had to give preference to low-income areas, to densely populated areas (for modernization projects), to poverty areas (for outpatient facility construction), to safety hazard elimination projects, and to comprehensive care entities. The state agency administering the State Medical Facilities Plan had to be the same one that administered the state health planning program.

Comments on the National Health Planning and Resources Development Act of 1974

The wording of the Act clearly indicated a Congressional intent to remedy many of the defects and strengthen many of the weaknesses of the federal, statewide, and local areawide planning mechanisms that were in effect under the provisions of the predecessor 1966 legislation.

Some points that deserve particular attention regarding this legislation follow:

1. The Congressional "findings and purpose" reaffirmed, at least implicitly, the acceptance of universal access to medical care as a right, declaring its attainment to be a "priority of the Federal Government." But in the absence of national universal and comprehensive health insurance it could not in and of itself guarantee "the achievement of equal access to quality health care at a reasonable cost. . . . " The Act proclaimed equal access to quality health care to be a desirable "purpose" or goal but the provisions addressing both access and quality were not accompanied by enforcement provisions adequate to guarantee them as a right. While the state and local health planning agencies, if properly financed, could have been expected to point out unmet needs, there was no provision for them or any other agency to act directly to remedy the discovered deficiencies. On the other hand, if inefficiency in the form of excess capacity were uncovered, state mechanisms of licensing and federal reimbursement existed that could be used to force contraction or at least prevent further expansion of facilities. Thus, from the beginning the Act was tilted toward resource containment to meet only the effective demand under existing insurance (mostly private) coverage, government welfare medicine and direct-service government programs and away from seriously planning for any expansion that might be required to meet the need, especially of underserved areas, despite the pronouncements of the findings and purpose in the Preamble and Guidelines. The tension between the two avowed purposes of the Act, cost containment and improving service to the underserved, under the conditions of the lack of reimbursement coverage for a large number of persons, were to provide the principal background for much of the later confrontations and disagreements over the funding levels and proper functions of the state and especially the local health planning agencies.

Equal access to quality health care, insofar as it might result from federal actions, would still depend in the first instance on whether universal national health insurance were passed, but then also on the success of the health personnel programs being funded by the federal government in producing a proper number and specialty distribution of health personnel and assuring their proper geographic distribution, and the success of the PSROs and PROs in assuring an adequate minimum level of quality and uniformity of health care.

2. The local planning agencies were now to be fully subsidized by the federal funds would no longer have to depend on local health providers (especially the local hospital councils) for any portion of their operating funds as they had under the 1966 legislation. However, the composition of the boards of these agencies came to consist of representatives of local providers to an important extent. The idea that HSAs should be strictly governmental (state and local) agencies had been incorporated in another bill that did not pass. Thus the public interest was expected to be served by nonpublic local planning bodies and a state agency needing full cooperation from the local nongovernmental agencies, in which the boards were often provider-dominated and the staff for the most part was not protected by civil service.

3. The Act did increase the clout of planning agencies in enforcing compliance with areawide plans as noted above, but not substantially. The only federal penalties for providers who did not supply requested information to or abide by the HSA's areawide plan was the denial of requested government funds for construction or modernization, and small reductions in Medicare and Medicaid reimbursement rates. As has been noted, the first sanction was not effective under the later Hill-Burton legislation because these grants were no longer needed by community hospitals to raise capital for expansion or modernization—the cost reimbursement methods used by Medicare and Blue Cross in effect supplied capital as needed. And with respect to the second sanction—that under Section 1122 of the Social Security Act (pp. 459–460) the Medicare reimbursement rate of a noncomplying hospital would be reduced—the increased clout was more a potential than an actually realized consequence of the Act because the size of the federal penalties for noncompliance were so modest as often to be inconsequential. The gaining of more clout by the HSAs in enforcing planning decisions awaited the passage and enforcement of stronger state certificate-of-need legislation

tied to health planning agency recommendations.

4. While the development of expert local and state health planning bodies was hoped for, little in the Act indicated that these bodies were to be guaranteed access to the information needed on a continuing basis to develop objective criteria for planning recommendations. In particular, the submission by hospitals of patient origin information,[23] classified by admitting physician and patient residence, was not mandated. Thus, the call for development of health planning expertise would seem to have offered an opportunity for the rapid development of objective methodology, but because plans were not actually put into operation with the force of law, the basic determinant for the development of useful technique, feedback from operations with iterative corrections of the methodology to reflect the results, was lacking.

STATE GOVERNMENT LEGISLATION AND ITS EFFECT ON HEALTH PLANNING AGENCIES

Paralleling the federal efforts to establish a nationwide network of local health planning agencies coordinated by their respective states, a movement was growing to establish regulatory state bodies that would use the data and analyses of the local planning agencies to control the proliferations of excess hospital beds. I have given examples of the growing advocacy of hospital franchising to control facility proliferation such as Ray E. Brown's 1959 remarks (p. 458). Bodenheimer also cited such advocacy by Mc-Nerney and Riedel (1962) and he himself stated that "A truly comprehensive system of regionalization cannot by completely voluntaristic" (1969). By 1964, the concern with controlling the growth of "excess" beds in the interest of hospital cost containment and the currency of views such as those cited above had become sufficiently widespread for the New York legislature to pass a law prohibiting the construction, expansion, or alteration of any health facility or its equipment without state approval. As noted earlier, this type of law was known as certification-of-need (CON) legislation, and by 1972 it had been adopted in some form by twenty

states and introduced into the legislatures of nineteen others, where it had either been defeated or not yet acted upon (Curran, 1973). In most of the twenty states that had passed such laws by 1972, all types of health facilities were included under the legislation. In three states, only hospitals were covered and in one state, only nursing homes. Also, all the laws required certificate-of-need approval for proposed changes in existing facilities as well as new construction. The procedure for enforcing these laws varied from state to state. In many states, the areawide B agencies and the statewide A agency played central roles in the administration of these laws under the 1966 CHP planning act. Later the HSAs and state agencies played similar but explicitly mandated roles under the 1974 Health Planning Act.

In most of these states, the "regulatory programs . . . [were] being engrafted upon the comprehensive health planning programs" (Curran, 1973). In many, the local areawide CHP agencies, the state CHP agency, and the state health agency[24] were all involved in the process, but details varied from state to state. Where the local CHP B agency was given the responsibility for initial review of applications for certificates of need, its recommendations were usually advisory to either the state CHP A or the health agency that actually granted the certificate. In Arizona and Kentucky, however, the B agency decision was binding on the state agency, while in five states no local review was provided for. In some states, the process started at the top with the application going first to the state agency, and in other states the procedure was reversed, starting with the local CHP B agency. Various provisions were made in the state laws for hearings, presentations or findings, and appeal (Curran, 1973; AHA, 1972).

As was noted earlier, considerable disagreement was registered over the advisability of combining the regulatory and planning functions in the same agency. Apparently many legislatures thought it a good idea, but some commentators (Havighurst, 1973; Cohen, 1973; Krause, 1973), opposed this trend, arguing that such a combination subverts the planning process because of the all-consuming demands on staff resources to analyze and make recommendations on requests for certificated of need. Curran merely posed it as an unanswered question (1973). Havighurst (1973) argued against use of certificate-of-need legislation altogether, largely on the basis of what he asserted were the bad effects of regulating airlines,[25] radio and television outlets, and public utilities. Others advanced other arguments. The main arguments for and against certificate-of-need legislation boiled down to the following:

For

The existing strong provider control of utilization in the health field required it.

There were serious distortions of open-market mechanisms by third-party payers.

An abysmal lack of consumer knowledgeability existed about appropriate medical care.

Open-market mechanisms also failed to operate with respect to the theoretically expected effects of a surplus of supply (of beds) on reducing prices. And although the presence of excess beds did not, in general, act to induce price competition among hospitals, in the relatively infrequent cases where it did, there were often bad effects on medical quality through inappropriate price competition.

Community interests transcend those of providers.

The experience with lack of leverage of withholding capital funds on constraining the growth of excess beds indicated that regulation was needed.

Klarman (1971) expanded on these and other arguments from the "for" side.

Against

Fear of cartelization.

Low technical state of the planning art.

Behavior of regulating agencies as seen in other regulated industries.

There are better ways to control costs such as encouragement of HMOs and inducing price competition.

As noted, Havinghurst (1973) expanded on these from the "against" side. While these controversies were swirling about, the actions being taken by the states led to the state and local areawide CHP agencies playing central roles in the regulatory activities associated with certificate of need by 1975, the year the new planning act

went into effect. The trend had been to give them more power, if for no other reason than the lack of any other body the states could turn to for quick evaluation of expansion proposals submitted by hospitals. If the CHP agencies and their successor HSA agencies were to satisfy the cost containment expectations to any considerable degree they would have had to hone their areawide planning methodology very substantially. It would have to be sharp enough to enable the drafting of plans that accurately represented the demands, needs, and resources of their areas along with a comprehensive set of data-based criteria by which to judge objectively and consistently the appropriateness of proposed changes. And very importantly, the HSA's methodology would have had to stand up well in court upon appeal. Failing the resources to formulate such plans and criteria at the necessary level of technical excellence, the decisions of the CHP and HSA agencies were often too easy to characterize as contrived, and the opposition, mostly by provider interests, to increasing their regulatory leverage was partially based on such technical assertions of faulty technique.[26] There was a curious circularity in this criticism because in large measure the failure to grant the HSAs and/or the state health planning agency the resources and powers needed to expeditiously obtain the necessary data and expertise (both health planning and legal) was perhaps the underlying reason for their falling short of effectively containing unnecessary capital expansion in the first place. In any case it is interesting to note that the state CON programs outlived the repeal of the federal health planning act at the end of 1986. As of March 1989, thirtynine states were still conducting reviews of hospital capital expenditures (Today in Health Planning, April 14, 1989).

SOME LATER DEVELOPMENTS AND REVIEW OF ISSUES IN THE FEDERAL PLANNING PROGRAM

The Reagan administration took office in 1981 determined to dismantle the federal health planning program. The very idea of a federal network of local planning agencies setting goals and objectives for health service resource de-

velopment in conformity with federally proclaimed policy expressed in regulations and
guidelines, and based on an overall aim of better
aligning resources and accessibility with health
service needs through regulation was an almost
perfect formulation of everything that was
anathema to the administration. The ideology of
unquestioning and unqualified support for untrammeled market competition found receptive
ears in many circles of the health service industry, and no countervailing body of public opinion was strong enough to inspire effective Congressional opposition to the proposed planning
program reductions.

There was no loud outcry against the proposed cuts in the health planning program coming from consumers and populist activists as
there was when Community Health Centers and
Migratory Health Centers faced severe fund reductions because there was no similar constituency for community-based health planning. At
first social reform and consumer activists became involved in the formation and governance
of the HSAs being formed in 1975 and 1976.
Many of them seemed to be under the impression, after reading the Act, that these agencies
would make decisions that would be followed
by improving access to local health services.
When it became clear that most of the activity
would revolve around arguments over the best
way to reduce bed complements, and that in any
case the end products were areawide plans that
were largely theoretical, the consumerists and
other interested activist constituencies were
largely lost to the HSAs. Federal funding for the
national comprehensive health planning program was first severely reduced under the Reagan Administration, and finally the program was
dismantled. From a peak of some 212 local
HSAs, the number fell to 100 by 1983 with
funding set at $63 million, about the same as for
1982. The peak appropriation had been $158
million in 1980 and in 1981 it was still $116
million.

However, for a time substantial support developed among some business leaders and portions of the hospital industry for continuing
some form of the planning program. They
seemed to appreciate the potential of the general
cost-cutting orientation that the agencies were
increasingly adopting. This support was also re-

flected in some Congressional quarters with the
question of continuing the program persisting as
a point of contention in Congress. In 1982 the
Senate Labor and Human Resources Committee
asked the Congressional Budget Office (CBO)
to examine the background and effects of the
federal health planning program in connection
with Congressional consideration of reauthor-
izing the program. The resulting study found
that "cost containment has been the focus of
most health planning." The overall conclusion
drawn from examining the reports of pertinent
investigations was that CON review had not
shown an unambiguously measurable effect on
a national basis in reducing hospital costs, utilization, total hospital investment, or the number
of hospital beds. However, the report continued,
the time elapsed since the 1975 initiation of the
newest health planning act had been much too
short for clearly showing such results. Hospital
investment was reported to have been constrained by CON review in some states, one of
which was Massachusetts. The evidence adduc-
ing this, however, was called "weak" by the
CBO study. Overall, the confounding efffects of
the many variables other than the measures
taken by the planning program itself, that are
presumed to have contributed to the observed
end results—such as saturation of the market,
changes in reimbursement procedures, and the
use of other regulatory devices—leaves us without clear-cut evidence of the extent to which the
reduction in the rate of hospital expansion was
attributable to the effect of CON tied to planning
as a controlling device for containing excess
capital expansion.

The CBO report provided a trenchant and perceptive review and analysis of the progress made
by the federal planning program and the problems it faced. Many of the issues the report presented had featured for many years in the debates about the role of government in health
planning. In particular, ever since the formal inception of the government local areawide comprehensive health planning program in 1966 and
its major expansion in 1975, a number of unre-
solved policy questions had persistently surfaced. These issues were debated over and over
again with vigor or even acrimony, particularly
during appropriation or reauthorization deliber-
ations.

The first of these issues, the one underlying the others, was a lack of public consensus on a clear-cut *mission definition* for the planning agencies. Widespread agreement was never achieved even on the basic question of whether it is desirable to have comprehensive health planning under government auspices at all, and among those who did favor some form of planning, there was even less consensus about what mode of planning should be followed. The issue had been framed in the form of questioning whether it is desirable for "them" (government) to tell "us" what to do, scarcely a new question to public health professionals. Although it has been recognized since the earliest days of public health that individual behavior must be legally circumscribed in some manner for the collective benefit, many people subscribe to this proposition only in general. They are quick to complain about the intrusive character of public health regulation if it stops them personally from doing something they like or find profitable. A particularly revealing indication of the perception of public health as societal control appears in its early history in Germany, where sanitation inspection and enforcement personnel were called "sanitary police" (Rosen, 1958).

The contemporary version of this question is whether enforcement powers (clout) in health matters, even if one grants their applicability to issues affecting the environment, are appropriately extended to substantial authority over the therapeutic health service system, i.e., "medical care." And if it is appropriate to so extend it, should these powers be restricted to measures of rudimentary quality assurance like licensing and facility inspection or do they include arranging for access to medical care for all who need it but cannot obtain it? Is access to medical care a right to be enforced by government? If it is an obligation of government to ensure universal access to medical care, does that imply that government must take action to guarantee that the care is of good quality and efficiently delivered?

The expressed intent of the law framing the federal health planning program answered these questions in 1974 with a resounding "yes."

The text of the 1974 act setting up the largest of the federal health planning programs explicitly expressed the intent of assuring access to health care for populations that needed it and of

regulating much of our health system to operate with greater cost efficiency: access *and* efficiency, *a two-branched goal.* If successfully implemented it should have established two strongly loyal constituencies actively supporting the health planning program: those persons urgently desiring improved access for underserved populations and those urgently wanting cost containment and efficiency, That these were indeed the two main aims of the framers and Congressional supporters of the health planning program is attested to both by the preamble to the 1974 act itself and by the 1982 policy analysis of the CBO, which stated:

> The health planning program is intended to improve the distribution of health services to ensure that they are available to those who need them *and* to restrict investment in unnecessary facilities and services. Problems of medically underserved areas *and* investments in duplicate facilities that are rarely used were factors motivating Federal participation in planning activities [emphasis added].

However, ambivalent messages were sent to local health planning agencies. While the legislation under which the agencies operated asserted the dual goals of planning for improved access *and* for efficiency, the federal administration and Congress were stressing only one of them—efficiency. Eliminating excess and duplicative health service resources, expenditures and utilization was virtually the sole preoccupation of federal health planning de facto policy. As the local organizational structure called for by the 1974 act lumbered into place by 1976, this emphasis became ever more overriding, dictated by the federal focus on cost containment. It became virtually the sole federal criterion for judging the effectiveness of the program, diverting attention from resource development in underserved areas.

The boards of local HSAs, however, were in many instances composed of local persons who took the need-based access development charge of the planning act seriously; they wanted their HSA plans to target improved access to health care by underserved populations.

An important facet of this confusion is that cost containment has been a much more important goal for the Federal government than for most state and local agencies. Many state CON laws are intended to improve the distribution of health services rather than limit investment and total costs. HSAs often emphasize planning goals—developing preventive and primary services, for example—rather than the regulatory function of advising CON review decisions. On the average, less than 20 percent of HSA budgets were used for project review, including CON review. Over half the budgets are allocated to plan development and implementation, data management, and public education (CBO, 1982).

The funding would have been inadequate to do the need-based resource planning job properly even if the HSAs and state planning agencies could have used their entire appropriations for that single function alone. But the one-sided federal emphasis on pressing the agencies to show results in constraining resource expansion, a pressure that reached its peak during the Carter Administration, further contributed to the HSAs' failure to develop a strong positive program for comprehensive, needs-based planning. Despite the CBO's finding about less than 20 percent of HSA budgets being used for project review on average, it proved impossible for them, with their limited funding, to pay sufficient attention to the *positive* task of indentifying the need for more resources and services in underserved areas while being forced to devote so much staff time to the *negative* task of indicating where reductions should be made or requests for expansion denied. In some communities, especially those that were poorly served medically, the planning program came to have an overwhelmingly negative public image. The outcome was that the local health agencies were driven to attempt both tasks, the regulatory task of controlling capital expansion and the planning task of making good, comprehensive, population-based plans, with insufficient funding to do even one of these well. The constituencies of both these aims were thus dissatisfied with the program's performance, each for its own reasons.

The second major issue raised in the report was the *lack of authority to enforce planning decisions*. If the one-sided emphasis by the Administration and Congress on cost containment had been accompanied by granting the local agencies (or the state agency acting on their behalf) adequate powers and resources to enforce

decisions that would contain excess resource growth, it is conceivable that at least this half of the HSA mission might have been accomplished. But this was not the case. Although the federal administration attempted to turn the planning act into a single-purpose regulatory mechanism for containing hospital resource expansion, the limited powers and resources given to local health planning agencies for performing this function ensured that their efforts would fail to implement this goal, especially when many of the agencies' staffs were obliged to concentrate so heavily on area plan development to satisfy their local boards. Since the reimbursement systems of both private insurance (especially the Blues) and Medicare-Medicaid were based essentially on paying providers their costs or charges, capital costs were for the most part amply reimbursed. Along with tax exemptions granted to individuals and employers for private health insurance premiums and for interest income from hospital bond issues, this ensured an ample flow of capital to many private health services institutions. With so much capital available, and the competitive pressures on hospitals for plant and equipment expansion and improvement so persistent, the HSAs and the state health planning agencies were not strong enough to withstand the unrelenting litigation and political pressure used by the powerful hospital industry to obtain approval for spending it.[27]

The plans of the local and state planning agencies to bring about changes in the health system, then, were implemented very spottily. The lack of effective enforcement authority became a major source of frustration for the HSAs as they wondered what could be done to implement the plans, not only to reduce excess capacity but also to improve access in underserved areas. The CBO analysis described it well:

The limited authority of state and local planning agencies under the Federal planning program is a serious obstacle to implementation of their health plans. HSAs and state planning agencies have no direct authority to enforce their health plans, but must rely on encouraging voluntary actions by health-care providers, state and local health agencies, and other community organizations. CON review is the only regulatory tool available, and it is a negative authority. Although planning agencies could sometimes influence the content of local grant requests because they were required, until recently, to review proposed use of Federal funds for grant applications, they were not the decision makers. Similarly, HSAs were required to review the appropriateness of existing facilities, but had no authority to act on their findings unless a facility proposed to expand or replace its facilities or services. Planning agencies usually lack the authority to close unneeded facilities, and cannot require the development of needed ones. (The 1974 Planning Act authorized funding for area health resources development, which was meant to be seed money used by HSAs to start projects and attract further financial support. No funds were ever appropriated for this purpose.) They cannot take direct action to improve access to care for those who cannot afford it (1982).

As in the case of the issue of "mission ambiguity," the problem of "lack of authority" prevented the planning agencies from developing a strong and united constituency among the forces that were pushing primarily for improved cost containment. And the supporters of public planning did not widely disseminate the facts about the amount of public money that lay behind private operations when questions about the propriety of enforcing public planning decisions on the private sector were raised. These facts were not well known in the early 1970s and certainly even less before then. It seems now that it was not then generally recognized just how extensive and pervasive the funding and subsidization of the health care system by the public purse was.

The third major issue raised in the report concerned questions dealing with the structure and composition of *local sponsorship* of the HSA and the composition of its governing board.

The rationale underlying the [health planning] program structure was that health resources allocated by representatives of a cross-section of the community would provide better health services at less cost than those allocated only by providers. In seeking to provide the best care for their patients, physicians and other medical professionals do not necessarily consider the total costs or the distribution of services. Planning agencies were expected to consider these factors, which are not always relevant to decisions made independently by providers. For example, planning may encourage development in rural or other needy areas (1982).

The 1974 planning law and its regulations provided that the formation of an HSA be initiated by nonprofit groups in a local health plan-

ning area who form an association and apply to HEW for designation as the area's official HSA. In practice, virtually all of these applicants were private community groups because the Act made it very difficult for the local government to be designated as the HSA. (Of the peak number of 212 HSAs, only about four were sponsored by local government.) In all cases the HSA board was required to be composed of at least 51 percent health care consumers and was supposed to represent, in some fair manner, the composition of the population over which the HSA had jurisdiction. How to ensure this eluded many HSAs, however. There were frequent complaints from local people about disproportionate representation of provider groups despite the 51 percent consumer proviso.[28] The lack of local incentives for cost control and the potential for providers to dominate the planning process were considered to be the two main problems of locally based planning in the CBO analysis. It considered the "local structuring" of health planning to have been inappropriate for cost-containment actions, asserting that local consumers are often interested only in obtaining more resources and more services, especially when these are paid for by third parties, and that the concern with cost containment is more likely to appear at more global levels, such as the state or nation. But the analysis did not comment on whether the local, consumer-based structure of the HSAs was good or bad for developing need-based plans for resources in underserved areas. Presumably that was good, but again, since cost containment became so overriding an imperative, the main expected advantage of community participation, better targeting of resource development on underserved areas, was never given a fair trial, nor was it balanced in the CBO analysis against the asserted tendency to push for excess resources.

Of the four options suggested to Congress in the CBO report for changing the health planning program, one was abolishing the program (identified as the "Administration Proposal"). The other three alternatives all called for *abandoning the goal of improving access* and concentrating only on the cost-containment goal—frankly and with determination. It would seem, therefore, that support for continuing the health planning program in Congress as of mid-1982 was primarily confined to use of the program only as a cost-containment measure and abandoning the resource development goal even as an aspiration.[29]

This view of the health planning program's future proved agreeable to some business groups and to some conservative political leaders who had previously opposed government planning vigorously and now came to support the realigned program. The leading business group was the Washington Business Group on Health, a membership group of the nation's largest employers, and among the changing conservative supporters were Senator Dan Quayle, Representative Edward Madigan, and David Stockman, Director of the Office of Management (Western Center for Planning, 1983).

With the sharp reduction in federal support for local HSAs in 1981 also came a change in the structuring of the funding. Under the legislation passed after 1981 the HSAs were to be permitted to continue only if they could raise their own operating funds in the community. This opened the doors for employer and provider groups to fund the HSAs and consequently have a dominant voice in the planning. Many of the HSAs that briefly survived the demise of the federally funded program were now substantially funded by such groups and rapidly became the paid professional planning and research staffs of the employer coalitions that supported them. They were, therefore, entirely focussed on cost reduction and soon lost their character as government agencies altogether. A few other HSAs continued to operate with state funding, among these being HSAs in the states of New York, Florida, and Ohio.

SUMMARY COMMENTS AND A LOOK AT SOME POSSIBLE FUTURES FOR A FEDERALLY SPONSORED, STATE COORDINATED AND LOCALLY ORIENTED HEALTH PLANNING PROGRAM

The nation at the end of 1983 stood at a fork in the road with respect to the national health planning program. One path led to continuing it by strengthening its public health orientation, increasing its emphasis on improving the avail-

ability of needed health services or resources and in the course of that process also identifying excess services or resources that make the system inefficient. That Congress would take this direction in that year was realistically inconceivable. The other road led toward using the program only to contain costs by reducing capital expansion and downplaying the public health emphasis or perhaps discontinuing it altogether. The second road was taken. By 1986 funding for the planning act had been ended and as of January 1, 1987 it was repealed.

Many strong advocates of public health (defined in the broad sense) did not view this decision point as of great import. The federal emphasis in the planning program on achieving broadside capital reductions and the neglect of equitable health services development had convinced them that the planning program was not relevant to their concerns for better protection of the health of all the public. Yet it is reasonable to argue that local areawide health planning is a fundamental public health function and that somewhere in the federal government structure there needs to be an office or program devoted to building a nationwide *structure* that will develop local health planning agencies charged with tying together the personal and environmental health activities in each locality. This would seem to duplicate much of the federal system of public health agencies described in Part I of this book, but the federal public health agency system has dealt seriously only with some aspects of the environmental issues and a few categorical personal health problems. It remains quite outside the main channels of the general personal health services system. Many local health departments are too subject to idiosyncratic and other undue interference from powerful local forces that are able to forestall local applications of good national health policies and have led to chaotic jurisdictional assignments.[30] They need the support of a powerful national program. How to bring about a system of local health planning (and development) agencies that will display a proper mix of sensitivity to local needs and desires and also appropriate dedication and authority to effectuate national objectives is the problem.

If in the future there were to be a return to an emphasis on needs-based planning, one would hope that many of the unsolved problems from the past efforts would be faced with the added wisdom of accumulated experience. The CBO report of 1982 identified these as ambiguity of mission definition, lack of authority to enforce planning decisions, and local sponsorship.

These problems might have been soluble had there been a comprehensive-service, universal-access national health insurance system in place. This is especially true for the second issue—the lack of authority to enforce decisions. Our old friend, the problem of clout, would have been vastly reduced because compliance with planning decisions could have been directly and effectively tied to reimbursement for services and capital outlays to nearly all providers. It would seem that for a national system of local health planning agencies to work, universal medical care coverage is a prerequisite. However, certain types of problems faced in the previous programs would continue to need much work, including the proper balance between local, state and federal authority and function; the composition of local boards; and the relationship between preventive and curative services. But it would then be possible for health planners and planning boards to work on these problems in a more meaningful way because estimates for services would be constrained by overall national budgets and not by inequitable rules of access that distribute health services according to the financial condition of people rather than the condition of their health.

NOTES

1. Management literature currently uses the term "strategic planning" to define non-short-term planning for the "firm."

2. Corporate planning that is overly centralized is opposed by some libertarians and others who subscribe to antitrust legislative controls. In addition to the unanswerable question of how central does planning have to be before it becomes "in restraint of trade," the plain fact is that antitrust control has proven to be a chimera in practice.

3. This process is represented by boxes "C" and "D" (Fig. 15–2) without the reference to small-area planning. See Cartwell and Last, 1980, for discussion of the epidemiological terms.

4. It will be recalled that the GMENAC report

(Chapter 13, p. 406) used a similar method, dubbed a "delphi technique" in the usage of later years, to estimate 1990 needs for physicians.

5. See Chapter 9 and Ellwood, 1985, for a discussion of the majority and minority recommendation of the report.

6. This class of public hospital is discussed in Chapter 7 where the findings of the American Hospital Association's Commission on Public Hospitals appear.

7. The resource expansion aspects of the program are treated in Chapter 12. As its title implies, this chapter deals with the planning features of the legislation. Some of the material in this chapter unavoidably overlaps with some of Chapter 12.

8. This term did not have the same meaning in this 1946 law as it was to have in the Comprehensive Health Planning Act of 1966. The 1946 meaning was closer to the designation *public* member or representative, meaning a person, preferably knowledgable or concerned about the subject matter of the advisory council, selected at large and not formally representing an identified interest group, than to the later populist or activist meaning of the term consumer. The exact wording was "representatives of the consumers of hospital services selected from among persons familiar with the need for such services."
This assumption was especially expressed in the Mountin regionalization plan.

9. While there has been some evidence that there may be a substantial degree of match between a patient's diagnosis and the type of hospital he or she is hospitalized in Elaimey, 1969, I know of no studies that investigated whether the operation of the Hill-Burton construction grant program increased this type of patient "regionalization" in actual practice.

10. However, the "special consideration to rural and poor areas" factor was rarely effective in obtaining Hill-Burton grants for such areas because of the provisions of the law that required local agencies or other sponsors applying for funds to provide one-third of the construction costs from their own resources after state and federal governments each had provided their required thirds. Poor areas could not raise their required one-third of the construction costs and were consequently generally unable to field an acceptable application for a Hill-Burton grant (see Chapter 12).

11. This is a good example of the effects of health services research results on national health policy. See Chapter 14 for a discussion of this point.

12. The availability of capital through cost reimbursement also fueled a proliferation of new for-profit hospitals beginning in the mid-1960s.

13. As noted below, no hierarchical arrangements were found.

14. These were categorical public health grants earmarked for the formation of local health planning agencies. See Chapter 12.

15. Brown did not make clear what approval by these areawide planning councils implied. The review

and comment provisions of some federal legislation passed after 1965 is discussed later (see pp. 459, 461).

16. These amendments were to the Public Health Service Act of 1944.

17. Not just planning *for* local areawide communities, but also to some degree *by* local communities.

18. About one-fourth of the regions were poorly defined because of the existence of too many medical schools or the absence of any medical schools at all in the area.

19. The Congressional OTA study on technology transfer (1982) (see Chapter 14) noted that Congress understood the purpose of the RMP law mainly in this one way.

20. The law changed Section 314 of the Public Health Service Act to have five sections. We are concerned here only with the first three (A, B, and C), dealing with local comprehensive health planning. The remaining two sections dealt with the revision of the system of federal grants to state and local health departments described in pages 97–98. As noted there, the placing of the planning legislation and the public health grant structure revision into the same law was not entirely coincidental. It was thought in some quarters that the new planning structure might help coordinate the large number of federal categorical health grants that were being given. But as noted below, the work of the local planning agencies was diverted early and permanently from any major concern with coordinating governmental public health programs.

21. These included Medicare, Medicaid, and maternal and child care programs funded under Title V of the Social Security Act. Capital expenditures that required planning agency approval were those over a given amount, originally $100,000, or those that would have resulted in changes in bed capacity or that would substantially have changed the services provided by the institution; modernization was included in these types of expenditures.

22. Some of these technical goals were partially achieved many years later with the databases collected by HCFA with respect to Medicare and Medicaid utilization and costs and the setting of new forms of provider reimbursement based on this data. There was also the Medical Care Expenditure Survey and the work on the number of uninsured done in 1977 and subsequently. These were, however, federally executed without the involvement of local health planning except in the preventive and health promotion areas. (See Chapter 10.)

23. A listing of the home address of every patient admitted by each hospital in the area. See Shonick, 1986, for more details. In later years, a number of states passed laws requiring the routine submission of such lists to the state health planning agency.

24. That is, the SHA of Chapter 3, which in many states was called the State Health Department. This agency should not be confused with the Designated Planning Agency or the "State Agency," which were what the statewide operating health planning agencies were called under the health planning acts of 1966 and 1974 respectively.

25. Havighurst had been active in achieving the deregulation of the airlines.

26. While it is true that many of the HSAs' decisions to reject expansion proposals by hospitals were overturned more often than need be because of some shortfall in technical expertise, it is also true that the states were heavily out-gunned by the legal resources the hospitals were able to field against them in the courts.

27. Trying to limit capital expenditures in the face of the flow of capital provided the hospitals by federal reimbursement and tax policies was akin to attempting to stanch the flow of water from a high-pressure hose without shutting the wide-open spigot. It was only later that the idea of turning off the spigot first by changing reimbursement and tax laws gained currency, but by that time the federal planning program was all but dead.

28. The definition of a consumer with respect to health services has long been elusive. The intent, as in this case, is always to differentiate professional and interested business representatives from truly lay persons, but this often proves to be very difficult. Is a drug store clerk a provider? Is his or her spouse? A corporate executive's wife who volunteers in a hospital?

29. Some contrary views on desirable future directions stressing planning that would identify population needs were heard but these came from state or local levels. One example is the contents of the 1983 report to the Governor and State Legislature made by the California Health Planning Law Revision Committee. It called for defining the essence of local areawide planning as health service needs assessment and needed resource development. It recommended that some of the cost-containment functions that had been given to HSAs in California be taken over by the state health planning agency that would administer the CON program and foresaw other cost-control functions being addressed by impending changes in federal law dealing with reimbursement methods and tax exemption provisions.

30. For example, the existing situation has led to dual and overlapping networks of local public health departments responsible to their local governments and local branches of specialized environmental agencies responsible to state and federal specialized agencies. This is noted in the chapters on public health.

V

Reflections and Comments

16

Recapitulation and Reflections

WHAT HAS IT ALL MEANT?

Do the events and policy formulations delineated in the preceding chapters support some generalizations about United States health policy—what it has been over the almost fifty-year period 1935–1980, what forces shaped it, and where it is going? I believe they do, and this chapter will present them.

It should be borne in mind that while this book deals mainly with the development of *public* policy about health services, the content of this policy has not been limited to the public sector of health services. Rather the *total* system for protecting the public health has been shaped by this evolving policy. The components of governmental policy on health services that were described in the preceding chapters have involved both public and private agencies as well as both personal and nonpersonal services. Overall protection of the health of the public is what I take to be the modern meaning of the term "public health." Environmental controls, particularly with the restricted scope encompassed in the older, classical definition of "public health," constitute an important subset, but only a subset, of the totality of modern public health concerns.

Large- and Small-Focus Investigation

Research on public policy formation and implementation in the health services field—health policy analysis, for short—has been increasingly concerned in the last thirty years or so with the details of particular mechanisms by which one aspect or another of our health system operates as viewed through the lens of a given cognate[1] disciplinary paradigm. Many of these studies have been well done and have provided instructive insights into numerous facets of our health services system. However, this trend has perforce involved an increased narrowing of focus as researchers dedicated to the use of the paradigms currently dominant in their respective medical, behavioral, and social science cognate disciplines immersed themselves ever more deeply in aspects of the health services system seen from their special points of view. In many instances their research has focused on the high-priority ("cutting edge") methodological problems of their discipline itself (e.g., econometrics, sociometrics, biometrics, survey research, meta-analysis) rather than the substantive priorities of health services research.[2] The technical and small-focus monographs provide the indispensable underlying material for wider, integrative analyses, but they frequently do not by themselves provide a broad enough view of our health services system for general understanding and debate.[3] This has contributed to the growth of an attitude among decision makers and other interested citizens that much existing health services research is little more than the application of information processing through administrative-statistical computer-driven techniques, useful for limited in depth analysis of specific measures by professional policy analysts but offering no guidance on longer-term trends along broader fronts.

There have, of course, been integrative analyses but not enough of them. This book is meant to be such an analysis. Throughout the earlier chapters I have used a transdisciplinary synthesis of health services literature to address a large, basic question: What has been the role of government in forming the existing U.S. health services system? Because many of the developments in health services policy were also taking place in other subfields of social welfare—education, housing, cash assistance, unemployment insurance, retirement, and discrimination—I have suggested that developments in these other subfields and in health services may have been responding to some of the same underlying historical influences and have therefore had recourse to the literature in these areas and their histories. Furthermore, developments similar to those occurring in the United States during 1935–1980 had already taken place in other industrially developed countries and were still being modified, albeit always with important individual differences. It seemed reasonable to view a phenomenon that arched across different social welfare subfields and comparable types of countries as a systemic response to similar underlying developments in the politico-economic system common to all these countries rather than as happenstance or as essentially peculiar to the United States.

The most basic phenomenon underlying the development of the U.S. health system between 1930 and 1980 has been the U.S. version of the development of the *capitalist welfare state* in industrialized countries with an accelerated spurt after 1945. The advent of the welfare state meant a changing conception of the role of the state in a democratic capitalist society.

The Belief Framework of the Social Welfare State and the Actual Role of Government in United States Health Services

The role of government in a developed capitalist state has been the subject of an enduring and often heated argument among politicians, political writers, intellectuals, and other public[4] commentators. The argument has not only been about what this role should be, but also about what it actually has been and what the outcomes were.

Viewpoints on the appropriate role of government in a democracy have ranged from wanting it absolutely minimal to wanting it as extensive as practicable. The minimal-government view has customarily, but not always, been associated with a position labeled "right-wing," asserting or implying that the condition of private business determines the country's economic and social soundness and government's role should therefore be essentially limited to policies that

facilitate profitable business operation. In this view, social welfare will largely be taken care of by the full employment that will result and by private philanthropy, which will be more munificent if industry operates at full capacity and taxes are less onerous. The maximal-government view has customarily, but again not always, been associated with the position labeled "left-wing" because it asserts that only government can act for all the people. In this view, private industry, if left entirely to itself, must by the very definition of its "bottom line" orientation, follow the road of single-minded self-interest.

In between the polar minimum and maximum positions are a large variety of compromise views, which during the period 1930–1980 came increasingly to cluster around a centrist view that wants to retain the advantages it sees as accruing from the competitive and entrepreneurial elements of Capitalism but also wishes to restrain overly vigorous competition and untrammeled entrepreneurship, which it sees as resulting in two adverse outcomes: it produces unacceptable numbers of human casualties as well as an unacceptable number of business casualties. The latter leads to a concentration of business in ever fewer hands and thereby damps the very competition that is at the heart of the economic benefits provided by a truly competitive capitalist society. To avoid damaging the very kernel of the avowed aim of capitalism, the maintenance of a free and competitive economy, competitive practices must be monitored and controlled to keep the system from destroying itself. This centrist view is the core of the ideology of the capitalist welfare state. It seeks to preserve and enhance the capitalist system by controlling conditions that undermine it and to do so within the framework of democratic capitalist structures. It is indeed one of the ironies of history that the corrective measures the advocates of the welfare state propose should so often have been attacked as "socialistic." Some of these proposals have come from clearly identified conservative governments, and no indigenous overthrow of a capitalist system has ever occurred under a well-functioning social welfare state.

Looking at these components of the philosophy of the social welfare state, it is not surprising to find that its adherents' positions on specific social welfare proposals are usually based more on pragmatic judgments about the need for them—within the context of the currently most pressing social problems and their political manifestations—than on ideological generalizations about what they imply for changing the role of government. The centrists' belief framework rests on two footings: society must be structured to provide an equitable and humane distribution of goods and services, and this must be done by democratic means, including a market structure that allows reasonable opportunity for all to enter it. Their view of whether government should run the health services system, for example, will vary over time depending on how well the existing health services system appears to be meeting its mission and their resulting preference may not apply to all types of services. This centrist position, with its pragmatic flexibility about the mix of private and public involvement in administering social welfare (and otherwise regulating the economy), was the prevailing philosophy of the developed capitalist countries during 1945–1980 and provided the underpinning for the political support of the modern social welfare state. This position was less well developed in the United States, however, than in European capitalist states for reasons discussed below.

The central notions of social welfare capitalism that were the prevailing views in U.S. national policy formulations from 1933 through 1980 (they were the dominant views through 1968), never included the idea that all persons were entitled to economic equality. They did hold that in the competition to succeed, everyone was entitled to a fair race from an even start[5] regardless of ethnicity, race, income, origins, gender, or region of upbringing. To have an even start and a fair race for success persons should not be handicapped by poor health; hence the growing support for universal access to all needed health care. Those who fell by the wayside, the casualties of the system, were entitled to dignified succor and support even if they could not return to the race. Those who had run the complete race through to the finish line but were now too old to run any longer were entitled to an honored and comfortable old age, even if their lifetime earnings were not enough to provide for it. An indispensable part of an at least tolerable old age, with its advancing indispositions, was access to good medical care.

While the view of modern capitalism as a social welfare state was gaining currency in the United States during these fifty years, the overwhelming majority of the population always clung strongly, much more strongly than in capitalist Europe, to the idea that private for-profit industry operating in an openly competitive market is unquestionably the best mechanism yet devised for the efficient production of commodities and services. Socialist ideas never gained any substantial currency in the United States even in their heyday during the 1930s. This contrasts sharply with the European experience, where socialist parties had large memberships, especially in Italy and France, and sizable contingents in parliament. But in the United States government did not come to be widely regarded as the best mechanism for protecting people's security and preserving their quality of life.

Despite this history, the concept of the social welfare state has often been characterized in the United States by its opponents on the right as a ''left'' view,[6] a characterization that muddies the waters. Support for the capitalist social welfare state in the United States has been and is a centrist view because it defends the basic tenets of capitalist organization of society, whereas a ''left'' view does not. The centrist view does want government to control the content, pace, and extent of industrial development, but only when these threaten to create unacceptable levels of health and other types of social casualties; it does not advocate that government operate the economic system. This distinction has often been overlooked or confounded in the arguments over proposed changes in the system of medical care. Government operation of health facilities or even paying for medical care in the private sector has often been loosely referred to as ''socialized medicine,'' a term used more as a slogan than a description and quickly transformed to ''socialism'' by opponents of this aspect of the capitalist social welfare state. In the United States the centrist view advocating the social welfare state has more generally come to be labeled as ''liberal,'' and that of its right-wing opponents as ''conservative.'' Both these terms have grown to be rather fuzzy as descriptors of the ideas they represent, but with respect to the social welfare state, a "liberal"[7] is now generally assumed to be a person who supports the social welfare state form of capitalism while a "conservative" is assumed to be one who opposes it. In what follows I shall use these terms in this sense unless further specification is required. With the advent of the Nixon/Ford administrations the underlying tenets of the welfare state began to be eroded; they were totally and actively rejected by the Reagan administration. The latter used "liberal" as a pejorative epithet describing "failed" social welfare programs on which enormous sums had been spent for which the public had been heavily taxed. Not only did the programs fail, but the economy had been thereby ruined. As the 1980s progressed, the right frequently attempted and often succeeded in establishing the perception that leftists and liberals were synonymous despite the heated disagreements, often including vilification, that took place between them.

The De Facto Government Policy for Building a National Health Services System in the United States

With the possible exception of old age pensions, in no area was the implementation of the ideas of United States social welfare capitalism better exemplified than in the health services. Reviewing the phases of governmental (mostly federal) action that fostered the development and guided the design of a national health services system presented in earlier chapters of this book, we see that the health services policy of the federal government during 1935–1980 was to establish a complete system, including a plan to provide universal access to resources needed to protect the public's health.[8] The enunciated policy included a system of high caliber medical care, but the implementation of the enunciated policy (i.e., the de facto policy) fell short of this goal. While some components of the resultant system were excellent, others had serious deficiencies.

Throughout the evolution of public health services in the United States, the goal of federal health policy was to protect the health of the people, with due concentration on reducing the health casualties of a burgeoning industrialization by controlling its detrimental effects on

health as well as by helping meet the personal health service needs of its economic casualties. The early concentration on sanitary ordinances and cleaning_up of nuisances, on quarantine, food and milk inspection, and clean water supplies was in large part prompted by the threats to health and the casualties actually produced by a too loosely fettered enterprise system sending its ships to foreign shores, dumping its wastes into the rivers and streams, cutting corners in guaranteeing the safety of food and the safety and healthfulness of living quarters and work places. As American industry and business grew in sophistication and size, the role of occupationally associated illness, as well as air, water, and solid waste pollution in threatening health and producing health casualties, greatly extended the tasks of public health. At every point, much governmental health policy was inspired by the ideal of the social welfare state that it is a public responsibility to care for the casualties caused by excesses of the competitive system and to reduce their number by maintaining reasonable controls over tendencies toward unbridled entrepreneurism.

When medical science advanced to the point at which medical care came to be generally regarded as efficacious and desirable, again the ideal of the social welfare state impelled the view that access to *medical care* should be considered a public good based on a natural right. In the United States, government actions began to implement this ideal nationally after 1935.

This social welfare philosophy motivated the passage of legislation and the development of many programs, most of which were highly successful in terms of carrying out their missions within the constraints of the resources allotted them. The particulars of these legislative acts and the programs they established form much of the substance of the fourteen Chapters 2 through 15 and are briefly reviewed on pages 481 and 482. They constitute examples of governmental policy formulation (either enunciated or de jure policy) and policy implementation (de facto policy).

By 1980 the United States health services system had in place extensive government-supported preventive services, environmental services, and medical care programs. This structure was similar to that of the European[9] social welfare states, but there was a glaring difference. There was no national health insurance system providing for *universal* access to comprehensive personal health services. The motor needed to drive the entire system lacked horsepower. This weakness was the most important feature that differentiated the government's role in the U.S. medical care system from those of its European industrialized counterparts, reflecting the different development of the U.S. health system from the European ones.

Most European systems had begun with arrangements for health insurance covering physicians' ambulatory services while the practice of medicine was still in a relatively primitive technological stage. These arrangements were made, for the most part, by guilds and later by trade unions and other types of consumer and cooperative groups, such as benevolent societies that dealt with individual physicians or organized groups of physicians. Hospitals were largely owned at first by religious orders and later either by government or by religious or lay philanthropic organizations. They, too, were well established as societal institutions before the advent of modern medical technology. As medical science and technology developed and various European countries instituted national systems of health care, they added resource development to their existing programs to meet the requirements of modern medical practice. This accelerated the trend toward hospitals being increasingly owned by government and lay philanthropic entities, with government predominating. European hospitals generally employed their own physicians and were for the most part free to the patient or later were included in national health insurance benefits. The salaried hospital physicians were mostly specialists and a breed apart from the practicing community physicians who were mostly general practitioners with no hospital admission privileges for their patients.

It was quite different in the United States, where a national politically powerful medical profession developed before there was any widespread government involvement in medical care. This entrepreneurially oriented organization of the medical profession, which had by 1920 emerged as a strong political power, was built on local guild-type organizations of pri-

vately practicing individual physicians banded together in a national organization, selling their services on a fee-for-service basis and fiercely opposing anything that smacked of working for nonphysicians for contracted prices or having to negotiate with organized groups of nonphysicians for terms of payment. This professional organization had emerged the winner from the long and fierce battle among competing schools of medicine as *the* unquestioned medical profession, and the only group whose members were legally permitted to hold themselves out as physicians. They were adamant about having the full say about what constituted a properly trained physician and how medicine was to be organized and practiced. They controlled the policies of hospitals to which they admitted their patients; there was no separate category of "hospital doctors," as in Europe, employed by the hospitals to assume the management of the office doctors' patients when they were hospitalized. Yet despite their control of hospital policy and their collection of fees from their paying patients in the hospital, they took no official responsibility, except as individuals, for the financial condition of the hospital itself. The responsibility for financing the hospital was borne by a self-selected and self-perpetuating board of lay or religious philanthropic leaders. Physicians had no tradition of group negotiation with consumers for fee schedules, and what experience they did have with salaried or contracted service ("contract medicine") they rightly considered to have provided a very poor milieu for good medical practice or for properly paying the physicians.

Above all, the medical profession brooked no challenge to the total hegemony of physicians from any "outside" quarter. Organized medicine at first opposed all health insurance that was not physician-society-sponsored, and later, after having accepted other private insurance, it narrowed its opposition to government health insurance for physicians' services. When government-sponsored health insurance was finally legislated in 1965, albeit only for the elderly, in the face of swelling political support, organized medicine still insisted and was able to have inserted in the law a "no interference" proviso guaranteeing that the government would simply pay for what the physician ordered and raise no questions relating to the medical content of the treatment it was being asked to pay for. The medical profession vehemently opposed universal national health insurance every step of the way. In the course of this successful opposition the profession relied heavily on the assertion that national health insurance was a socialist measure. This diverted the public's attention from the basic problem of lack of access for a substantial segment of the American people, which the existing reimbursement system had been unable to solve despite patching with many gap-filling measures. Promising attempts to pass general government health insurance were defeated in 1920, in 1935, and all through the mainly liberal Democratic years during 1935–1980.

Until 1960, organized medicine also strongly opposed the organization of medical practice into prepaid group practices. In many states it was instrumental in making this form of practice organization illegal by getting laws passed forbidding the "corporate practice of medicine." The government-led development of the social welfare structure in medical care thus consisted of generous resource development, based on expert estimates of need, on the supply side, but was restricted to disjointed gap-filling measures, which left many persons not covered, on the demand side.

The "mainstream" physician payment structure developed along lines that were purported to be more compatible with basic American ideas about how services should be bought and sold—in the open and free market. But the market of reality was hardly the market of standard economic theory. The actual market for medical care was largely without the self-adjusting factors that were still discernible in varying degree in many other commodity markets. In some markets both supply and demand still showed substantial sensitivity to price changes with considerable price competition among suppliers. But in the mainstream fee-for-service medical care market, price competition was severely constrained by the medical societies, as was entry into the medical profession. For example, price advertising was prohibited as professionally unethical while state governments helped reinforce the professional monopoly exerted by the medical societies over who could practice medicine and how they could practice it. Until 1968,

even the total number of physicians was controlled by the medical societies' influence over the admissions policies of medical schools. This background contributed significantly to causing social welfare ideas about medical care to be less firmly established in the United States than in other, older capitalist societies and accounted for much of the differences in their national systems.

The unique history of the development of U.S. medical services helps explain the unique outcome—the building of a national medical resources development program and a government support system for providing medical services to some special populations before the creation of a national health insurance system rather than the other way around. The outcome is also and perhaps even more strongly explained by the late development of the entire social welfare system in the United States compared with the European systems. To a great extent this was so because the European systems were older and their economic depressions had become more severe earlier than they did in the United States. The U.S. system also had the safety valve of the western frontier until about 1890. The young and most energetic among the unemployed and low-wage earners (provided they were white) were not so severely confined to their depressed areas as were most European workers.

The major social welfare measures were introduced in Europe during periods when the capitalist governments faced serious electoral and even revolutionary challenges from the left—the true left, not the misnamed centrist liberals. In the 1880s the conservative chancellor of Prussia, facing a strong socialist party in the elections, engineered passage of a series of social welfare laws, including health insurance. In 1911 a rudimentary national health service was legislated in Great Britain as the government faced a labor movement demand for reforms. These movements, led by strong labor and socialist organizations, especially in Britain and in Germany, were responses to increased unemployment and poverty resulting from economic downswings. The government answer was to develop the capitalist social welfare state, with national health insurance as one of its social welfare measures.

In the United States there were similar depressions around the end of the century following the particularly severe depression of 1873. They produced an upsurge of left-wing advocacy exemplified by the Socialist Party of Eugene V. Debs, who in 1912 polled one million votes for the presidency. The response in the United States was also to increase government social welfare activities. Some consumer protection laws were passed, the eight-hour workday was decreed for federal workers, and about thirty states passed Workmen's Compensation Laws. In 1916, the income tax amendment to the Constitution gave promise of requiring corporations and affluent persons to pay a share of their income to help support social welfare. But all these measures were weaker and less comprehensive than their European counterparts. The early (1915–1920) movement for state-sponsored health insurance failed as the upturn in the economy following the outbreak of World War I in 1914 arrested all further development until the Great Depression forcefully reopened the issue in 1932. The full flowering of the capitalist welfare state began shortly after World War II when fully universal and comprehensive national health insurance (or service) systems were introduced in many European capitalist countries and became the established goal of the federal administration under President Truman on the heels of twelve years of national leadership on social welfare thinking and action under Franklin D. Roosevelt (who himself never supported a universal bill).

The ideas of the social welfare state were by then widely held in and out of government, more extensively in government circles than out. Having first gained currency during the years 1932–38 in reaction to the ravages of the Great Depression, these ideas continued as dominant federal policy through 1968 even though the United States experienced unparalleled prosperity after 1945.

By 1945 government involvement in the older, more limited concept of public health was widely perceived as having been substantially accomplished. The newer challenges of an extended view of public health lay mostly in the future, but one aspect of this extended view had already surfaced as a problem—guaranteeing access to medical care to all who needed it. For the years 1945–1970 this became perhaps the central issue of public policy on health services in this country. It remained a pivotal issue after

1970 but was joined by a rising interest in the health threats posed by the new types and alarming scale of environmental despoliation.

The United States emerged from World War II economically powerful and ideologically more unified than it would be in later years. Strong national leaders enunciated a health services policy that called for a compulsory, universal, comprehensive national health insurance system. Although such a system had been a topic of national interest since 1932, there had never been such strong support for it in high places. In particular, never before had a President of the United States been one of its strong backers. Truman's support was formalized in a series of Congressional bills for national health insurance drafted over a number of years, and several included a complete program of health service resource development. The resource development was to prepare the system to accommodate the expected increase in demand if, as expected, the *enunciated* policy of President Truman and others in favor of national health insurance were to become law (i.e. de jure public policy) and de facto public policy upon its implementation. None of the bills passed. The reasons that the enunciated public policy failed to become the de jure, let alone de facto, public policy have already been discussed at length in this book.

Although the universal national health insurance bills failed to pass in Congress after Congress, the federal government nevertheless proceeded to enact and implement laws from 1945 until 1980 aimed at putting into place many of the supply-increasing components that would be required to meet the demand if a bill for universal insurance did pass. There was expansion of

Facility supply, initiated by the passage of the Hill-Burton Act in 1945, which signaled the federal government's commitment to fostering health facility construction. During the next thirty years many hospitals, public health centers, and other health facilities were built or remodeled until bed supply so far exceeded existing demand that a halt had to be called (Chapter 12).

Physician and other personnel supply, brought about by the health "manpower acts" (Chapter 13)

Biomedical research support (Chapter 14) to increase the effectiveness of medical care, and health services research support to increase the efficiency of operating medical care services.

Mental health support (Chapter 6) to include care for psychological problems.

Support for health planning (Chapter 15) to establish and develop a potential for rational local areawide planning.

By contrast, the demand-increasing measures were relatively modest and narrowly focused on gaps in access for specially defined populations whose needs had come to national attention. These programs consisted mainly of Medicare and Medicaid but also included federally financed neighborhood health centers, the National Health Service Corps, and other measures designed to meet the needs of special classes of persons not adequately protected by the private health insurance systems.

In the 1970s a federal commitment was also made to expand support for protection against the newer and more massive environmental threats to health. Stronger support was enacted for consumer product (especially food and drug) protection and for workplace protection. There was also an increased recognition of the importance of promoting healthful personal behavior in protecting people's health.

Again, what has been missing in this comprehensive federal effort is a *universal access* component, the driving motor of the entire system proposed as public policy in 1945. The record shows that when the postwar supply-increasing measures were passed one by one while at the same time the national health insurance bills of 1945–52 were being ignored one by one, the linchpin of the entire system proposed by enunciated public policy was pulled. Private insurance and the gap-filling measures taken together were not enough to make full use of the additional hospital facilities and medical personnel that were made available, and the utilization patterns of the personal health service system became very unbalanced. The perfectly reasonable assumption on which the estimates guiding the supply-increasing measures had been based did not come to pass. No universal national health insurance had been passed to raise the demand

to the need levels used in these estimates and much of the increased supply of beds and physicians wound up as surpluses in well-insured areas while the uninsured continued to suffer an effective "shortage" of medical care. Thus, the effects of a de facto public policy that boldly supplied public support for supply and technology expansion but left the financing of consumption mainly to private health insurance had by 1980 resulted in a medical care system that was operating at a low level of effectiveness in underserved areas and at a low level of efficiency in overserved ones—without being both effective *and* efficient almost anywhere.

The Reining In of the Social Welfare State: Retrenchment in Governmental Sponsorship of Health Services—Some Notes on the Reagan Years

By the 1970s the American economy had begun a downward trend. It did not perform well with respect to any of three economic goals held by "every administration," as important indicators of the state of the economy—price stability, high employment, and economic growth (Sawhill and Stone, 1984). The move toward social welfare measures as the answer to increasing economic insecurity was being replaced by a widespread concern for the rising costs of social programs, especially medical care (Stone, 1981, chapter four). It was reflected politically in an erosion of social welfare state ideas under the Nixon, Ford, and Carter administrations, and culminated in their outright rejection by the Reagan administration. The Reagan administration revived the pure "right"-wing version of the proper role of the state under Capitalism, taking it as its enunciated policy. All progress in reducing the number and alleviating the condition of the casualties of industrialization and business reorganization would come from revitalized industries spurred on by the lure of large after-tax profits. This would minimize unemployment and enhance the ability of private philanthropy to care for the small unavoidable residual of "worthy" casualties, in tandem with a minimal "safety net" of government aid largely administered by the states. All social welfare programs, by contrast, demean their beneficiaries, destroying their self-reliance and perpetuating their dependence on government subsistence, thereby destroying the self-respect of the recipients and hurting the economy at the same time.

The turnabout in enunciated policy on social welfare generally was reflected specifically in government de facto health services policy. A main point in the Reagan administration policy formulation[10] was that social welfare costs were too high and were adversely affecting the ability of American industry to compete with foreign products because of the high taxes and direct employer expenditures required to finance them. Medical care costs, both private and public, were singled out as particularly excessive, and it was therefore necessary to lower them by reducing both the unit price of services and the volume of utilization. This was to be done not by reliance on the regulation typical of the social welfare state, but by promoting the competitive market in the functioning of the health care system.

For the first two years of the Reagan administration much was heard of competition that was to be induced through federal legislation on fiscal and health insurance matters. Conservative economists and private policy analysis institutes were formulating the details of a grand strategy to convert the health care system into a strongly market-driven sector of the economy. Consumers were to be made price conscious by increasing insurance cost sharing and by making their health benefit premiums taxable. During the first administration, proposals were advanced to promote competitiveness among health providers, and some of their features were incorporated into national health insurance bills that were introduced in Congress, but they never advanced to hearings or a vote. Interest in this type of proposal waned in Reagan's second administration, and efforts to promote price competition in the health services system were mostly supplanted by changing the reimbursement procedures of Medicare and Medicaid and facilitating the adoption of self-insurance by private industry.

Paralleling the changes in federal and state reimbursement methods, private insurance payers were also instituting changes in organization and payment methods. The large corporations that had not seemed much concerned over paying sharply accelerating premiums for health benefits for their employees during the years of the booming economy after World War II were becoming determined to lower these costs beginning with about 1970. They were putting increasing pressure on insurers, both the Blues and commercials, to lower the cost of medical care premiums or at least to substantially moderate the rate of increase.

There was also an increase in the use of self-insurance by corporations, with many of them contracting with hospitals and physicians to obtain discounted prices. Employees were given incentives or compelled to use these discounting providers. In a number of cities, the local representatives of national corporations banded together to form cost containment coalitions that were expected to be more effective in bargaining as a group (collectively!) with individual providers or groups of physicians and hospitals for discounted fees.

The effects of the phenomena triggered by the growth of self-insurance began to make themselves felt mainly during and after 1983. Price competition among hospitals eroded the financial cushions provided by higher charges to paying patients that many private hospitals had used to pay for the care of uncovered persons, causing an increased burden to fall on municipal hospitals that they were ill-equipped to handle. Employers were substantially increasing the cost sharing and premium sharing of their employee health benefits.

The 1981–82 recession and the weak recovery following it increased unemployment, and many persons lost their private health insurance benefits. Local public hospitals were reeling from the effects of the "tax revolt" against local taxation, and community health centers were suffering from the declining support given by the federal government. Medicaid benefits were steadily being reduced. The number of persons not protected by any third-party coverage continued to grow, and the benefits of those covered by government programs were reduced. A number of studies showed that the health status among persons with no third-party coverage was measurably lower than that of the rest of the population.

While the Reagan administration's main effort in the health field was directed at reducing medical care costs, largely because many of these costs were paid by the Federal government, its agenda also called for reductions in environmental protection and occupational safety and health programs. Proceeding from the same ideological rationale used to justify medical care cost reductions, the argument was that environmental protection and occupational safety and health programs were excessively restrictive, handicapping industry in its need to be price competitive with foreign companies. In a succession of appointments, heads of the environmental and occupational safety and health agencies were chosen who were openly opposed to the agencies' missions and whose close relationships with leaders of the industries that needed most to be regulated were widely known. Support for such programs as toxic waste control and clean air control was sharply reduced, and public pronouncements vigorously attacked environmentalists' warnings as exaggerated alarms unsupported by fact. Until the very end of his administration, President Reagan refused to fully acknowledge the extent of the threat from acid rain, for example, or the disadvantages and even dangers of felling stands of ancient trees.

Some commentators even thought that a major objective of the Reagan administration might have been not only to undo the social welfare state that had been crafted in the fifty years after 1930, but to render it very difficult, and perhaps impossible, for subsequent governments to reinstate it.[11]

WHAT MIGHT THE FUTURE LOOK LIKE?

Has the progression toward completing and maintaining the social welfare state been permanently halted, or at least halted for a long period? What may the answer to this question mean for the future of the health services system in the United States? The historian Arthur Schlesinger, Jr., in his contribution to a discussion of the future of American politics just before the 1984 elections, saw the Reagan administration as merely an expected phase of an oscillation he detected in U.S. history between periods of "public action" and periods of "private interest." However some commentators observed that part of the Reagan strategy was to ensure that the sharp reductions made after 1980

in social welfare programs did not turn out to be just another periodic and transitory "private action" phase that some subsequent administration, elected as the result of a cyclical return of a "public action" phase, will reverse. As Walter Dean Burnham, professor of politics at MIT, put it in the same discussion: "The basic domestic purpose of Reagan's second term would be to reorganize the federal government in order to make sure that nothing like the Great Society programs can ever happen again" (Burnham in New York Review of Books 1984). The main obstacle erected against future attempts to implement a "public action" phase at levels equal to or exceeding prior government involvement was the increase in the national debt. It was raised astronomically during Reagan's eight years in office, by more than the cumulative total under all previous presidents from George Washington through Jimmy Carter. It will indeed be exceedingly difficult for future governments to find enough money to pay even the interest on this debt, let alone amortizing it, and also substantially restore the level of social welfare activity. The national debt is a long step toward making "sure that nothing like the Great Society programs can ever happen again."

Because of this, a prediction of a return to high levels of social welfare activities cannot be based solely on a straightforward extrapolation of the observed past cyclical behavior of government policy between "public action" and "private interest" phases. The program erosion has been deep enough and the mortgaging of future federal revenues serious enough to make tenable the assertion that they have destroyed any underlying cyclical pattern that may have existed. If a forecast that government activity to assure better health services is bound to return to pre-Reagan or even higher levels is to be at all believable, it has to be justified with arguments additional to, or even entirely other than, reliance on any "natural" swings of the political pendulum. The main defense of such a hypothesis must rest on the argument that government-sponsored social welfare measures, and health care measures in particular, are essential to the viability of our society.

The current health problems that are worsening and are bound to compel federal action include the increasingly deleterious effects of a rapidly accelerating concentration of business control and its greater mobility in avoiding local and even state controls; the proliferation and sharply increasing toxicity of polluting technology; the explosive growth and urbanization of populations, especially of the poor; the accelerated development of automated work processes and unsafe worksites; and the enduring persistence of a population that has little access to needed health care, especially during times of high unemployment and other features of recession. The observed exacerbation of these problems in recent years strongly suggests that they will not be controlled without vigorous government regulation and support and that they cannot be ignored without serious threat to our entire social structure.

The minimal-governmentalist reply to this continues to be that the above scenario is unlikely. The arguments of the social welfare state protagonists are invalid on three major counts: first, the so-called empirical observations on which they are based are not objective; they largely reflect the exaggerated fears of weak and nervous alarmists and if listened to will kill the goose that lays the golden eggs—vigorous economic growth. Second, those criticisms that have some merit—there are indeed persons who cannot afford decent health care (or food and housing)—can best be met by a vigorous private economy that will provide more jobs and therefore more goods and services to more persons. Private philanthropy will also be strengthened by the economy and will readily be able to take care of most of the persons who cannot benefit directly from the competitive world. And third, for the small number of persons who remain out of the reach of the opportunities provided by the private entrepreneurial world or private philanthropy, government can and should provide a small, a very small, safety net. All this can happen only if entrepreneurial activity is not interfered with.

Empirical support for the view that underlying social pressures will compel federal action to improve health services is provided by experiences under the Reagan administration itself. Witness the passing of a long-term care law as an amendment to Medicare (even though it was repealed shortly thereafter), the mounting of a drive to improve child health and child care conditions, and the increasing seriousness with which the Administration began to address the AIDS issue after initially dragging its feet. Witness also the increasing support for some form of government health insurance by employers and the movement by some states to pass compulsory health insurance of some sort during the tenure of President Reagan.

These and other developments, especially the fact that every developed country, including our strongest economic competitors, has a universal health care system, support an informed guess that the government role in developing health services cannot be gainsaid and that events will compel a restoration of the badly damaged system of government health protection.

If this hypothesis holds up, the central corollary question relates to the organizational structure of the restored medical services: Will we use our past experience to avoid repeating past mistakes? The most serious of these mistakes has been to initiate programs of increasing resource supply without first ensuring a universal demand of determined magnitude. With respect to public health, we recall that a committee of the Institute of Medicine noted in its 1988 report *The Future of Public Health,* that the existence of a population with no coverage for medical care has been a major barrier to the effective organization of public health agencies in their battle against the manifold threats to the health of the public. Early passage of universal coverage would lift the albatross of worrying about almost 40 million people having no coverage from the necks of national health policy makers and public health administrators who will then be freed to concentrate on building the nation's health defenses.

Strengthening environmental, occupational, and consumer protection would include increasing support for and more clearly defining the role of the cooperative network of local health departments, state health agencies, and the United States Public Health Service, including unflagging monitoring and control of epidemic disease. An important part of this task would be defining the relationship between the official multipurpose health agencies (i.e., local health departments, state health departments, and the U.S. Public Health Service) and specialized environmental, occupational, mental health, and similar agencies.

If improving the health-related behavior of individuals (health promotion) is to benefit from the passage of a national universal access bill, aspects of the program will have to be integrated more closely with general medical practice. In today's pattern of practice there is little incentive for medical practitioners to concentrate on health promotion, but with a universal system of health insurance the payment and quality assurance mechanisms could be used to enhance the health promotion (behavior-changing) programs.

And with respect to medical care we recall that the past and present fragmentation of access to care among special populations was largely the result of the lack of a national system of universal access. We can avoid many of the previous mistakes if the universal access system is among the earliest of the new health measures enacted, thereby providing early entitlement to to medical care for mothers and children, veterans, poor and elderly people, American Indians, and all other populations now served by special programs as well as those with no present access at all. It will then become possible to effectively plan for the amount, type, and location of needed health resources and much of the call for efficiency in delivery will be at last possible of achievement while serving all persons according to need. The existing categorical programs will no longer be needed in all their present byzantine complexity—difficult and expensive to administer and still leaving many needy persons without service.

Universal access to care will not only make it possible to greatly improve the effectiveness and efficiency of the delivery of medical care services and the maintainance of an appropriate resource supply. It will also clarify the priorities for research support and the mission of local areawide planning; guide the content and operations of an adequate national health information system; and promote the required personal prevention services.

Developments during the Reagan (and Bush) years may have greatly increased the potential for widening the support for national health in-surance. Increasing segments of various sectors of society—consumers, industry, many hospitals and physicians, and Congress—are beginning to have their fill of the complexity, turmoil, and confusion that have resulted from the development of complicated reimbursement schemes, the administration of segmented gap-filling programs, and the continually growing nuisance and distraction to business of being administratively involved in all this instead of "paying attention to business." Many persons who are less than very affluent have difficulty in being adequately insured for medical care, and anxiety about not receiving needed care or becoming impoverished in paying for it is increasingly widespread.

How a needed health program would be financed under the circumstances of the huge deficit passed down from the Reagan-Bush years is an enormously intricate question, both ethically and technically. It is beyond the scope of this book or the expertise of its author. One can only say that it must be done—the problem can only get worse and consequently more difficult to solve. Furthermore, it does seem reasonable to assume that what is still the wealthiest country in the world, can, objectively speaking, install a health services system at least as good as the best of those presently in place in other developed countries even with a dark cloud of enormous debt hanging over its head. What is required is the political will, for even after considering the huge questions of ethics and techniques, the underlying task is the political one of achieving a strong enough consensus.

A major obstacle to forming this political will has been a mindset among many voters based on misconceptions about the evils of the social welfare state. A main objective of this book has been to trace and explain the actual nature of the transition of the nation's public policy on health during the years 1932–1980 from an almost single-track emphasis on laissez faire to one that encompasses the capitalist social welfare state and emphasizes strengthening the weak points of the unfettered entrepreneurial society, with its tendency toward runaway competition, while often forgetting the side effects of turning up the power of its productive engines too high and too fast for human or ecological tolerances.

NOTES

1. A discipline "cognate" to the field of health services policy analysis is a discipline whose subject matter and methodology are frequently used in health services research, e.g., economics, sociology, statistics, political science, etc.

2. This is often a necessity for the researcher, who wants to and indeed may need to be in good standing with his or her peers in one of the established cognate disciplines. See Kuhn (1970).

3. Another way of saying this is that social research is done in *fields* of study that very often use the results of *several disciplinary* studies as their underlying data. Examples of scholarly fields are transportation, housing, urban studies, education, social welfare, health services, and police protection.

4. As well as many not-so-public ones declaiming in bars and classrooms, at dinner tables, and in other accommodating venues. It should be noted that this discussion does not deal with the question of controlling freedom of expression.

5. See Thurow (1980) for an elaboration of this abbreviated formulation of the "even start" notion.

6. It has also often been characterized by portions of the left as a "right" view, as nothing more than a use of social reform to strengthen capitalism at its weakest points and thereby increase its viability (which, of course, was precisely its avowed aim). But discussion of this charge is outside the scope of matters I wish to address in this book.

7. The meaning should not be confused with the eighteenth- and nineteenth-century meaning of the word, especially in Great Britain. In the United States the present day "libertarians" most nearly approximate the views of the nineteenth century British liberals.

8. See, for example, the description of the 1938 National Health Program on page 271 (which, however, did not include the programs for expanding health personnel, research, and health planning discussed in Chapters 13, 14, and 15.)

9. I include here those industrialized capitalist states which, although geographically non-European, have modeled their social welfare system on the European model. Examples are Canada, Australia, New Zealand, and to a lesser degree, Japan.

10. It is difficult to say precisely what the component points of the Reagan program were because they never appeared in complete form in a single or even a few documents. The Reagan program must be deduced from general statements made in addresses by the President and by his advisers and top administrators in congressional testimony, speeches, and documents. Most of the health policy positions were enunciated by David Stockman, the Director of the Office of Management and Budget. Some Congressmen, such as Jack Kemp, introduced legislation that was said by the Republican leadership to embody "the White House" position, but it is difficult to determine just who in the White House was advocating it. However, the general ideology of the Reagan position came to be clearly established through the actions and speeches of the main administrators in the government—taxes must be reduced, especially on industry, federal spending for social programs must be reduced drastically and their administration turned over to the states, regulation of the private sector must be sharply diminished and competition among companies (including health services companies) increased, and the private market in health care must be expanded.

11. See, for example, reference to Professor Burnham's remarks on page 484.

References

Aaron, H. J. *Politics and the Professors: The Great Society in Perspective.* Washington, DC: The Brookings Institution, 1978.

Abdellah, F. G. Overview of Nursing Research 1955–1968, Part II. *Nursing Research,* 3–4/1970, 19: 2, 151–162.

Accreditation Study (b). *Study of Accreditation of Selected Health Educational Programs (SASHEP), Staff Working Papers.* Washington, DC: The Commonwealth Fund, Feb. 1972.

Advisory Commission on Intergovernmental Relations. *Intergovernmental Problems in Medicaid.* Washington, DC: Advisory Commission on Intergovernmental Relations, Sept. 1968.

Agency for Health Care Policy and Research. *Carotid Endartectomy* (revised), Health and Technology Reports, 1990, No. 5R. Washington: DC: Department of Health and Human Services, July 1991.

Alford, R. *Health Care Politics: Ideological and Interest Group Barriers to Reform.* Chicago: The University of Chicago Press, 1975.

Alinsky, S. D. *Reveille for Radicals.* Chicago: University of Chicago Press, 1945.

Allen, J. R., M.D., and Curran, J. W., M.D. Prevention of AIDS and HIV Infection: Needs and Priorities for Epidemiologic Research. American Journal of Public Health, April 1988, 78:4, 381–386.

Allied Health Subommittee. *Education for the Allied Health Professions* (Allied Health Professions Subcommittee of the National Advisory Council, Public Health Service Publication No. 1600). Washington, DC: GPO, 1967.

AMA Council on Medical Education. *Medical Education in the United States 1971–72.* American Medical Association, 1972.

AMA/AAMC. Joint AMA-AAMC Statement on Health Manpower. *Journal of Medical Education,* 1968, 43, 506–7, 1009–1010.

American Academy of General Practice. The Core Content of Family Medicine (Committee on Requirements for Certification). In *Transactions of the American Academy of General Practice.* Kansas City, MO: American Academy of General Practice, 1966.

American Health Planning Association. Updated Survey of State Certificate of Need Programs. *Today*

in Health Planning, April 14, 1989, Volume 12, No. 1

American Hospital Association. *Report of the Committee on American Hospital Association Program.* Chicago: American Hospital Association, 1967.

———. "Guide" Issue (years as indicated). *Hospitals.*

———. Plight of the Public Hospital. *Hospitals,* July 1, 1970, 44:13, 40–92.

———. *Invitational Conference on Comprehensive Health Planning (Papers from the Conference held October 24–25, 1968).* Chicago: American Hospital Association, 1969.

———. *Survey Report: Review of 1971 State Certification-of-Need Legislation.* Chicago: American Hospital Association, 1972.

———. *Hospital Statistics (for indicated years).* Chicago: American Hospital Association.

———. *The Operation of State Hospital Planning and Licensing Programs (Hospital Monograph Series No. 15).* Chicago: American Hospital Association, 1965.

———. *Outpatient Health Care* (A report and recommendation of a conference on hospital outpatient care, March and June 1968). Chicago: American Hospital Association, 1969.

American Medical Association. *Distribution of Physicians in the United States 1970* (Report by the Center for Health Services Research and Development). Chicago: American Medical Association, 1971.

———. Public Health (Position Statement of the House of Delegates, AMA). *Journal of the American Medical Association,* Dec. 8, 1962, 182:10, 35–36.

———. Medical Education, 1932 Editorial. *Journal of the American Medical Association,* Aug. 27, 1932, 99, No. 9.

American Nurses' Association. American Nurses' Association's First Position on Education for Nursing. *American Journal of Nursing,* Dec. 1965, 65:12, 106–111.

American Public Health Association. An Official Declaration of Attitude of the American Public Health Association on Desirable Standard Minimum Functions and Suitable Organizations of Health Activities. *American Journal of Public Health,* Sept. 1940, 1099–1106.

———. An Official Declaration of Attitude on Desirable Standard Minimum Functions and Suitable Organization of Health Activities. Adopted Oct. 9, 1940—suppl. Dec. 19, 1941, and January 29, 1943. *American Journal of Public Health,* 1940, 30, 1099–1106.

———. The Local Health Department and Responsibilities. An official statement of the American Public Health Association, adopted November, 1950. *American Journal of Public Health,* 1951, 41, 302–307.

———. Policy Statement (Adopted November, 1963). *American Journal of Public Health,* 1964, 54, 131–139.

———. The State Public Health Agency. *American Journal of Public Health,* Dec. 1965, 55:12, 2011–2020.

———. The State Health Department—Services and Responsibilities (official statement of the association adopted November 11, 1953). *American Journal of Public Health,* Feb. 1954, 44, 235–252.

———. The State Health Department (policy statement of the governing council of the association, November 13, 1968). *American Journal of Public Health,* Jan. 1969, 59:1.

Anderson, O. W. Influence of Social and Economic Research on Public Policy in the Health Field: A Review. In D. Mainland (Ed.), *Health Services Research.* New York: Milbank Memorial Fund, 1967.

———. *The Uneasy Equilibrium: Private and Public Financing of Health Services in the United States, 1875–1965.* New Haven, CT: College & University Press, 1968.

APHA Committee on Administrative Practice. *Survey of 100 Largest Cities in the U.S. (Public Health Bulletin #164)* Washington, D.C.: U.S. Public Health Service, 1925.

Archibald, K. A. *The Supply of Professional Nurses and Their Recruitment and Retention by Hospitals.* New York: The New York City Rand Institute, July 1971.

Armstrong, G. E. The Medical Program of the Veterans Administration. *Journal of the American Medical Association,* Oct. 1959, 171:5, 50–54.

Ashford, N. A. (Summary of Crisis in the Workplace: Occupational Disease and Injury (A Report to the Ford Foundation). Cambridge, MA: The MIT Press, 1975.

Association of American Medical Colleges. *Planning for Medical Progress Through Education.* Evanston, IL: Association of American Medical Colleges, 1965.

———. Datagrams from issues indicated. *Journal of Medical Education.*

———. *Meeting the Challenge of Family Practice (Report of the Ad Hoc Committee on Education for Family Practice of the Council on Medical Education).* Chicago: American Medical Association, 1966a.

———. *The Graduate Education of Physicians (Report of the Citizens' Commission on Graduate Medical Education).* Chicago: American Medical Association, 1966b.

Assocation of State and Territorial Health Officials. *Services, Expenditures and Programs of State and Territorial Health Agencies, Fiscal Year 1978.* Washington, D.C.: 1980.

Bardach, E. *The Implementation Game: What Happens After a Bill Becomes a Law.* Cambridge, MA: The MIT Press, 1977.

Barger, S. D., Hillman, D. G., and Garland, H. R. *The PPO Handbook.* Rockville, MD: Aspen Systems Corporation, 1985.

Baughman, L. N. Child Nutrition Programs Amended by Budget Reconciliation Bill. *Washington Social Legislation Bulletin,* Jan. 26, 1981, 27:2.

Beck, E. M., Horan, P. M., and Tolbert, C. M. Stratification in a Dual Economy: A Sectoral Model of Earnings Determination. *American Sociological Review,* Oct. 1978, 43:5, 704–720.

Becker, A., and Schuelberg, H. C. Phasing Out State Hospitals—A Psychiatric Dilemma. *New England Journal of Medicine,* Jan. 29, 1976, 294:5, 255–261.

Behney, C. J., *The Turning Outward of the National Institutes of Health,* paper presented at the Annual Meeting of the Association for the Advancement of Medical Instrumentation (Cited in Office of Technology Assessment (1982). Washington, DC: April 1, 1978.

Bell, D. *The Coming of the Post-Industrial Society.* New York: Basic Books, 1973.

Bennett, D. Deinstitutionalization in Two Cultures. *Milbank Memorial Fund Quarterly/Health and Society,* Fall 1979, 57:4, 516–532.

Bensman, D. Solidarity Under Siege. *The Nation,* Sept. 14, 1985, 241:7, 213.

Bernstein, B. J. What Happened to Ghetto Medicine in New York State? *American Journal of Public Health,* July 1971, 61:7, 1287–93.

Blake, E., and Bodenheimer, T. *Closing the Doors on the Poor: The Dismantling of California's County Hospitals (A Health/PAC Report).* San Francisco: Health Policy Advisory Center, 1975.

Bodenheimer, T. S. Regional Medicine Programs: No Road to Regionalization. *Medical Care Review,* Dec. 1969, 26, 1125–1166.

Bovbjerg, R. R., and Davis, B. A. States' Response to Federal Health Care "Block Grants": The First Year. *Milbank Memorial Fund Quarterly/ Health and Society,* Fall 1983, 523–560.

Brandt, A. M. AIDS in Historical Perspective: Four Lessons from the History of Sexually Transmitted Diseases. *American Journal of Public Health,* 1988, 78:4, 367–371.

Breining, B. M. Blessings of a Doctor "Surplus." *Health Pathways* (State of California Office of Statewide Planning & Development), 3–4/1984, 6: 10.

Brodeur, P. *Expendable Americans.* New York: Viking Press, 1974.

Brook, R. H. *Quality of Care Assessment: A Comparison of Five Methods of Peer Review* (DHEW Publication No. (HRA) 74–3100). Rockville, MD: Department of Health, Education and Welfare, July 1973.

Brown, D. R. The Process of Area-Wide Planning: Model for the Future? *Medical Care,* Jan.–Feb. 1973, 11:1, 1–11.

Brown, E. L. Nursing and Patient Care. In F. Davis (Ed.), *The Nursing Profession: Five Sociological Essays.* New York: John Wiley and Sons, 1966.

Brown, E. R. *Rockefeller Medicine Men: Medicine and Capitalism in America.* Los Angeles: University of California Press, 1979.

Brown, R. E. Let the Public Control Utilization Through Planning. *Hospitals,* December, 1959, 33:23, 34–39.

———. The Public Hospital. *Hospitals,* July 1, 1970, 44:13.

Buchanan, J. M. *The Public Finances: An Introductory Textbook* (3d ed.). Homewood, IL: Richard D. Irwin Inc., 1970.

Bureau of Medicine and Surgery. *Statistics of Navy Medicine* (years as indicated). Washington, DC: Department of the Navy.

Burlage, R. K. *New York City's Municipal Hospitals: A Policy Review.* Washington, DC: Institute of Policy Studies, 1967.

Burns, E. M. The Role of Government in Health Services. *Bulletin of the New York Academy of Medicine,* July 1965, 41:7, 753–794.

Burrow, J. G. *AMA: Voice of American Medicine.* Baltimore: The John Hopkins Press, 1963.

Butter, I. Health Manpower Research: A Survey. *Inquiry,* Nov. 1967, 4:4.

California Department of Health. *Health Care Costs and Services in California Counties (Report to the Legislature in Response to Senate Concurrent Resolution No. 117.* Sacramento: Planning and Policy Analysis Office, 1978.

California Health Planning Law Review Commission. *Statewide Health Planning and Development in California (Report to the Legislature and Governor).* Sacramento: Feb. 13, 1983.

Cameron, C. M., and Kobylarz, A. Nonphysician Directors of Local Health Departments: Results of a National Survey. *Public Health Reports,* July/Aug. '80, 95:4, 386–397.

Carlson, R. J. Health Manpower Licensing and Emerging Institutional Responsibility for the Quality of Care. *Law and Contemporary Problems, Health Care, Part II,* Autumn 1970, 35:4.

Carnegie Commission on Higher Education. *Higher Education and the Nation's Health: Policies for Medical and Dental Education (A special report and recommendations).* New York: McGraw-Hill Book Company, Oct. 1970.

Carroll, M. S., and Arnett, R. H. Private Health Insurance Plans in 1978 and 1979: A Review of

Coverage, Enrollment, and Financial Experience. Health Care Financing Review, Sept. 1981, 3:1, 55–88.

Carson, R. *Silent Spring.* New York: Fawcett Crest, 1962.

Cartwell, P. E., and Last, J. M. Epidemiology. In J. M. Last (Ed.), *Maxcy-Rosenau: Public Health and Preventive Medicine.* New York: Appleton Century Crofts, 1980.

Cavanaugh, J. H. Comprehensive Health Planning and Public Health Service Act of 1966 (P.L. 89-749). *Indicators,* (Department of Health, Education and Welfare), Jan. 1967, 9–18.

Chapman, C. B., and Talmadge, J. M. The Evolution of the Right to Health Concept in the United States. *The Pharos of Alpha Omega Alpha,* Jan. 1971, 34:1.

Chase, E. T. The Politics of Medicine. *Harper's,* Oct. 1960, 221:126 (special supplement).

Child Welfare League of America. *Washington Social Legislation Bulletin (issues as indicated).*

Churchman, C. W. *The Systems Approach.* New York: Dell Publishing Co., 1968.

Clarke, G. J. In Defense of Deinstitutionalization. *Milbank Memorial Fund Quarterly/Health and Society,* Fall 1979, 57:4, 461–479.

Cline, J. W. The Physician's Point of View on Regional Organization of Hospitals. *California Medicine,* July 1948, 69:1, 12–15.

Cohen, F. S. *Handbook of Federal Indian Law.* GPO, Washington, D.C., 1941.

Cohen, H. S. Regulating Health Care Facilities: Certificate-of-Need Process Reexamined. *Inquiry,* Sep. 1973, 8:3, 3–9.

Cohn, B. *Los Angeles County Merger of Governmental Health Agencies: A Case Study.* Unpublished. Xeroxed copy on file with author, Dec. 1977.

Coll, B. D. *Perspectives in Public Welfare.* Washington, DC: Department of Health, Education and Welfare, Social & Rehabilitation Service, 1969.

Commission on Hospital Care. *Hospital Resources and Needs—Report of the Michigan Hospital Survey.* Battle Creek, MI: W.K. Kellogg Foundation, 1946.

Commission on Hospital Care. *Hospital Care in the United States.* New York: 1947. The Commonwealth Fund. (Reprinted in 1937 by Harvard University Press)

Commission on Services Integration. *Commissioned Papers (Volume IV of Health Services Integration: Lessons for the 1980s, a study of the Institute of Medicine).* Washington, DC: National Academy of Sciences, June 1982a.

———. *Case Reports (Volume III of Health Services Integration: Lessons for the 1980s, a study of the Institute of Medicine).* Washington, DC: National Academy of Sciences, June 1982b.

———. *Report of a Study (Volume I of Health Services Integration: Lessons for the 1980s, a study of the Institute of Medicine).* Washington, DC: National Academy of Sciences, June 1982c.

Commission on Workmen's Compensation *Report of the National Commission on State Workmen's Compensation Laws.* Washington, DC: 1972.

Committee of Consultants on Medical Research. *Federal Support of Medical Research; Report to the Subcommittee on Departments of Labor and HEW and of the Committee on Appropriations,* U.S. Senate, 86th Congress—2nd Session). 1960, GPO, Washington, DC

Committee on Costs of Medical Care. *Medical Care for the American People.* Chicago: University of Chicago Press, 1932. (Reprinted 1970 by HEW)

Committee on Metropolitan Planning. *Tentative Draft of Report* (mimeo). Chicago: American Hospital Association, 1960.

Comptroller General of US. *Report to the Congress: Are Neighborhood Health Centers Providing Services Efficiently and to the Most Needy? (HRD–77–124).* Washington, DC: General Accounting Office, June 20, 1978.

Congressional Budget Office. *Health Planning: Issues for Reauthorization.* Washington, DC: U.S. Congress, March 1982.

———. *Options for Change in Military Medical Care.* Washington, DC: Congress of the United States, March 1984.

Connery, R. H. *The Politics of Mental Health, Organizing Community Mental Health in Metropolitan Areas.* New York: Columbia University Press, 1965.

Cooney, J. P., Roemer, M. I., and Ross, M. B. *The Contemporary Status of Large Urban Public Hospitals—Ambulatory Services (Summary report).* Los Angeles: School of Public Health, UCLA, Nov. 1971.

Cooper, B. S. Medical Care Spending for Three Age Groups. *Social Security Bulletin,* May 1972, 35: 5, 3–16.

Cooper, H. M. *The Integrative Research Review: a Systematic Approach* (Applied Social Research Methods Series, Vol 2.). Beverly Hills: Sage Publications, 1984.

Corning, P. A. *The Evolution of Medicare: From Idea to Law.* Washington, DC: Department of Health, Education and Welfare, 1969.

Council of State Govternments. *Book of the States 1976–1977.* Lexington, Kentucky: Council of State Governments, 1976.

Cowen, D. L. Denver: Neighborhood Health Centers, Operations Within an Integrated System Provide Dignified Comprehensive Care for All. *Hospitals,* July 1, 1970, 44:13.

———. Community Health—a Local Government Responsibility. *American Journal of Public Health,* Oct. 1971, 61, 2005–2009.

Crawford, R. You are Dangerous to Your Health: The Ideology and Politics of Victim Blaming. *International Journal of Health Services,* 1977, 7:4, 663–680.

Curran, W. J. *National Survey and Analysis of Certificate-of-Need Laws: Health Planning and Regulation in State Legislatures, 1972.* Chicago: American Hospital Association, 1973.

———. Health Planning Agencies: A Legal Crisis? *American Journal of Public Health,* 1970, 60, 359–360.

Cutler, J. C., M.D., M.P.H., and Arnold, R. C., M.D. Venereal Disease Control by Health Departments in the Past: Lessons for the Present. *American Journal of Public Health,* 1988, 78:4, 372–380.

Daggett, E. L. Los Angeles County's New Health Services Super-Agency. *California's Health,* March 1973, 9–12.

Darley, W. Allied Health Personnel and Their Employment for the Improvement of Medical Care. *The New England Journal of Medicine,* Aug. 21, 1969, 281:8, 443–445.

Darley, W., and Somers, A. R. Medicine, Money, and Manpower, Challenge to Professional Education. II. Opportunity for Excellence. *The New England Journal of Medicine,* 1967, 276, 1291–1296.

Davis, F., Ed. *The Nursing Profession: Five Sociological Essays.* New York: John Wiley and Sons, 1966.

Davis, K. *Primary Care for the Medically Underserved: Public and Private Financing* (Paper presented for the 1981 American Health Planning Association and National Association of Community Health Symposium.) Leesburg, VA: Oct. 1981.

———. Community Hospital Expenses and Revenues: Pre-Medicare Inflation. *Social Security Bulletin,* Oct. 1972, 35:10, 3–19.

Davis, K., Gold, M., and MaKuc, C. Access to Health Care for the Poor: Does the Gap Remain?. *Annual Review of Public Health,* 1981, 2, 159–182.

Davis, K., and Rowland, D. Uninsured and Underserved: Inequities in Health Care in the United States. *Milbank Memorial Fund Quarterly/ Health and Society,* 1983, 61:2, 149–176.

Davis, K., and Schoen, C. *Health and the War on Poverty: A Ten-Year Appraisal.* Washington, DC: The Brookings Institution, 1978.

Department of Health, Education and Welfare. *Health Insurance Statistics (DHEW Publication No. (SSA) 74–11702).* Washington, DC: Department of Health, Education and Welfare, 1973.

———. *Medicare: Health Insurance for the Aged, 1971, Section 2: Enrollment (DHEW Publication No. (SSA) 73–11704).* Washington DC: GPO, Aug. 1973.

———. *NIOSH Fact Sheet.* Rockville, MD: Public Health Service, Centers for Disease Control, undated.

Department of Health and Human Services. *Report on the Status of Health Personnel in the U.S.,* years as indicated.

Department of HEW Social Security Administration.

Health, Education, and Welfare Trends, 1966–67, Part 1, National Trends, 1966–67.

Dillingham, W. P. *Federal Aid to Veterans 1917–1941.* Gainsville: University of Florida Press, 1952.

Dixon, J. P., M.D. Integration of Public Health and Hospital Services in Denver. *American Journal of Public Health,* Aug. 1950, 40, 973–977.

Dodds. Adventures in Medical Education. *Journal of Medical Education,* 1957, 32, 781, 787–88.

Donabedian, A. Evaluating the Quality of Medical Care. *Milbank Memorial Fund Quarterly,* 1966, 44:3–4.

———. *Medical Care Appraisal.* Washington, DC: American Public Health Association, 1969.

Donabedian, A., and Thorly, J. A. The Systemic Impact of Medicare. *Medical Care Review,* June 1969, 26:6, 567–584.

Dubos, R. *Mirage of Health: Utopias, Progress, and Biological Change.* Garden City, NY: Anchor Books, Doubleday and Co., 1959.

———. *Man Adapting.* New Haven, CT: Yale University Press, 1965.

Earle, V. Current State Practices with Regard to Hospitalization of Indigent Patients. *Public Welfare,* April 1952. (Cited in Blake and Bodenheimer, 1975).

Edelman, M. *The Symbolic Uses of Politics.* Urbana: University of Illinois Press, 1964.

Eilers, R. D., and Moyerman, S. S. ed. *National Health Insurance: Proceedings of Conference on National Health Insurance held at University of Pennsylvania, 1970.* Richard D. Irwin, Inc, Homewood, Ill. 1971.

Elaimey, W. M. *Regionalization of Hospital and Health Services: A Dr.P.H. Dissertation.* School of Public Health, UCLA. Los Angeles: 1969.

Elliot, C. M., and Vaughan, E. J. *Fundamentals of Risk and Insurance.* New York: John Wiley & Sons, Inc., 1978.

Elliott, R. H. E. The Current Nursing Situation. *Journal of Medical Education,* March 1969, 44.

Ellwood, D. A. Medicare Risk Contracting. *Health Affairs,* 1985, 5:1, 183–189.

Ellwood, P. M., and Hoagberg, E. J. Problems of the Public Hospital. *Hospitals,* July 1, 1970, 44:13, 51 ff.

Emerson, H. *Local Health Units for the Nation.* New York: The Commonwealth Fund, 1945.

Enthoven, A. C. *Health Plan: The Only Practical Solution to the Soaring Cost of Medical Care.* Reading, MA: Addison-Wesley Publishing Co., 1980.

Epstein, J. The Political and Economic Basis of Cancer. *Technology Review,* 1976, 78:8, 1–7.

Etzioni, A. *The Semi-Professions and their Organization: Teachers, Nurses, Social Workers.* New York: The Free Press, 1969.

Falk, I. S. Preface to the Reprint in *Medical Care for the American People.* The Final Report of the Committee on the Cost of Medical Care, 1932. U.S. Dept. of Health Education and Welfare. Reprinted 1970, Washington, D.C. p. x.

Falkson, J. L. *HMOs and the Politics of Health System Reform.* Bowie, MD: American Hospital Association & J. Brady Co., 1980.

Federation of American Hospitals. *1981 Directory of Investor-Owned Hospitals and Hospital Management Companies.* Little Rock, AR: Federation of American Hospitals, 1981.

Feia, R. The New National Health Spending Policy. *New England Journal of Medicine,* Jan. 17, 1974, 290:3, 137–140.

Fein, R. *The Doctor Shortage: An Economic Diagnosis.* Washington, DC: The Brookings Institution, 1967.

Feldstein, P. J., and Waldman, S. The Financial Position of Hospitals in the First Two Years of Medicare. *Inquiry,* March 1969, 6:1, 19–27.

Ferrell, J. A., Wilson, G. S., Covington, P. W., and Mead, P. A. *Health Departments of States and Provinces of the United States and Canada* (Public Health Bulletin, #124). GPO: U.S. Public Health Service, April 1, 1929.

Flexner, A. *Medical Education in the United States and Canada.* New York: Carnegie Foundation for the Advancement of Teaching, 1910.

Flook, E. Health Services Research and Development. *Public Health Reports,* April 1969, 84:4, 358–362.

Foreman, G. *Indian Removal, the Emigration of the Five Civilized Tribes of Indians.* Norman, OK: University of Oklahoma Press, 1953.

Forgotson, E. H., Roemer, R., and Newman, R. W. *Legal Regulation of Health Personnel in the United States* (Report of the National Advisory Commission on Health Manpower, Vol. III, Appendix VII). Washington, DC: GPO, Nov. 1967.

Fox, P. D., Goldbeck, W. B., and Spies, J. J. *Health Care Cost Management: Private Sector Initiatives.* Ann Arbor, MI: Health Administration Press, 1984.

Freeman, H. E., Kiecolt, K. J., and Allen, H. M. Community Health Centers: An Initiative of Enduring Utility. *Milbank Memorial Fund Quarterly/Health and Society,* Vol. 60, No. 2, Spring 1982, 245–267.

Friedman, I. Freedom of Contract and Occupational Licensing, 1890–1910: A Legal and Social Study. *California Law Review,* 1965, 53:48.

Gage, L. S. *Statement of Larry S. Gage, President National Association of Public Hospitals, before the Subcommittee on Health, Committee on Ways and Means.* Washington, DC: Feb. 15, 1983.

Galbraith, J. K. *The Affluent Society.* Boston: Houghton Mifflin, 1958

———. *The New Industrial State.* New York: Times Mirror, 1968.

Garland, J. E. *An Experiment in Medicine: A History*

of the First Twenty Years of the Pratt Clinic and the New England Center Hospital of Boston. Cambridge, MA: Riverside Press, 1960.

Geiger, H. J. The Meaning of Community Oriented Primary Care in the American Context. In E. Connor and F. Mullan (Eds.), Community Oriented Primary Care: New Directions for Health Services Delivery (Proceedings of Conference in Washington, D.C.). Washington, DC: National Academy Press, 1983.

Gerber, A. Our Growing Dependence on Foreign Physicians. Los Angeles Times, Aug. 26, 1973.

Gibson, R. M., and Waldo, D. R. National Health Expenditures, 1980. Health Care Financing Review, Sept. 1981, 3:1, 1–54.

Gilbert, B., Moose, M., and, and Miller, C. A. State-Level Decision Making for Public Health: the Status of Boards of Health. Journal of Public Health Policy, March 1982, 3:1.

Ginsburg, P. B. Resource Allocation in the Hospital Industry: The Role of Capital Financing. Social Security Bulletin, Oct. 1972, 35:10, 20–30.

Ginsburg, P. B., and Hackbarth, G. M. Alternative Delivery Systems and Medicare. Health Affairs, 1986, 5:1, 6–22.

Glaser, W. A Medical Organization and the Social Settings. New York: Atherton Press, 1970.

———. Paying the Doctor: Systems of Remuneration and Their Effects. Baltimore: The John Hopkins Press, 1970.

———. Lessons from Germany: Some Reflections Occasioned by Schulenburg's ''Report.'' Journal of Health Politics, Policy and Law, Summer 1983, 8:2, 352–365.

Glasscote, R. M. The Mental Health Center: Portents and Prospects. American Journal of Psychiatry, Jan. 1971, 127:7, 940–941.

Glogow, E. Community Participation in Sharing in Control of Public Health Services. Health Services Reports, May 1973, 88:5, 442–448.

GMENAC. Report to the Secretary, Department of Health and Human Services Washington, DC: Graduate Medical Education Advisory Committee, 1980.

Goldbeck, W. B. Health Care Coalitions. In W. B. Goldbeck and J. J. Spies (Eds.), Health Care Cost Management: Private Sector Initiatives. Ann Arbor, MI: Health Administration Press, 1984.

Goldberg, J. H. The Power Struggle at Cook County Hospital is Boiling Over. Hospital Physician, Feb. 1972, 31–32.

Goldmann, F. Public Medical Care: Principles and Problems. New York: Columbia University Press, 1945.

Gooding, R. E. Reasons for Welfare: The Political Theory of the Welfare State. Princeton: Princeton University Press, 1988.

Goodrich, C. H., M.D., Olendzki, M. C., and Crocetti, A. Hospital-based Comprehensive Care: Is It a Failure? Medical Care, 7–8/1972, 10:4, 363–368.

Gossert, D. J., and Miller, C. A. State Boards of Health, Their Members and Commitments. American Journal of Public Health, June 1973, 63:6, 486–493.

Grad, F. P. Public Health Law Manual: A Handbook on the Legal Aspects of Public Health Administration and Enforcement. New York: American Public Health Association, 1970.

Green, R. Assuring Quality in Medical Care. Cambridge: MA: Ballinger Press, 1976.

Greenberg, S. The Troubled Calling: Crisis in the Medical Establishment. New York: The Macmillan Company, 1965.

Greenfield, M. Medicare and Medicaid. The 1965 and 1967 Social Security Amendments. University of California at Berkeley: Institute of Governmental Studies, 1968.

———. Medi-Cal: The California Medicaid Program (Title XIX) 1966–1967. Berkeley, CA: University of California, 1970.

———. Medical Care for Welfare—Basic Problems. U.C. Berkeley, CA: Bureau of Public Administration, Sept. 1958.

Greer, E. Black Power in the Big Cities. The Nation, July 23, 1974, 525–529.

Gregorieff, P., and Kell, D. Initial Description of the National AHEC Program. Cambridge, MA: Abt Associates Inc., May 28, 1976.

Greve, C. H. and Campbell, J. R. Organization and Staffing for Local Health Services (Public Health Services Publication #682). Washington, DC: GPO, 1961.

Gruenberg, E. M., and Archer, J. Abandonment of Responsibility for the Seriously Mentally Ill. Milbank Memorial Fund Quarterly/Health and Society, Fall 1979, 57:4, 485–506.

Hadley, J., Feder, J., and Mullner, R. Care for the Poor and Hospital's Financial Status: Result of a 1980 Survey of Hospitals in Large Cities. Chicago: American Hospital Association, 1983.

Hall, T. L., Rudolph, S., and Parsons, W. B. Schools of Public Health: Trends in Graduate Education. Washington, DC: U.S. Department of Health and Human Services, 1980.

Hamilton, J. A. Patterns of Hospital Ownership and Control. Minneapolis: University of Minnesota Press, 1961.

Hamlin, R. H., M.D., Kisch, A. I., M.D., and Geiger, J. H., M.D. Administrative Reorganization of Municipal Health Services—The Boston Experience. New England Journal of Medicine, July 1, 1965, 273:1, 26–29.

Handel, G. Social Welfare in Western Society. New York: Random House, 1982.

Hanlon, J. J. Principles of Public Health Administration. St. Louis, MO: C.V. Mosby Company, 1969.

————. *Public Health Administration and Practice.* St. Louis, MO: C.V. Mosby Company, 1974.

————. Is There a Future for Local Health Departments? *Health Services Report,* Dec. 1973, 88: 10.

Hansen, W. L. An Appraisal of Physician Manpower Projections. *Inquiry,* March 1970.

Havighurst, C. C. Regulation of Health Facilities and Services by "Certificate of Need." *Virginia Law Review,* Oct. 1973, 59:7, 1143–1232.

Hilleboe, H. E., and Barkhuus, A. Health Planning in the United States: Some Categorical and General Approaches. *International Journal of Health Services,* 1971, 1:2, 134–148.

Hiscock, I. V. The Development of Neighborhood Health Services in the United States. *Milbank Memorial Fund Quarterly,* Jan. 1935, 13, 50–51.

Hitt, D. H. The Hospital's Role in the Planning Process (from Invitational Conference on Comprehensive Health Planning held October 24–25, 1968). In (Hitt, D.H., Ed.), *Papers from the Invitational Conference on Comprehensive Health Planning.* Chicago: American Hospital Association, 1969.

Health Care Financing Administration. *Health Care Financing Review* (issues as indicated). Washington, DC: Health Care Financing Administration.

Health Insurance Council. *HICHAP Inventory of Community Health Planning Agencies.* New York: Health Insurance Council, March 1969.

Health Policy Advisory Center. *Health PAC Bulletin* (issues as indicated). New York: Health Policy Advisory Center.

Hoffer, C. R., et al. *Health Needs and Health Care in Michigan.* Lansing, MI: Michigan State College, 1950, (Cited in Anderson, 1967)

Hoffer, C. R., and Schuler, E. A. Measurement of Health Needs and Health Care. *American Sociological Review,* Dec 1948, 13, 719–724 (Cited in Anderson, 1967).

Hofstadter, R. *Social Darwinism in American Thought.* New York: George Braziller, Inc., 1959.

Hollister, R. M., Kramer, B. M., and Bellin, S. S. *Neighborhood Health Centers.* Lexington, MA: Lexington, 1974.

Horowitz, L. A. Medical Care Price Changes in Medicaid's First Five Years. *Social Security Bulletin,* March 1972, 35:3.

Hospitals. AHA House Approves Financial Statement. *Hospitals,* March 1, 1969, 43:23.

Hospital Research and Education Trust. *The Future of the Public-General Hospital: An Agenda for Transition (Report of the Commission on Public-General Hospitals).* Chicago: Hospital Research and Education Trust, 1978a.

————. *Readings on Public-General Hospitals (Prepared for the Commission on Public-General Hospitals).* Chicago: Hospital Research and Education Trust, 1978b.

House Committee on Ways and Means. Hearings on HR1, 1971 to amend Social Security Act (Medicare and Medicaid), 6 volumes.

Hunter, R. *Poverty.* New York: Macmillan Company, 1907.

Hurley, R. The Health Crisis of the Poor. In H. P. Dreitzel (Ed.), *The Social Organization of Health.* New York: Macmillan Company, 1971.

Hyde, D. R., Wolff, P., Gross, A., and Hoffman, E. L. The American Medical Association: Power, Purpose, and Politics in Organized Medicine. *The Yale Law Journal,* 1954, 63, 938–1022.

Illich, I. *Medical Nemesis: The Expropriation of Health.* New York: Pantheon Books, 1973.

Indian Health Service. *FY 1985 Appropriation ("Chart Series" Tables).* Rockville, MD: Office of Planning, Evaluation and Legislation, April 1984.

Ingraham, H. S. Federal Grants Management: A State Health Officer's View. *Public Health Reports,* Aug. 1965, 80:8, 670–676.

Institute of Medicine. *Graduate Medical Education and Military Medicine.* Washington, DC: National Academy of Sciences, 1981.

————. *Health Services Research: Report of a Study.* Washington, DC: National Academy of Sciences, 1979.

————. *Community Oriented Primary Care: New Directions for Health Services Delivery* (Conference proceeding ed. by Eileen Connor and Fitzhugh Mullan). Division of Health Care Services within IOM. Washington, DC: National Academy Press, 1983.

————. *Responding to Health Needs and Scientific Opportunity: The Organizational Structure of the National Institutes of Health.* Washington DC: National Academy Press, 1984.

————. *The Future of Public Health.* (A report by the Committee for the Study of the Future of Public Health of the IOM.) Washington, DC: National Academy Press, 1988.

Interstudy. *National HMO Census 1984.* Excelsior, MN: Interstudy, 1985.

Isaacs, M. R., Lichter, K. G., and Lipschultz, C. M. *The Urban Public Hospital: Options for the 1980s.* Bethesda, MD: Alpha Center, 1982.

Jeffers, J. R., Bognano, M. F., and Bartlett, J. C. On the Demand Versus the Need for Medical Service and the Concept of "Shortage." *American Journal of Public Health,* 61:54, January 1971.

Journal of the American Medical Association. Medical Education in the United States. *Journal of the American Medical Association,* issues as stated.

Johnson, J. O. *Big Merger in Big Government: The Los Angeles County Department of Health Services,* (Ph.D. dissertation). Los Angeles: University of Southern California, 1977.

Johnson, W. L. Personnel Shortages in the Health Field and Working Patterns of Women. *Public Health Reports,* Jan. 1957, 72:1, 61–66.

Jordan, E. O., Whipple, G. C., and Winslow, C. A. *A Pioneer of Public Health, William Thompson Sedgwick.* New Haven, CT: Yale University Press, 1924.

Kane, R. L., and Kane, R. A. *Federal Health Care (With Reservations!).* New York: Springer Publishing Company, 1972.

Kaufmann, H. *The New York City Health Centers.* Indianapolis: Bobbs-Merrill Company, 1959.

Kenadjian, B. Appropriate Types of Federal Grants for State and Community Health Services. *Public Health Reports,* Sept. 1966, 81:9.

Kershaw, J. A. *Government Against Poverty.* Chicago: Markham Publishing Co., 1970.

Kesey, K. *One Flew Over the Cuckoo's Nest.* New York: The Viking Press, 1962.

Kessel, R. A. The A.M.A. and the Supply of Physicians. *Law and Contemporary Problems, Health Care, Part I,* Spring 1970, 35:2.

Keyssar, A. *Out of Work: The First Century of Unemployment in Massachusetts.* Cambridge, MA: Cambridge University Press, 1986.

Klarman, H. E. Analysis of the HMO Proposal—Its Assumptions, Implications, and Prospects. In *Health Maintenance Organizations: A Reconfiguration of the Health Services System.* (Proceedings of 13th Annual Symposium on Hospital Affairs). Graduate Program in Hospital Administration and Center for Health Administration Studies, Graduate School of Business, University of Chicago, May 1971.

———. Approaches to Moderating the Increases in Medical Care Costs. *Medical Care,* May–June 1969, 7:3, 175–190.

———. Effect of Prepaid Group Practice on Hospital use. *Public Health Reports,* Nov. 1963, 78:11, 955–965.

Knowles, J. H. The Quantity and Quality of Medical Manpower: A Review of Medicine's Current Efforts. *Journal of Medical Education,* Feb. 1969, 44, 81–118.

Knutson, J. W. Ferment in Public Health. *American Journal of Public Health,* Dec. 1957, 47:12, 1487–1492.

Koleda, M., and Craig, J. *The Long Range Viability of Municipal Hospitals.* Washington, DC: Center for Policy Studies, National Planning Association, July 1976.

Kracke, R. P. The Medical Care of the Veteran. *Journal of the American Medical Association,* Aug. 12, 1950, 143:15, 1321–1331.

Kramer, M. Patients in State and County Mental Hospitals.: National Institute of Mental Health. Department of Health and Human Welfare, GPO, 1969.

Kratz, F. W. The Present Status of Full-Time Local Health Organization. *Public Health Reports,* 1–6/1962, 47, 194–196.

Krause, E. A. Health Planning as a Managerial Ideology. *International Journal of Health Services,* Summer 1973, 3, 445–464.

Kuhn, T. *The Structure of Scientific Revolutions.* Chicago: University of Chicago Press, 1970.

Last, J. M. Epidemiology and Health Information. In Last 1986, Ch. 2.

Last, J. M. *Maxcy-Rosenau. Public Health and Preventive Medicine* (11th ed.). New York: Appleton-Century-Crofts, 1980.

———. Maxcy-Rosenau. *Public Health and Preventive Medicine* (12th ed.). New York: Appleton-Century-Crofts, 1986.

Lee, R. J., and Jones, L. W. *The Fundamentals of Good Medical Care (Publications of the Committee on Costs of Medical Care).* Chicago: University of Chicago Press, 1933.

Leiby, J. *A History of Social Welfare and Social Work in the United States, 1815–1972.* New York: Columbia University Press, 1978.

Lentz, E. A. Changing Philosophy and Role of the Health Facilities Planning Agencies. In (American Hospital Association, 1968) American Hospital Association, 1969.

Levine, R. A. *The Poor Ye Need Not Have With You: Lessons from the War on Poverty.* Cambridge, MA: The MIT Press, 1970.

Levitan, S. A. *The Great Society's Poor Law: A New Approach to Poverty.* Baltimore, MD: The John Hopkins Press, 1969.

Lewis, B. J. *VA Medical Program in Relation to Medical Schools* (House Committee Print No. 170, 91st Congress, 2nd Session). Washington, DC: GPO, 1970.

Lindblom, C. E. The Science of Muddling Through. *Public Administration Review,* Spring 1959, 79–88.

Lloyd, W. B., and Wise, H. B. The Montefiore Experience. *Bulletin of the New York Academy of Medicine,* No. 1968, 44:11.

Lohr, K. N. *Peer Review Organizations: Quality Assurance in Medicare.* Santa Monica, CA: The RAND Corporation, 1985.

Los Angeles Times. "Cranston Assails VA Hospitals' Lack of Care: Tragic Conditions Held Result of False Economy Measures by Government. *Los Angeles Times,* Jan. 10, 1970.

———. "We Are Going to Practice Medicine: County Hospital Threat to Health," Doctors Say. *Los Angeles Times,* Jan. 13, 1970.

———. Medical Center Report Urges Broad Changes. *Los Angeles Times,* Jan. 17, 1970.

———. Proposals to Ease Crowding at County Hospital Held "Piddling." *Los Angeles Times,* Jan. 20, 1970.

———. New VA Facilities (editorial). *Los Angeles Times,* Jan. 26, 1972.

———. "Big General": A Hospital That's Now Too Small. *Los Angeles Times,* Feb. 3, 1970.

———. Board and Care: New Approach to Mental Illness; State Hospitals Closing, but Value of Community Homes is Still Undecided. *Los Angeles Times,* May 13, 1972.

———. Improving Veterans' Medical Care (editorial). *Los Angeles Times,* Aug. 20, 1970.

———. Two Doctors Hit Care at Veteran Hospital Here. *Los Angeles Times,* Aug. 29, 1970.

———. Patients Still Dying of Neglect at County Hospital, Group Says. *Los Angeles Times,* Dec. 16, 1970.

———. Poor Bombard County Health Commission. *Los Angeles Times,* Nov. 6, 1970.

Lowell, J. S. *Public Relief and Private Charity.* New York: G.P. Putnam's Sons, 1884. (As cited in Coll, 1969).

Lowenstein, R. Early Effects of Medicare on the Health Care of the Aged. *Social Security Bulletin,* Apr. 1971, 34:4, 3–20.

Majone, G., and Wildavsky, A. Implementation as Evolution (1979). In J. L. Pressman and A. Wildavsky (Eds.), *Implementation: How Great Expectations in Washington are Dashed in Oakland,* Second Edition. Berkeley, CA: University of California Press, 1979.

Malmberg, C. *140 Million Patients.* New York, NY: Reynal and Hitchcock, 1947.

Marcus, I. *Dollars for Reform: The OEO Neighborhood Health Centers.* Lexington, MA: Lexington, 1981.

Marshall, D. R. Attempting a Merger: Reorganizing Health Services in Los Angeles County. *HSMHA Health Reports (U.S. Public Health Service),* Oct. 1971, 86:10, 967.

May, J. J. *Health Planning: Its Past and Potential (Health Administration Perspective Number A5).* University of Chicago: Center for Health Administration Studies, 1967.

McGeary, M., et al. *Case Studies* (Volume II of *Health Services Integration: Lessons for the 1980s,* a study of the Institute of Medicine, Division of Health Care Services). Washington, DC: National Academy of Sciences, June 1982.

McGraw-Hill. *Washington Report on Medicine and Health* (issues as indicated). Washington, DC: McGraw-Hill.

McKeown, T. An Historical Appraisal of the Medical Task. In T. McKeown and G. McLachlan (Eds.), *Medical History and Medical Care: A Symposium of Perspectives.* London: Oxford University Press, 1971.

McKinlay, J. B., and McKinlay, S. M. The Questionable Contribution of Medical Measures to the Decline of Mortality in the United States in the Twentieth Century. *The Milbank Memorial Fund Quarterly/Health and Society.* Vol. 55 No. 3, Summer 1977.

McLaughlin, M. C., Kavaler, F., and Stiles, J. Ghetto Medicine Program in New York City. *New York State Journal of Medicine,* 10/1/71, 2321–2325.

McNeil, R., Jr., and Schlenker, R. E. HMOs, Competition and Government. *Milbank Memorial Fund Quarterly/Health and Society,* Spring 1975.

McNerney, W. H., and Riedel, D. C. *Regionalization and Rural Health Care: An Experiment in Three Communities.* Ann Arbor, MI: The University of Michigan, 1962.

McNerney, W. J., and Study Staff, *Hospital and Medical Economics.* Chicago: Hospital Research and Education Trust, 1962.

McWilliams, C. *North from Mexico.* New York: Greenwood Press, 1949.

Medical World News. Hospitals Divide Control to Multiply Their Funds. *Medical World News,* March 14, 1969, 10:11, 28.

Medicaid in New York: Utopianism and Bare Knuckles in Public Health. *American Journal of Public Health,* May 1969, 59:5, 814–831.

Medicine and Health. Continuation of the weekly newsletter, "Washington Report on Medicine and Health" after October 1986. Published by McGraw-Hill until Oct 1989 and then by Faulkner and Gray's Health Information Center, Wash. D.C.

Medicine and Health Perspectives. Published as a weekly supplement to "Washington Report on Medicine and Health" and then to "Medicine and Health." (Dates and issues are given in text citations.) Published by McGraw-Hill until Oct. 1989 and then by Faulkner and Gray

Meeks, L. G., and Merwin, E. P. A Rebuttal. *Health Pathways,* 3–4/1984, 6: 10.

Miller, A. E. Remodeling the Municipal Health Services for a Unified System of Ambulatory Medical Care in the Central City. *Medical Care,* 9–10/1972, 10:5, 395–401.

Morehead, M. A., Donaldson, R. S., and Seravalli, M. R. Comparisons between OEO Neighborhood Health Centers and Other Health Care Providers of Ratings of the Quality of Health Care. In R. M. Hollister, B. M. Kramer and S. S. Bellin (Eds.), *Neighborhood Health Centers.* Lexington, MA: Lexington, 1981.

Moses, E. R. Nursing's Economic Plight. *American Journal of Nursing,* Jan. 1965, 65:1, 68–81.

Mott, F. D., and Roemer, M. I. *Rural Health and Medical Care.* New York: McGraw-Hill Book Company, 1948.

Mountin, J. H. *Health Service Areas: Requirements for General Hospitals and Health Centers.* Washington, DC: GPO, 1945.

———. Administration of Public Medical Service by Health Departments. *American Journal of Public Health,* Jan. 1940, 30, 138–144.

Mountin, J. W., and Greve, C. H. *The Role of Grants-in-Aid in Financing Public Health Programs (Public Health Bulletin #303).* Washington, DC: U.S. Public Health Service, 1949.

Mountin, J. W., Hankla, E. K., and Druzina, G. B. *Ten Years of Federal Grants-in-Aid for Public Health, 1936–1946 (Public Health Bulletin #300).* Washington, DC: U.S. Public Health Service.

Mountin, J. W., Pennell, E. H., and Flook, E. E. *Experience of the Health Department in 811 Coun-*

ties, 1908–34 (Public Health Bulletin #230). Washington, DC: GPO, U.S. Public Health Service, Oct. 1936.

Mountin, J. W., and Townsend, J. G. Observations on Indian Health Problems and Facilities (Public Health Service Bulletin No. 223). Washington, DC: GPO, 1936.

Moynihan Maximum Feasible Misunderstanding: Community Action in the War on Poverty. New York: Free Press, 1969.

Muse, D. N., and Sawyer, D. The Medicare and Medicaid Data Book, 1981, Department of Health and Human Services, Health Care Financing Administration, Office of Research and Demonstrations, Baltimore, 1982

Mustard, H. S. Government in Public Health. New York: The Commonwealth Fund, 1945.

Myrdal, G. Objectivity in Social Research. New York: Pantheon Books, 1969.

Mytinger, R. E. Innovations in Local Health Services. Arlington, Va.: Department of Health, Education and Welfare, 1968.

————. What Thirteen Local Health Departments are Doing in Medical Care. U.S. Public Health Service Publ. No. 1664, GPO, June, 1967.

Nader, R. Unsafe at Any Speed. New York: Grossman, 1972

National Academy of Sciences. Study of Health Care for American Veterans (Senate Committee Print No. 4, 5th Congress, 1st Session). Washington, DC: GPO, June 6, 1977.

National Advisory Commission on Health Manpower. Report. Washington, DC: GPO, Nov. 1967.

National AHEC Bulletin. Dates as indicated. 5110 E. Clinton Way, Fresno, CA 93727

National Center for Health Statistics. Monthly Vital Statistics Report (issues as indicated). Hyattsville, MD, National Center for Health Statistics.

National Commission on Community Health Services. Health Manpower Action to Meet Community Needs (Report of the National Commission on Community Health Services). Washington, DC: Public Affairs Press, 1967a.

————. Health is a Community Affair. Cambridge, MA: Harvard University Press, 1967b.

————. Report of the Task Force on Health Manpower. Bethesda, MD: National Commission on Community Health Services, Feb. 1966.

National Commission on Health Occupations. Federal Regulation of Health Occupations. Washington, DC: The Commission, 1982.

National Institute of Mental Health. The Cost of Mental Illness—1971 DHEW Publication No. (ADM) 76–265. Washington, DC: GPO, 1975.

————. The Characteristics of Persons Served by the Federally Funded Community Health Centers Program. Series A, No. 20, 1974 DHEW Publication No. (ADM) 79–771. Washington, DC: GPO, 1979.

————. Economics of Mental Health DHHS Publication No. (ADM) 81–114. Washington, DC: GPO, 1981.

National Institutes of Health. National Institutes of Health Research Plan, FY 1982–1984—Draft July 1980. Washington DC: NIH, 1980.

————. NIH Data Book. Washington, DC: Department of Health and Human Services.

New England Journal of Medicine. Boston's Department of Health and Hospitals (editorial). New England Journal of Medicine, March 24, 1966, 274:12, 687–689.

New York Review of Books. The [1984] Election and After. New York Review of Books, August 16, 1984, 31:13

Newhouse, J. P., Williams, A. P., Schwartz, W. B., and Bennett, B. W. Does the Geographic Distribution of Physicians Reflect on Market Failure? Bell Journal of Economics, 1982a, 13:2, 493–505.

Newhouse, J. P., et al. Where Have All the Doctors Gone? Journal of the American Medical Association, 1982b, 247, 2392–2396.

NIHS Study Comm. of HEW. Biomedical Science and Its Administration: A Study of the National Institutes of Health (This is the Wooldridge Committee.) Washington, DC: The White House, 1967.

Nunemaker, J. C. The Veterans Administration–Medical School Relationship. Journal of Medical Education, Feb. 1959, 34:2, 77–83.

Odegaard, C. E. Area Health Education Centers: The Pioneering Years, 1972–1978. Berkeley: Council on Policy Studies in Higher Education, 1979.

Office of Technology Assessment. Technology Transfer at the National Institutes of Health: A Technical Memorandum. Washington, DC: Congress of the U.S., Office of Technology Assessment, 1982.

Ozarin, L. D., Feldman, S., and Sparer, F. E. Experience with Community Mental Health Centers. American Journal of Psychiatry, 1971, 127, 912–916.

Ozarin, N., and Feldman, S. Implications for Health Services Delivery: The Community Mental Health Centers Amendments of 1970. American Journal of Public Health, Sept. 1971, 61:9, 1780–1784.

Pace, W. G., and Schweikart, R. B. OMEN: 1966–1967: Ohio Medical Education Network, originating at Ohio State, Now Has Outlets in 54 Ohio and Neighboring-State Hospitals. Ohio State Medical Journal, Jan. 1967, 63: 1, 30–32.

Page, J., and O'Brien, M. Bitter Wages. New York: Grossman Publishers, 1973.

Palmer, J. L., and Sawhill, I. V. The Reagan Experiment: An Examination of Economic and Social Policies Under the Reagan Administration. Washington, DC: The Urban Institute Press, 1982.

Pennsylvania Economy League. Coordinated Plan-

ning for Hospitals. Pittsburgh: Pennsylvania Economy League, 1959.

Pestana, C. *The Rejected Medical School Applicant: Options and Alternatives.* San Antonio, TX: Pub. by author, 1984.

Pettengill, J. H. Trends in Hospital Use by the Aged. *Social Security Bulletin,* July 1972, 35:7, 3–15.

Philadelphia Mayor's Committee. *Report of the Mayor's Committee on Municipal Hospital Services.* Philadelphia: Feb. 1970.

Pickett, G., M.D., *The New Federalism and Local Government* (A paper presented at the closing session of 101st Annual Meetng of APHA.) San Francisco, CA: 1973.

Pickett, G., and Hanlon, J. J. *Public Health: Administration and Practice (1990).* Times Mirror/Mosby, St. Louis. College Publishing, Ninth Edition.

Piel, G. *Comprehensive Community Health Services for New York City* (Report of Mayor's Commission on the Delivery of Personal Health Services). New York: 1969.

Piven, F. F., and Cloward, R. A. *Regulating the Poor: The Functions of Public Welfare.* New York: Pantheon Books, 1971.

Poland, E., and Lembcke, P. A. *Delineation of Hospital Service Districts: A Fundamental Requirement in Hospital Planning.* Kansas City, MO: Community Studies, 1962.

Polk, L. D. The Comprehensive Health Planning Laws from the Local Viewpoint. *Public Health Reports,* Jan. 1969, 84, 86–90.

President's Biomedical Research Panel. *Report of the President's Biomedical Research Panel DHEW pub. No. (OS) 76–500.* Washington, DC: Department of Health, Education and Welfare, April 30, 1976.

President's Commission on Heart Disease, Cancer, and Stroke. *A National Program to Conquer Heart Disease, Cancer, and Stroke (A Report to the President).* Washington, DC: GPO, 1964–1965.

Pressman, J. L., and Wildavsky, A. *Implementation: How Great Expectations in Washington are Dashed in Oakland.* Berkeley, CA: University of California Press, 1973.

Price, D. N. Workers' Compensation: Coverage, Benefits and Costs, 1980. *Social Security Bulletin,* May 1983, Vol 46, No. 5.

Price, W., and Cohn, B. *Development of the Denver Department of Health and Hospitals.* Los Angeles: Feb. 1978. Unpublished manuscript in author's files. Part of the research conducted in connection with Shonick (1980).

Public Law 89-749. *Comprehensive Health Planning and Public Health Services Amendments of 1966 (89th Congress).* :, Nov. 3, 1966.

Rabe, B. G. The Eclipse of Health Departments and Local Governments in American Environmental Protection. (Paper delivered at annual meeting of APHA, New Orleans, Oct. 20, 1987).

———. *Fragmentation and Integration in State Environmental Management.* Washington, DC: The Conservation Foundation, 1986.

Rayack, E. *Professional Power and American Medicine: The Economics of the American Medical Association.* Cleveland, OH: The World Publishing Company, 1967.

Redburn, T. Budget Deficits to Restrict Social Programs for Years: ''Used Up All the Resources.'' *Los Angeles Times,* Aug. 26, 1988.

Redick, R. W. *Patterns in the Use of Nursing Homes by the Aged Mentally Ill.* HEW Statistical Note #107, Washington, D.C. Alcohol, Drug Abuse, and Mental Health Administration, June 1974.

———. *Referral of Discontinuations from Inpatient Services of State and County Mental Hospitals, United States, 1969,* Statistical Note No. 58. Rockville, MD: National Institute of Mental Health, November 1971.

Redick, R. W., Witkin, M. J., Bethel, H. E., and Manderscheid, R. W. Changes in Inpatient, Outpatient, and Partial Care Services in Mental Health Organizations, 1970–1980. Mental Health Statistical Note #168, Washington, D.C.: National Institute of Mental Health, August 1985.

Redick, R. W., Witkin, M. J., Atay, J. E., Fell, A. S., and Manderschied, R. W. *Patient Care Episodes in Mental Health Organizations, United States: Selected Years Between 1955 and 1986.* NIMH Statistical Note #192 Washington, DC: National Institute of Mental Health, Aug. 1990.

Reinhardt, U. W. Health Insurance and Health Policy in the Federal Republic of Germany. *Health Care Financing Review,* Dec. 1981, 3:2, 1–14.

Reizen, M. S. *State Control: The State Health Department and Comprehensive Health Planning (A paper presented at the 102nd annual APHA meeting).* New Orleans, LA: 1974.

Renthal, A. G. Comprehensive Health Centers in Large U.S. Cities. *American Journal of Public Health,* 61 (1971) 324–336.

Revenue Advisory Service. *Revenue Sharing Bulletin* (issues as indicated). Washington, DC: Revenue Advisory Service.

Reynolds, R. A. Improving Access to Health Care Among the Poor—The Neighborhood Health Center Experience. *Milbank Memorial Fund Quarterly/Health and Society,* Volume 54, 47–82, No. 1, Winter 1976.

Rochester Regional Hospital Council. *The Rochester Regional Hospital Plan.* New York: Rochester Regional Hospital Council.

Roemer, M. I. *The American Public Health Association as a Force for Change in Medical Care* (An address before the 100th annual meeting of the American Public Health Association, Atlantic City, NJ.). *Medical Care,* Vol. 11, No. 4, pp 338–351, July–August 1973.

———. *Ambulatory Health Services in America:*

Past, Present, and Future. Rockville, MD: Aspen Systems Corporation, 1981.

————. Bed Supply and Hospital Utilization: A Natural Experiment. *Hospitals,* Nov. 1960, 35:21, 36–42.

Roemer, M. I., and Mera, J. A. "Patient-Dumping" and Other Voluntary Agency Contributions to Public Agency Problems. *Medical Care,* Jan./Feb. 1973, 11:1, 30–39.

Roemer, M. I., and Shain, M. *Hospital Utilization Under Insurance.* Chicago, IL: American Hospital Association, 1959

Roemer, R. Social Regulation of Health Manpower. In A. N. Charters (Ed.), *Fostering the Growing Need to Learn,* Vol. 1. Monographs. Rockville, MD: Department of Health, Education and Welfare, 1973.

Roemer, R., Kramer, C., and Frank, J. E. *Planning Urban Health Services: From Jungle to System.* New York: Springer, 1975.

Roemer, R., and Shonick, W. *Private Management of California County Hospitals* (published for the California Policy Seminar, Monograph No. 4, Institute of Governmental Studies). Berkeley, CA: University of California, 1980.

Rorkey, L. Health-Care Crisis in Chicago. *Chicago Sun-Times,* April 26, 1970.

Rose, S. M. Deciphering Deinstitutionalization: Complexities in Policy and Program Analysis. *Milbank Memorial Fund Quarterly/Health and Society,* Fall 1979, 57:4, 429–460.

Rosen, G. *A History of Public Health.* New York: MD Publications, Inc., 1958.

————. The Impact of the Hospital on the Physician, the Patient and the Community. *Hospital Administration,* 1964, 9, 15–33.

————. The First Neighborhood Health Center Movement—Its Rise and Fall. *American Journal of Public Health,* Aug. 1971, 61:8, 1620–1637.

Rowe, M. J., and Ryan, C. C. Comparing State-Only Expenditures for AIDS. *American Journal of Public Health,* 1988, 78:4, 424–429.

Sade, R. M. Medical Care as a Right: A Refutation. *New England Journal of Medicine,* Dec. 2, 1971, 285, 1288–1292.

Sadler, A. M., Sadler, B. L., and Sadler, A. L. *The Physician's Assistant—Today and Tomorrow.* New Haven, CT: Trauma Program Department of Surgery, Yale University, 1972.

Sale, K. *Power Shift: The Rise of the Southern Rim and Its Challenge to the Eastern Establishment.* New York: Random House, 1975.

Sanders, B. S. Local Health Departments: Growth or Illusion? *Public Health Reports,* Jan. 1959, 74, 13–20.

Sawhill, I. V., and Stone, C. F. *The Economy: The Key to Success.* In Palmer, J. L. and Sawhill, J. V. (Ed.) *The Reagan Record,* Cambridge, MA: Ballinger Publishing Company, 1984 (Chapter 3)

Schloss, E. P. Beyond GMENAC—Another Physi-

cian Shortage from 2010 to 2030? *New England Journal of Medicine,* 1988, 318:17, 920.

Schofield, J. R. *New and Expanded Medical Schools, Mid-Century to 1980s.* San Francisco: Jossey-Boss, 1984.

Schorr, L. B., and English, J. T. Background, Context, and Significant Issues in Neighborhood Health Center Programs. *Milbank Memorial Fund Quarterly,* 1968, 46, 289–296.

Schulenburg, J. M. Report from Germany: Current Conditions and Controversies in the Health Care System. *Journal of Health Politics, Policy and Law,* Summer 1983, 8:2, 320–351.

Schwartz, D. A. Community Mental Health in 1972: An Assessment. In *Progress in Community Mental Health.* Barten H. H. and Bellak L. (Eds.). Vol 2, pp 3–34, New York: Grune and Stratton, Inc., 1972.

Schwartz, W. B., Sloan, F. A., and and Mendelson, D. N. Why There Will Be Little or No Physician Surplus Between Now and the Year 2000. *New England Journal of Medicine,* August 7, 1988, 318:17, 892.

Schwartz, W. B., et al. The Changing Geographic Distribution of Board-Certified Physicians. *New England Journal of Medicine,* 1980, 303, 1032–1038.

Shannon, F. A. *America's Economic Growth (3d Ed.).* New York: The Macmillan Company, 1951.

Shepard, W. P. Public Health and Socialized Medicine. *American Journal of Public Health,* Nov. 1951, 41:11, 1333–1341.

Sherman, J. F. The Organization and Structure of the National Institutes of Health (Cited in Office of Technology Assessment, 1982). *New England Journal of Medicine,* 1977, 297(1).

Shonick, W. *Elements of Planning for Personal Health Services.* St. Louis, MO: C.V. Mosby, 1976.

————. The Public Hospital and Its Local Ecology in the United States: Some Relationships Between the "Plight of the Public Hospital" and the "Plight of the Cities." *International Journal of Health Services,* 1979, 9:3.

————. Health Planning. In J. M. Last (Ed.), *Maxcy-Rosenau Public Health and Preventive Medicine (11th Ed.).* New York: Appleton-Century-Crofts, 1980.

————. Health Planning. In J. M. Last (Ed.), *Maxcy-Rosenau, Public Health and Preventive Medicine (12th Ed.).* Norwalk: Appleton-Century-Crofts, 1986.

————. Mergers of Public Health Departments with Public Hospitals in Urban Areas, Findings of 12 Field Studies. *Medical Care,* Aug. 1980, 18:8 Supplement.

Shonick, W., and Price, W. Organizational Milieus of Local Public Health Units in the United States: Analysis of a Questionnaire Response. *Public Health Reports,* Nov. 1978, 93, 648–665.

Shonick, W., and Price, W. Reorganizations of Health

Agencies by Local Government in American Urban Centers: What Do They Portend for Public Health? *Milbank Memorial Fund Quarterly/ Health and Society,* Spring 1977, 55:2, 233–271.

Shonick, W., and Roemer, R. *Public Hospitals Under Private Management: The California Experience (California Policy Seminar, Institute of Governmental Studies).* Berkeley, CA: University of California, 1983.

Shyrock, R. *Licensing in America 1650–1965.* Baltimore, MD: The Johns Hopkins Press, 1967.

————. *The Development of Modern Medicine, an Interpretation of the Social and Scientific Factors Involved.* Madison, WI: The University of Wisconsin Press, 1979.

Shubick, H. J., and Wright, E. O. *Composite Study of Fifty Health Department Organizational Charts Representing Forty-nine States and the District of Columbia (1961).* (An unpublished report—cited in (Hanlon, 1969).

Sieverts, S. A Review of J. Joel May's Health Planning: Its Past and Potential. *Health Services Research,* Fall 1968, 3:3, 251–256.

Sigmond, R. M. Health Planning. *Milkbank Memorial Fund Quarterly,* 1968, 46.

Snoke, A. W. The Unsolved Problems of the Career Professional in the Establishment of National Health Policy. *American Journal of Public Health,* Sept. 1969, 59:9, 1575–1588.

Somers, A. R. Comprehensive Prepayment Plans as a Mechanism for Meeting Health Needs. *Annals of the American Academy of Political and Social Science.,* Sept. 1961, 337:85, 81–92.

Somers, H. M., and Somers, A. R. *Workmen's Compensation.* New York: John Wiley & Sons, Inc., 1954.

————. *Doctors, Patients, and Health Insurance.* Washington, DC: The Brookings Institution, 1961.

Sparer, E. V. *Medical School Accountability in the Public Hospital: The University of Pennsylvania Medical School and the Philadelphia General Hospital.* Philadelphia: Health Law Project, 1974.

Sparer, G., and Anderson, A. Cost of Services at Neighborhood Health Centers—A Comparative Analysis. In R. M. Hollister, B. M. Kramer, and S. S. Bellin (Eds.), *Neighborhood Health Centers.* Lexington, MA: Lexington, 1974.

Sparer, G., and Johnson J. Evaluation of OEO Neighborhood Health Centers. *American Journal of Public Health,* May 1971, 61:5, 931–942.

Starfield, B. Measurement of Outcome: A Proposed Scheme. *Milbank Memorial Fund Quarterly,* 1974, 51, 39–50.

Starr, P. *The Social Transformation of American Medicine.* New York: Basic Books, 1981.

Stern, B. J. *Medical Services by Government: Local, State and Federal.* New York: The Commonwealth Fund, 1946.

Stevens, R. *American Medicine and Public Policy.* New Haven, CT: Yale University Press, 1971.

Stimmel, B. and Graettinger, J. S. Medical Students Trained Abroad and Medical Manpower. *New England Journal of Medicine,* January 26, 1984, 310: 230–235

Sturm, H. M. Technological Developments and Their Effects Upon Health Manpower. *Monthly Labor Review,* Jan. 1967, 90:1, 1–8.

Subcommittee on Health of the Elderly. *Medical Assistance for the Aged: The Kerr-Mills Program 1960–1963.* A Report by the Subcommittee to the Special Committee on Aging, United States Senate. GPO, October 1963

Sunshine, J. H., Witkin, M. J., Atay, J. E., Fell, A. S., and Manderschied, R. W. *State and County Mental Hospitals, United States and Each State,* National Institute of Mental Health, DHHS, Washington, DC: GPO, 1990.

Surgeon General, USAF. *Annual Reports of USAF Medical Service* (years as indicated). Washington, DC: Office of the Surgeon General, U.S. Air Force.

Surgeon General, U.S. Army. *Annual Reports* (years as indicated). Washington, DC: Office of the Surgeon General, Department of the Army.

Szasz, T. S. *The Manufacture of Madness: A Comparative Study of the Inquisition and the Mental Health Movement.* New York: Delta, 1970.

Terenzio, J. V., and Manning, H. E. Case Study: New York City. *Hospitals,* July 1, 1970, 44:13, 65–75.

Terris, M. Hermann Biggs' Contribution to the Modern Concept of the Health Center. *Bulletin of the History of Medicine,* Oct. 1946, 20:3, 387–412.

Testoff, A., Levine, E., and Siegel, S. E. Analysis of Part-Time Nursing in General Hospitals. *Hospitals,* Sept. 1, 1963.

Thurow, L. C. *The Zero-Sum Society: Distribution and the Possibilities for Economic Change.* New York: Penguin Books, 1980.

Tilson, D., Reader, J., and Morison, R. The Federal Interest (Cited in *Office of Technology Assessment,* 1982). In G. Gordon and G. L. Fisher (Eds.), *The Diffusion of Medical Technology.* Cambridge, MA: Ballinger Publishing Co., 1975.

Times-Picayune. Public Hospitals: A Comparison. *The Times-Picayune (New Orleans),* Dec. 28, 1969 through January 8, 1970.

Tobin, J. Reaganomics and Economics. *The New York Review of Books,* Dec. 2, 1981.

Treloar, A. E., and Chill, D. *Patient Care Facilities: Construction Needs and Hill-Burton Accomplishments* (Hospital Monograph Series No. 10). Chicago: American Hospital Association, 1961.

Trussell, R. E. *The Quality of Medical Care as a Challenge to Public Health* (The Fourth Bronfman Lecture). Washington, DC: American Public Health Association, 1965.

Tuchman, B. W. *A Distant Mirror: The Calamitous 14th Century.* New York: Ballantine Books, 1978.

Tuler, S. L. *A History of Indian Policy.* Washington, DC: Department of Interior, Bureau of Indian Affairs, 1973.

U.S. Bureau of the Census. *Historical Statistics of the United States Colonial Times to 1957.* Washington, DC: U.S. Department of Commerce, Bureau of the Census, 1960

————. *Historical Statistics of the United States Colonial Times to 1970.* Washington, DC: U.S. Department of Commerce, Bureau of the Census, 1975

————. *State Government Finances in [years as indicated].* Washington, DC: GPO,

————. *Statistical Abstract of the United States 1981 (101st Ed.).* Washington, DC: U.S. Department of Commerce, Bureau of Census, 1980.

————. *Statistical Abstract of the United States 1988* (108th Ed.). Washington, D.C., U.S. Department of Commerce, Bureau of the Census, 1987

U.S. Chamber of Commerce. *Analysis of Workmen's Compensation Laws.* Washington, DC: Chamber of Commerce of the U.S., 1983

U.S. Congress and Senate Committee on Indian Affairs. *Survey of Conditions of the Indians in the U.S. (Hearings, Part 17).* Washington, DC: GPO, 1931.

U.S. Department of the Army. *A Decade of Change in U.S. Hospitals 1953–1963: A Study Comparing Utilization, Staffing and Cost Trends in Civilian and CONUS Army Hospitals.* Office of the [Department] Surgeon General, Washington DC, GPO:, May 1965.

U.S. Department of Commerce. *Statistical Abstract of the United States* (issues as indicated). Washington, DC: Bureau of the Census.

U.S. Department of Defense and Department of Health, Education and Welfare. *Civilian Health and Medical Programs of the Uniformed Services (CHAMPUS).* Washington, DC: GPO, Jan. 10, 1977.

U.S. Department of Defense, Department of Health, Education and Welfare, and Office of Management and Budget. *Report of the Military Health Care Study.* Washington, DC: GPO, Dec.1975.

U.S. Department of Health, Education and Welfare. *Statistical Notes,* National Institute of Mental Health, various issues, Rockville, MD, years as indicated.

————. *The National Institutes of Health Almanac.* (years as indicated). Washington, DC: Office of Information, National Institute of Health.

————. *Health, Education and Welfare Indicators.* (Dates and pages as indicated), Office of Program Analysis, GPO, Wash. DC.

————. *Health Services for American Indians* (Public Health Service Publication no. 531). Washington, DC: GPO, 1957.

————. Public Health Service. *The Hospital Association Evaluates Hospital Planning: Principles for Planning the Future Hospital System (Publication no. 721).* Washington, DC: Department of Health, Education and Welfare, 1959a.

————. *A Report on Proceedings of Four Regional Conferences to Develop Principles for Planning the Future Hospital System.* Washington, DC: GPO, 1959b.

————. *Area-Wide Planning for Hospitals and Related Health Facilities (Report of the Joint Committee of the American Hospital Association and Public Health Service, PHS Publication no. 855).* Washington, DC: GPO, July 1961.

————. *Procedures for Areawide Health Facility Planning—A Guide for Planning Agencies* (PHS Publication no. 930–B–3). Washington, DC: GPO Sept. 1963.

————. Office of Program Analysis. *Health, Education and Welfare Trends 1966–67 Part 1 National Trends,* 1966–67, United States Dept. of Health, Education and Welfare, Wash. DC

————. *Vital Statistics Rates in the United States 1940–1960 (Chapter I).* GPO: Department of Health, Education and Welfare, National Center for Health Statistics 1968.

————. *Health Resources Statistics: Health Manpower and Health Facilities,* 1969. Washington, DC: Department of Health, Education and Welfare, 1970.

————. *Report on Licensure and Related Health Personnel Credentialing* (Office of Assistant Secretary for Health and Scientific Affairs, Publication No. HSM 72–11). Washington, DC: Department of Health, Education and Welfare, June 1971.

————. *Directory of State, Territorial and Regional Health Authorities 1971–1972.* Washington, DC: Department of Health, Education and Welfare.

————. Health Resources Statistics: Health Manpower and Health Facilities, 1971, Washington, DC, DHEW, 1972.

————. *Federal Assistance Review: A Special Report from the Department of Health, Education and Welfare* (DHEW Publication no. OS 72–38). Washington, DC: Department of Health, Education and Welfare, June 1972.

————. *Hill-Burton Program Progress Report, July 1, 1947–June 30, 1971* (HEW Pub. no. HSM 73-4001). Rockville, MD: U.S. Public Health Service, 1972.

————. *Section 1122 of the Social Act: Limitation of Federal Participation for Capital Expenditures—Some Questions and Answers (DHEW Publication No. (HRA) 74–14002).* Washington, DC: Department of Health, Education and Welfare, 1973.

————. *Source Book of Health Insurance 1972–73.* New York: Health Insurance Institute, 1973.

————. *Bureau of Medical Services* (HEW Publication no. HSA 77–2004). Washington, DC: Department of Health, Education and Welfare, 1977.

———. *Indian Health Trends and Services* (DHEW Publication no. HSA 78–12009). Washington, DC: Department of Health, Education and Welfare, 1978.

———. *Selected Vital Statistics for Indian Health Service Areas and Service Units, 1972–1977* (DHEW Publication no. HSA 79–1005). Washington, DC: Department of Health, Education and Welfare, 1979.

———. *Training Health Manpower for Underserved Areas, 1973–79* DHEW Pub. no. HRA 79–58. Hyattsville, MD: U.S. Public Health Service, 1979.

———. *Healthy People (The Surgeon General's Report on Health Promotion and Disease Prevention).* Washington, DC: Department of Health, Education and Welfare, 1979a.

———. *Healthy People (The Surgeon General's Report on Health Promotion and Disease Prevention, Background Papers, 1979).* Washington, DC: Department of Health, Education and Welfare, 1979b.

———. *Health United States 1979.* Hyattsville, MD: Public Health Service, 1980

U.S. Department of Health and Human Services. Earlier published in the predecessor Department of Health, Education and Welfare. Issues as indicated. *Social Security Bulletin.*

———. *Statistical Notes,* National Institute of Mental Health, (various issues) Rockville, MD

———. *NIH Almanac.* Washington DC. Issues as indicated.

———. *National Plan for Fiscal Years 1981–84: The Indian Health Care Improvement Act, P.L. 94–437.* (Department of Health, Education and Welfare Pub. no. 80–1021)—Public Health Service, Indian Health Service. Rockville, MD:, 1980.

———. *Promoting Health/Preventing Disease; Objectives for the Nation.* GPO: Public Health Service, Fall, 1980.

———. *Indian Health Service Chart Series Book—* Public Health Service, Indian Health Service. GPO:, April 1988.

———. *NIH Advisory Committees.* Bethesda, MD: National Institutes of Health, April 1991.

———. *NIH Public Advisory Groups* (Public Health Service, National Institutes of Health, NIH Publication no. 83–11). Bethesda, MD:, Jan. 1983.

———. *National Center for Health Statistics: Organization and Activities Monitoring the Nation's Health* Public Health Service Pub. no. PHS 92–1200. Hyattsville, MD: Public Health Service, Centers for Disease Control, National Center for Health Statistics, 1992.

U.S. Department of the Navy. *Medical Statistics U.S. Navy (109th Annual Summary, NAVMED P-5027),* Naval Medical Command, Naval Medical Data Services Center. Washington, DC: 1978 and 1979.

U.S. Department of the Treasury. *Annual Report of the Secretary of the Treasury: Combined Statement of Receipts, Expenditures and Balance of the United States Government.* Washington, D.C., Financial Management Service (Stated years).

U.S. Environmental Protection Agency. *A Progress Report.* Washington, DC: Environmental Protection Agency, Nov. 1972.

U.S. General Accounting Office. *Returning the Mentally Disabled to the Community: Government Needs to Do More* (Report to Congress by the Comptroller General of the United States). Washington, DC: General Accounting Office, Jan. 7, 1977.

———. *Are Neighborhood Health Centers Providing Services Efficiently and to the Most Needy?* (Report to the Congress.) Washington, DC General Accounting Office:, 1978.

U.S. Office of Management and Budget. *Restoring the Balance of Federalism* (Second Annual Report to the President on the Federal Assistance Review, Executive Order of the President, Office of Management and Budget, June 1971). Washington DC:.

U.S. Public Health Service. *Contagious and Infectious Diseases Among the Indians* (Senate Document no. 1038, 62nd Congress, 3rd Session). Washington, DC: GPO, 1913.

———. *Directory of State and Areawide Agencies Under Section 314 of the Public Health Service Act, July 1972.* Washington, DC: Department of Health, Education and Welfare, July 1972.

———. *Distribution of Health Services in the Structure of State Government, 1950* (Public Health Service Publication no. 184, Part 1). Washington, DC:, 1952.

———. *Toward Quality in Nursing: Needs and Goals (Report of the Surgeon General's Consultant Group on Nursing* [the "Eurich Report"] PHS Pub. no. 992). Washington, DC: GPO, 1963.

———. *Hill-Burton Program 1946–1966, Two Decades of Partnership for Better Patient Care* (Public Health Service Publication no. 930–F–8). Washington, DC: GPO, Aug. 1966.

———. *Physicians for a Growing America* (Report of the Surgeon General's Consultant Group on Medical Education, PHS Publication no. 709). Washington, DC: GPO, 1959.

U.S. Senate. *Department of Defense Appropriation Bill 1983* (Senate Report 8, 97-580). Washington, DC: Sept. 8, 1982.

U.S. Senate Commitee on Finance. *Summary of Social Security Amendments of 1972, Public Law 92-603 (H.R.1).* : Joint publication of U.S. Senate Committee on Finance and Committee on of the Surgeon General's Consultant Group on Medical Education, PHS Publication no. 709). Washington, DC: GPO, 1959.

U.S. Senate. *Department of Defense Appropriation Bill 1983* (Senate Report 8, 97-580). Washington, DC: Sept. 8, 1982.

U.S. Senate Commiteee on Finance. *Summary of Social Security Amendments of 1972, Public Law 92-603 (H.R.1).* : Joint publication of U.S. Senate Committee on Finance and Committee on Ways and Means of U.S. House of Representatives, November 17, 1972, GPO.

———. *Medicare and Medicaid: Problems, Issues and Alternatives* (Report of the Committee Staff, Russell B. Long, Chairman). : The Committee, Feb 9, 1970.

Vaughan, E. J., and Elliott, C. M. *Fundamentals of Risk and Insurance.* New York: Wiley/Hamilton, 1978.

Vaughan, H. F. City Health Administration. In H. Emerson (Ed.), *Administrative Medicine.* Baltimore: Williams and Wilkins, 1951.

———. Local Health Services in the United States: The Story of the CAP. *American Journal of Public Health,* Jan. 1972, 62:1, 95–111.

Veteran Administration. *Administrator of Veteran Affairs, Annual Report.* (years as indicated). Washington, DC: GPO.

———. *VA History in Brief* (VA pamphlet 06–77–1). Washington, DC: GPO, May 1977b.

———. *The Vietnam Veteran in Contemporary Society: Collected Materials Pertaining to the Young Veterans.* Washington, DC: Department of Medicine and Surgery, May 1972a.

Veterans Administration Department of Medicine and Surgery. *Transition of the Presidency, DM and S Section.* : U.S. Veterans Administration, Nov. 1976.

Vear, A. J. Emergence of the Medical Care Section of the American Public Health Association, 1926–1948. *American Journal of Public Health,* Nov. 1973, 63:11, 986–1007.

Volkenburg, V. A. Local Health Administration: Rural. In H. Emerson (Ed.), *Administrative Medicine.* Baltimore: Williams and Wilkins, 1951.

Wald, L. D. *The House on Henry Street.* New York: Henry Holt and Co., 1915.

Waldman, S. *National Health Insurance Proposals: Provisions of Bills Introduced in the 93rd Congress as of October 1973* (DHEW Publication no. SSA 74–11916). GPO: Social Security Administration Office of Research and Statistics, 1973.

Wallack, S. S. Financing Care for the Chronically Mentally Ill: The Implications of the Various Approaches. In NIMH (Ed.), *Economics and Mental Health (DHHS Publication no. ADM 81–114)).* Wasington, DC: Department of Health and Human Services, 1981.

Ward, M. J. *The Snakepit.* New York: Random house, 1946.

Washington, Rept on Medicine and Health. McGraw-Hill's Health Information Center, Wash D.C. (issues and dates as indicated). For later issues see Medicine and Health. See also *Washington Report on Medicine and Health Perspectives (Supplement to Washington Report on Medicine and Health).*

Weber, M. *The Protestant Ethic and the Spirit of Capitalism.* New York: Charles Scribner's Sons, 1958.

Weick, K. Educational Organizations as Loosely Coupled Systems. *Administrative Science Quarterly,* 1962, 6, 395.

Weinstein, I. Eighty Years of Public Health in New York City. *Bulletin of the History of Medicine,* April 1947, 221–237.

Wennberg, J., and Gittelson, A. Variations in Medical Care Among Small Areas. *Scientific American,* 1982, 246, 120–134.

Wert, H. Five Years of Medicare—A Statistical Review. *Social Security Bulletin,* Dec. 1971, 34:12, 17–27.

Western Center for Planning. *Statewide Briefing Memo 18.* San Francisco: Western Center for Health Planning, Sept. 19, 1983

White, K. L. *Health and Health Care: Personal and Public Issues* (The 1974 Michael M. Davis Lecture, The Center for Health Administration Studies, Graduate School of Business, The University of Chicago.) Chicago: 1974.

Wilensky, G. R. Filling the Gaps in Health Insurance: Impact on Competition. *Health Affairs,* Summer 1988, 133–149.

Williams, A. P., et al. How Many Miles to the Doctor? *New England Journal of Medicine,* 309, 958–963, 1983.

Williams, C. A., Barth, P. S., and Rosenbloom, M., Ed. *Compendium on Workmen's Compensation* (Issued by the National Commission on State Workmen's Compensation Laws). Washington, DC: National Commission on State Workmen's Compensation Laws, 1973.

Williams, S. J., and Torrens, P. R. *Introduction to Health Services (3d ed.).* New York: John Wiley & Sons, 1988.

Wilson, F. A., and Neuhauser, D. *Health Services in the United States.* Cambridge, MA: Ballinger Publishing Company, 1982.

———. *Health Services in the United States (2d ed.).* Cambridge, MA: Harper & Row, 1985.

Winslow, C. A. *The Evolution and Significance of the Modern Public Health Campaign.* New Haven, CT: Yale University Press, 1923.

———. *The Life of Hermann M. Biggs: Physician and Statesman of the Public Health.* Philadelphia, PA: Lea and Febiger, 1929.

———. *The Conquest of Epidemic Disease: A Chapter in the History of Ideas.* Madison, WI: The University of Wisconsin Press, 1978.

Wolf, S., and Sherer, H. P. *Public General Hospitals in Crisis: An Overview of National Trends with a Specific Look at Baltimore, Philadelphia,*

St. Louis and New York City. Washington, DC: Coalition of American Public Employees, 1977.

Wolkstein, I. Medicare 1971: Changing Attitudes and Changing Legislation. *Law and Contemporary Problems,* Autumn 1970, 35:4.

Worcester, D. L. W. Public Health and Private Doctors. *Survey Graphic,* April. 1934, 23:4, 149 ff.

Yett, D. E. The Chronic Shortage of Nurses: A Public Policy Dilemma. In H. E. Klarman (Ed.), *Empirical Studies in Health Economics.* Baltimore, MD: The John Hopkins Press, 1970.

———. Lifetime Earnings for Nurses in Comparison with College Trained Women. *Inquiry,* Dec. 1968, 35–70.

———. The Supply of Nurses: An Economist's View. *Hospital Progress,* Feb. 1965, 83–103.

———. The Causes and Consequences of Salary Differentials in Nursing. *Inquiry,* March 1970, 79–98.

Zwick, D. I. Some Accomplishments and Findings of Neighborhood Health Centers. *Milbank Memorial Fund Quartery,* 50:4 (1972).

———. Project Grants for Health Services. *Public Health Reports,* Feb. 1967, 82:2, 131–138.

Index

Burlage, R. K., 215, 218, 219–20, 226
Burlage Report (1969), New York City, 225–26
Burnham, Walter D., 484
Burns, E. M., 247
Burrow, J. G., 22
Butter, I., 374, 375
Butterfield v. Forrester, (1809), 283n1

Cameron, C. M., 66
Campbell, J. R., 36, 37t
Capitalism
    health threats in early, 3–6
    industrial revolution, 6–9
Carlson, R. J., 369, 371, 404
Carnegie Commission on Higher Education report
    (1970), 397–98, 402–3
Carrol, James, 17
Carson, Rachel, 39
Carter administration
    initiatives for national health insurance, 327–28
    mental health field activity during, 208–9
    public health goals, 104–10
Catastrophic Health Insurance and Medical
    Assistance Reform Act (proposed 1973), 320–
    21
Cavanaugh, J. H., 97
Centers for Disease Control (CDC), 105–6
Chadwick, Edwin, 10, 15, 55
Chapin, Charles V., 24, 25
Chapin study (1915), 24, 25
Chapman, C. B., 130
Charity Organization Society (COS), 252
Children's Bureau, 83, 91–92
Chill, D., 451
Civilian Health and Medical Program of the
    Uniformed Services (CHAMPUS)
    cost effectiveness, 178–81
    health insurance plan, 176–77
Clarke, G. J., 206, 207
Cline, J. W., 458
Clinics
    Children and Youth, 349
    Maternal and Infant Comprehensive Care, 349
    for migrant workers, 349
    rural, 349
    Urban Health Initiative, 349
Coal Mine Health and Safety Act (1969), 118
Cohen, F. S., 160, 162, 163
Cohen, H. S., 464
Cohn, B., 229
Coll, B. D., 248, 249–57
Collier, John, 165, 167
Commission on Costs of Medical Care (1932), 368
Commission on Hospital Care report (1947), 358
Commission on Public–General Hospitals report
    (1978), 237–40

Commission on Workmen's Compensation (1972),
    267
Committee on the Costs of Medical Care report
    (1932), 268–69, 430–31, 442–44
Communicable Disease Center, 105. *See also*
    Centers for Disease Control (CDC)
Community Action Program, 342, 343–45
Community–based services, 202–3
Community Health Centers (CHCs), 347–48, 350
Community Mental Health Centers Act (1963). *See
    also* Mental hospitals; Mental Retardation
    Facilities and Community Mental Health
    Centers Construction Act
provisions from other programs and legislation,
    200–3
Community Mental Health Centers (CMHCs)
    federal funding for, 205–6
    provisions of, 200
Community Oriented Primary Care concept, 350–51
Community rating, 280
Community Support Program (CSP), 208
Community Support Systems (CSS), 208
Comprehensive Employment and Training Act of
    1973 (CETA), 102
Comprehensive Health Assessment and Treatment
    for Poor Children (CHAP), 104
Comprehensive Health Insurance Act (proposed
    1974), 318–19
Comprehensive Health Planning and Public Health
    Service Amendments (1966, 1967), 75–76, 97–
    98, 201, 456, 457–60
Comprehensive National Health Insurance Act
    (proposed 1974), 319–20
Connery, R. H., 74; 188, 190, 191, 195
Contagionist theory, 5
Contracting out, 255
Contributory negligence doctrine, 262–63, 283n1
CONUS. *See* Army Continental United States
    (CONUS)
Cooney, J. P., 47, 215, 220
Cooper, B. S., 292
Corning, P. A., 268, 270, 271, 272, 273
Corporations. *See also* Employer health care
    coalitions; Self–insurance systems
Corporations, health benefit structures (1980s), 330–
    32
Cost containment
    in Carter administration, 327–28
    during Nixon, Ford, Carter, and Reagan
        administrations, 80, 404–5
    growing concern of corporations, 330–32
    post–1972 focus, 321–23
Cost sharing
    employer increases in (1980s), 330
    in proposals for financing national health
        insurance, 309